Fundamentals of ORTHOPAEDICS

Fundamentals of ORTHOPAEDICS

N.V. SINGH

M.B.B.S., D.ORTH., M.S.C.S., M.I.O.A.

PGDORT (Std), Dundee University, U.K.

Junior Consultant, Orthopaedics

Sitaram Bhartia Institute of Science & Research

New Delhi

PUBLISHING FOR ONE WORLD

NEW AGE INTERNATIONAL (P) LIMITED, PUBLISHERS

New Delhi • Bangalore • Chennai • Cochin • Guwahati • Hyderabad

Jalandhar • Kolkata • Lucknow • Mumbai • Ranchi

Visit us at **www.newagepublishers.com**

Published by New Age International (P) Ltd., Publishers
First Edition: 2011

Branches:

- No. 37/10, 8th Cross (Near Hanuman Temple), Azad Nagar, Chamrajpet, **Bangalore**-560 018. Tel.: (080) 26756823, Telefax: 26756820, E-mail: bangalore@newagepublishers.com
- 26, Damodaran Street, T. Nagar, **Chennai**-600 017. Tel.: (044) 24353401, Telefax: 24351463 E-mail: chennai@newagepublishers.com
- CC-39/1016, Carrier Station Road, Ernakulam South, **Cochin**-682 016. Tel.: (0484) 2377004, Telefax: 4051303. E-mail: cochin@newagepublishers.com
- Hemsen Complex, Mohd. Shah Road, Paltan Bazar, Near Starline Hotel, **Guwahati**-781 008. Tel.: (0361) 2513881. Telefax: 2543669, E-mail: guwahati@newagepublishers.com
- No. 105, 1st Floor, Madhiray Kaveri Tower, 3-2-19, Azam Jahi Road, Nimboliadda, **Hyderabad**-500 027. Tel.: (040) 24652456, Telefax: 24652457, E-mail:hyderabad@newagepublishers.com
- RDB Chambers (Formerly Lotus Cinema)106A, 1st Floor, S.N. Banerjee Road, **Kolkata**-700 014. Tel.: (033) 22273773, Telefax: 22275247, E-mail:kolkata@newagepublishers.com
- 16-A, Jopling Road, **Lucknow**-226 001. Tel.: (0522) 2209578, 4045297, Telefax: 2204098 E-mail: lucknow@newagepublishers.com
- 142C, Victor House, Ground Floor, N.M. Joshi Marg, Lower Parel, **Mumbai**-400 013. Tel.: (022) 24927869. Telefax: 24915415, E-mail: mumbai@newagepublishers.com
- 22, Golden House, Daryaganj, **New Delhi**-110 002. Tel.: (011) 23262370, 23262368, Telefax: 43551305. E-mail: sales@newagepublishers.com

ISBN : 978-81-224-3065-3

Rs. 325.00

C-10-06-4671

Printed in India at Ajit Printers, Delhi.
Typeset at Goswami Associates, Delhi.

PUBLISHING FOR ONE WORLD
NEW AGE INTERNATIONAL (P) LIMITED, PUBLISHERS
4835/24, Ansari Road, Daryaganj, New Delhi-110002
Visit us at **www.newagepublishers.com**

Dedicated

to

My wife Dr. Kamna

for giving me strength & support

Foreword

It gives me great pleasure to write foreword to this book on Orthopaedics and Trauma written by Dr. N. V. Singh with a lot of dedication and hard work. I have scanned through the pages of manuscript and am impressed with it's simplicity and brevity. I feel it should prove useful for a student of the subject particularly at undergraduate level as well as a young trainee in Orthopaedics.

Dr. N. V. Singh has been working as Junior Consultant in Orthopaedics at Sitaram Bhartia Institute of Science and Research, New Delhi. His efforts in bringing out this book are truly laudable. I feel this book will serve the young aspiring Orthopaedic Surgeons as well.

J. P. MANOCHA

Head of Deptt. of Orthopaedics at

Sitaram Bhartia Institute of Science & Research

New Delhi

Ex. Asst. Prof. Orthopaedics, AIIMS

Preface

This book starts from basic knowledge of bone physiology, structure of bone, growth of bone, types of joints and fractures. This basic knowledge is always required before proceeding to trauma and cold pathology in Orthopaedics.

Each chapter starts with applied anatomy so that student can recall his knowledge of anatomy. Most of the chapters contain hand made diagram prepared by author. Suitable X-ray plates have been added in chapters.

Commonly accepted classifications of various fractures have been given in corresponding chapter. Chapters also contain unanimously accepted treatment plan of fractures and other pathology. Latest treatment of corresponding pathology has been added if it exists.

Chapter on tuberculosis covers all joints and tuberculous osteomyelitis without joint involvement. Recent treatment of osteoarthritis, rheumatoid arthritis, ankylosing spondylitis and osteoporosis has been added.

Approach to a case of arthritis (excluding osteoarthritis) has been discussed in chapter 35. Chapter on arthroscopy covers basic knowledge of arthroscope, its basic instruments, irrigation system and triangulation technique of arthroscope.

Chapter on joint replacement includes THR, TKR, total shoulder replacement and total elbow replacement. This chapter gives basic and concise knowledge of replacement which is required at undergraduate level.

For the revision of Orthopaedics mainly before exam time, 60 commonly asked questions are given in chapter. For practical purpose most commonly given clinical cases and clinical methods of examination are covered.

Chapter on implants and instruments contains basic instruments and implants in Orthopaedics. A few latest implants have also been added just to have awareness about the same.

Last but not the least, chapter 47 contains multiple choice questions asked in AIIMS and various PG entrance exams, so that students can assess themselves.

Although all the sincere efforts have been done to verify accuracy of text and answers of MCQs, yet there may be chance of human error. Any correction, suggestion or improvement will be highly appreciated and duly acknowledged.

drnvsingh.2007@yahoo.co.uk

N.V. SINGH

Acknowledgement

It gives me immense pleasure to express my gratitude to every person who helped me to bring this book forward.

I am thankful to Dr. J. P. Manocha not only for he wrote foreword for this book also for giving me of tips of Orthopaedics. He also taught me perfection in Orthopaedic surgery. He is not only an excellent Orthopaedician but also a good human being for everyone.

I express my gratitude to Dr. Abhishek Kumar Mishra who helped me to shape this book. He devoted his precious time to go through the contents of this book.

I am also thankful to Dr. Suraj Prakash, Dr. R. Grover, Dr. Nithiraj Oberoi, Dr. Biren Nadkarni and Dr. Gurinder Bedi.

I am also thankful to Dr. Sanjay Sarup whose company gave me an opportunity to understand hidden aspects of Paediatric Orthopaedics. Company of Prof. B.K. Dhaon is always fruitful for every Orthopaedician. I express thank to him for the same. I am also thankful to Prof. Surya Bhan, as through him I have learnt indirectly. I also express my gratitude to Ex. Additional Prof. of Orthopaedics at AIIMS, J. Maheshwari with whom I have learnt not to leave any stone unturned during clinical assessment of patient and every new patient is a challenge for every surgeon. I thank all my teachers who taught me Orthopaedics during my postgraduation.

I also admire my school time English teacher Sri S. N. Gupta. The person like him is a priceless gift for every student. He is not only a teacher but also a guide and mentor. I am also thankful to my Biology teacher Sri Umesh Parasher. Such teachers are always a great guide for one's life and students remember them throughout life.

I am also thankful to entire team of New Age International Publishers, specially Mr. Saumya Gupta (Managing Director) and Dr. R. C. Gupta (Academic Director) to bring this book forward.

N. V. SINGH

Contents

CHAPTER

1 Introduction

INTRODUCTION

Word Orthopedics was coined by Dr. Nicholas Andrey in 1741. This word comprises of 2 Greek words—orthos (straight) and padion (child). Speciality of orthopaedics is divided into sub-branches as follows:

- Sports Medicine
- Traumatology (Accidental services)
- Cold Orthopaedics
- Hand and foot surgery
- Joint replacement surgery
- Spinal injuries unit
- Rehabilitation Medicine.

FRACTURE

Definition: This is a breech in the continuity of cortex of bone.

TYPES OF FRACTURES

Fractures have been classified on the basis of their etiology, clinical picture, displacement and on radiological features.

1. **Aetiological**
   a. Traumatic
   b. Pathological
2. **Clinical**
   a. Simple
   b. Compound
3. **Displacement**
   a. Displaced
   b. Undisplaced
4. **Radiological**
   a. Transverse
   b. Oblique
   c. Spiral
   d. Segmental

e. Comminuted

f. Greenstick

Traumatic Fracture

It can occur due to assault, road traffic accidents or hanging.

Pathological Fracture

Patient may have pathology in the bone, e.g. Tumor, cyst or secondaries. Usually this fracture occurs due to trivial trauma.

Simple Fracture

Patient does not have wound over fracture site i.e. fracture is not communicating to exterior.

Compound Fracture

When fracture communicates to exterior, it is called as compound fracture. It can be from within, (internal compound) where sharp fracture end protrudes out through skin. It can be from outside (external compound) where object striking over bone, pierces skin and soft tissue overlying it.

Displaced Fracture

Fractured bone looses its anatomical alignment. It may be shifted or angulated. It may undergo rotation or over-riding. It is respectively known as shift angulations and rotation or overriding. (See Fig. 1.1 (*a*), (*b*), 1.2 and 1.3)

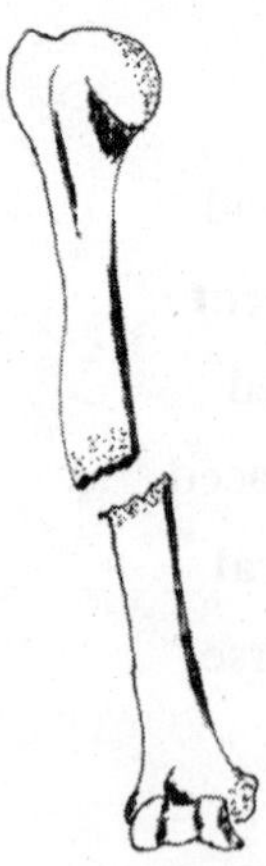

Fig. 1.1 (*a*) Displaced fracture

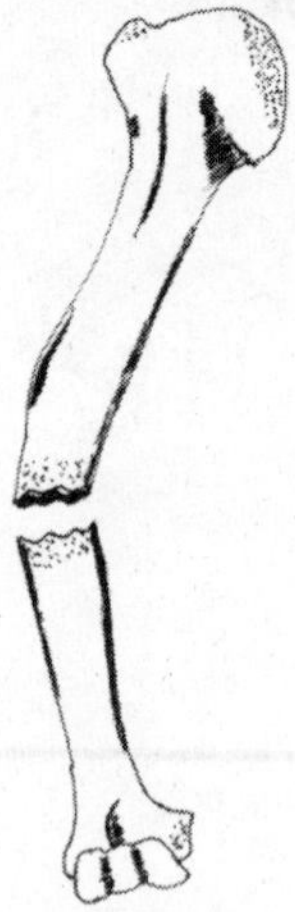

Fig. 1.1 (*b*) Angulated fracture

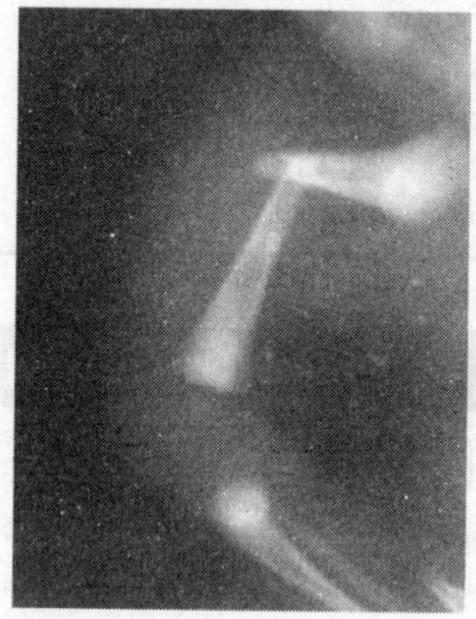

Fig. 1.2 Angulated and displaced fracture of shaft femur

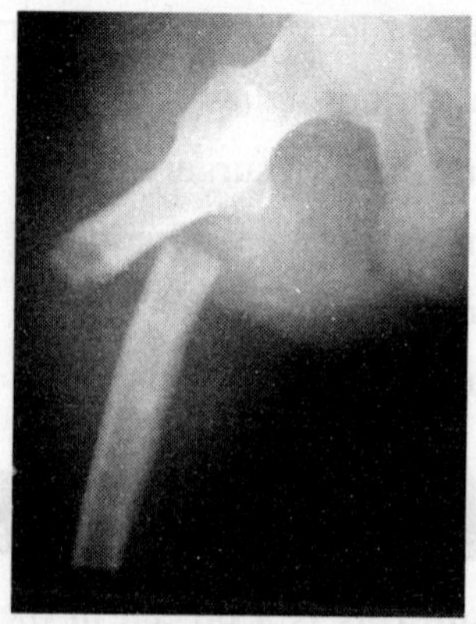

Fig. 1.3 Transverse and displaced fracture of shaft femur

Transverse Fracture

Fracture line is perpendicular to long axis of bone. (See Fig. 1.4)

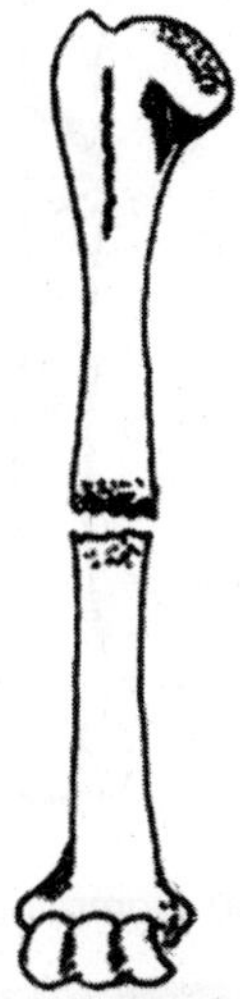

Fig. 1.4 Transverse fracture

Oblique Fracture

Fracture line runs obliquely. (See Fig. 1.5 and 1.6)

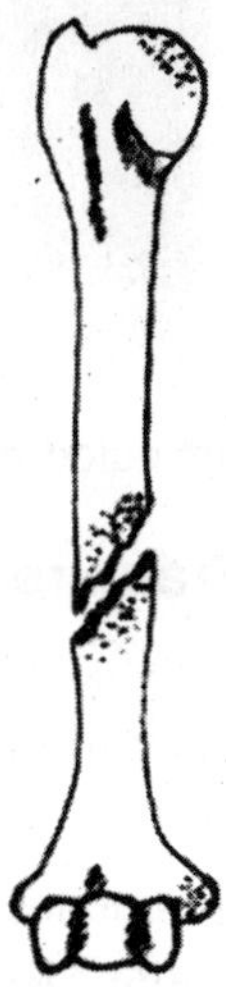

Fig. 1.5 Oblique fracture

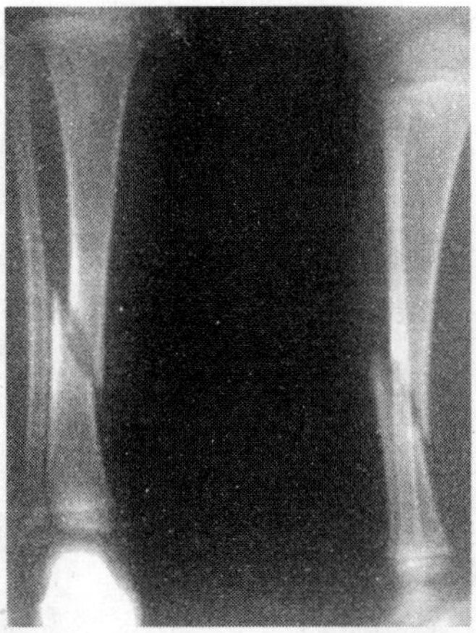

Fig. 1.6 Oblique fracture of shaft tibia

Spiral Fracture

Fracture exists in more than one plane. (See Fig. 1.7 and 1.8)

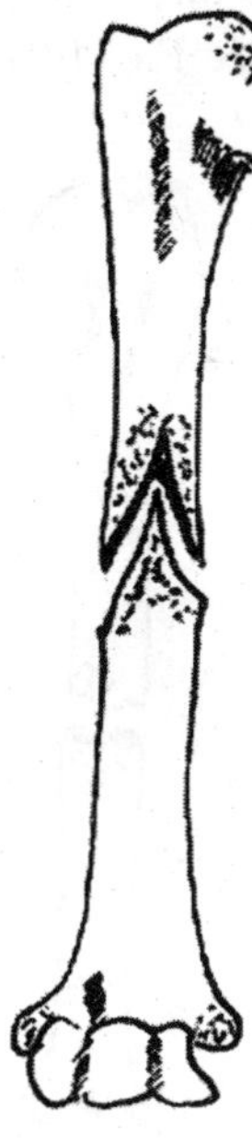

Fig. 1.7 Spiral fracture

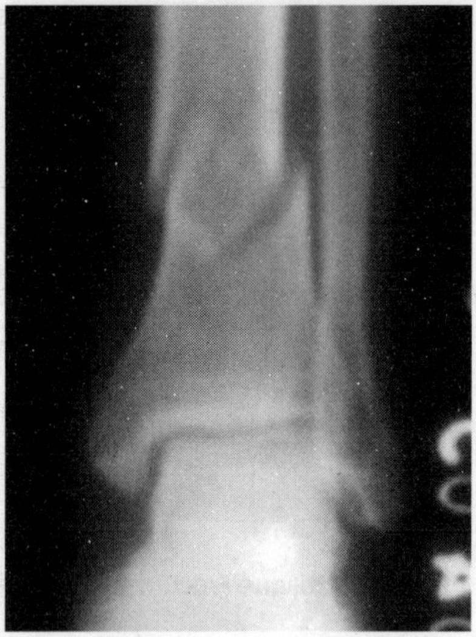

Fig. 1.8 Spiral fracture of lower end of tibia

Segmental Fracture

Two or more fractures are present in a bone at different level. (See Fig. 1.9)

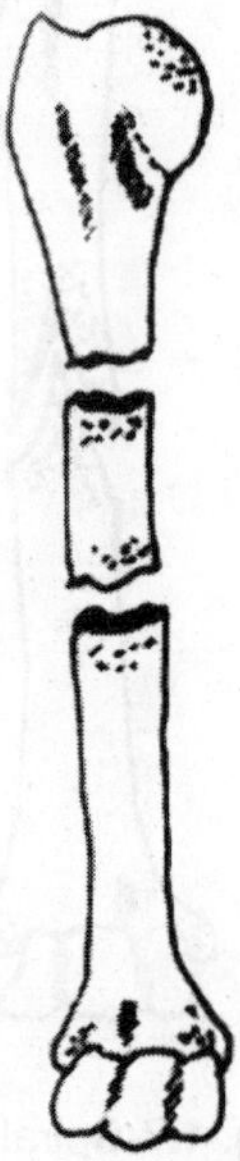

Fig. 1.9 Segmental fracture

Comminuted Fracture

This type of fracture has more than two fragments in number. (See Fig. 1.10 and 1.11)

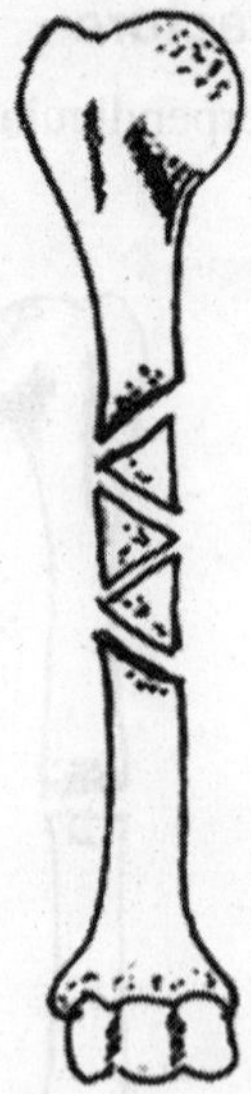

Fig. 1.10 Comminuted fracture

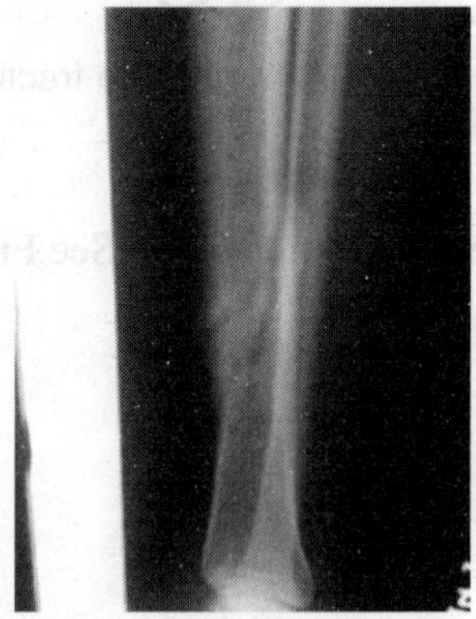

Fig. 1.11 Comminuted fracture of shaft tibia

Pathological Fracture

Osteogenesis imperfecta is an important cause of pathological fracture up to five years of age. (Fig. 1.12)

Osteoporosis is commonest cause of pathological fracture in old age. Bone cyst or chronic osteomyelitis are a common cause of pathological fracture in children. Secondaries can also cause fracture in old age persons. Osteopetrosis (**Marble bone disease** or **Albers Shonberg disease**) starts during gestation and progresses till growth stops. It presents with frequent fractures which heal slowly. Rickets, Scurvy, Osteomalacia, Multiple myeloma, Fibrous dysplasia, Eosinophillic granuloma, Paget disease, Histiocytosis X and Gaucher's disease are other causes of pathological fracture. (See Fig. 1.12)

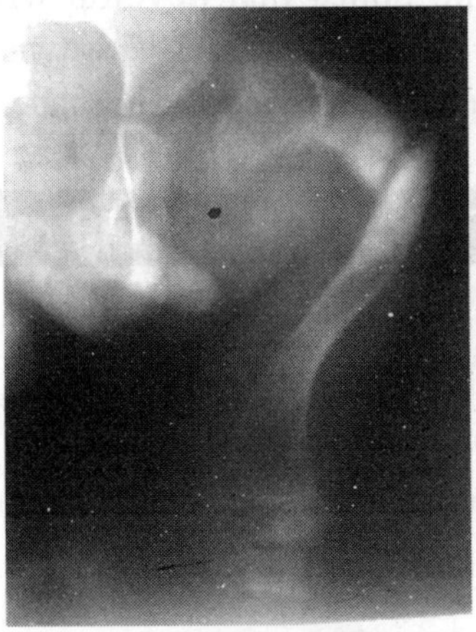

Fig. 1.12 Pathological fracture of femur in osteogenesis imperfecta

Dislocation

When the articular surface of a joint are completely displaced from each other, joint is said to be dislocated. Joints that commonly undergo dislocation are hip, shoulder, elbow, knee and patella. Other joint may also dislocate depending on mode of trauma. Chopart (intertarsal) dislocation and Lisfranc (tarsometatarsal) dislocation are uncommon. (See Fig. 1.13 (*a*), (*b*) and 1.14)

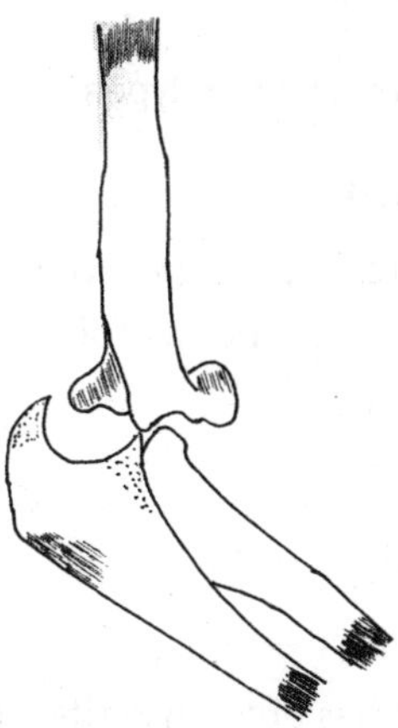

Fig. 1.13 (*a*) Dislocation of elbow (lateral view)

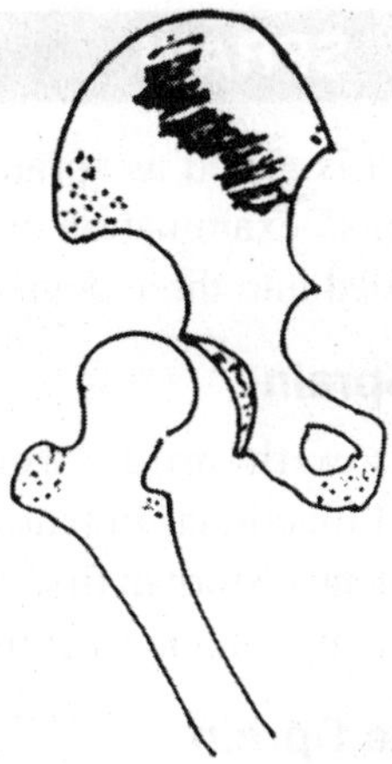

Fig. 1.13 (*b*) Dislocation of hip joint

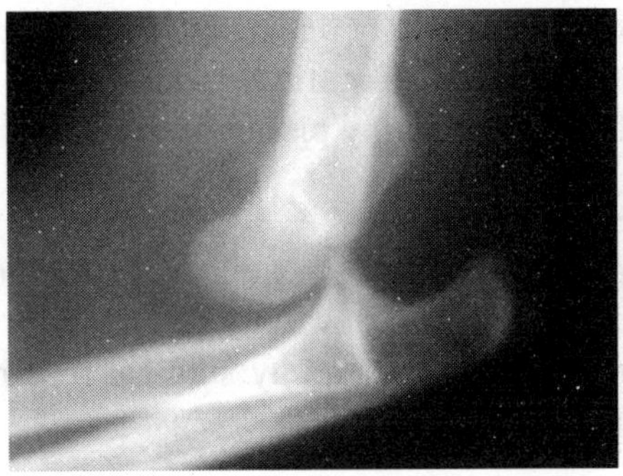

Fig. 1.14 Dislocation of elbow

Subluxation

When the articular surface of a joint are partially displaced, it is said to be subluxated. (See Fig. 1.15)

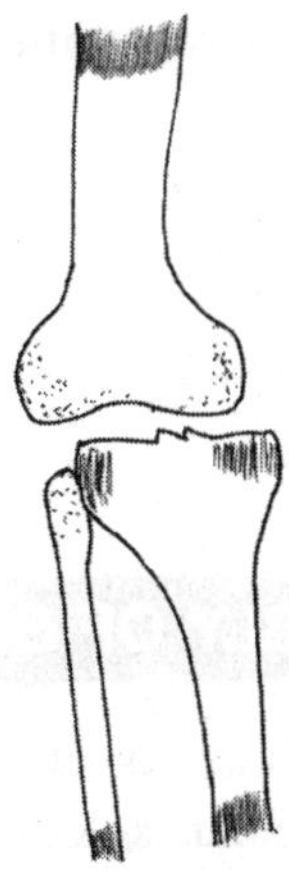

Fig. 1.15 Subluxation of knee

SPRAIN

A tear in ligament is called as sprain and can be diagnosed by clinical examination and stress test. It has been classified into three degree as follows:

First Degree Sprain

Patient presents with mild swelling, local tenderness and no functional impairment. Only a few fibres of ligament are torn in first degree sprain. In this condition symptomatic treatment is given.

Second Degree Sprain

Patient presents with pain, swelling and inability to use limb. Joint movements are within normal limit. Most of the fibres of ligament are torn sparing only few fibres. Treatment is given by immobilizing the joint by plaster application.

Third Degree Sprain

Patient presents with gross swelling. Pain is less. Joint movements may show talar tilt in ankle. All fibres are torn. It is treated by surgical repair of ligament.

Strain

Strain means tear in muscle and is commonly seen in young athletes.

BLOOD SUPPLY OF LONG BONES

Long bones are mainly supplied by following vessels:

1. Nutrient artery
2. Epiphyseal vessels
3. Metaphyseal vessels
4. Periosteal vessels

ASSEMBLY OF BONE

Human body has been assembled into axial skeleton and appendicular skeleton. Axial skeleton has got 80 bones forming upright axis of body. Whereas appendicular skeleton has got 126 bones forming appendages and girdles that connect them to axial skeleton.

Sesamoid Bone

These are the bones that develop within the substance of a tendon or fascia. This type of bone is small, rounded and triangular in shape.

TYPES OF JOINTS

Joints have been classified into three types as follows:

1. Fibrous Joint (Synorthosis)
2. Cartilaginous Joint (Amphorthosis)
3. Synovial Joint (Diarthrosis)

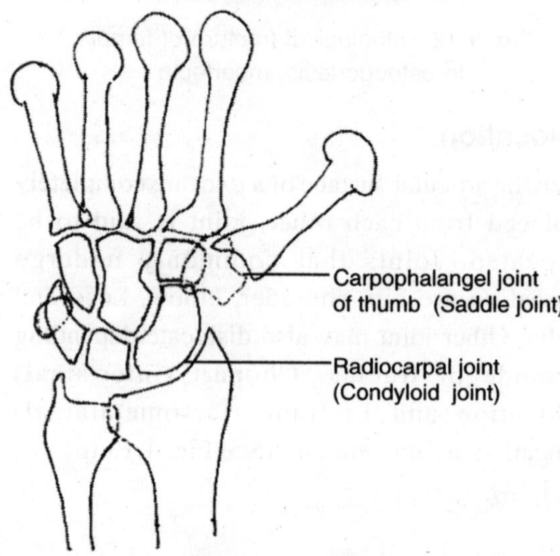

Fig. 1.16 Different types of joint

1. Fibrous Joint

Fibrous joints are immovable joints and further divided into three subtypes as follows:

a. Syndesmosis

b. Sutures

c. Gomphosis

a. Syndesmosis

This kind of joint has got dense fibrous membrane which holds the articular surface close and tight to each other. Distal tibiofibular joint is an example of such kind of joint.

b. Sutural joint

Sagittal, coronal and lambdoid sutures of skull come under this type of joint. Bone margins are united by jagged interlocking process.

c. Gomphosis

This kind of joint has one socket into which conical part of bone fits itself e.g., teeth and socket of jaw bones.

2. Cartilaginous Joint

This kind of joint is made up of either hyaline cartilage (synchondrosis) or fibrous cartilage (symphysis). This joint provides slight movement. Symphysis pubis is an example of fibrocartilaginous joint whereas articulation between ribs and sternum is an example of synchondrosis.

3. Synovial Joint

Synovial joints are lined by **synovial membrane** which secretes **synovial fluid** that keeps the joint lubricated and provides nourishment to articular cartilage. Synovial joints has fibrous capsule outside, holding the articulating bones together. These joints are most mobile joint in body.

Synovial membrane

This is the membrane in a joint which lines capsule of synovial joint, bursae and tendon sheath. Synovial cells lining, have abundant fenestration capillaries which facilitate diffusion of fluid and plasma proteins between circulation and joint. Hyaluronan, chondroitin sulphate, type VI collagen and tenascin are found in intercellular matrix.

Two types of cells are found in this membrane.

Type-A Macrophage like phagocytic cell

Type-B Fibroblast like cell

These two cells produce synovial fluid.

Synovial fluid

Synovial fluid has two main functions in a joint. It provides lubrication to the joint and nutrition to avascular cartilage. Synovial fluid is nothing but an ultrafiltrate of plasma containing locally secreted hyaluronan and lubricin. Hyaluronan provides viscoelastic properties, while lubricin provides lubrication to the joint.

Synovial fluid has following features:

1. This is viscous fluid which is pale yellow in colour.
2. Intra-articular pressure is minus 8 cm to minus 12 cm H_2O.
3. Its specific gravity is 1.008–1.015.
4. Synovial fluid contains 2 g of protein (albumin, globulin and mucin).
5. A : G ratio in synovial fluid is 20 : 1.
6. Albumin is present in larger quantity in synovial fluid in comparison to senum.
7. Fibrinogen is not present in synovial fluid.
8. This also contains certain enzymes e.g., amylase, lipase and protease.

Articular cartilage

This cartilage is present at the joint line of long bones and consists of chondrocytes. Articular cartilage is avascular structure which even does not have nerves. Tensile strength of articular cartilage is provided mainly by type-II collagen. Aggrecan is main proteoglycan in articular cartilage and consists of a protein core with side chains of chondroitin and keratin sulphate. Certain degradative enzymes are also found in articular cartilage e.g. collagenase, gelatinase, aggrecanase and stromelysin. Tissue inhibitor of metalloprotienases (TIMP) is also found.

Types of Synovial Joint

Synovial joints are divided into three types as follows:

a. Uniaxial

b. Biaxial

c. Multiaxial

a. Uniaxial joint

It provides movement in one axis; either in horizontal (elbow joint) or vertical axis (atlantooccipital joint) known as Hinge and Pivotal joints respectively.

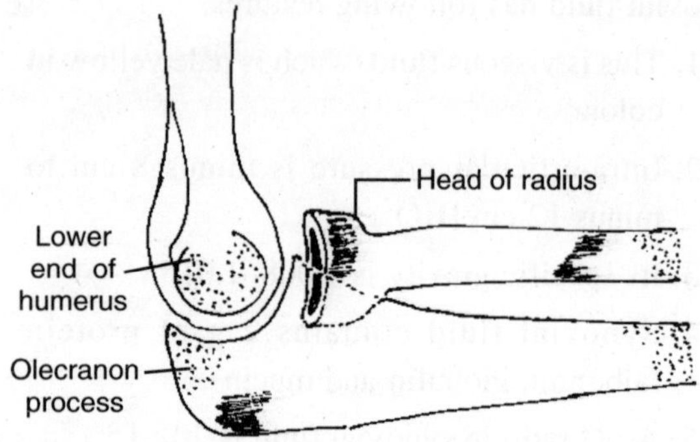

Fig. 1.17 Elbow joint (Hinge joint)

b. Biaxial joint

It provides movements in two axes and two plains at 90 degree. These joints have two subtypes as follows:

i. Saddle joint: Articular surface of saddle joint is concave in one direction and convex in other direction whereas the articulating surface of opposite bone is exactly opposite. Carpophalangeal joint of thumb, joints between C1 and C2, the atlantoaxial joint are this kind of joint.

ii. Condyloid joint: It has one condyle that fits into a socket e.g., Radiocarpal joint.

Knee joint

Knee joint is a compound synovial joint which has 2 condylar joint between femoral and tibal condyles and another saddle joint between femur and patella.

c. Multiaxial joint

These joints provide movement in more than two axis. It is subdivided into two types as follows:

i. Ball and socket joint: For example, Hip, knee and shoulder joint.

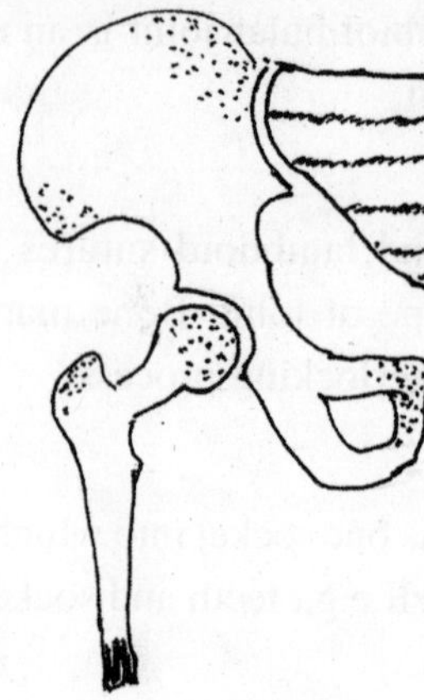

Fig. 1.18 Ball and Socket joint

ii. Gliding joint: This joint provides gliding movement in all planes. For example, joints between carpal bone and tarsal bone, joint between articular processes of vertebrae.

BONE PHYSIOLOGY

Bone is a kind of connective tissue with a collogen framework impregnated with calcium and phosphate salts particularly hydroxyapatite which have general formula of $Ca_{10}(PO_4)_6(OH)_2$.

Total blood flow in bone is 200–400ml/min in adults.

Calcium turnover rate is 100% in infant and18% in adults.

Bone Types I

Human bone structure is compared of the following two types:

1. Compact bone (cortical bone)
2. Trabecular bone (spongy bone)

Compact bone

This bone is predominantly found in diaphyseal area of long bones.

This bone has following characteristic features:

a. It accounts for 80% of bone in body.

b. It makes outer layer of bone in body.

c. Bone cells lie in lacunae.

d. Collagen is arranged in concentric layers around the Haversian canal known as **Osteon** or **Haversian system**.

e. Surface to volume ratio is low.

Trabecular bone

This bone is predominantly seen at the ends of long bones (epiphysis) and vertebral bodies. This bone has following characteristic features:

a. It accounts for 20% of bone in the body.

b. It lies inside cortical bone.

c. It is made up of spicules or plates. Many cells are sitting on surface of plates.

d. Nutrition is provided via bone ECF into trabeculae.

e. Surface to volume ratio's high.

f. This bone is more quickly remodelled than cortical bone due to having greater surface area.

90% of protein in bone matrix is type 1 collagen. This collagen is as strong as steel and is made up of helix of three polypeptides bound tightly together. Two of these are alpha-1, polypeptide encoded by one gene and other is alpha-2 polypeptide encoded by different gene.

Structure of Bone

Basic structural unit of compact bone is Haversian system also known as Osteon. This system consists of lamellae which are arranged concentrically about the haversian canal. Haversian system is present along the long axis of bone. Haversian canals connect with each other and with Volkman's canal. Volkman's canals run horizontally from endosteal to periosteal surface.

Sharpey's fibres are very important structure as they fix the periosteum to outer surface of bone specially at the attachment site of muscle and tendon.

Growth of Bone

First appearance of bone is seen after 7th embronic week. Bone grows by enchondral and intramembranous ossification. In enchondral ossification (***cartilaginous bone***) bones are modelled in cartilage and transformed into bone. When mesenchymal cells form bone directly, it is called as intramembranous ossification (membranous bone) e.g. clavicle, mandible and certain bones of skull.

Cartilage first appears at 5th embryonic week. It is of three types. (hyaline, elastic and fibrous)

Bone increases in length by epiphyseal plate which lays down new bone on the end of shaft of bone. Width of bone is markedly affected by pituitary growth hormone and IGF-1.

Types of Bone

Our human body has 3 types of bone: long, flat and small bone.

Long bone

Middle portion (shaft) of long bone is known as diaphysis. This has medullary cavity inside. Diaphysis is made up of compact bone.

Ends of long bone is known as epiphysis, are madeup of spongy bone which is covered by thin layer of compact bone.

Area of spongy bone just beneath the epiphyseal plate is known as metaphysis.

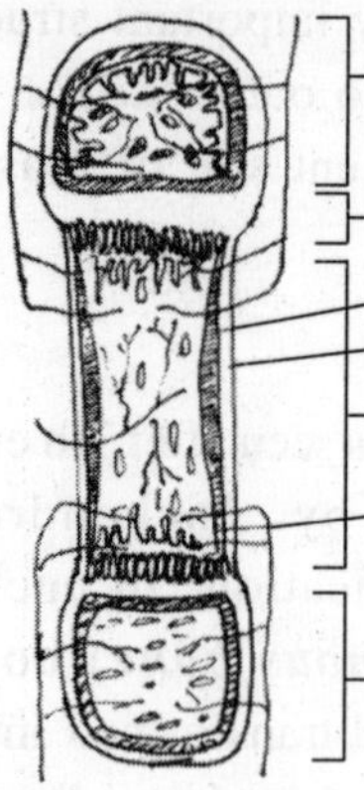

Fig. 1.19 Structure of long bone prior to epiphyseal closure

Flat bone

Outer and inner table of skull are example of flat bone.

Small bone

Carpals and metacarpals are small bones.

COMPONENTS OF BONE

Bone is composed of periosteum and osteogenic cells.

Periosteum

This is a tough membrane which covers outer surface of bone. This is made up of 2 layers. Outer layer is thin fibrous layer which contains fibroblasts. Inner layer is osteogenic layer which contains osteogenic cells. These osteogenic cells differentiate into osteoblast, chondroblast and perhaps osteoclast and osteocyte.

Osteoblast

This is an osteogenic cell and has following features:

a. Osteoblasts are modified fibroblast.

b. Bone formation is done by osteoblast.

c. Osteoblast lay down type-1 collagen and form new bone.

d. Osteoblast regulates the process of osteoclast formation via RANKL-RANK and M-CSF-OPG mechanism.

e. Osteoblast contains following enzymes e.g. alkaline phosphatase, phosphorylase and glycolate.

Osteoclast

This is also an osteogenic cell and has following features:

a. Osteoclasts are member of monocyte family.

b. Osteoclasts are attached to bone via integrins in sealing zone.

c. Osteoclasts erode and absorb previously formed bone.

d. Pyridinoline is a breakdown product of collagen, which is used to measure in urine as an index of rate of bone resorption.

e. Parathyroid hormone accelerates bone resorption where as estrogen hampers bone resorption.

f. First osteoclast resorbs bone, then osteoclast lay down new bone. This cycle takes 100 days.

Osteocyte

Osteocytes are synthesized by osteoblast. Osteocyte has large oval nucleus with large chromatin granules. Its cytoplasm is faintly basophilic. Glycogen and PAS positive granules are abundantly found in osteocytes.

PHYSIOLOGY OF WALKING

Normal walking comprises of two phases: stance phase and swing phase. Both of these phases are further divided into 3 phases as follows:

Stance phase

1. Heel stroke (heel strikes the ground) [Fig. 1.20 (*a*)]

2. Mid stance (foot is kept flat on ground) [Fig. 1.20 (*b*)]

3. Push off (foot is off the ground) [Fig. 1.20 (*c*)]

Swing phase

1. Acceleration phase (leg comes infront of body) [Fig. 1.21 (*a*)]
2. Swing through (leg is swinging forward) [Fig. 1.21 (*b*)]
3. Deceleration phase (swinging becomes slow and heel becomes ready to strike the ground) [Fig. 1.21 (*c*)]

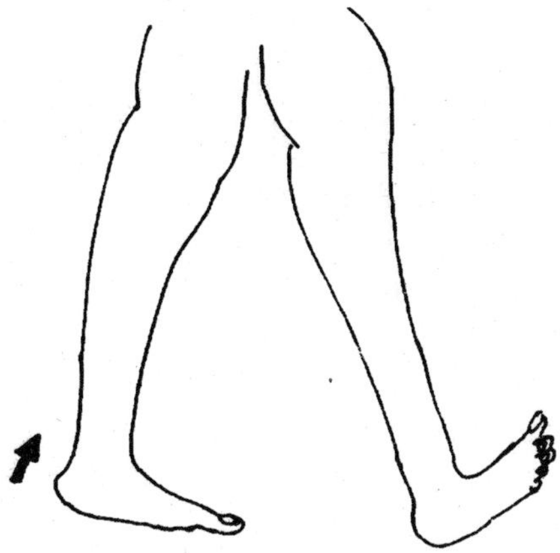

Fig. 1.20 (*c*) Push off

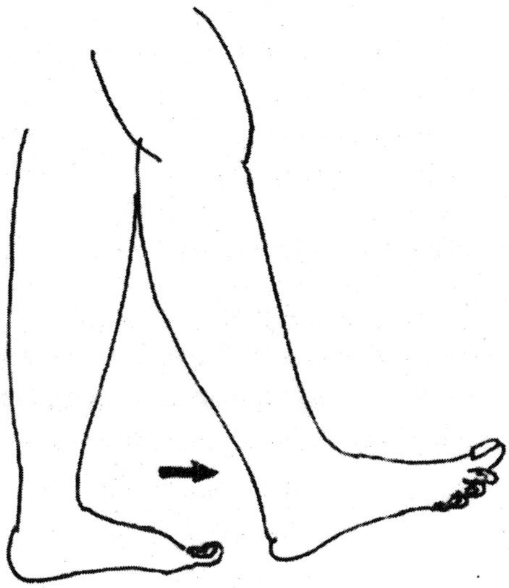

Fig. 1.20 (*a*) Heel stroke

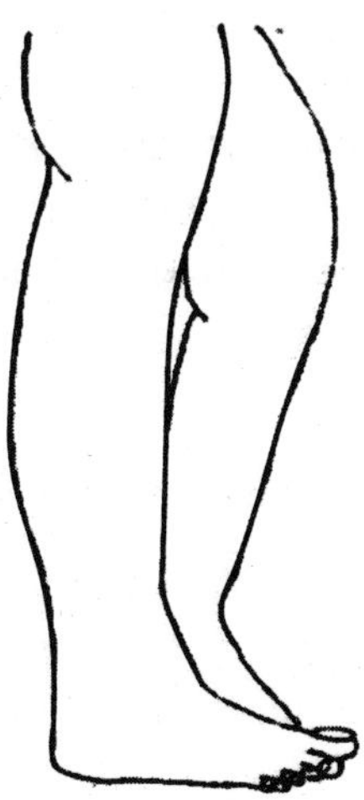

Fig. 1.20 (*b*) Mid stance

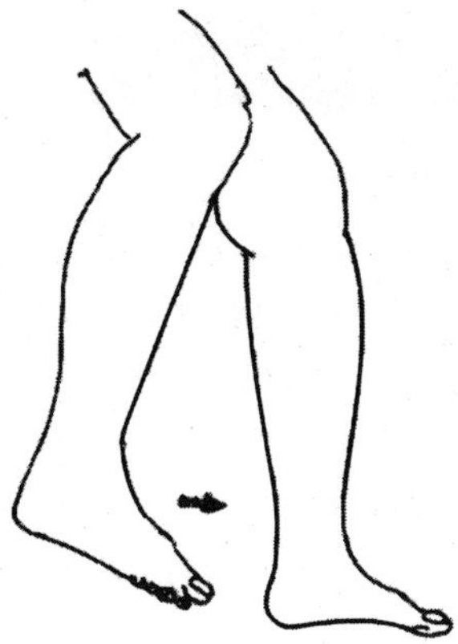

Fig. 1.21 (*a*) Acceleration phase

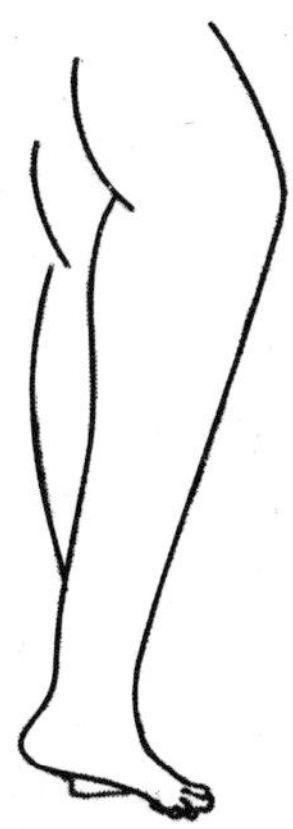

Fig. 1.21 (*b*) Mid swing phase

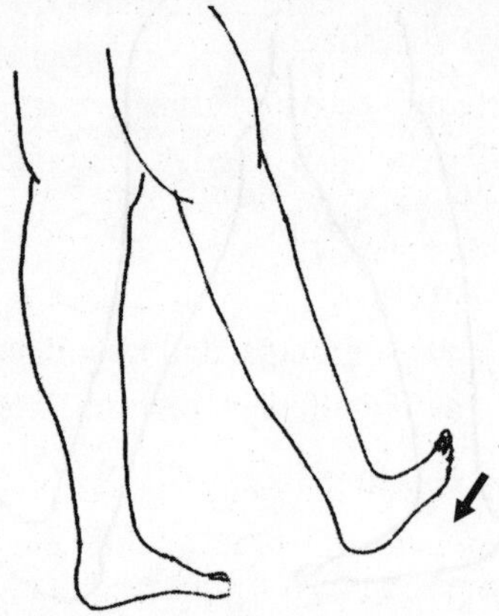

Fig. 1.21 (c) Deceleration phase

FRACTURES WITH EPONYMS

Fracture of necessity

This is Galeazzi fracture i.e. fracture of lower end of radius with subluxation or dislocation of inferior radioulnar joint. Galeazzi fracture is also known as reverse monteggia fracture.

Chauffer's fracture

This is fracture of radial styloid process.

Bennet's fracture

This is an intraarticular fracture of base of first metacarpal bone.

Monteggia fracture

This is fracture of upper 1/3rd of ulna with dislocation of head radius.

Colles's fracture

This is a transverse fracture of lower end of radius within 3/4th of an inch from it's distal articular margin at the corticocancellous junction occurring as a result of fall on outstretched hand leading to dinner fork deformity; commonly seen in postmenopausal elderly females.

Chopart fracture-dislocation

This is fracture-dislocation through inter-tarsal joint.

Burst fracture

This is comminuted fracture of vertebral body where its fragments burst out in different direction. This fracture manifests in 5 pattern (discussed in chapter of spinal injuries).

Straddle fracture

This is fracture of superior and inferior pubic rami on both sides.

Rolando fracture

This is an extraarticular fracture of base of first metacarpal bone.

Essex-Lopresti fracture

This is fracture head of radius with dislocation of inferior radioulnar joint.

Night stick fracture

This is fracture of shaft of ulna.

Smith fracture

This is reverse of colles's fracture, i.e. fracture of lower end of radius with palmar displacement.

Volar barton fracture

This is anterior marginal fracture of lower end radius.

Dorsal barton fracture

This is posterior marginal fracture of lower end of radius.

Base ball finger

This is also known as **Mallet finger.** This is an avulsion of extensor tendon of distal interphalangeal joint from it's insertion at the base of terminal phalanx.

Whiplash injury

This is a ligamentous injury of neck.

Malgaigne's fracture

This is disruption of pelvic ring associated with injury to pubic symphysis and sacroiliac joint on same side.

Holstein-Lewis fracture

This is an oblique fracture of distal third of humerus associated with radial nerve injury. Radial nerve is entrapped between fracture ends.

Mallet thumb/finger

This is an avulsion of extensor pollicis longus insertion into base of disal phalanx, leading to flexion deformity of thumb/finger.

Jersy finger

This fracture is seen in adolescent and young adults. Instead of more common avulsion of FDP from its metaphyseal insertion on volar aspect of distal phalanx, a metaphyseal fragment with variable amount of physis may accompany the tendon.

Gamekeeper's thumb

This is also known as **Skier thumb.** This is partial or complete disruption of ulnar collateral ligament and volar plate, is caused by valgus stress applied to metacarpophalangeal joint of thumb.

Boxer's fracture

This is a fracture neck of 5th metacarpal that is ventrally displaced. It is commonly seen in boxers.

Jefferson's fracture

This is a fracture of first cervical vertebra.

Hangman fracture

This is a fracture of second cervical vertebra that occurs through its pedicle. This is not associated with any neurological deficit.

Chance fracture

This is a type of seat belt injury. This is a horizontal avulsion fracture of vertebral body.

Clay shoveller's fracture

This is a fracture of spinous process of first thoracic vertebra, caused by strong muscular action. It is commonly seen in shovelling by labourers.

Bumper's fracture

This is fracture of lateral condyle of tibia, occurs as a result of hit by bumper of a car or truck.

Dash board fracture

This is a fracture of patella that occurs as a result of knee striking to dash board of a car due to sudden application of brake.

Pott's fracture

This is a fracture of medial and lateral malleoli and also known as bimalleolar fracture.

Side-swipe fracture

This fracture is seen in elbow, while projecting out of a car and side swept by other vehicle. This injury involves fracture of distal humenus, proximal end of radius and or ulna.

Cotton's fracture

This is a fracture of medial, lateral and posterior malleoli also known as trimalleolar fracture.

Aviator's fracture

This is a fracture of neck of talus, caused by forced dorsiflexion of ankle and commonly seen in air craft crash.

Jone's fracture

This is a fracture of base of 5th metatarsal.

March fracture

This is fatigue fracture of second metatarsal caused by repeated stress and commonly seen in soldiers.

Hoffa's fracture

This is a fracture of femoral condyle in coronal plane.

Massonaise's fracture

This is an ankle injury associated with fracture neck of fibula.

IMPORTANT SIGNS

Reisser's sign

This sign is seen in scoliosis. Iliac apophysis fuses with the iliac bone at maturity, i.e., growth is completed and there is no chance of worsening of spinal curve. This is called as Reisser's sign and seen on X-ray.

Trethowan sign

This is seen in slipped capital femoral epiphysis. If we draw a line along the superior surface of neck, it remains superior to head of femur.

Hawkin's sign

This sign is seen in avascular necrosis of talus. This is best radiographic indication of viability of talus. Avascular necrosis can be seen radiologically 6–8 weeks after fracture-dislocation. Disuse atrophy can be seen in bones of foot and lower end of tibia. Subchondral atrophy of talus rules out avascular necrosis.

Scottish dog sign

This is seen in spondylolisthesis. In oblique view of spine, pars interarticularis area looks like a Scottish dog. If it looks like a Scottish dog wearing a collar it means that defect is in the pars interarticularis (isthmus) of vertebra and patient has spondylolysis (without slippling of vertebra). If dog's head is separated from neck it means there is slip of vertebra and called as spondylolisthesis.

Aneurysmal sign

This is seen in anterior type of spinal tuberculosis.

MOVEMENTS AT THE JOINTS

Movements at various joints in degrees are as follows:

HIP	
-Flexion (with knee extended)	0–90
-Flexion (with knee flexed)	0–120
-Extesion	0–20
-Abduction	0–45
-Adduction	0–30
-External rotation	0–45
-Internal rotation	0–30

KNEE	
-Flexion	0–135
-Extension	135–0
ANKLE	
-Dorsiflexion	0–25
-Plantarflexion	0–45
SHOULDER	
-Flexion	0–90
-Extension	0–45
-Adduction	0–45
-Abduction	0–180
-External and Internal rotation (with arm in neutral position, hanging by the side of chest)	0–70
ELBOW	
-Flexion	0–145
-Extension	145–0
RADIOULNAR JOINT	
-Supination	0–90
-Pronation	0–80
WRIST	
-Dorsiflexion	0–70
-Palmar flexion	0–90
-Radial deviation	0–20
-Ulnar deviation	0–30
MP JOINT	
-Flexion	0–90
-Extension	0–40

CHAPTER

2 Fracture Healing

FRACTURE HEALING

Fracture healing starts from the day of trauma. Fracture healing has been differentiated into five stages. (*See Fig. 2.1 on next page*)

1. Stage of Haematoma

As the fracture occurs, bleeding starts from minor vessels in the base leading to haematoma formation. Ischaemic necrosis at the fracture ends occur due to stripping of periosteum. Osteoclasts die due to lack of blood supply but few are survived and sensitized to differentiate into daughter cells thus helping in healing process.This stage lasts for 7 days.

2. Stage of Granulation Tissue Formation

Fibroblasts, osteoblasts and blood vessels are formed from their precursor cells. All of these collectively form soft granulation tissue. Later this tissue forms a soft tissue callus. This stage lasts for 14 days.

3. Stage of Callus Formation

Granulation tissue further differentiates in osteoblast. Intercellular matrix is formed by osteoblast that becomes impregnated with calcium salt. This makes a woven bone. Callus formation is quicker in children and cancellous bone. Callus becomes visible after 3 weeks of fracture.

4. Stage of Remodelling

This is also known as stage of consolidation. Woven bone turns into mature bone which has lamellar structure.

This lamellar bone is formed by multicellular unit based remodelling of callus. It may take 1-2 years to complete the process.

5. Stage of Modelling

Weight bearing forces and muscle strength provide a good stimulus for maturation of bone. In this process bone becomes strong. This process takes years to develop. Shape formation of endosteal and periosteal surface occurs in such a way that the fracture becomes indistinguishable from the normal bone.

Features	Period	Stages
• Necrosis occurs at fracture ends. • Precursor cells are sensitized.	< a week	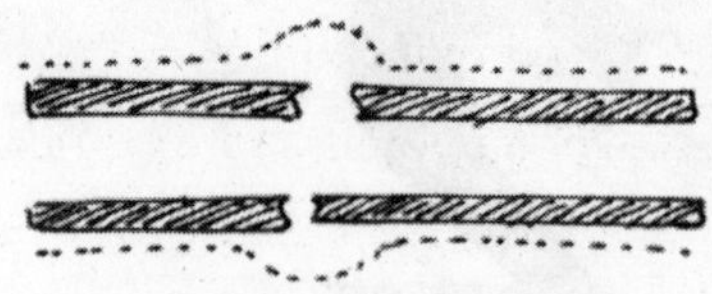 Stage of haematoma
• Daughter cells are proliferated and differentiated into fibroblast and osteoblast vesels. • Mobility is still present at fracture site.	2–3 weeks	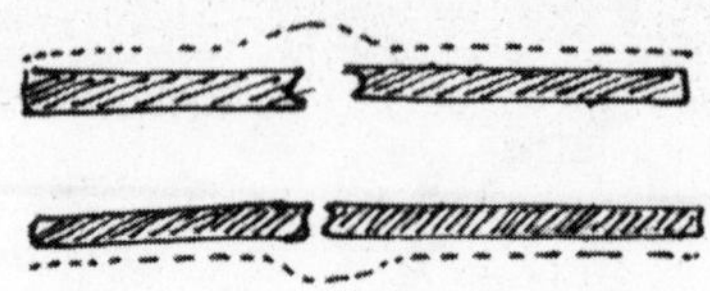 Stage of granulation tissue formation
• Callus is formed and radiologically visible. • Fracture union takes place.	1–3 months	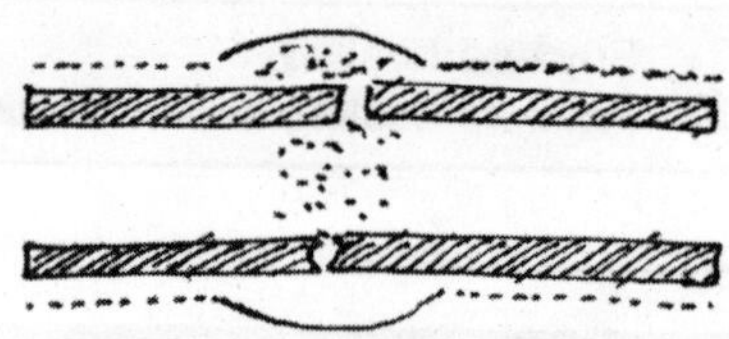 Stage of callus formation
• Typical lamellar pattern of bone develops. • Callus is sharply defined.	1–2 years	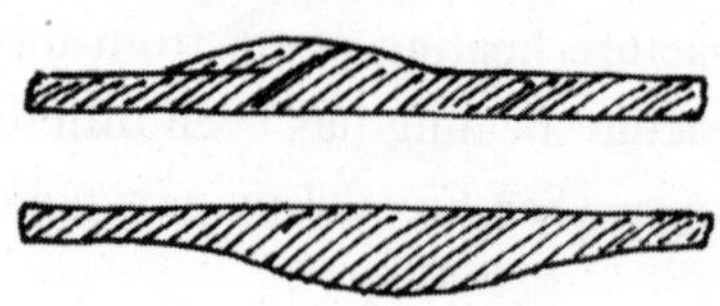 Stage of remodelling
• Fracture site is invisible due to modelling at endosteal and periosteal surfaces.	> 2 years	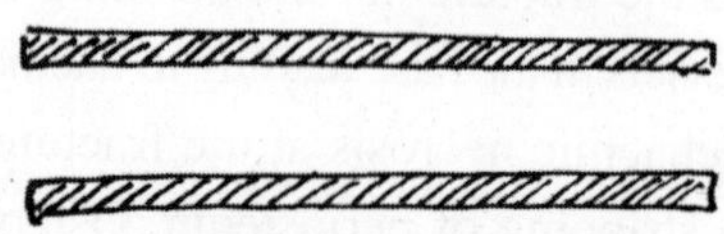 Stage of modelling

Fig. 2.1 Fracture healing

FRACTURE HEALING IN CANCELLOUS BONE

In cancellous bone stage of callus formation is missing. Rest of the process of healing is same as in cortical bone.

PREDISPOSING FACTORS FOR HEALING

There are certain factors which promote healing:

1. Young age
2. Flat and cancellous bone

3. Spiral fracture
4. Comminuted fracture
5. Good reduction
6. Compression and electrical stimulation at fracture site

FACTORS DELAYING FRACTURE HEALING

Factors which delay fracture healing are as follows:

1. Old age
2. Tubular and cortical bone
3. Transverse fracture
4. Soft tissue interposition
5. Ischaemic necrosis of fracture ends
6. Compound fracture

CHAPTER

3 Open Fractures

- Introduction
- Gustillo and anderson classification
- Treatment
- Complications

INTRODUCTION

This is also known as compound fracture. This is a fracture that communicates to external environment due to break in soft tissue and skin. **Gustillo** and **Anderson** have classified open fracture into three types.

GUSTILLO AND ANDERSON CLASSIFICATION

Gustillo and Anderson have classified compound fractures into three types as follows:

Type 1: Wound is less than 1 cm size.

Type 2:

- Wound ranges between 1–10 cm.
- Soft tissue is not devitalized
- Little contamination is present

Type 3:

- Wound is more than 10 cm
- Soft tissue is devitalized and contaminated.

A. Extensive soft tissue injury but adequate soft tissue is available to cover the fracture site.

B. Extensive soft tissue loss. Bone is exposed and can not be covered.

C. Compound fracture is associated with arterial injury.

Investigations

- Hb must be sent in all compound fractures.
- BT/CT
- Blood grouping
- Urine examination for benzidine reaction (indicative of myoglobinuria), albumin, creatinine and pigmented granular cast (seen in crush syndrome) and x-ray of local part should be done.

TREATMENT

Fresh compound fractures of less than 6 hours duration should undergo thorough cleaning of wound with either normal saline or running tap water. It is followed by dressing of wound and splintage application.

Airway, breathing and circulation should be checked and restored.

Intravenous fluid/blood/plasma expander should be given depending on requirement to treat the shock.

Neurovascular status of the limb should be examined in following points: pulse, colour, capillary filling, pin prick, temperature.

Wound older than six hours should be debrided. Debridement includes exploration of wound, excision of dead and devitalized tissue, freshening of wound margin and removal of foreign material.

First six hours since the time of trauma are supposed to be crucial because bacteria (that are lodged into wound through contamination) take hours to grow and multiply within the tissue.

Inside out wound is more dangerous as the fractured bone that comes out, gets contaminated and goes inside. Infection settles deep inside the bone. Drainage of wound becomes difficult as the wound size is small in these wound.

Injection of tetanus must be given in all compound fractures.

Injection of tetglobe can be given in old cases.

A.G.G.S. (Anti Gas Gangrene Serum) is given if gas gangrene develops.

Broad spectrum antibiotics e.g., Ceftriaxone, Gentamicin/Amikacin and Metronidazole should be given by intravenous route.

Later fracture can be fixed by external or internal method, depending on depth of infection.

COMPLICATIONS

Compound fracture may have following complications:

1. Tetanus
2. Gas gangrene
3. Neurovascular deficit
4. Osteomyelitis
5. Delayed union
6. Non-union
7. Fat embolism
8. Hypovolaemic shock
9. Crush syndrome
10. Avascular necrosis
11. Compartment syndrome
12. Myositis ossificans
13. Sudeck's dystrophy
14. Stiffness of joint

CHAPTER

4 Complications

- Classification
- Hypovolemic shock
- Malunion
- Nonunion
  - Electrical stimulation method
- Role of Illizarov in nonunion
  - Types of bone grafting
  - Cancellous bone graft
  - Cortical bone graft
- Fat embolism
- Deep vein thrombosis
- Crush syndrome
- Compartment syndrome
- Gas gangrene
- Traumatic myositis ossificans
- Myositis ossificans progressiva
- Avascular necrosis of bone
- Histological changes in AVN
- Sudeck's dystrophy

CLASSIFICATION

Complications of fractures have been classified on the basis of their duration i.e. immediate, early and late:

Immediate complications

Immediately after the fracture, patient can have following complications:

1. Hypovolaemic shock
2. Neurovascular injury
3. Injury to soft tissue and joint

Early complications

These complications occur sometime after the fracture:

1. Hypovolaemic shock
2. Crush syndrome
3. Fat embolism
4. Septicaemia
5. Compartment syndrome

Late complications

These complications occur when significant time has passed, i.e., weeks to months.

1. Delayed nonunion
2. Nonunion
3. Malunion
4. Synostosis
5. Limb shortening
6. Joint stiffness
7. Avascular necrosis
8. Osteomyelitis
9. Traumatic myositis ossificans
10. Sudeck's dystrophy

Most common complication of a fracture is hypovolemic shock. We should always keep this in our mind during management of a fracture.

HYPOVOLEMIC SHOCK

Most common cause of death in fracture is hypovolaemic shock and seen in fracture of major bones e.g., fracture pelvis and fracture of femur. An adult may loose 1000–1500 ml blood in fracture shaft femur and 1500–2000 ml in fracture pelvis.

MALUNION

When fracture does not unite in normal position, it is known as malunion.

Aetiology

Certain fractures may undergo malunion due to various causes. Most common causes of malunion are as follows:

1. Inadequate blood supply
2. Inadequate immobilization
3. Grossly contaminated fracture

Common Fractures Prone to Undergo Malunion

Not all bones undergo malunion. Common bones known for malunion are as follows:

1. Supracondylar fracture of humerus
2. Colles's fracture
3. Clavicle fracture
4. Intertrochanteric fracture

Types of Malunion

Fracture can have three types of malunion:

1. Length malunion
2. Rotatory malunion
3. Angulatory malunion

Length malunion

This type of malunion gives rise to shortening of limb.

Rotatory malunion

External or internal rotation deformities are the outcome of this type of malunion.

Angulatory malunion

This malunion causes valgus or varus deformity.

Clinical Features

Patient presents with bony deformity and impaired function. Certain associated features like shortening of limb or muscle may be present.

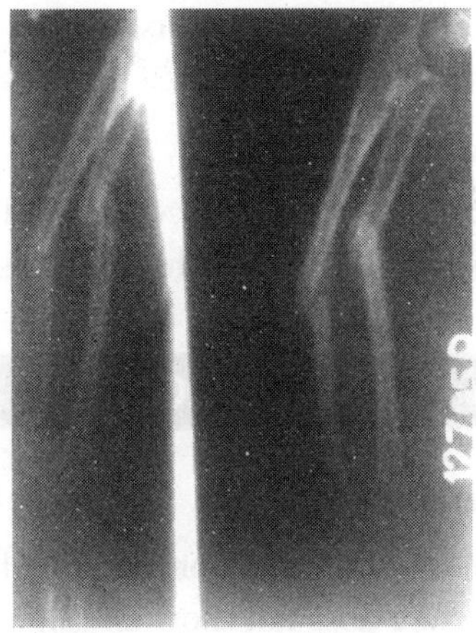

Fig. 4.1 Malunited fracture both bones forearm

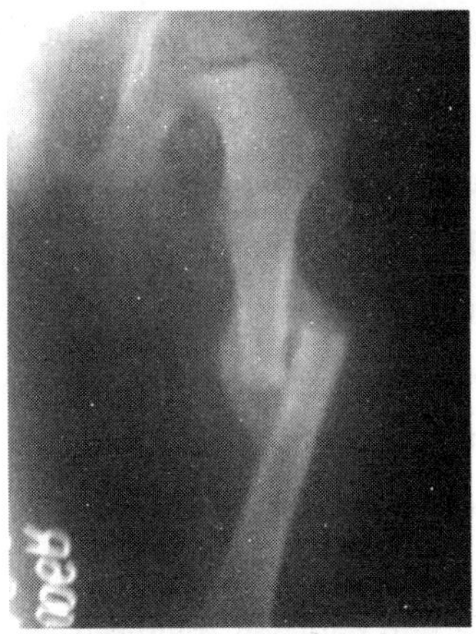

Fig. 4.2 Rotatory malunion

Modes of Treatment

Different modes of treatment are used depending on site of fracture.There are three following treatment that can be used.

CHAPTER 4

1. Osteoclasis
2. Osteotomy
3. Arthrodesis

Osteoclasis

This mode of treatment is used in children to correct angular deformity. In this method we break the intact cortex, e.g., Green stick fracture.

Osteotomy

This is a corrective osteotomy used in malunited fracture supracondylar humerus e.g., Lateral closed wedge osteotomy. This is also known as **French osteotomy.**

Arthrodesis

Only indication of this procedure is to provide relief from pain. In this method joint is fused.

NONUNION

Definition

When the normal time of bone healing has passed and still fracture dose not show any sign of clinical and radiological union, then it is said to be nonunion. In other words, biological process of bone healing has stopped in nonunion.

Aetiology

Common causes of nonunion are as follows:

1. Inadequate immobilization
2. Inadequate blood supply
3. Infection
4. Poor internal fixation
5. Intact companion bone
6. Soft tissue interposition
7. Bone gap between fractured ends.

Clinical Features

Patient with ununited fracture may present with the following features:

1. Patient gives old history of trauma.
2. Bony tenderness is absent.
3. Bony crepitus is absent.
4. Frank painless abnormal mobility at fracture site.
5. Loss of transmitted movements.

X-ray Findings

X-ray may show following findings:

1. Sclerosis and smoothened fractured ends.
2. Breach in continuity of bone.

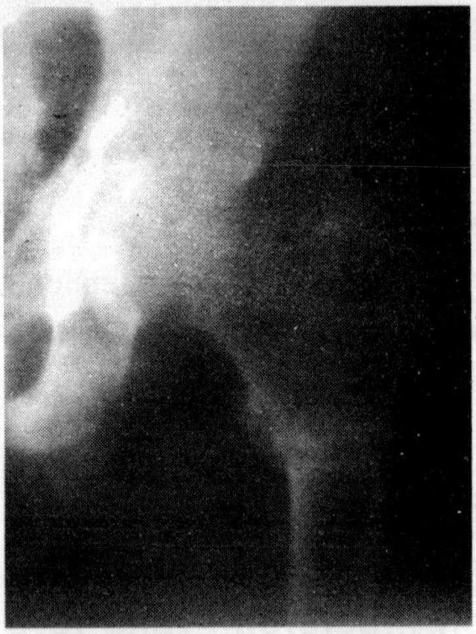

Fig. 4.3 Nonunion of fracture subtrochanteric femur

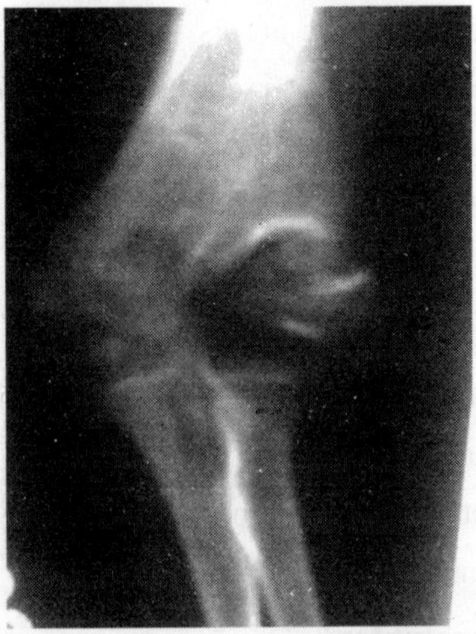

Fig. 4.4 Nonunion lateral condyle humerus

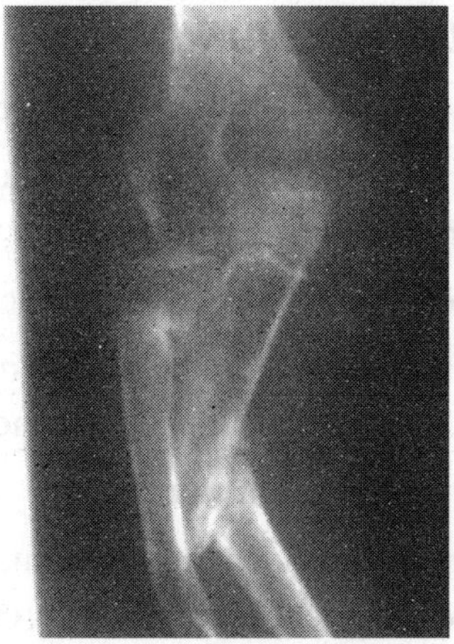

Fig. 4.5 Nonunion fracture head radius and shaft of ulna

3. Bone marrow cavity is obliterated.
4. Area around the fracture site shows osteoporosis.

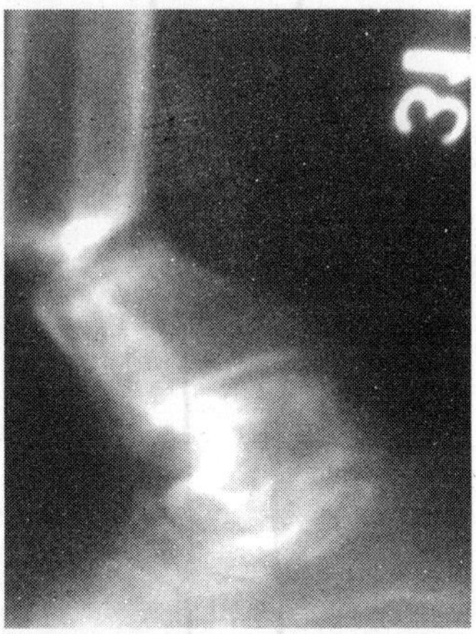

Fig. 4.6 Nonunion lower end tibia

Muller and Weber Classification of Nonunion

Muller has classified nonunion into two types, which are further subdivided into subtypes.

1. **Hypervascular nonunion**
   a. Hypertrophic
   b. Horsehoof
   c. Oligotrophic
2. **Avascular nonunion**
   a. Torsion wedge nonunion
   b. Atrophic nonunion
   c. Defect (Gap) nonunion
   d. Comminuted nonunion

Paley's Classification

Paley has classified nonunion into two types, depending on amount of bone loss.

Type A: In this type bone loss is less than 1 cm.

Type B: In this type bone loss is more than 1 cm.

Hypervascular Nonunion

This type of nonunion has following characteristics:

1. In this type of nonunion fractured ends are viable.
2. Biological reaction is seen at fracture site.
3. This type of nonunion can be managed by stable internal fixation. Bone grafting is not required.

a. Hypertrophic nonunion

This type of nonunion occurs due to poor fixation of fracture and early weight bearing. Exuberant callus is formed in this type. This is also known as **elephant foot nonunion.** [See Fig. 4.7 (*a*)]

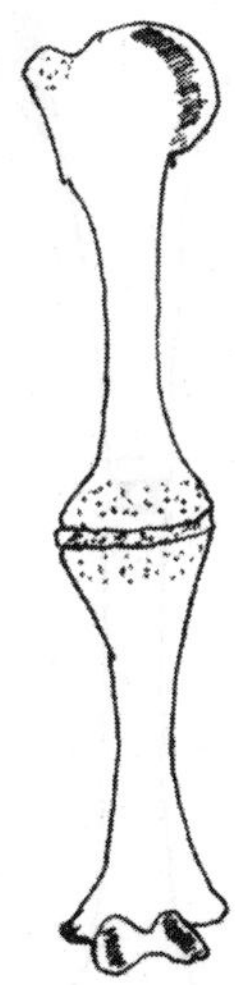

Fig. 4.7 (*a*) Elephant foot nonunion (Hypertrophic nonunion)

b. Horsehoof nonunion

This is seen in inadequate fixation with plates and screws. Callus is formed in less quantity. [See Fig. 4.7 (*b*)]

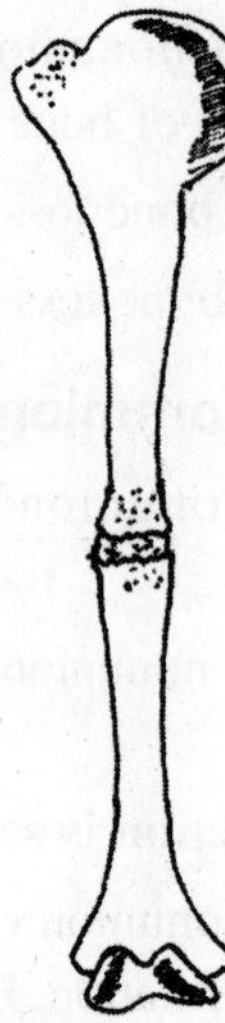

Fig. 4.7 (*b*) Horsehoof nonunion

c. Oligotrophic nonunion

Grossly displaced and distracted fractures are likely to undergo this type of nonunion. Very poor callus is formed. [See Fig. 4.7 (*c*)]

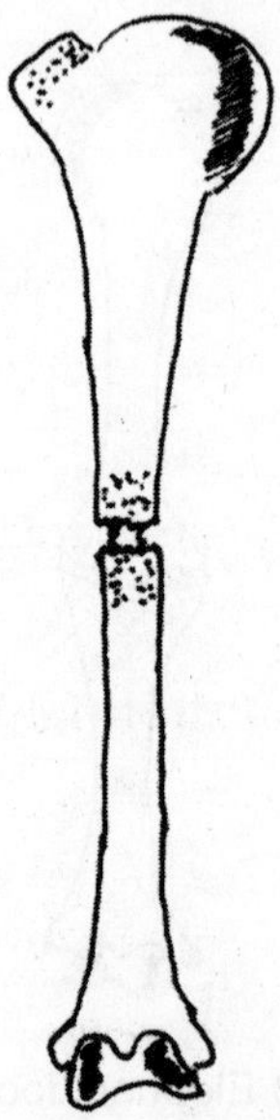

Fig. 4.7 (*c*) Oligotrophic nonunion

AVASCULAR NONUNION

This type may show following features:

1. Due to poor blood supply fracture ends undergo ischaemic necrosis.
2. This does not show any biological reaction.
3. This type of nonunion can be managed by rigid internal fixation with bone grafting.

a. Torsion wedge nonunion

This is commonly seen in segmental fracture. Intermediate fragment has healed at one end and not at the other.

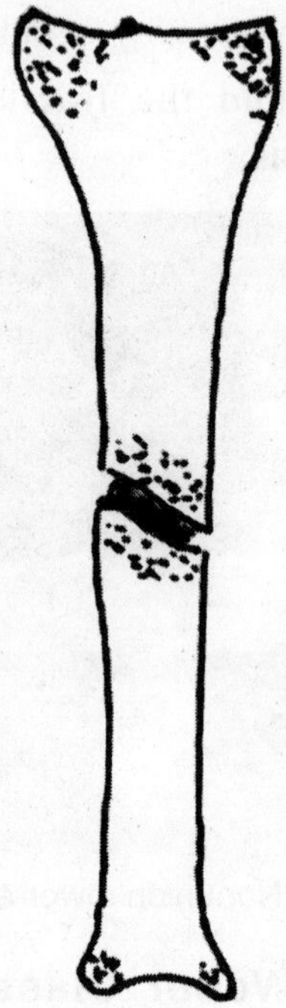

Fig. 4.8 (*a*) Torsion wedge nonunion

b. Atrophic nonunion

Fracture ends become tapered, thin and sclerosed. A lot of scar tissue is formed in between the ends. [See Fig. 4.8 (*b*)]

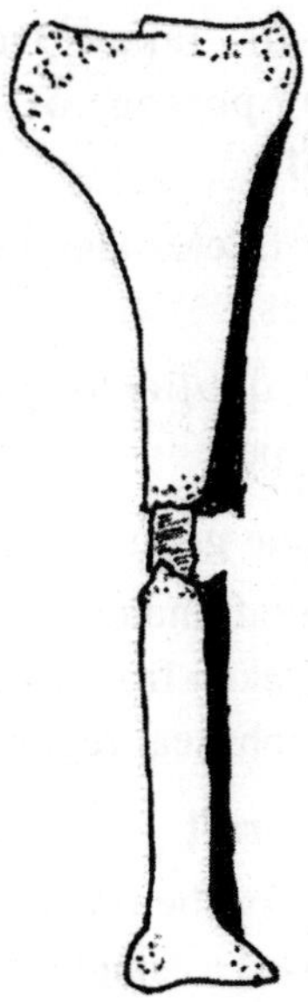

Fig. 4.8 (*b*) Atrophic nonunion

c. Defect (Gap) nonunion

In this type bone fragment is lost. It is commonly seen in compound fracture and osteomyelitis. [See Fig. 4.8 (*c*)]

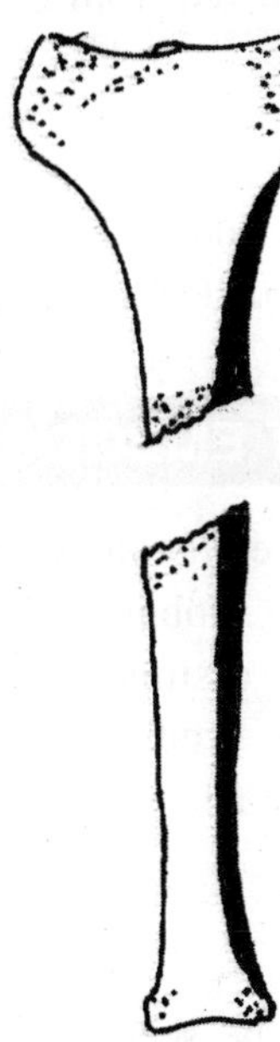

Fig. 4.8 (*c*) Gap nonunion

d. Comminuted nonunion

Proper callus is not formed in this nonunion. It is commonly seen in comminuted fracture. [See Fig. 4.8 (*d*)]

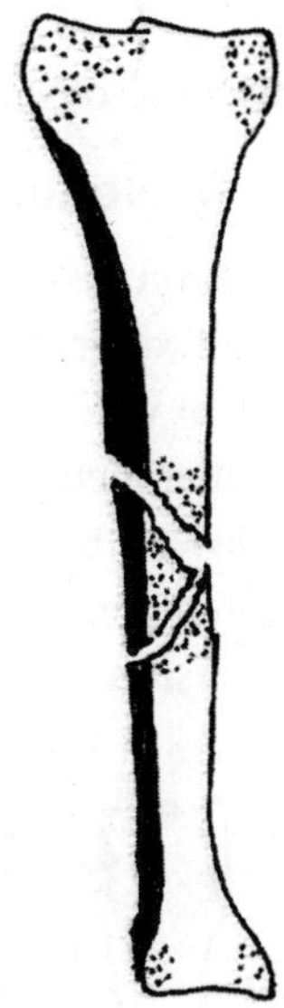

Fig. 4.8 (*d*) Comminuted nonunion

Treatment

Different types of nonunion can be treated by different plans as follows:

1. Open reduction and rigid internal fixation is mainstay of treatment in atrophic nonunion.
2. Open reduction and rigid internal fixation is sufficient in hypertrophic type.
3. **Electric stimulation, Illizarov** and interlocking nail are other modes of treatment.

Electrical Stimulation Method

In this method 20 mA of electric current is used by a cathode that converts fibrous tissue to fibrous cartilage, which undergoes ossification by enchondral ossification.

This cathode can be used as:

1. Invasive (inside the fracture site)
2. Semi invasive (subcutaneously)
3. Non invasive (incorporated into a plaster externally)

This method has become obsolete in these days.

Role of Illizarov in Nonunion

This acts on the basis on distraction histogenesis. This is a kind of ring fixator consisting of 1.5 mm diameter stainless steel wire. Corticotomy (cortex is cut in such a way that medullary cavity remains intact) is done; followed by distraction of bone ends at the rate of 1mm per day. Natural bone fills the gap (created by distraction of bone ends).

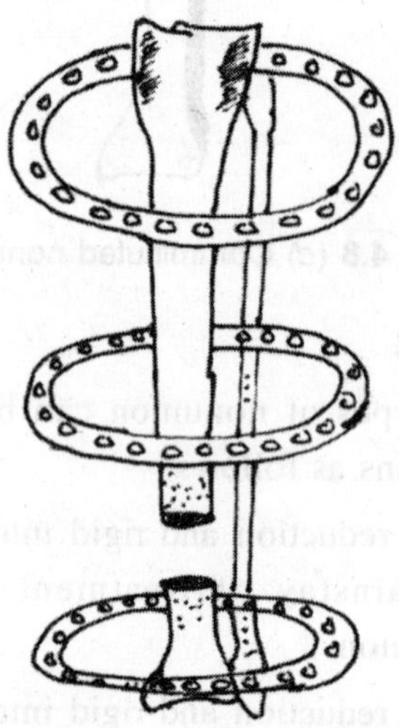

Fig. 4.9 Distraction osteogenesis by Illizarov

Types of Bone Grafting in Nonunion

Fresh autogenous, cancellous bone graft is most appropriate for nonunion. Graft induces osteogenesis. Graft is also useful in filling up bone gap and also provides stability.

On the basis of type of donor, bone grafts are of three types as follows:

1. Auto graft is taken from patient itself.
2. Allograft is taken from genetically dissimilar person of same species. **(Homograft)**
3. **Xenograft (Heterogenous)** is taken from other species.

On the basis of quality of bone, graft is of following three types:

1. Cancellous bone graft

Cancellous bone graft induces better osteogenesis. This graft can be taken from iliac crest and upper end of tibia (metaphyseal region).

2. Cortical bone graft

This graft is used for the fracture of shaft of long bones. It can be used as single onlay graft (placed on one surface) or dual onlay graft (placed on both surface) or as a sliding graft (bone graft is brought from above to fracture site in a sliding manner). Cortical bone graft is taken from middle third of medial surface of tibia and middle third of fibula.

3. Cortico cancellous graft

This graft can be taken from iliac crest, ribs and fibula.

Delayed union

When fracture has taken more than the expected time to unite, it is called as delayed union.

FAT EMBOLISM

This is a clinical entity in which small vessels are occluded by fat globules. This is also known as post traumatic distress syndrome or acute respiratory distress syndrome. It occurs with in 72 hours of trauma and usually manifests within 24–48 hours.

Aetiology

Fat embolism can be seen in following clinical conditions:

1. Multiple fracture

2. Fracture shaft femur
3. Fracture pelvis
4. Multisystem injuries.

Pathogenesis

Fat globules can come from bone marrow and uncommonly from agglutinated chylomicron (from plasma acting as an embolus). These fat globules enter the small vessels and transmitted to various sites of body e.g., brain and small pulmonary vessels, where they produce respective symptoms.

Clinical Features

Fat embolism can give two types of manifestation, Cerebral and Pulmonary.

A. Cerebral type

Patient may show following features:

1. Patient is confused, drowsy and restless.
2. Patient may present in coma.
3. Sometimes seizure may be one of the manifestations.
4. Petechial rash over lower lid conjunctiva is diagnostic.
5. Petechial rash can also be seen at infra and supraclaviclar area and retina.
6. Tachycardia >140/min.
7. Tachypnoea.
8. Pyrexia.

B. Pulmonary type

Patient may present with following features:

1. Tachypnoea and tachycardia are more prominent features.
2. Respiratory failure and death may occur.
3. Petechial rash.
4. Pyrexia.

Other features of rash

1. Rashes are periodic in nature and come with attack of coma.
2. These are fleeting type and fades quickly.
3. Retinal rash can be diagnosed by fundoscopy.

Investigations

Following investigations can be done to confirm fat embolism:

1. Thrombocytopenia shows platelet count less than 1.5 lacs.
2. PaO_2 is between 60–65 mmHg.
3. ECG shows S wave.
4. X-ray chest shows snow storm appearance.
5. Fat emboli can also be isolated from blood by **Gurd test.**

Treatment

Patient can be treated as follows:

1. First of all, secure the airway and give respiratory support to the patient in terms of oxygen.
2. Blood volume should be restored.
3. Dehydration and electrolyte imbalance should be corrected.
4. Fracture should be immobilized by cast.
5. Careless handling of fracture site must be avoided.
6. Corticosteroid should be given to reduce inflammation in lungs.
7. Lomodex (low molecular weight dextran) is given to increase plasma volume.
8. Heparin acts as lipolytic and antiplatelet agent.
9. Some physicians prefer to give 5% Dextose with alcohol. It helps in emulsification of fat globules.

DEEP VEIN THROMBOSIS

Virchov's triad is clinical presentation of deep vein thrombosis. It has following components:

1. Venous stasis
2. Vascular damage
3. Hypercoagulability.

Causes of DVT

Deep vein thrombosis can be encountered in various conditions. Some of them common conditions are as follows:

1. Fracture pelvis
2. Fracture shaft femur
3. Fracture shaft tibia
4. Surgical procedure
5. Prolonged immobilization
6. Oestrogen intake
7. Pregnancy
8. Hypercoagulable conditions
9. Obesity
10. Behcet's disease
11. T.A.O.

Clinical Features

Patient of deep vein thrombosis can be diagnosed on the basis of following clinical features:

1. Pain and swelling in calf muscle.
2. Difficulty in standing and walking.
3. Local temperature is raised.
4. Superficial veins are enlarged.
5. Pitting oedema.
6. **Homan's sign:** Passive forceful dorsiflexion of foot with extended knee will produce pain in calf muscle. This is a positive Homan sign and pathognomonic of DVT.

Treatment

Patient of DVT should be treated on the following lines of action:

1. Limb elevation.
2. Patient should be ambulated.
3. Heparin is drug of choice.
4. Aspirin can be given.
5. Low dose Warferin to be given orally.
6. Low molecular weight dextran is also given.

Sequelae of DVT

Pulmonary embolism

- If patient presents with severe dyspnoea which can not be explained by any reason is suggestive of pulmonary embolism.
- Patient also presents with chest pain increased respiratory and heart rate.
- Cor pulmonale may also be a presentation.
- Heparin is given as a drug of choice.

CRUSH SYNDROME

Crushing of muscles due to prolonged compression leads to extensive muscle necrosis and release of large quantity of myoglobin and potassium into systemic circulation. This condition is known as Crush syndrome. This may become life threatening.

Pathology

Patient with crush syndrome will show following pathological findings:

1. Muscles become necrotic, friable and blanched. Muscle looks like a fish flesh.
2. **Kidney** is grossly swollen and enlarged in size. Distal convoluted tubules show large hyaline cast and brown pigment material.

Distal convoluted tubules are blocked by precipitated myoglobin that leads to tubular necrosis. Cloudy swelling and desquamation is seen in proximal convoluted tubule.

Clinical Features

Patient may present with following clinical features:

1. Most common presentation is shock.
2. Extremities are pale and cold. Skin is moist.
3. Hypotension and dehydration are also seen.
4. Peripheral pulses are usually absent.
5. Extremities show patchy anaesthesia.
6. Vesicle, bullae and petechae may appear 4-5 days after trauma.

Investigations

1. Urine is highly acidic and show positive benzidine reaction that is indicative of myoglobinuria.
2. Urine also shows albumin creatinine and pigmented granular cast.
3. Increased blood urea nitrogen is indicative of **Crush kidney**. (Myoglobin renal failure)
4. Phosphate concentration is also increased.
5. CO_2 combining power is reduced.
6. CPK is raised upto 14000 I.U. almost 11 times of it's normal value.
7. Hyperkalemic metabolic acidosis is seen.

Treatment

Patient can be treated on following lines:

1. Principles of treatment is to correct hypovolemic shock. It can be corrected by giving plasma, isotonic sodium citrate or sodium lactate (1/6 molar), oral bicarbonate (30–40 gm). Injectable calcium gluconate can be given if tetany is induced.
2. **Avoid** whole blood transfusion as the patient is already suffering from haemoconcentration.
3. **Avoid** potassium salt.
4. Decompression of compartment can be done by epimysiotomy of all muscles and by neurolysis.
5. Necrotic muscles are excised.
6. Antibiotics are given to treat the infection as it is a common cause of death.
7. Manitol (250 mg/kg) infusion can be given stat; followed by with continuous intravenous drip of manitol.
8. Haemodialysis is done in case of raised serum K^+ and raised BUN. Haemodialysis is effective in first two days.
9. Monitoring of serum K^+ and BUN level should be done frequently.

COMPARTMENT SYNDROME

Raised pressure of more than 40 mm of water in osseofascial-compartment is known as compartment syndrome. This condition hampers the blood supply to muscles and nerves leading to ischaemia of muscle. Later muscles are grossly swollen.

Causes

1. Supracondylar fracture of humerus
2. Fracture both bones forearm
3. Crush injury of leg and forearm
4. Fracture of shaft tibia.

Pathology

There are three main factors which can lead to compartment syndrome, odema of muscles, fracture haematoma and ischaemia of muscles. In compartment syndrome a vicious cycle is developed which continues until vascular supply of entire oseofascial compartment is hampered.

Raised pressure hampers blood supply of muscles and nerve which leads to ischaemia of muscles. Ischaemia causes swelling of muscles which inturn reduces blood supply. Ischaemic muscles become necrotic and heal by fibrosis. Later muscle contractures are developed. This condition can also lead to nerve damage which can cause motor and sensory loss. In severe cases, gangrene can also develop.

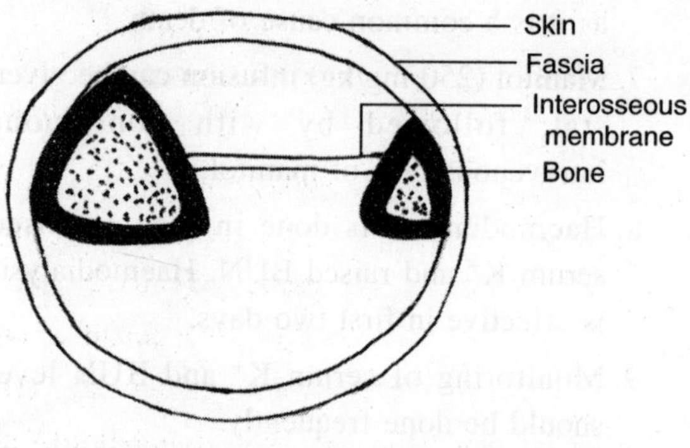

Fig. 4.10 (*a*) Osseofascial compartment

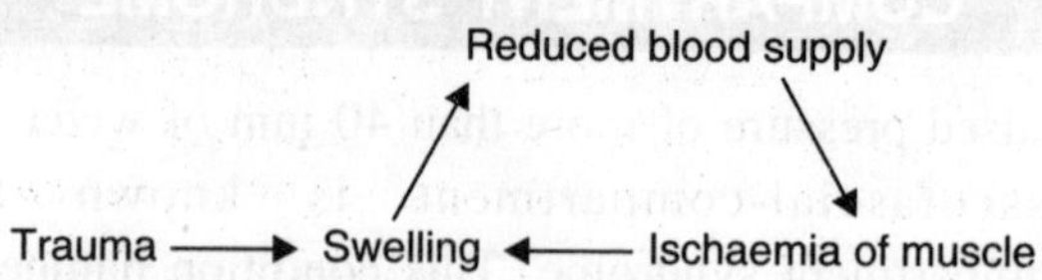

Fig. 4.10 (*b*) Vicious cycle of compartment syndrome

Clinical Features

Patient can be diagnosed with following features:

1. Excessive pain in a limb which is not relived even by usual dose of analgesics.
2. Grossly swollen and tense limb.
3. Stretch test is positive. Passive extension of fingers causes pain in forearm.
4. Hpoaesthesia of the limb.
5. Muscles are weak.

Management

Limb should be strictly elevated. Plaster should be opened. Patient is adviced to do active movement of fingers or toes.

If condition is not improved patient will require following methods:

Fasciotomy

Deep fascia of forearm should be slit in a longitudinal direction. This will release the pressure inside the osseofascial compartment.

Fibulectomy

This method is applicable to compartment syndrome of leg. In this surgery middle third of shaft of fibula is excised. This will release the pressure inside the osseofascial compartment.

GAS GANGRENE

This is a fatal complication of road traffic accidents. This is mainly caused by **Clostridium welchii**. Clostridium septicum and oedematiens are other organism which may cause gas gangrene. Clostridium is found in intestine and soil. Patient presents with pain in wound, grossly swollen muscle, toxaemia and vomiting. Crepitations can be felt over muscle. Exposed muscles become brick-red. Toxins released by clostridium act on adrenal glands leading to low blood pressure. X-ray is confirmatory which shows gas bubbles.

TRAUMATIC MYOSITIS OSSIFICANS

This is a reactive lesion seen in soft tissue and sometimes near bone and periosteum. This is also known as ossifying haematoma, characterized by fibrous, osseous and cartilaginous proliferation and by metaplasia.

Types

1. Extraosseous
2. Periosteal
3. Parosteal

Common muscles to be involved

1. Brachialis

2. Quadriceps femoris
3. Adductor muscle (**Prussian disease**)
4. Deltoid muscle (common in foot soldiers).

Joint involved

1. Elbow
2. Ankle
3. Knee
4. Shoulder
5. Hip

Pathology

1. Changes start in ground substance of connective tissue that shows remarkable proliferation of undifferentiated mesenchymal cells.
2. Fibroblast and mesenchymal cells show intense cellular proliferation histologically resembling with fibrosarcoma or myosarcoma.
3. Three peculiar zones are seen in histology.
   a. Central highly cellular zone.
   b. Zone of fibroblastic tissue surrounding the previous zone.
   c. Zone of new bone formation (outermost layer).

Aetiology

Traumatic myositis ossificans can be caused by various conditions as follow:

1. Trauma is commonest cause leading to haematoma formation in soft tissue. Later it undergoes ossification.
2. Vigorous massage
3. Repeated minor trauma
4. Dislocation and avulsion injuries.

Clinical Features

Patient of traumatic myositis ossificans may present with the following clinical features:

1. Patient presents with pain, localized swelling and loss of movement.
2. In elbow dislocation, brachialis is commonest muscle to undergo ossification.
3. In foot soldiers, repeated trauma is caused by carrying a rifle leading to ossification of deltoid muscle.
4. In horse riders, constant pressure of saddle against adductor causes ossification of adductor muscle known as **Prussian disease.**
5. **Post traumatic osteochondroma.** When myositis ossificans becomes mature, it is usually covered by a cartilaginous cap which is known as post traumatic osteochondroma.

Investigation

Biopsy will show the zone effect.

Treatment

1. First step is to immobilize the part by splintage.
2. Active physiotherapy.
3. Manipulation should be done under general anaesthesia. All the adhesions should not be broken slowly but it should snap abruptly.
4. Calcitonin, biphosphonate and analgesics can be tried.
5. Growth should be removed in mature stage.

Differential Diagnosis

Osteosarcoma is main tumor that can be included in it's differential diagnosis.

MYOSITIS OSSIFICANS PROGRESSIVA

This is a **congenital condition and not caused by trauma**. It has been mentioned here due to resemblance with the name of **Traumatic myositis ossificans.**

It may be associated with microdactyly, brachydactyly and klippel-feil syndrome.

Ossification commonly starts in trapezius and latissimus dorsi.

It has repeated episodes of sudden extension of ossification in muscle, fascia, tendon and aponeurosis.

Death may occur due to intercurrent infection. Only laboratory finding is raised eosinophil count. Blood chemistry is normal. It spreads distally in body. All the joint movements are lost.

AVASCULAR NECROSIS OF BONE

This is also known as aseptic necrosis of bone. Death of bone occurs due to lack of blood supply.

Aetiology

Avascular necrosis is not very uncommon entity and can be seen in following conditions:

1. Fracture dislocation
2. Excessive stripping of periosteum from bone during surgery
3. Caisson (Dysbaric) disease
4. Prolong intake of corticosteroid
5. Prolong intake of alcohol
6. Bone transplantation
7. Organ transplantation
8. Exposure to X-rays and radioactive substances
9. Metal erosion and ionization
10. Excessive reaming of intramedullary cavity, prior to insertion of nail.

Common Sites of AVN

1. Head of femur
2. Scaphoid
3. Talus

Other Sites of AVN

1. Capitellum
2. Segmental fractures

Head of femur

In fracture neck of femur blood supply to head of femur is disrupted. It later causes ischaemic necrosis of head of femur.

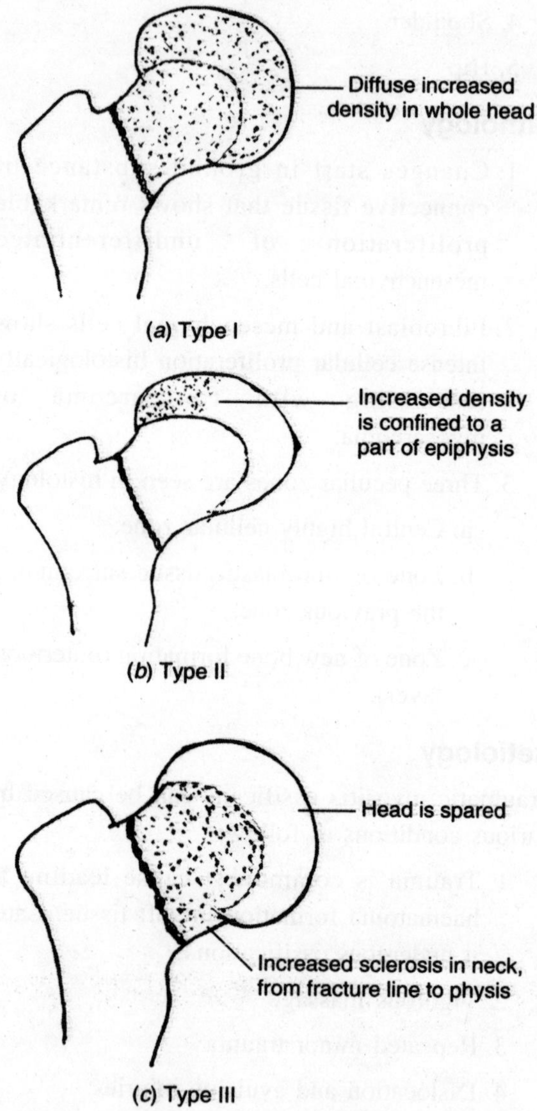

Fig. 4.11 Types of avascular necrosis of head of neck femur in children

Scaphoid

Avascular necrosis is more likely to develop in scaphoid if fracture is more proximal in it.

Talus

Fracture through the neck of talus or tarsal tunnel is more prone to develop avascular necrosis. Complete dislocation and excessive stripping can also cause AVN.

Capitellum, Head radius, Lateral femoral condyle

These bones can also develop AVN but it is not so common.

Segmental fracture

Due to separation of fragment from its shaft it deprives of blood supply. So it develops avascular necrosis later.

Histological Changes in AVN

Histology of AVN will show following findings:

- Lacunae are empty due to autolysis of osteocytes.
- Reactive hyperemia is seen in adjacent bone. Early demineralization and trabecular thining is seen.

Investigations

Following investigations should be done:

- X-ray of local part.
- Bone scan and Radioisotope study can detect AVN in early stage.
- It is visible as cold area on bone scan.

X-ray Findings

- Osteoporosis is seen in adjacent bone.
- Zone of sclerosis is observed at necrotic bone.
- Bone is deformed.
- Osteoarthritic changes are also present.

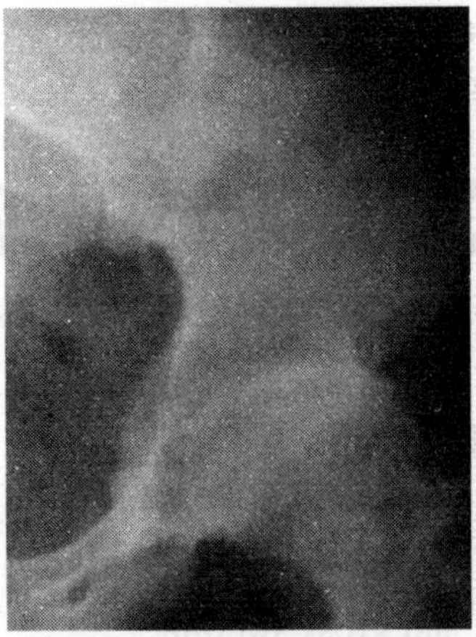

Fig. 4.12 AVN head femur

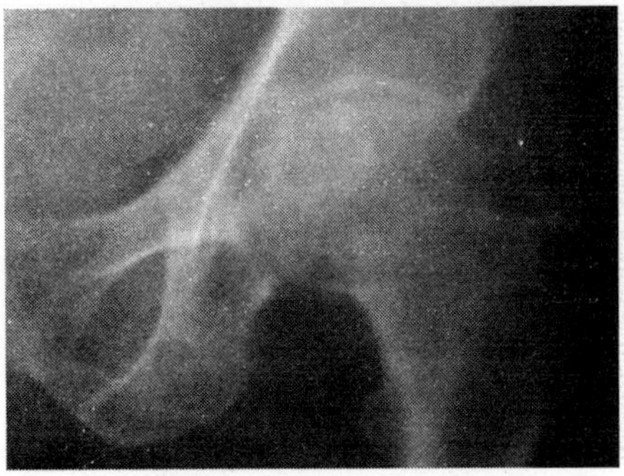

Fig. 4.13 AVN head femur

Treatment

AVN of head of femur, scaphoid and talus can be treated as mentioned below:

Head of Femur

- Avoid weight bearing.
- Excision of head femur followed by replacement arthroplasty.
- Avoid all predisposing factor to osteonecrosis.
- AVN head of femur due to fracture neck femur can be managed by ORIF by multiple screws and vascularised muscle pedicle bone graft, taken from quadratus femoris muscle.

Scaphoid and Talus

- Avascular segment can be excised.

SUDECK'S DYSTROPHY

This is also known as reflex sympathetic dystrophy. This condition is a sequalae of trauma.

Clinical Features

Patient presents with the following clinical features:

1. Pain and gross swelling.
2. Skin is red, shiny and warm in early stage.
3. In late stage, atrophic changes are seen in skin, muscle and nails.
4. Joint becomes stiff and deformed.

X-ray Findings

Spotty rarefaction is seen in X-ray.

Treatment

1. Prolonged physiotherapy gives best result.
2. In some cases beta blockers or sympathetic blockers are also helpful.

CHAPTER

5 Plaster, Traction and Splint

- Plaster of paris
- Types of plaster
- Period of immobilization in plaster
- Splints
- Traction

PLASTER OF PARIS

Chemical formula of powder of plaster is calcium sulphate hemihydrate. When it is dissolved in water, it converts into Calcium sulphate dihydrate by an exothermic reaction as follows:

$2(CaSO_4 \frac{1}{2}H_2O) + 3H_2O \leftrightarrow 2(CaSO_4.2H_2O) + Heat$

This is hard in consistency. Word 'Cast' or POP is used to denote complete plaster.

TYPES OF PLASTER

1. Above elbow POP with shoulderhood
2. Above elbow POP
3. Below elbow POP
4. Scaphoid cast
5. Below elbow volar slab
6. Above knee POP
7. Above knee cylinder POP
8. Sarmiento POP (patellar tendon bearing plaster)
9. Below knee POP
10. Shoulder spica
11. POP Hip spica
12. Whitman POP hip spica
13. One and half POP hip spica.

AEPOP with Shoulderhood

This plaster is applied in diaphyseal fracture of humerus. It extends proximally from base of neck, and distally to mid 1/3 of forearm. Elbow is kept at 90 degree flexion.

AEPOP

This plaster is indicated in following conditions:

1. Fracture both bones forearm
2. Monteggia fracture
3. Galeazzi fracture
4. Fracture supracondylar humerus
5. Fracture intercondylar humerus
6. Fracture lateral or medial condyle of humerus
7. Fracture head radius

8. Fracture olecranon
9. Fracture dislocation elbow

It extends proximally from insertion of deltoid and distally just proximal to MP joint (dorsal aspect) and on palmer aspect till distal or middle palmar crease. Elbow is kept in 90 degree flexion. Forearm is kept in midprone position in fracture of mid third of both bones. Forearm is kept in full supination in fracture upper third of both bones. Forearm is kept in full pronation in fracture of lower third of both bones of forearm. Wrist is kept in 10–15 degree of dorsiflexion.

BEPOP

At volar aspect it extends proximally 1 inch below the elbow crease and on dorsal aspect just distal to tip of olecranon. Lower extent is same as in AEPOP.

Scaphoid Cast

This cast is applied in scaphoid fracture. It extends proximally from middle of forearm and distally as in BEPOP with incorporation of thumb just proximal to interphalangeal joint. Wrist is kept in 20–30 degree dorsiflexion and little radial deviation. Thumb is kept in flexion and abduction. This position is known as cup holding position.

BEPOP Volar Slab

This plaster is applied in fractures of metacarpal and phalanx. This applied on volar aspect of palm and forearm. It extends proximally from 1 inch below elbow crease to tip of fingers. Wrist is kept in 10–15 degree of dorsiflexion. MP joints are kept at 90 degree of flexion. IP joints are fully extended. This plaster takes the shape of cobra hood in palm.

AKPOP

This is applied in fracture of both bones of leg. It extends proximally from the junction of upper and middle third of thigh and distally up to toes on plantar aspect, while on dorsal aspect it extends just proximal to metatarsophalageal joint. Knee is kept in 5–10 degree of flexion to avoid post reduction stiffness at knee. Ankle is kept in neutral position.

AKPOP Cylinder Cast

This plaster is applied in fracture of patella. Proximal extent is same as in AKPOP, while distal extent is just above the malleoli. Knee is kept in full extension.

BKPOP

This is applied in fracture of malleoli, talus, calcaneum, tarsal and metatarsal bone. Proximally it extends from the junction of upper and middle third of leg. Distal extent is same as in AKPOP.

POP Hip Spica

This is applied in children and young adults, when fracture shaft femur becomes sticky after reduction on Thomas knee splint. It extends proximally from subcostal margin and distally upto the same level as in AKPOP. Ankle is kept at five degree of plantarflexion, knee at 10 degree of flexion, hip at 20 degree abduction and 40 degree flexion. It can also be applied in one and half POP hip spica including opposite hip and lower one third of thigh.

Whitman POP Hip Spica

Proximally it extends from contralateral axilla and ipsilateral subcostal margin. Distal extent is same as in POP hip spica. This is applied in post operative phase of fracture neck femur where osteotomy is done.

Shoulder Spica

This plaster is applied in fracture shaft humerus and tuberculosis of shoulder joint. This plaster extends upward from subcostal margin and fixes shoulder and elbow joint. It extends up to middle 1/3 of forearm.

PTB Plaster

This plaster is applied when adequate callus is present in fracture both bones leg and patient is encouraged for walking. This is applied with heel. Upper part of this plaster is moulded in such a way that it takes the shape of patellar tendon. Proximally it extends from superior margin of patella on anterior aspect while at lowest margin of popliteal fossa at posterior aspect.

PERIOD OF IMMOBILIZATION IN PLASTER

Fracture	Adult	Children
Shaft humerus	2-3 months	1-1½ month
Surgical neck of humerus	3-4 weeks	3-4 weeks
Supracondylar humerus		3 weeks
Dislocation elbow	3 weeks	3 weeks
Head radius	3 weeks	
Neck radius		2-3 weeks
Clavicle	3-6 weeks	3 weeks
Dislocation shoulder	3 weeks	
Monteggia	2-3 months	1½ -2 months
Galleazi	3 months	
Green stick fracture		1½ -2 months
Scaphoid	3-4 months	
Colles's	6 weeks	
Neck femur	3-4 months	
Intertrochateric femur	3-4 months	
Dislocation hip	3-6 weeks	
Shaft femur	3-4 months	2-3 months
Patella	3-6 weeks	
Both bones leg	4-5 months	2-3 months
Potts	2-3 months	
Calcaneum	6-8 weeks	
Meatatarsal	3-4 weeks	
Talus	6-8 weeks	

SPLINTS

Splint is a kind of support used to immobilize the fracture.

Types of Splints

Wooden splints

1. **Long liston splint:** It is indicated in fracture neck femur, intertrochanteric femur and dislocation of hip.
2. **Posterior leg splint:** It is indicated in fracture both bones of leg, pott's and patella. It can be used with long liston splint in fractures around knee joint.
3. **Short posterior leg splint:** It is indicated in fracture of talus, calcaneum and metatarsal.
4. **High lateral elbow splint:** It is indicated in fracture shaft humerus.
5. **Lateral elbow splint:** It is indicated in fracture of both bones of forearm, supracondylar and intercondylar fracture humerus, lateral condyle humerus, monteggia fracture, galeazzi fracture, colles's fracture and dislocation of elbow.
6. **Airplane splint:** It is indicated in brachial plexus injury with fracture upper end humerus.

Metallic splint

1. **Thomas knee splint:** Sir Hugh Oven Thomas had invented this splint. He is also

CHAPTER 5

known as **father of orthopaedic surgery**. Earlier Thomas knee splint was used for tuberculosis of knee as an ambulatory treatment. Upper part of splint has a circular ring, which is connected by two parallel bars. Its lower end has a notch. This is **indicated** in fracture intertrochanteric femur, shaft femur and dislocation of hip.

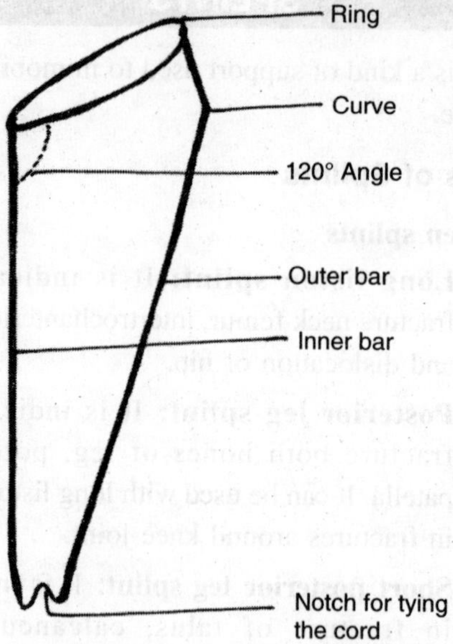

Fig. 5.1 Thomas knee splint

Following **precautions** should be taken while applying this splint:

a. Adequate padding should be done below popliteal fossa, over head of fibula (to prevent lateral popliteal nerve palsy) and around the ring to prevent pressure sores.
b. Limb should be kept in flexion and abduction to maintain reduction and to prevent pressure sores.

Complications of Thomas knee splint

- Lateral popliteal nerve palsy.
- Pressure sores
- Leukoplast reaction

Leukoplast contains zinc oxide that causes allergic reaction in skin beneath the leucoplast. Blisters develop in skin and later skin peels off. It should be treated by regular dressing of raw area by soframycin ointment and if required antibiotic coverage can be given.

2. **Crammer wire splint:** This is a mouldable splint and made up of galvanized iron. This is used in fracture patella and fracture surgical neck of humerus. It can also be used in radial nerve injury as an dynamic cock up splint.

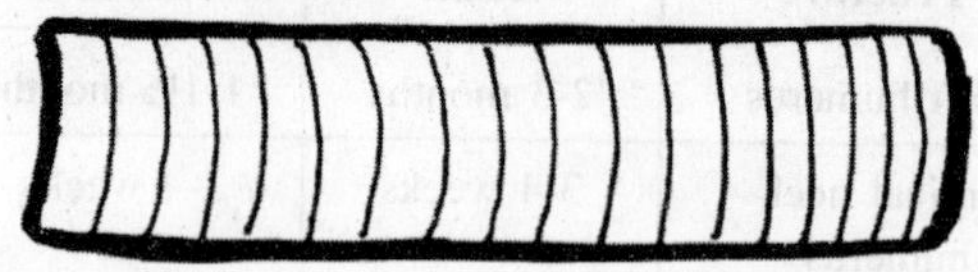

Fig. 5.2 Crammer-wire splint

3. **Dynamic cock up splint:** This is made up of crammer wire and used in radial nerve injury. Patient actively flexes his fingers while passive extension is done by finger loops attached to it.
4. **Bohler-Braun splint:** This is used in comminuted fracture of shaft femur and both bones leg.

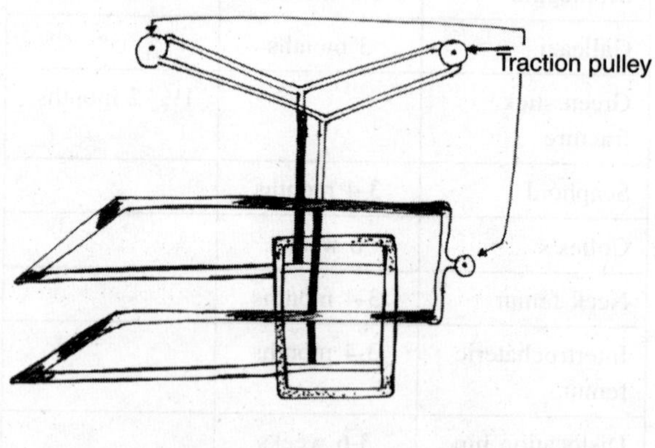

Fig. 5.3 Bohler-Braun splint

Other Splints

1. Pneumatic splint
2. Plaster splint

TRACTION

Force applied to a limb distal to fracture/ dislocation for reduction is known as traction. Apart from fracture/dislocation, traction is also applied in tuberculous arthritis, septic arthritis, flexion deformity of knee and hip.

Traction can be applied in following ways as follows:

- Manual traction
- Skin traction
- Skeletal traction

Traction can be applied between two fixed points, just to maintain the reduction. This is known as fixed traction e.g., in Thomas knee splint, traction is fixed to its notch.

When traction cord is passed through a pulley and weight is hanged through a pulley to counter the traction, it is known as balanced or sliding traction e.g., traction applied through Bohler Braun splint, below knee skin traction, Crutch field traction and Hamilton Russel traction.

Skin Traction

To apply skin traction, remove all the hairs from leg. Then tincture benzoin is applied on this shaved leg. Now a well measured leucoplast is taken on which sponge is fixed with tincture benzoin. At the centre of leucoplast strip a Spreader is attached with a hole in it's centre. This leucoplast strip is adhered to leg in such a way that gap of two fingers remains in between Spreader and heel. Now adequate padding is done by putting cotton at head of fibula and at malleoi (depending on above or below knee traction). Spiral bandage is applied over leucoplast. Traction is applied through central hole of Speader. Maximum of five pounds weight can be applied.

Disadvantages:

- Leukoplast reaction
- Pressure sores
- Lateral popliteal nerve palsy

Skeletal Traction

This traction is applied through bones by means of Steinman pin, calcaneal pin and K wires. Steinman pin is most commonly used for skeletal traction. It is passed from lateral to medial side (to prevent injury to lateral popliteal nerve) at upper end of tibia 2 cm below and behind tibial tuberosity. Steinman pin can also be passed through condyle of femur, lower end of tibia and calcaneum. This should be applied under full aseptic condition, otherwise pintrack infection is likely to occur which may cause osteomyelitis later.

CHAPTER

6 Peripheral Nerve Injuries

- Applied anatomy
- Wallerian degeneration
- Motor march phenomenon
- Seddon's classification of nerve injury
- Lateral popliteal nerve palsy
- Foot drop
- Radial nerve injury
- Median nerve injury
- Ulnar nerve injury
- Leprosy and peripheral nerve injuries

APPLIED ANATOMY

Peripheral nerve is made up of axons. Each nerve fibre is covered by endoneurium. Bunch of each nerve fibres collectively make a fasiculus. Each fasiculus is covered by perineurium. Multiple number of fasiculi are bound together by epineurium. (See Fig. 6.1)

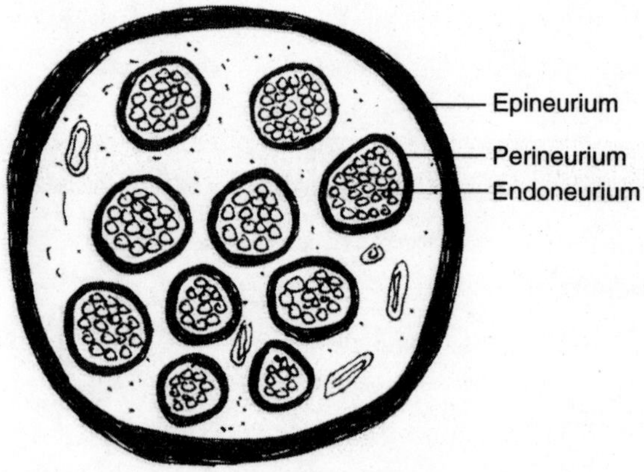

Fig. 6.1 Section of a nerve

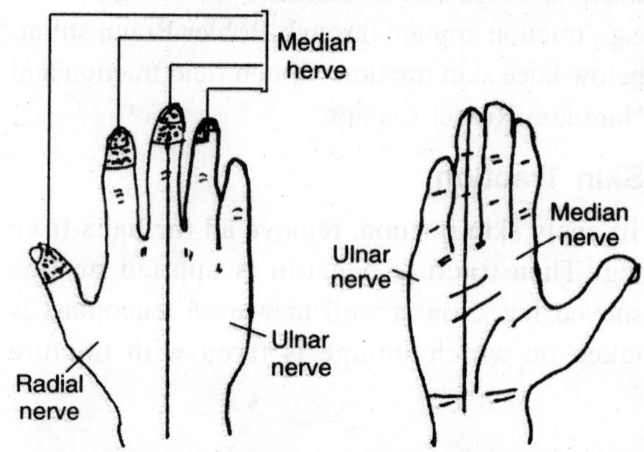

(*a*) Cutaneous nerve supply of dorsum of hand (*b*) Cutaneous nerve supply of palmar aspect of hand

Fig. 6.2 Sensory supply of hand

WALLERIAN DEGENERATION

Secondary degeneration of neuron occurring distal to site of injury in a nerve is known as Wallerian degeneration. Retrograde degeneration occurs in proximal part of nerve.

MOTOR MARCH PHENOMENON

Muscle which is nearest to the site of injury recovers first because reinnervation of muscle (by nerve) occurs from proximal to distal site.

Nerve regeneration occurs at the rate of 1 mm/day or 1 inch/month.

SEDDON'S CLASSIFICATION OF NERVE INJURY

Seddon's has classified three types of nerve injury as follows:

1. Neuropraxia
2. Axonotmesis
3. Neurotmesis

Neuropraxia

Physiological interruption of conduction of nerve fibre without any structural change is known as Neuropraxia. Complete recovery occurs in two weeks.

Axonotmesis

This type of injury presents with Wallerian degeneration. In this injury damage occurs to axon, maintaining the internal architecture intact. Complete recovery may not be possible. Recovery can occur with in few months.

Neurotmesis

Nerve is damaged by a sharp cut. This type of injury presents with Wallerian degeneration. This requires repair of nerve.

LATERAL POPLITEAL NERVE

Applied Anatomy (Sciatic Nerve)

1. This is thickest nerve of body.
2. Root value is L_{4-5}, $S_{1, 2, 3}$
3. Before dividing into branches it supplies biceps, semitendinosus, semimembranosus and adductor magnus.
4. Superficial peroneal nerve supplies peroneus longus and peroneus brevis.
5. Deep peroneal nerve supplies tibialis anterior, extensor hallucis longus, extensor digitorum longus and peroneus tertius.

Complete Sciatic Nerve Palsy

In addition to lateral popliteal nerve palsy, medial popliteal nerve is also paralysed. Patient will present with paralysis of intrinsic muscle of foot, loss of plantar flexion of ankle and toes. Patient also has sensory deficit over sole.

Sensory Supply of Foot

Lateral popliteal nerve gives it's sensory branches to following areas:

1. Lateral part of leg, skin over lateral malleolus and skin over dorsum of foot is supplied by superficial peroneal nerve.
2. First web space in dorsal aspect is supplied by deep peroneal nerve.
3. Medial border of foot is supplied by Saphenous nerve.
4. Lateral border of foot is supplied by Sural nerve.
5. Soles and tips of toes are supplied by posterior tibial nerve.

FOOT DROP

Foot drop has certain classical features as mentioned below:

1. It is caused by lateral popliteal nerve palsy also known as common peroneal nerve.
2. High stepping gait is characteristic.
3. Muscle wasting occurs at anterolateral aspect of leg.

4. **Motor paralysis** occurs in following muscles. (See table no. 6.1).

Table 6.1: Pattern of motor paralysis in foot drop

Muscles	Impairment
Tibialis anterior	Ankle dorsiflexion is lost
Extensor hallucis longus	Active extension of great toe is lost
Extensor digitorum longus	Active extension of toes is lost
Peroneus longus	Active eversion is lost
Peroneus brevis	Active inversion is lost

5. Sensory loss occurs at dorsum of foot i.e. autonomous zones.

Causes of Foot Drop

AT HIP

1. Posterior dislocation of hip.
2. Fracture acetabulum.
3. Deep intramuscular injection.

AT THIGH

1. Grossly displaced fracture shaft femur.
2. Stab or gun shot injury.

AT KNEE

1. Dislocation of knee.
2. Fracture neck of fibula.
3. Fracture medial condyle of tibia leading to varus stress on knee resulting on traction on nerve.
4. Overcorrection of gross genu valgum deformity.

Other Causes

1. Tight plaster without padding.
2. Incorrect skin traction.
3. Wrongly applied Thomas knee splint.
4. Leprosy is commonest general cause.

Treatment

In fresh case following conservative treatment is recommended:

1. Neurotropics can be given in terms of injections of methylcobalamine.
2. Toe raising appliance can be given to the patient by which he can passively move his toes.
3. Below knee caliper with a posterior check can be given to patient while walking. This foot drop appliance is of two types. One is dynamic spring shoe type and second is static with posterior check.
4. We should wait for recovery for 18 months. After this period chance of improvement in motor power is very low.
5. **Surgery.** Tibialis posterior can be transferred by interosseous route or circumtibial route as a substitute of tibialis anterior. Incomplete foot drop can be managed by transfer of tibialis posterior to EHL along with peroneus brevis transfer that checks excessive valgus deformity due to excessive eversion.

RADIAL NERVE INJURY

Applied Anatomy

1. Radial nerve arises from posterior cord of brachial plexus. Root value is $C_{5, 6, 7, 8}$ T_1.
2. It descends behind the third part of axillary artery and infront of subscapularis, latissimus dorsi and teres major.
3. Before radial groove this nerve gives rise to branch to medial head of triceps and posterior cutaneous nerve of arm.
4. In radial groove it gives rise to branches to lateral head of triceps, anconeus, cutaneous branch to arm and forearm.

5. Radial nerve pierces the lateral intermuscular septum at the junction of middle and lower third of arm.
6. It reaches to anterior compartment between brachialis on medial side and extensor carpi radialis longus and brachioradialis on lateral side.

Branches of Radial Nerve

Radial nerve divides into two branches before crossing elbow infront of lateral condyle.

Superficial sensory branches

This branch provides sensory supply to lateral part of dorsum of hand including lateral 3½ digits.

Deep branch (Posterior interosseous nerve)

This is primarily a motor nerve. Before piercing the supinator it gives rise branch to extensor carpi radialis brevis and supinator.

In posterior compartment of forearm it gives branches to following muscle:

1. Superficial muscles of forearm–ECRB, ED, EDM and ECU.
2. Deep muscles of forearm–supinator, APL, EPB, EPB, EPL and EI.

Aetiology of Radial Nerve Palsy

Radial nerve injury is commonly seen in orthopaedics OPD. It can be caused by following reasons:

1. Commonest cause of radial nerve injury is fracture shaft humerus
2. Crutch palsy
3. Saturday night palsy
4. Fracture dislocation of head radius (Posterior interoosseous nerve palsy)
5. Excision head radius (PIN palsy)
6. Monteggia fracture dislocation (PIN palsy)
7. During reduction of fracture shaft humerus
8. Post injection palsy.

High Radial Nerve Palsy

Triceps and anconeus are spared in high radial nerve palsy. This is seen when radial nerve is injured in radial groove. Rests of the muscles (supplied by radial nerve) are paralysed. In very high radial nerve palsy all the muscles including triceps are paralysed.

Clinically patient presents with loss of wrist extension, digital extension, and loss of radial abduction of thumb, loss of accessory forearm flexion and loss of accessory supination. Sensation is lost at lateral part of dorsum of hand including lateral 3½ digits.

Low Radial Nerve Palsy

All the muscles supplied by radial nerve in distal arm are paralysed except brachioradialis and extensor carpi radialis longus and brevis.

Crutch Palsy

Radial nerve injury caused by improper use of crutch or due to fracture dislocation of upper end humerus is known as crutch palsy.

Saturday Night Palsy

This radial nerve palsy occurs when patient takes deep sleep on a chair under the influence of alcohol (with arm hanging at the edge of chair).

Clinical Examination of Muscles Supplied by Radial Nerve

Brachioradialis

Ask the patient to flex his elbow from 90 degree onward against resistance. Forearm should remain in mid prone position. During examination contracted brachioradialis becomes prominent which can be felt.

Triceps

Ask the patient to extend his elbow against resistance. Contracted triceps becomes prominent that can be felt by examiner.

Management

Following investigations should be done prior to treatment of nerve injury:

1. Electromyography (EMG)
2. Nerve conduction velocity (NCV)
3. Strength duration curve.

Electromyography

In this procedure electrical activity of muscle is recorded on a graph during activity and rest.

EMG is indicated in following conditions:

a. To rule out nerve injury
b. To differentiate between complete and incomplete nerve injury
c. To find out regenerative changes in a nerve
d. To decide level of injury.

Nerve conduction velocity

Normal conduction velocity is approximately 70 meter/second. Measurement of conduction velocity of impulse generated between two points of nerve is known as nerve conduction velocity.

Strength duration curve

In this investigation, excitability of nerve and muscle is recorded on a graph.

Tinel sign

This is a clinical sign of recovery of nerve function. If we gently percuss the skin by hammer along the course of nerve from distal to proximal, a tingling sensation will be felt by the patient in the area supplied by nerve (not at the percussion site). This tingling sensation usually persists for a few seconds and known as positive Tinel sign.

Hitch-hiker's sign

Patient is unable to perform active extension of thumb, due to radial nerve palsy. This is known as Hitch-hiker's sign.

Treatment

1. Neurotropics should be started in the form of injection of methylcobalamine, Vitamin B1, B6, B12.
2. Gentle massage should be done at regu! interval.
3. Dynamic cock up splint is most useful device. This splint prevents contractures by keeping wrist joint in functional position. (15–20 degree) While using dynamic cock up splint patient actively flexes wrist and fingers but extension is done passively by the springs attached to splint. It also maintains the tone and nutrition of paralyzed extensor muscle.

Indications of surgery

1. Perineural fibrosis
2. Sharp cutting injury of nerve
3. Nerve injury producing gap between 2 ends of nerve.

Types of surgery in fresh injury

Among all nerves radial nerve has best chance of recovery. However following types of surgeries can be permormed:

1. Neurolysis
2. Neurorrhaphy
3. Nerve grafting.

Neurolysis

Nerve is freed from adjacent fibrosis or callus in this procedure.

Neurorrhaphy

In this surgical procedure both ends of nerve are sutured. Suturing can be done by three following methods: (See Fig. 6.3)

a. Epineural suturing

b. Perineural suturing

c. Epiperineural suturing.

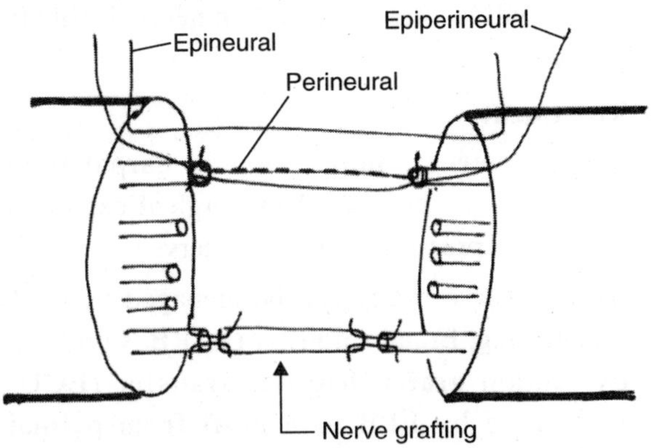

Fig. 6.3 Nerve repair techniques

Nerve grafting

A nerve graft can be taken from sural nerve to fill the gap between two ends of nerve.

Types of surgery in old cases

Old nerve injuries can be repaired by tendon transfer.

Jones tendon transfer

Three types of tendon transfer have been described by Jones

1. Pronator teres (PT) can be transferred to Extensor carpi radialis longus (ECRL) and brevis (ERCB).
2. Flexor carpi radialis (FCR) is transferred to Extensor pollicis longus (EPL) and abductor pollicis longus (APL).
3. Flexor carpi ulnaris (FCU) can be transferred to Extensor digitorum (ED) and Extensor pollicis longus (EPL).

Modified Jones transfer (Zachary's method)

1. Pronator teres (PT) can be transferred to ECRL and ECRB.
2. Palmaris longus can be transferred to Abductor pollicis longus (APL).
3. FCU is transferred to extensor digitorum (ED) and Extensor pollicis longus (EPL).

Other methods

1. Brand's transfer
2. Boye's transfer

MEDIAN NERVE INJURY

Applied Anatomy

1. Median nerve is formed by union of lateral and medial cord of brachial plexus.
2. In hand it passes deep to flexor retinaculum.
3. Median nerve terminates by dividing into 4-5 palmar digital branches.

Muscular branches in forearm

Median nerve gives following branches in forearm:

1. FDS (Flexor digiorum superficialis)
2. Lateral half of FDP
3. FPL (Flexor pollicis longus)
4. FCR (Flexor carpi radialis).

Muscular branches in hand

Following three muscle are supplied by median nerve in hand:

1. APB (Abductor pollicis brevis)
2. OP (Opponens pollicis)
3. First and second lumbricals.

Clinical Examination of Muscles Supplied by Median Nerve

Flexor digitorum superficialis and lateral half of FDP

Ask the patient to clasp his hand. If median nerve is injured, his index finger will remain straight, due to paralysis of finger flexor superficialis and profundus of index finger. This is known as **Pointing index or Oschner's clasping hand.** (See Fig. 6.10)

Benediction test

Ask the patient to lift his hand. Patient will be unable to flex index and middle finger, due to paralysis of flexor digitorum superficialis and lateral half of FDP. This is the position of clergyman's hand who uses to bless couple during marriage. (See Fig. 6.11)

Flexor pollicis longus

First stabilize the proximal phalanx of thumb then ask the patient to flex terminal phalanx of thumb. In median nerve injury he will not be able to do so. (See Fig. 6.9)

Flexor carpi radialis

If we ask the patient to palmar flex his wrist, it will deviate to ulnar side, if median nerve is injured.

Pen test (Abductor pollicis brevis)

Ask the patient to keep his hand flat on table with palm facing toward ceiling. Now a pen is held above the palm and patient is asked to touch the pen with the tip of thumb. In median nerve injury he will not be able to do so. (See Fig. 6.8)

Opponens pollicis

Patient is asked to count on fingers (opposition of thumb to fingers). In median nerve injury he will not be able to do so.

High Median Nerve Palsy

All the muscles supplied by median nerve are paralyzed and sensory deficit is present in skin of hand.

Low Median Nerve Palsy

All the muscles supplied by median nerve are paralyzed. Muscles of forearm are spared. Sensory deficit will be present at median nerve distribution in hand.

Treatment

Median nerve compression in carpal tunnel syndrome can be treated by surgical exploration and decompression of median nerve.

Median nerve injury can be managed by tendon transfer. e.g. Brand's transfer (ECRB is prolonged by tendon graft), Riordan transfer (ECU is prolonged by EPB or a graft from palmaris longus) or Brown's transfer (Transfer of ECRL is prolonged by a 4 tailed graft) to restore MP joint flexion.

ULNAR NERVE INJURY

Applied Anatomy

1. Ulnar nerve is a branch of medial cord of brachial plexus.
2. Root value is C_8T_1.
3. In axilla it lies on medial side of axillary artery.
4. In elbow it lies behind medial epicondyle along with superior ulnar collateral artery.
5. While entering in forearm it passes between two heads of Flexor carpi ulnaris.
6. In forearm it lies infront of flexor digitorum profundus.

7. In wrist it is superficial to flexor retinaculum.
8. It lies in between pissiform bone on lateral side and ulnar artey on medial side.
9. It terminates by dividing into two branches, superficial and deep.

Muscular branches

Ulnar nerve gives branches to following muscles:

1. Flexor carpi ulnaris and medial half of flexor digitorum profundus.
2. All interossei (Palmar and dorsal)
3. 3rd and 4th lumbricals
4. Hypothenar Muscles (Abductor digiti minimi, Flexor digiti minimi and opponens digiti minimi.)
5. Adductor pollicis
6. Flexor pollicis brevis (Deep head).

Sensory supply

Following parts of hand have been supplied by sensory branches of ulnar nerve:

1. Medial side of hand
2. Whole of little finger
3. Medial side of ring finger.

High Ulnar Nerve Palsy

Whenever we get a case of ulnar nerve injury, it becomes necessary to identify it as either high or low ulnar nerve injury. High ulnar nerve injury has following features:

1. FCU and medial half of FDP are paralyzed.
2. Paralysis of muscles supplied by ulnar nerve in hand.
3. Clawing of liltle and ring finger is minimum or absent.
4. Sensory deficit is seen in skin of hand.

Low Ulnar Nerve Palsy

Low ulnar nerve injury can be identified by following features:

1. Only the muscles of hand supplied by ulnar nerve are paralyzed. Muscles of forearm are spared.
2. Clawing of little and ring finger is more prominent.
3. Sensory deficit occurs in skin of hand.

Ulnar Paradox

High ulnar nerve palsy causes less deformity and known as Ulnar paradox. In high ulnar nerve palsy FDP (medial half) is paralyzed and does not work unopposed by interossei and lumbricals. This makes the deformity less obvious.

Claw Hand

In this deformity hyperextension occurs at MP joint and flexion occurs at PIP and DIP joint. It occurs due to paralysis of interossei and lumbricals (which cause flexion at MP joint and extension at PIP and DIP joint). Claw hand is seen in ulnar nerve injury. If at same time median nerve is also injured e.g. Klumpke's paralysis, this deformity becomes more prominent.

Clinical Examination of Ulnar Nerve

Card test

This test is done to check the function of palmar interossei. Insert a card in between 2 extended fingers and ask the patient to hold it tightly. Meanwhile examiner tries to pull out the card. Card can easily be pulled out in case of weakness of palmar interossei. (See Fig. 6.4)

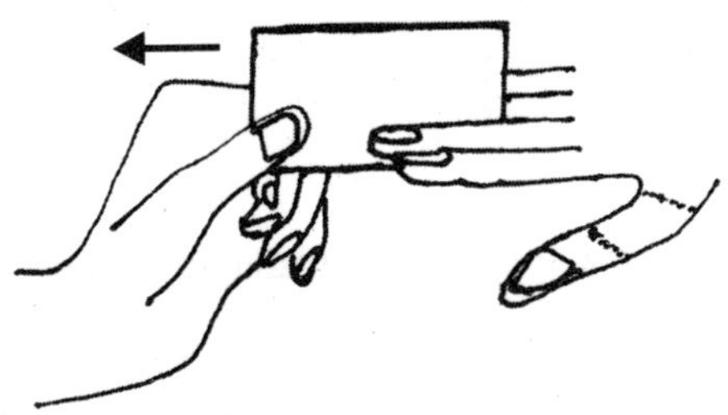

Fig. 6.4 Card test

Egawa test

This test is done to check the function of dorsal interossei. Dorsal interossei are abductors of middle finger. Ask the patient to keep his palm flat on table (palm facing downward). Now ask the patient to move his fingers sideways (abduction). In case of weakness of dorsal interossei he will not be able to do so. (See Fig. 6.5)

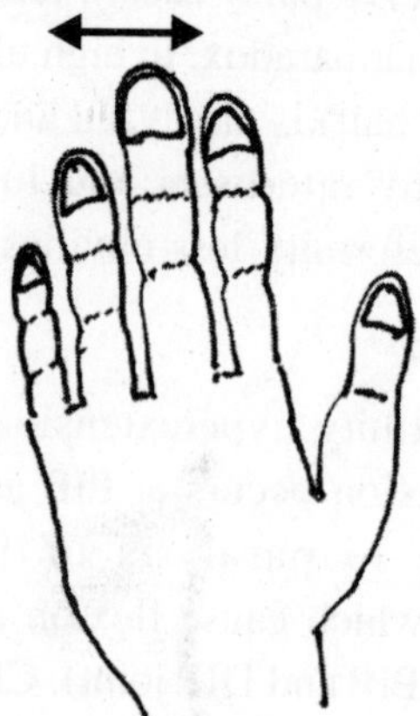

Fig. 6.5 Egawa test

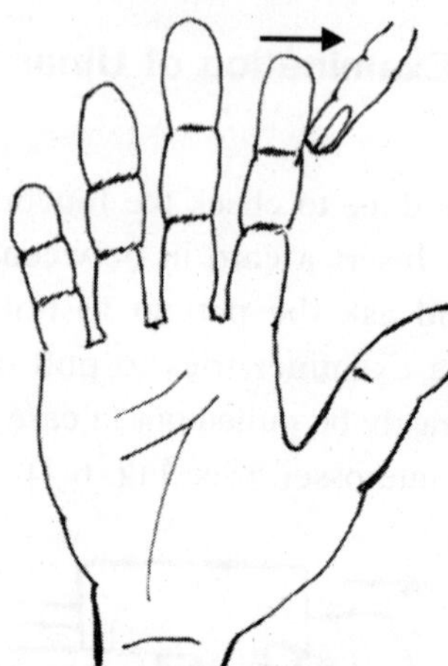

Fig. 6.6 Testing of first palmar interosseous

Froment sign

This test is done to check the strength of adductor pollicis. Ask the patient to hold a book firmly with extended thumb and fingers. In case of weakness of adductor pollicis patient will hold the book with flexion of thumb at interphalangeal joint. This flexon is caused by flexor pollicis longus, which is supplied by median nerve. (See Fig. 6.7)

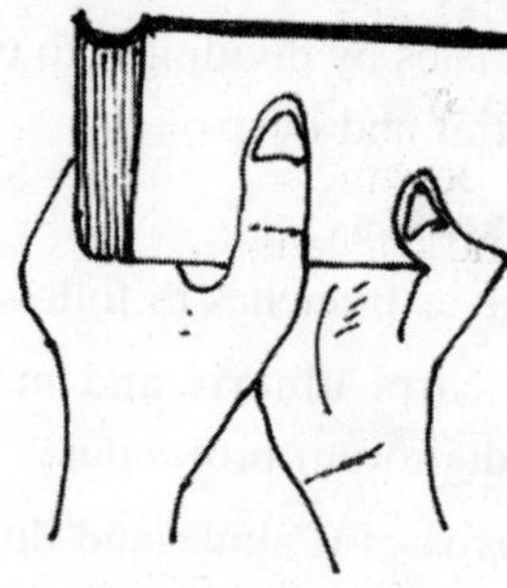

Fig. 6.7 Book test (Froment sign)

Flexor carpi ulnaris

This muscle can be tested by asking the patient to palmar flex the wrist against gravity, wrist will deviate toward radial side in case of weakness of FCU.

Abductor digiti minimi

To test this muscle, ask the patient to keep his hand flat on table, then ask to abduct the little finger against resistance. In case of weakness of this muscle he will not be able to do so.

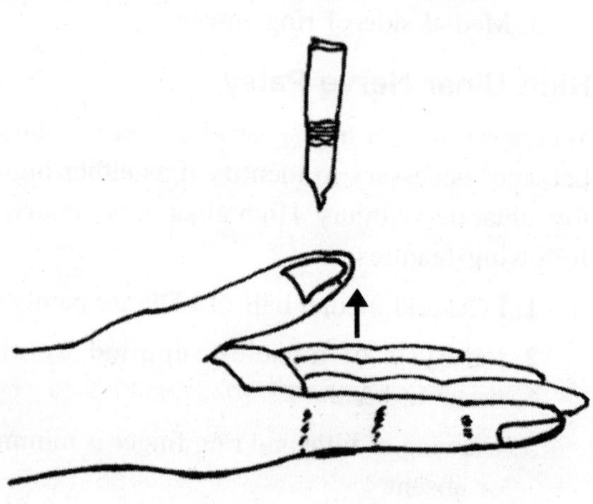

Fig. 6.8 Pen test

Tardy Ulnar Nerve Palsy

This is ulnar nerve palsy that appears late. It is commonly seen in fracture lateral condyle humerus leading to cubitus valgus deformity. It is also seen in fracture supracondylar humerus. This is managed by anterior transposition of nerve.

Causes of Ulnar Nerve Injuries

Immediate palsy

1. Most common cause is fracture supracondylar humerus.
2. Fracture medial condyle of humerus.
3. Lacerated injuries at wrist can also cause ulnar nerve injury.

Late (Tardy) ulnar nerve palsy

1. Cubitus valgus deformity in fracture lateral condyle of humerus and fracture supracondylar humerus.
2. Entrapment of ulnar nerve by callus formation, commonly seen in fracture supracondylar humerus.

Other Causes

Leprosy is commonest cause.

Tendon Transfer in Ulnar Nerve Injury

Brand's transfer

This is also known as Zancolli's capsulodesis. In this procedure volar capsule of MP joint is shortened.

Bunnell's transfer

Flexor digitorum superficialis of ring finger is transferred to radial aspect of all four fingers by dividing FDS into four slips.

LEPROSY AND PERIPHERAL NERVE INJURIES

Leprosy commonly affects three peripheral nerves:

1. Ulnar nerve
2. Lateral popliteal nerve
3. Posterior tibial nerve

Facial, trigeminal, median and radial nerves are less commonly affected.

Pathology

Nerve damage causes anhydrosis leading to development of cracks and ulcer. Anaeasthesia causes pressure sores and injury, leading to ulcer formation. Motor loss causes weakness and paralysis of muscles leading to contracture.

Deformities and Disabilities

Patient may present with deformities and disabilities according to type of nerve involvement as follows:

Ulnar nerve

1. Clawing of ring and little finger.
2. Anaesthesia and anhydrosis over little finger and inner half of ring finger.

Median nerve

1. Loss of abduction and opposition of thumb.
2. Anaesthesia over thumb, index, middle and lateral half of ring finger.

Radial nerve

1. Wrist drop
2. Anaesthesia and anhydrosis over back of hand.

Lateral popliteal nerve

1. Foot drop.
2. Anaesthesia over lower leg and dorsum of foot.

Posterior tibial nerve

1. Clawing of toes
2. Anaesthesia and anhydrosis over sole of foot.

Facial nerve

Patient is unable to close the eye (lagopthalmos).

Trigeminal nerve

Patient presents with anaesthesia over cornea.

Pauci Bacillary

If only one nerve is involved it is called as paucibacillary leprosy. Patient is given **six months therapy** of MDT regimen. Rifampicin (600 mg) is given once in a month for six months. Dapsone (100 mg) is given daily for six months.

Dose in children between 10–14 years age is different. Rifampicin is given 450 mg once in a month for six months. Dapsone is given 50 mg daily for six months.

Dose in children of less than 10 years of age is also different. Rifampicin is given 300 mg once in a month for six months. Dapsone is given 25 mg daily for six months.

Multi Bacillary

If more than one nerve are involved it is called as multi bacillary leprosy. Patient is given **12 months therapy of** MDT regimen. Rifampicin (600 mg) is given once in a month for 12 months. Dapsone (100 mg) is given daily for 12 months. Clofazamine (300 mg once in a month and 50 mg daily) is given for twelve months.

Dose in children between 10–14 years age is different. Rifampicin is given 450 mg once in a month. Dapsone is given 50 mg daily. Clofazamine is given 150 mg once in a month and 50 mg daily.

Dose in children below 10 years is also different. Rifampicin is given 300 mg once in a month. Dapsone is given 25 mg daily. Clofazamine is given 100 mg once in a month and 50 mg twice in a week.

Grading of Disabilities

Disabilities have been classified into three grades as follows:

Grade 0

No visible deformity/damage and no anaesthesia.

Grade 1

No visible deformity/damage but anaesthesia is present.

Grade 2

Visible deformity or damage is seen.

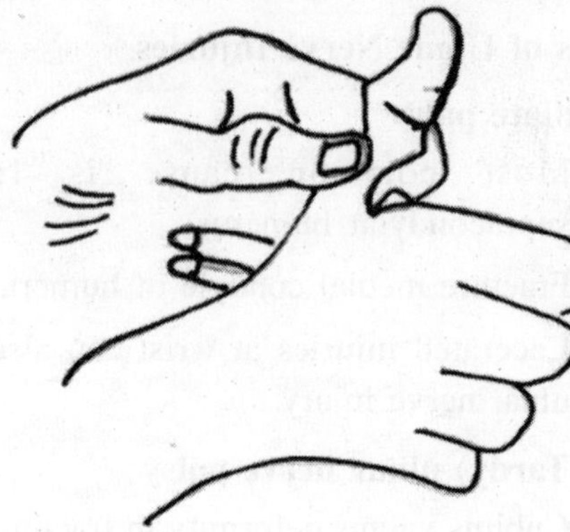

Fig. 6.9 Test for flexor pollicis longus

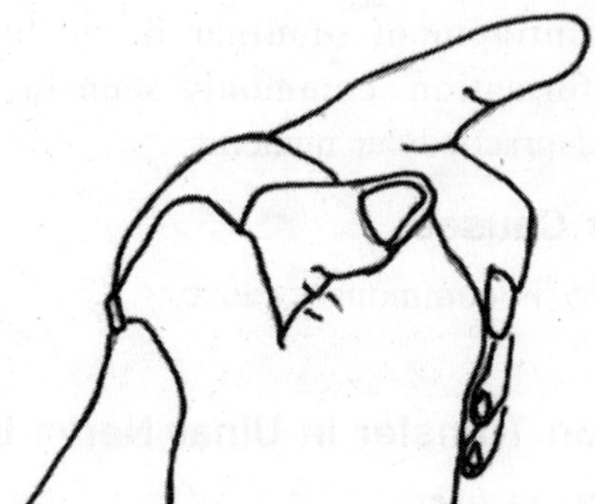

Fig. 6.10 Oschner's clasping hand

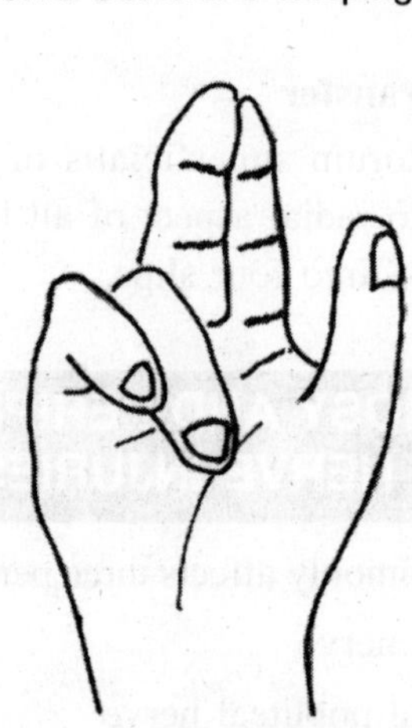

Fig. 6.11 Benediction test

CHAPTER

7 Injuries Around Shoulder

FRACTURE OF CLAVICLE

APPLIED ANATOMY

1. This is first bone to ossify in body (5th week of fetal life).
2. Clavicle ossifies from two primary centres.
3. Sometimes clavicle is pierced by middle supraclavicular nerve.
4. This is the commonest bone to be fractured in children.
5. This is the only long bone lying horizontally.
6. It ossifies from a membrane.
7. This bone is subcutaneous throughout.

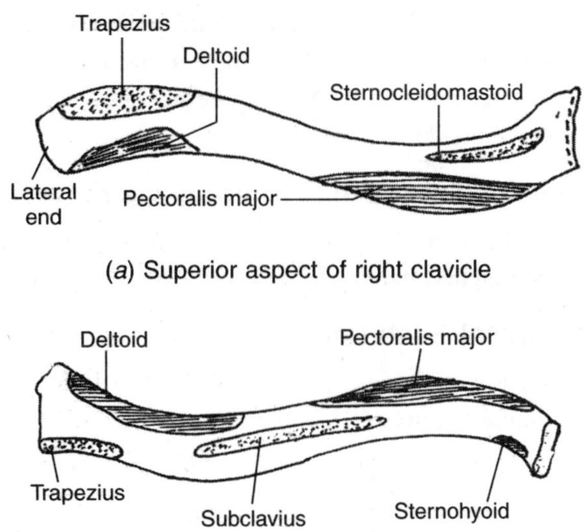

(b) Inferior aspect of right clavicle

Fig. 7.1 Applied anatomy of clavicle

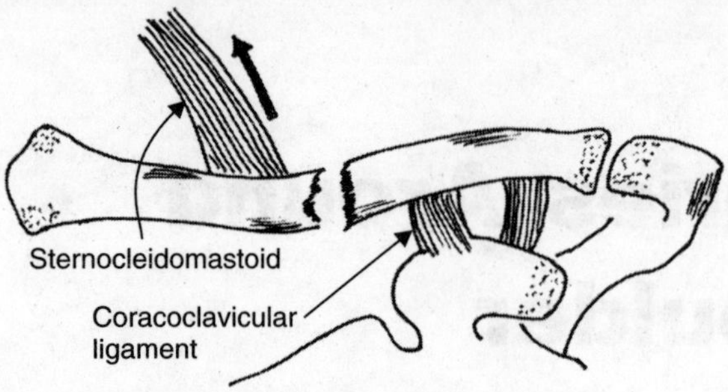

Fig. 7.1 (c) Fracture of clavicle

Allman's Classification

Allman has classified it into 3 groups as follows:

Group 1: Fracture of middle third.

Group 2: Fracture of distal third.

Group 3: Fracture of medial third.

Group 1 is most common type in adults and children (80%). It is at the junction of middle and distal third. Group 3 is least common.

Panclavicular Fracture

This is also known as **Traumatic floating clavicle.** In this condition there is no clavicular fracture, but two ligaments (sternoclavicular and coracoclavicular) are disrupted.

Mechanism of Injury in Clavicle Fracture

Most commonly it is caused by fall on outstretched hand.

Clinical Features

Fracture of clavicle can be diagnosed by following clinical features:

1. Pain, swelling and deformity at clavicle.
2. Difficulty in lifting the affected arm.
3. Bony tenderness, crepitus and abnormal mobility at fracture site.

Investigation

X-ray of shoulder AP view will show the fracture in clavicle.

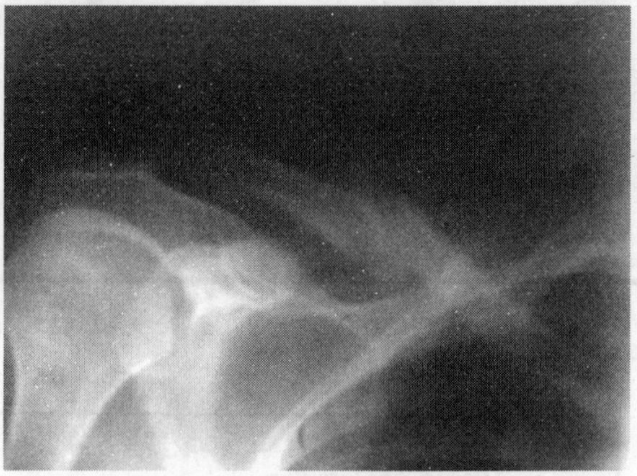

Fig. 7.2 Fracture clavicle

Treatment

This is treated by figure of eight bandage with cuff and collar sling. If we apply POP bandage over figure of eight bandage it is known as **Billington Yoke POP.**

New born and infants are treated by arm to chest bandage.

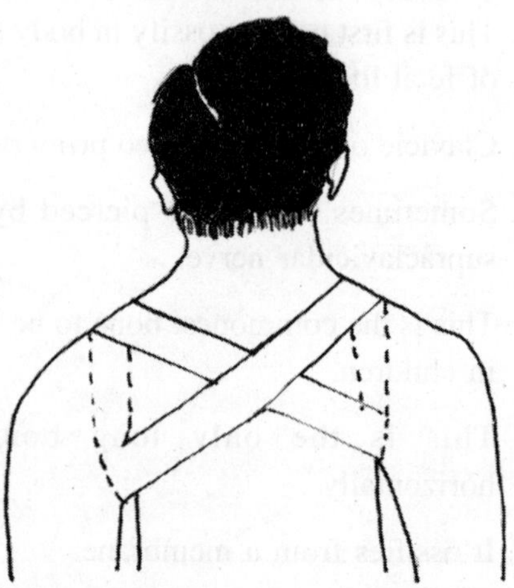

Fig. 7.3 Figure of eight bandage

Indications of ORIF

Surgical treatment of fracture clavicle is required in following conditions:

1. Neurovascular injury
2. Grossly displaced fracture
3. Compound fracture
4. Floating shoulder
5. Group 2 (distal clavicular) fracture.

ORIF can be done by dynamic compression plate or Steinman pin or knowle pin.

Complications

Fracture clavicle can have following complications:

1. Malunion
2. Nonunion (rare)
3. Neurovascular deficit
4. Post traumatic arthritis.

Floating Shoulder

This is fracture of clavicle and shoulder. This should be treated by open reduction and internal fixation of both fractures. Primarily clavicle should be stabilized.

Other Injuries at Shoulder

1. Acromioclavicular Injury
2. Costoclavicular Injury

Previous one is more common and caused by direct impact at shoulder. It can be treated by cuff and collar sling with adhesive or elastic strapping.

Costoclavicular injury is caused by indirect impact at shoulder. It can be treated by clavicular strapping or figure of eight bandage. If it fails, it can be fixed with K wire.

FRACTURE OF SCAPULA

Fracture of scapula is uncommon injury in orthopaedics. It constitutes 0.5% of all fracture.

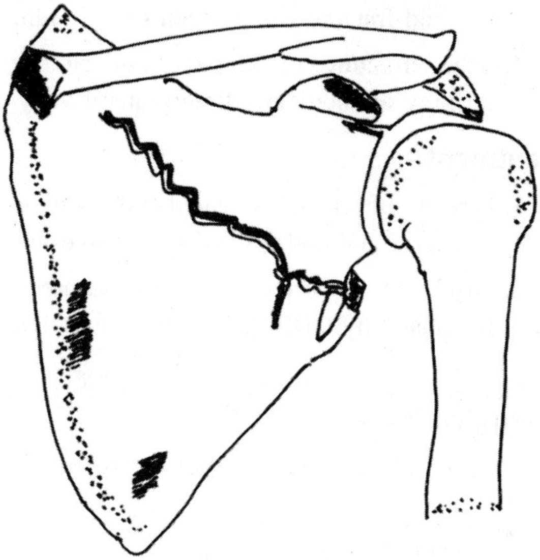

Fig. 7.4 Major scapular body fracture

Thompson's Classification

Thompson and colleagues have classified fracture of scapula into three types as follows:

Type 1: Coracoid, acromian and small fracture of body.

Type 2: Fracture of glenoid and neck.

Type 3: Major scapular body fracture.

Clinical Features

Fracture scapula can be diagnosed by following clinical features:

1. Patient presents with arm held in adduction.
2. Shoulder is flattened.
3. Echymosis is present at shoulder.
4. Patient complaints of pain on deep inspiration.
5. Bony tenderness and crepitus is present at fracture site.

X-Ray Findings

Different parts of scapula can be seen radiologically in certain views:

1. Coracoid fracture is seen in cephalic tilt or stryker notch view.

2. Glenoid fracture can be seen in CT scan.
3. Other fracture of scapula can be seen in x-ray of shoulder AP and lateral view.

Treatment

1. Fracture of scapula is treated conservatively with cuff and collar sling and analgesics.
2. Displaced intraarticular glenoid fracture can be treated by ORIF by 3.5 mm cannulated AO screw.

Complications

Fracture scapula can have following complications:

1. Fracture ribs on same side.
2. Pulmonary contusion.
3. Pneumothorax.
4. Brachial plexus injury.

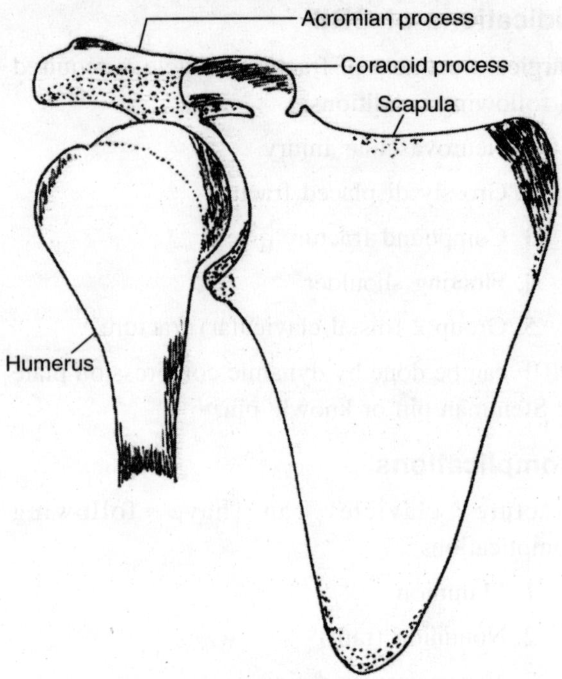

Fig. 7.5 Shoulder joint

FRACTURE OF PROXIMAL HUMERUS

Anatomy of Proximal Humerus

It has five parts humeral head, greater and lesser tuberosity, bicipital groove and proximal humeral shaft.

Anatomical fracture neck humerus is rare and likely to undergo avascular necrosis due to complete disruption of blood supply to humeral head. While fracture surgical neck humerus is more common. Blood supply is not hampered in this fracture.

Rotator cuff and deltoid muscles have main role in glenohumeral function. Rotator cuff consists of four muscles, subscapularis, supraspinatus, infraspinaus and teres minor. Teres minor and infraspinatus are external rotator while subscapularis depresses the head of humerus.

Blood Supply of Head of Humerus

Anterior circumflex humeral artery is the main arterial supply of humeral head.

Arterial Supply of Rotator Cuff

Rotator cuff is supplied by following arteries:

1. Anterior circumflex humeral artery
2. Posterior circumflex humeral artery
3. Subscapular artery
4. Suprascapular artery
5. Suprahumeral artery
6. Thoracoacromial artery.

Associated Nerve Injuries

In descending order of frequency associated nerve injuries are as follows:

1. Axillary nerve injury
2. Suprascapular nerve injury
3. Musculocutaneus nerve injury (rare).

Mechanism of Injury

Fall on outstretched hand from hight is usual mode of trauma.

Neer's Classification

Neer has classified 2, 3, and 4 part fracture. It is based on accurate identification of 4 major fragments and their relation to each other. More than 1 cm separation of fragment and angulation more than 45 degree from other fragment makes this fracture unstable.

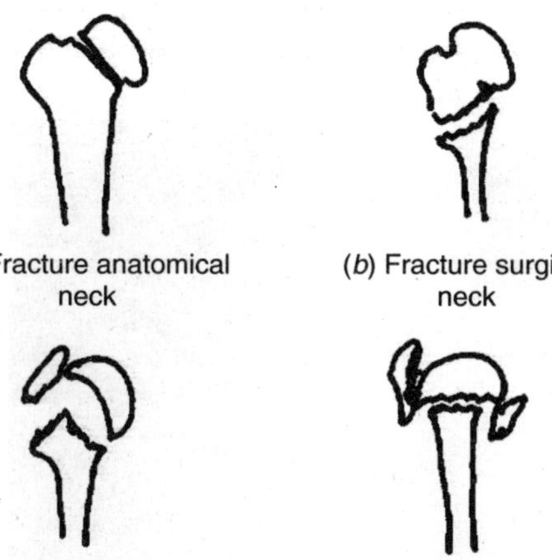

(*a*) Fracture anatomical neck

(*b*) Fracture surgical neck

(*c*) Three part humerus fracture

(*d*) Four part humerus fracture

Fig. 7.6 Fracture proximal humerus

A.O. Classification

A.O. has classified proximal humeral fractures into three types as follows:

A. This is least severe type. Avascular necrosis is not seen.

B. This is more severe than previous type. Partial separation of articular fragment creates less chance of avascular necrosis.

C. This is most severe type and associated with highest risk of avascular necrosis. This is intra articular type.

Clinical Features

Fracture of proximal humerus can be diagnosed by following clinical features:

1. Pain, swelling and deformity at shoulder.
2. Bony tenderness, crepitus is present at greater tuberosity.
3. Echymosis may be present at shoulder after 1-2 days of trauma.
4. Most common nerve injury seen in this fracture is axillary nerve injury. So sensation should be tested over deltoid.
5. Rarely chest injury may be associated with it. Pneumothorax can occur due to intrathoracic penetration of humeral head.

X-Ray Findings

X-ray will show the types of proximal humerus fracture. Following views of X-ray can be done:

1. AP and Lateral in scapular and axillary view.
2. Velpeau axillary view.

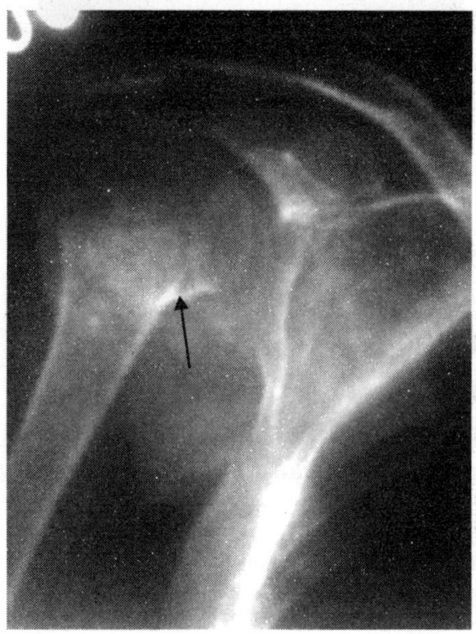

Fig. 7.7 Fracture surgical neck of humerus

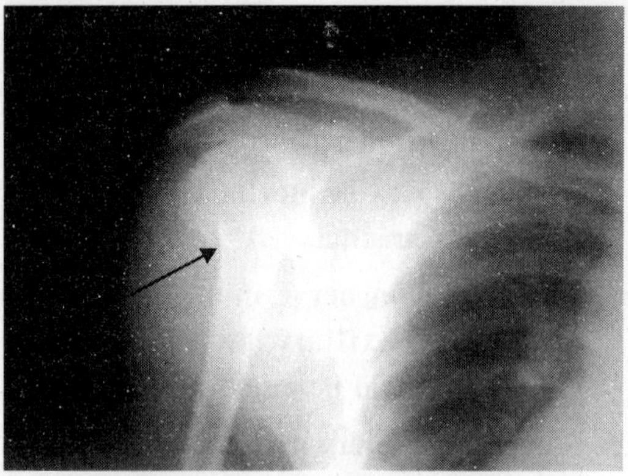

Fig. 7.8 Fracture surgical neck of humerus

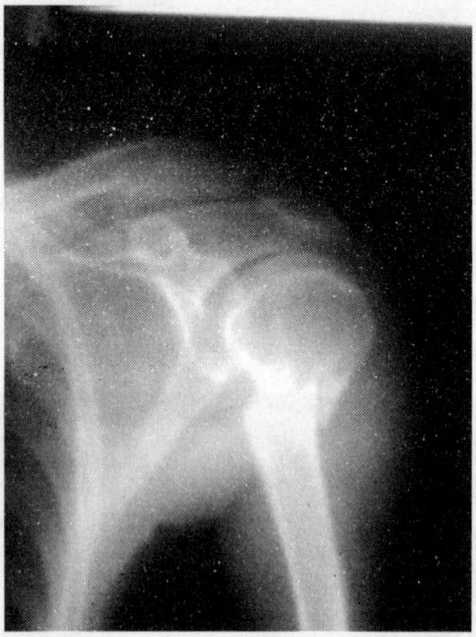

Fig. 7.9 Fracture proximal humerus

Treatment

Initially this fracture was treated by immobilization of shoulder. Arm was supported by a sling or velpeau strapping. After a week gentle motion exercise could be started.

Now treatment plan is decided according to type of fracture as follows:

Two part fracture of anatomical neck

This fracture can be managed by closed reduction.

Two part fracture of surgical neck

This fracture requires open reduction and internal fixation because of soft tissue interposition or due to unstable reduction. Open reduction and internal fixation can be done by A.O. buttress plate and screws.

Two part greater tuberosity fracture

This fracture can be managed by closed reduction. If it is displaced more than 1 cm, it will require open reduction and internal fixation by non absorbable suture.

Two part lesser tuberosity fracture

Undisplaced fracture is managed conservatively while displaced fracture requires open reduction and internal fixation with non absorbable suture.

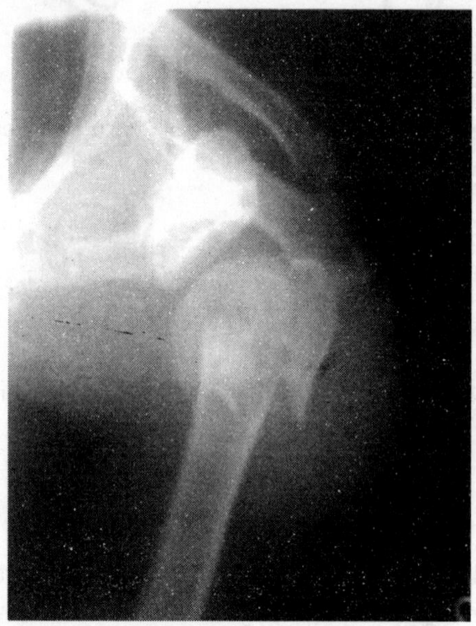

Fig. 7.10 Three part fracture of proximal humerus

Three part fracture

It is difficult to manage conservatively. Treatment of choice is open reduction and internal fixation by A.O. buttress plate or Cobra plate or **proximal humeral nail.**

Four part fracture

It has a very high risk of avascular necrosis. Malunion and degenerative arthritis are other likely complications. It can be fixed with multiple pins which can be left under skin subcutaneously.

Hemireplacement arthroplasty of shoulder is indicated in older patient where head of humerus cannot be salvaged.

Fracture dislocation

Two-three part fracture dislocation is treated by open reduction and internal fixation.

Shoulder Replacement (Neer's prosthesis)

It is used for fracture dislocation of proximal humerus. It has 2 head sizes 15 and 22 mm. Stem has 3 sizes 7, 9.5 and 12 mm. Stem length has 2 sizes 125 and 150 mm.

This is indicated in 4 part fracture, where head has lost it's soft tissue attachment thus creating high chances of avascular necrosis. This type of head cannot be salvaged so it needs hemireplacement arthroplasty.

Shoulder arthroplasty can also be done by Bigliani/Flatow shoulder prosthesis.

ANTERIOR DISLOCATION OF SHOULDER

Dislocation of shoulder is a common injury. It may dislocate by one of the followings mechanisms:

- A fall on outstretched hand with shoulder abducted and externally rotated.
- Sometimes it can dislocate due to a direct force pushing the humerus out of glenoid cavity.
- Posterior dislocation usually occurs due to an electrical shock or to epileptic fit.
- A direct blow on front of shoulder can also dislocate head of humerus posteriorly.

Classification

Dislocation of head of humerus has been classified into following three categories:

1. **Anterior:** Head comes out of glenoid cavity anteriorly. This type has been divided into following three subtypes:
   a. **Pre-glenoid:** Head comes out infront of glenoid.
   b. **Sub-coracoid:** Head dislocates below the coracoid.
   c. **Subclavicular:** Head comes out below the clavicle.

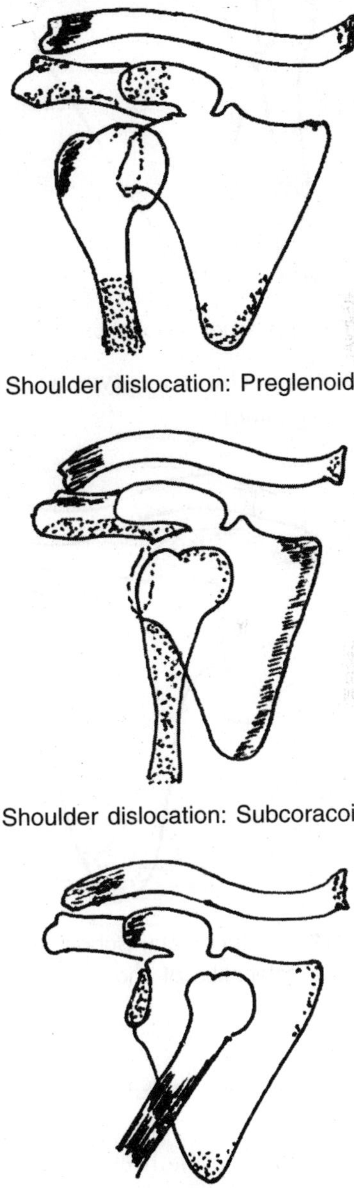

(*a*) Shoulder dislocation: Preglenoid type

(*b*) Shoulder dislocation: Subcoracoid type

(*c*) Shoulder dislocation: Infraclavicular type

Fig. 7.11 Types of anterior dislocation

2. **Posterior:** Head comes to lie posteriorly behind glenoid.

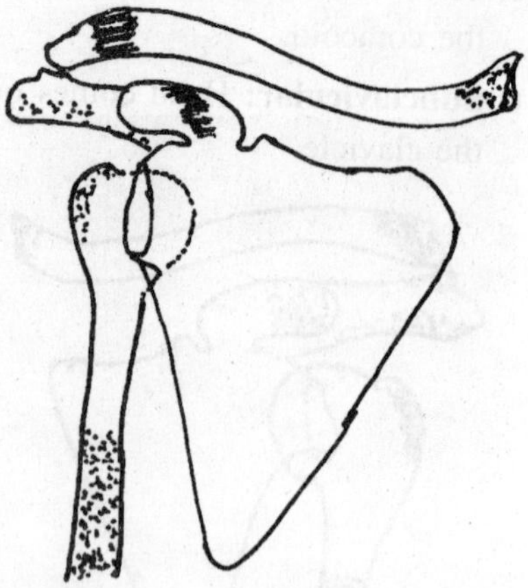

Fig. 7.12 Posterior dislocation of shoulder

3. **Luxatio erecta:** In this type head dislocates below glenoid.

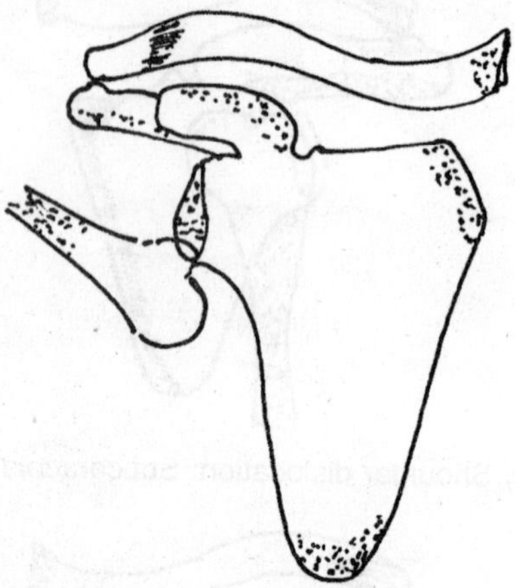

Fig. 7.13 Luxatio erecta: Subglenoid type dislocation of shoulder

Pathology

Head of humerus can dislocate due to following pathologies:

1. Stripping of capsule from inferior aspect of humeral head.
2. Disrupted glenohumeral ligament and stretched capsule (enclosing subscapular recess) cause dislocation of head humerus.
3. Shearing/tearing of glenoid labrum predisposes dislocation.
4. Rotator cuff tear mainly in subscapularis and supraspinatus also causes dislocation.
5. Displacement of biceps tendon from bicipital groove also plays an important role in aetiology.

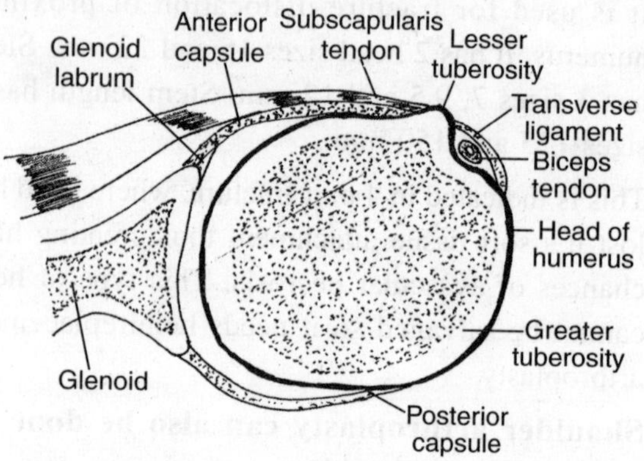

Fig. 7.14 Horizontal section of shoulder joint

Bankart's lesion

In this lesion glenoid labrum and periosteum are stripped from anterior surface of glenoid and scapular neck. This condition creates a pouch infront of scapular neck where head comes to lie.

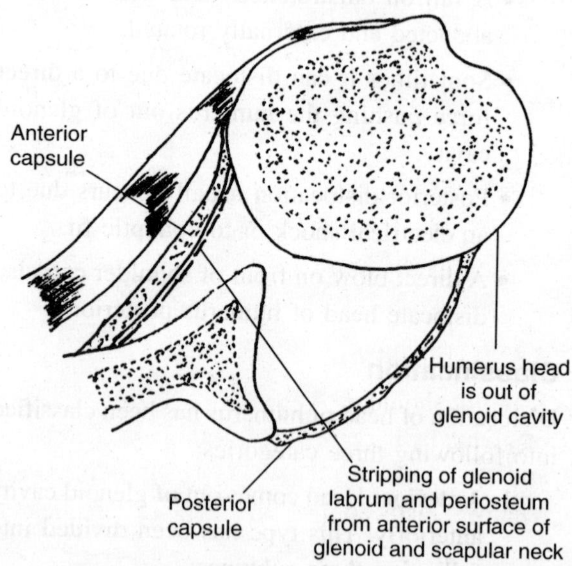

Fig. 7.15 Bankart's lesion

Hillsach's lesion

In this condition head of humerus is depressed in it's posterolateral quadrant due to impingement of anterior edge of glenoid.

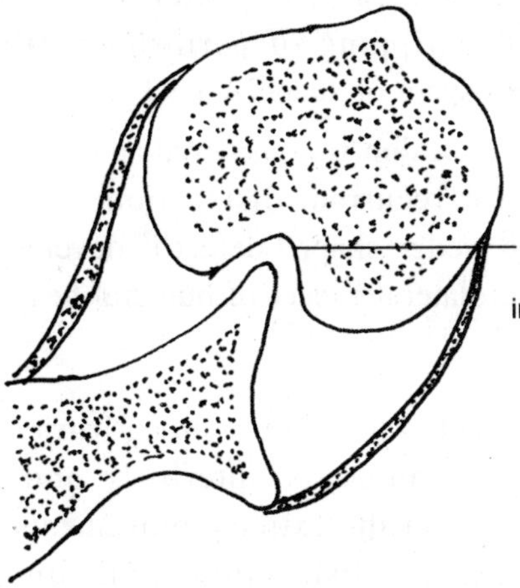

Fig. 7.16 Hillsach's lesion in dislocated humerus head

Clinical Features

Patient presents with the following features:

1. Patient presents with shoulder in abduction and external rotation. Dislocation is commonly seen in young adults of age 15–30 years.
2. Patient is unable to touch the opposite shoulder.
3. Anterior axillar fold is lowered down.
4. Shoulder is broadened.
5. Duga, Hamilton ruler, Callaway and Bryant tests are positive. (These tests have been described in Chapter No. 41)

X-Ray Findings

X-ray of shoulder (A.P. view) will show head out of glenoid cavity. Westpoint axillary lateral view and apical oblique view can be done in case of recurrent dislocation. Humeral head defect can be seen in Hermodsson's view (A.P. X-ray in 45 degree of internal rotation).

Vacant glenoid sign, Melony's line and trough line are seen in X-ray of posterior dislocation.

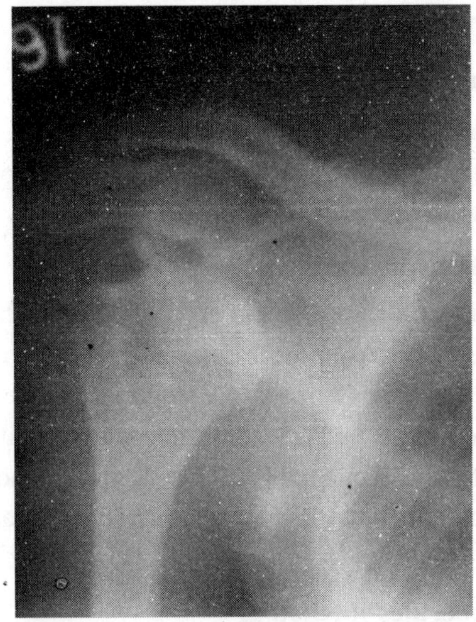

Fig. 7.17 Anterior dislocation of shoulder

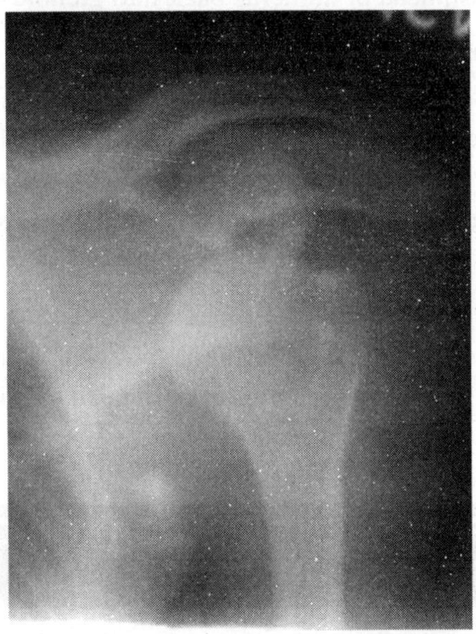

Fig. 7.18 Anterior dislocation of shoulder

Role of MRI

MRI is only indicated in case of recurrent dislocation. This is done to rule out cause of recurrence i.e. Hillsach's lesion, Bankart's lesion and rotator cuff tear.

Treatment

Dislocated head of humerus can be reduced under general anesthesia by one of the following methods:

Kocher's method

In this method traction is given along the shaft of humerus and counter traction is given through a folded towel in axilla. Now shoulder is externally rotated, adducted and then internally rotated in exactly this sequence (TERAI). Reduced shoulder is immobilized by a velpaeu arm to chest strapping for 3–4 weeks.

Hippocrates method

In this method a foot is kept in axilla which tries to push head of humerus back into glenoid cavity.

Stimson's method

This metod is used in prone position. Patient is asked to lie in prone position on the edge of table. Now a downward gentle traction is applied by hanging weight (5 pounds) at wrist. Head is reduced gradually in 15–20 minutes.

Milch's technique

This method is used in supine position. Thumb is kept in axilla which tries to push head of humerus back into glenoid cavity.

RECURRENT DISLOCATION OF SHOULDER

Recurrent dislocation is commonly seen due to following conditions:

1. Insufficient immobilization of shoulder following an initial episode is commonest cause of recurrent dislocation.
2. Improper healing of glenoid labrum and capsule provides a weak point for recurrent dislocation.
3. **Bankart's lesion** causes detachment of glenoid labrum from anterior rim of glenoid, stripping of periosteum from anterior aspect of scapular neck.
4. **Hillsach's lesion** is considered an essential lesion for recurrent dislocation. In this lesion a wedge shaped defect is developed in posterolateral aspect of humeral head.

Treatment

Aim of treatment is to create a strong barrier to exit of head of humerus anteriorly and to permanently restrict the extreme movements at shoulder that allow dislocation. This aim is achieved by shortening and reinforcing the capsule and short internal rotators infront of shoulder.

Operative methods

Head of humerus can be reduced by two following operative procedures:

1. Soft tissue repair
2. Bony repair.

Soft tissue repair

It can be done by following two methods:

1. Capsular repair

a. Staple capsulorrhaphy

b. Bankart's repair.

2. Subscapularis procedure

a. Puttiplate procedure

b. Magnuson's stock procedure

c. MacLaughlin's procedure.

Bony repair

It can be done by following two methods:

1. Bone block

a. Eden-Hypbbinette procedure

b. Oudard procedure.

2. Coracoid transfer

a. Bristow procedure

b. Trillat procedure

c. Laterjet procedure.

Puttiplate Operation

In this procedure proximal end of subscapularis is pulled across the overlapped capsule and sewn to scarified areas in greater tuberosity and bicipital groove.

Bristow Operation

In this procedure coracoid process is transferred to anterior rim of glenoid along with it's attached conjoint tendon. This is also known as **anterior bone block** procedure.

Arthroscopic Bankart's repair

This repair can be done by open as well as arthrosopic methods. In this procedure labrum is sutured back through holes drilled in rim of glenoid. Attenuated capsule is sutured to scarified glenoid margin and neck.

Other procedures

- Nicola's operation.
- Magnuson-stock operation.

POSTERIOR DISLOCATION OF SHOULDER

Posterior dislocation results following an electrical shock or epileptic fit. It can also be caused by trauma which creates anteromedial defect at head of humerus. Sometimes it is congenital in origin which is always bilateral. This is reduced by closed reduction under general anaesthesia. Unreduced dislocation can be reduced by surgical methods.

CHAPTER

8 Fracture Shaft Humerus

- Applied anatomy
- A.O./ASIF classification
- Clinical features
- Holstein-Lewis fracture
- Treatment
- Operative methods of fixation
- Complications of fracture shaft humerus

APPLIED ANATOMY

If fracture line is proximal to insertion of pectoralis major, proximal fragment of fracture will go in abduction and internal rotation due to pull of rotator cuff. Distal fragment goes medially by pull of pectoralis major. If fracture is distal to insertion of pectoralis major and proximal to deltoid insertion, proximal fragment will displace medially due to pull of pectoralis major, latissimus dorsi and teres major. While distal fragment is displaced laterally due to pull of deltoid. Fracture distal to insertion of deltoid muscle will lead to abduction and flexion of proximal fragment while distal fragment is displaced proximally.

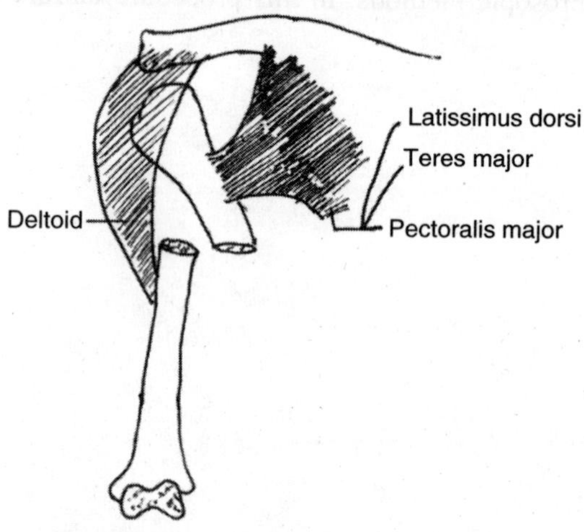

Fig. 8.1 Fracture between pectoralis major and deltoid. Deltoid displaces the distal fragment laterally, while proximal fragment is displaced medially by latissimus dorsi, teres major and pectoralis major

A.O./ASIF CLASSIFICATION

This classification is based on communition of fracture as follows:

Type A. This is simple and non-comminuted fracture.

Type B. This has a butterfly fragment.

Type C. This is comminuted fracture.

In other way this fracture is also classified in terms of proximal, middle and distal shaft fracture.

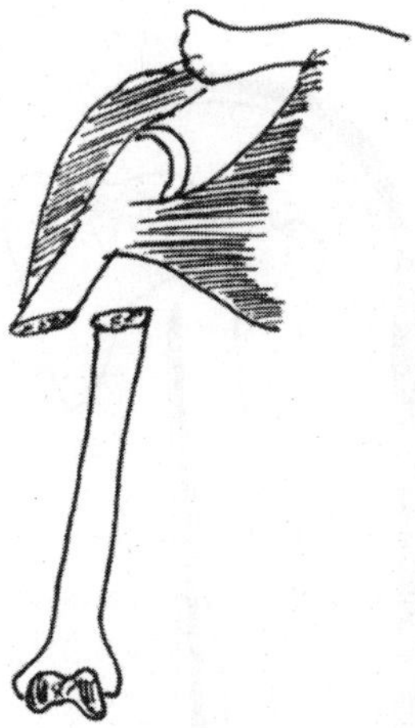

Fig. 8.2 Fracture distal to deltoid insertion. Distal fragment is proximally displaced, while proximal fragment is flexed and abducted

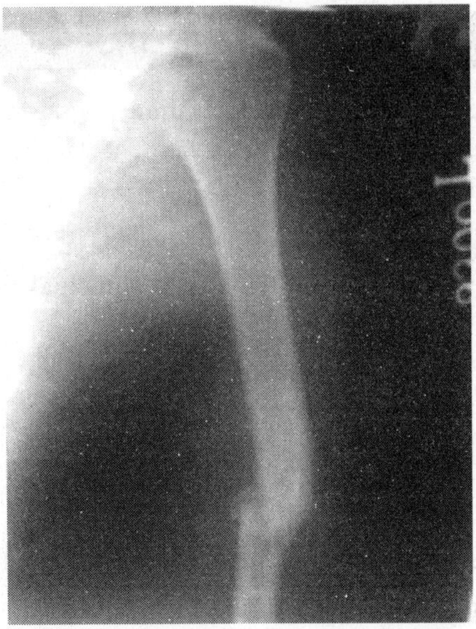

Fig. 8.3 Fracture shaft humerus with callus formation

CLINICAL FEATURES

Patient of fracture shaft humerus may present with the following clinical features:

1. Pain, swelling and deformity at arm.
2. Bony tenderness, crepitus and abnormal mobility at fracture site.
3. Radial nerve injury may be present in few cases. (18%)

HOLSTEIN-LEWIS FRACTURE

This is an oblique fracture of distal third of shaft of humerus associated with radial nerve injury.

In this fracture, nerve is entrapped in between fracture fragments.

X-Ray Findings

X-ray of arm AP and lateral view will show the type of fracture e.g. transverse, oblique, spiral, segmental and comminuted.

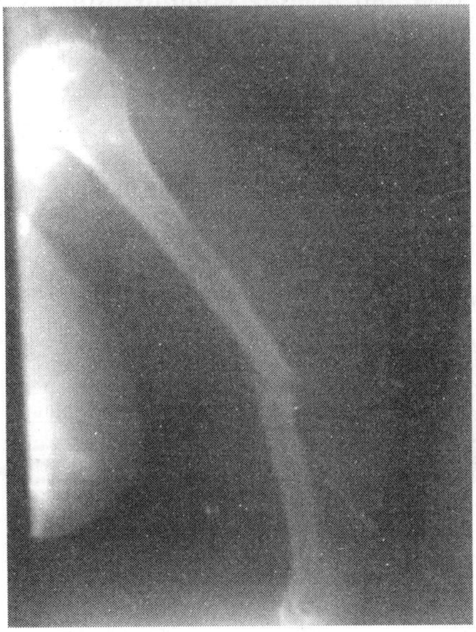

Fig. 8.4 Fracture shaft humerus with angulation

TREATMENT

Most of the humerus fractures unite conservatively (90%). Closed method of treatment can be done by following methods:

1. Hanging arm cast.
2. Coaptation or U-shaped brachial splint (U-slab).
3. Velpeau strapping with arm to chest bandage.
4. Shoulder abduction spica cast.
5. Skeletal traction.
6. Functional brace.

Hanging arm cast

This is applied in spiral fracture of mid shaft humerus with shortening. It is contraindicated in transverse fracture because it is more prone for distraction and healing complications. Cast is applied at least 2 cm proximal to fracture.

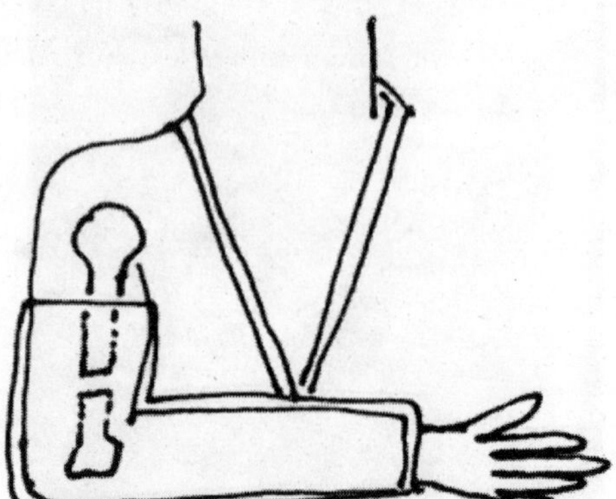

Fig. 8.5 Hanging cast

U-slab

This is applied in fracture shaft humerus with minimal shortening.

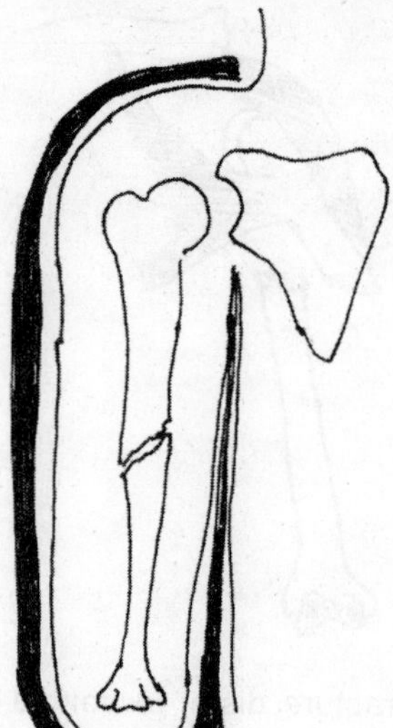

Fig. 8.6 U-slab in fracture shaft humerus

Velpeau strapping

This is applied in undisplaced or minimally displaced fracture in children. It can also be applied in elderly patients who do not accept another treatment.

Shoulder spica cast

When reduction becomes stable in abduction and external rotation of shoulder, this cast is applied in same position.

Skeletal traction

This is applied through tip of olecranon from medial to lateral side to reduce the risk of injury to ulnar nerve. This traction is rarely indicated in these days.

Functional brace (Sarmiento brace)

Sarmiento was the first person to describe this brace. This is an orthosis that helps in maintenance of reduction by closed method.

Indications of Surgery

These are the following indications in which surgery is required:

1. Compound fracture shaft humerus.
2. Fracture associated with neurovascular deficit.
3. Floating elbow.
4. Segmental and pathological fracture.
5. Bilateral fracture humerus.
6. Polytrauma.

OPERATIVE METHODS OF FIXATION

Locking Compression Plate (LCP)

This is latest method of fixation. When we insert a screw in hole of LCP, it becomes locked in the plate thus providing better fixation. In this fixation plate can not loose after the operation.

Dynamic Compression Plate (DCP)

DCP can be applied in diaphyseal fracture of humerus. 4.5 mm broad or narrow DCP can be used depending upon age of patient.

Intramedullary Fixation

Rush nail, Ender's nail and Hackenthal nails are flexible nail that can be inserted in retrograde manner through an entry portal located proximal to olecranon fossa. Antegrade insertion is done near rotator cuff.

Interlocking Nails

Aim of these nails is to prevent rotation of fragment and shortening of bone. When the fracture is 2 cm distal to surgical neck and 3 cm proximal to olecranon fossa, these nails become best choice of fixation.

Expandable Nails

These are of two types, interlocking and non interlocking. These are latest implants also known as **Israel nail.** (described in instrument section)

COMPLICATIONS OF FRACTURE SHAFT HUMERUS

This fracture has more chances of complications. It can have following complications:

1. Radial nerve injury (commonly seen in fracture middle third of humerus and at the junction of middle and lower third humerus)
2. Delayed union.
3. Non-union.
4. Malunion.

CHAPTER

9 Fracture Supracondylar Humerus

- Applied anatomy
- Classification
- Clinical features
- Treatment
- Complications
- Flexion type supracondylar fracture

This fracture is commonly seen in children of 5–8 years. This is most common fracture in children around elbow.

APPLIED ANATOMY

1. Most important aspect of this area is **3 bony point relationship**. It is formed by lateral epicondyle, medial epicondyle and tip of olecranon.
2. Normal **carrying angle** in males is 11 degree while in female it is 14 degree.
3. **C**apitulum, **M**edial condyle, **T**rochlea, and **L**ateral condyle ossify at 2, 6, 8, and 12 years respectively.
4. Head of radius and tip of olecranon ossify at 4 and 8 years of age respectively.

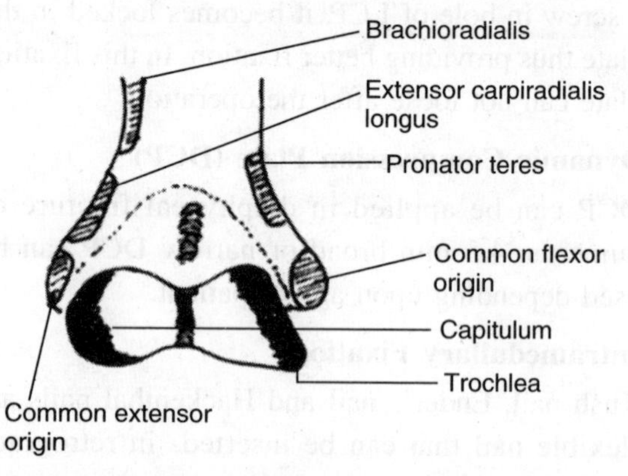

First appearance of epiphysis centre at :

Capitulum and lateral flange of trochlea	: 1st year
Medial flange of trochlea	: 9th year
Lateral epicondyle of humerus	: 12th year
Medial epicondyle of humerus	: 4–6 years

Fig. 9.1 Applied anatomy (fracture supracondylar humerus)

Mechanism of Injury

Supracondylar fracture occurs due to fall on outstretched hand with hyperextension of elbow.

CLASSIFICATION

Supracondylar fracture is of two types as follows:

1. Extension type.
2. Flexion type.

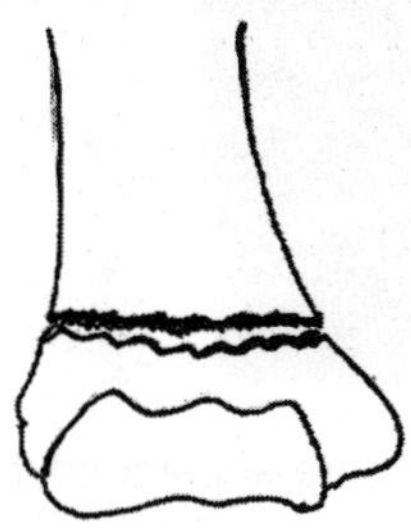

Fig. 9.2 (*a*) Fracture supracondylar humerus

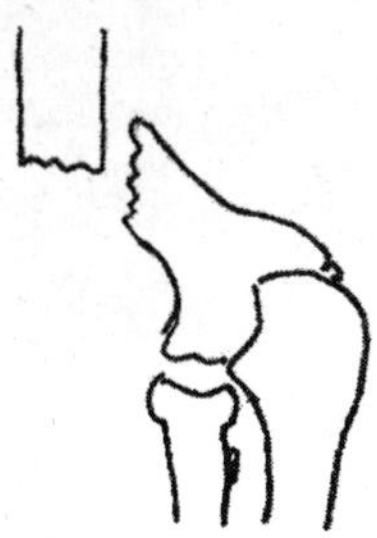

Fig. 9.2 (*b*) Extension type (more common)

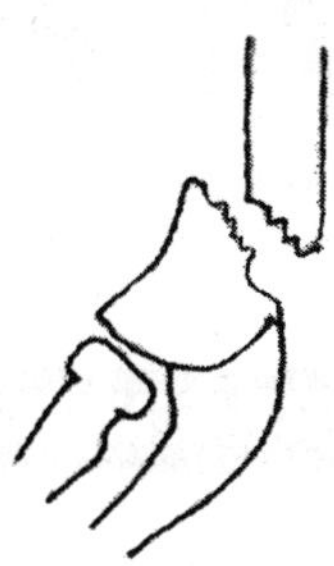

Fig. 9.2 (*c*) Flexion type

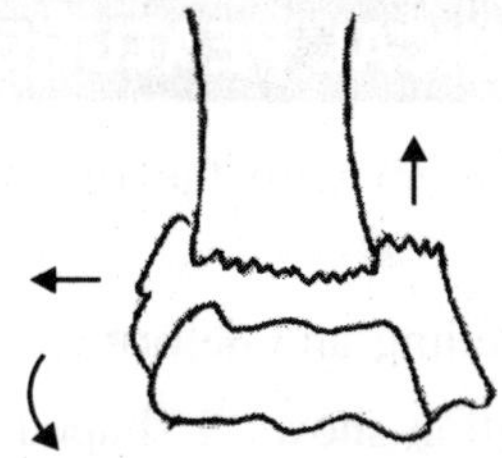

Fig. 9.2 (*d*) Types of displacement in A.P. view: It can go proximally; shift laterally, medially or it can tilt medially

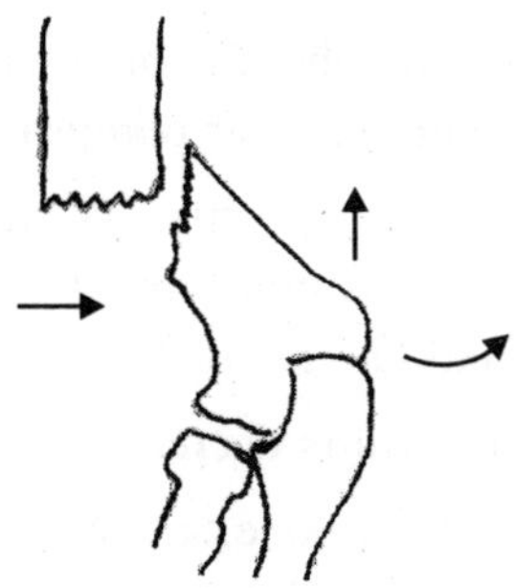

Fig. 9.2 (*e*) Types of displacement in lateral view: It can go proximally; shift and tilt dorsally

Extension type

1. This is most common type (97-98%).
2. Distal fragment goes posteriorly and proximally by pull of triceps.
3. This fracture is unstable.

Flexion type

1. This is very uncommon type. Approximately 2-3% supracondylar fractures are flexion type.
2. Distal fragment goes into flexion in relation to proximal fragment.

Displacement of fracture

Distal fragment is displaced **posteriorly, proximally** and **medially/laterally**. Distal fragment can be **rotated** and **angulated.**

CLINICAL FEATURES

Patient may present with the following clinical features:

1. Pain, swelling and deformity at elbow.
2. Examination shows S shaped deformity at supracondylar area. Tip of elbow becomes extraordinarily prominent.
3. Bony tenderness is present at supracondylar area.
4. Bony crepitus should not be elicited due to risk of neurovascular compromise.
5. Three bony points relationship is maintained. (Among tip of olecranon and medial and lateral condyle).
6. Length of arm is decreased.
7. We should also examine for signs of neurovascular compromise as there are chances of compression of brachial artery and radial nerve.

X-ray Findings

X-ray of elbow (AP and Lateral view) shows fracture at supracondylar area.

Fracture supracondylar humerus can be diagnosed by following radiological signs:

1. Distal fragment may show
   (a) Posterior, proximal, medial or lateral shift.
   (b) Posterior or medial tilt.
   (c) Internal rotation.
2. Tear drop sign is disturbed.
3. Normally a fat pad is present at olecranon fossa. Distension of capsule causes visualization of fat pad on X-ray as a radiolucent gap. It is known as **Fat pad sign**.
4. **Fish tail sign.** Anterior border of proximal fragment is visible as a sharp spike due to rotation of distal fragment.
5. **Crescent sign.** It indicates varus or valgus tilt of distal fragment. Overlapping of capitulum over olecranon masks the normal radioluscent gap of elbow joint thus makes Crescent sign positive.

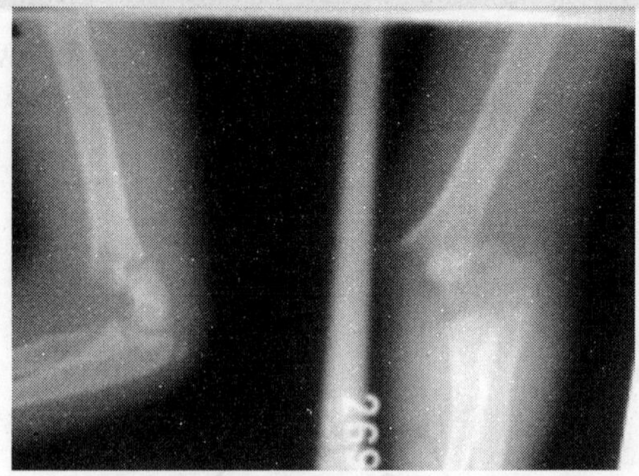

Fig. 9.3 Fracture supracondylar humerus

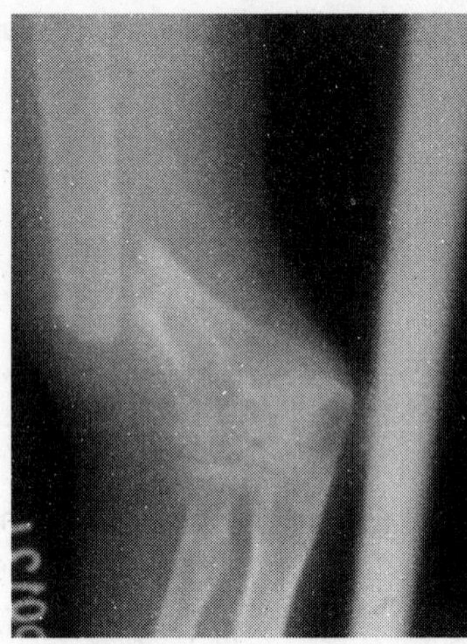

Fig. 9.4 Fracture supracondylar humerus (extension type)

TREATMENT

Closed reduction followed by AEPOP slab in flexed elbow with forearm in pronation is tried as a conservative treatment. Traction is given at forearm with 30–40 degree of flexion at elbow. Counter traction is given at arm. Elbow is fixed in traction with the thumb pushing the olecranon forward into flexion. During reduction, radial pulse is felt. Flexion is done to an angle where pulse disappears, now extend the elbow until pulse reappears. Slab is applied in this position.

Check X-ray should be done after 2 days and to be repeated again after one week to rule out displacement of fracture.

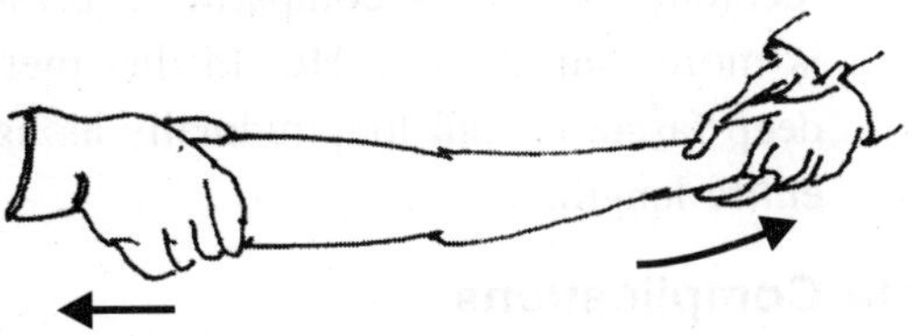

(*a*) Traction

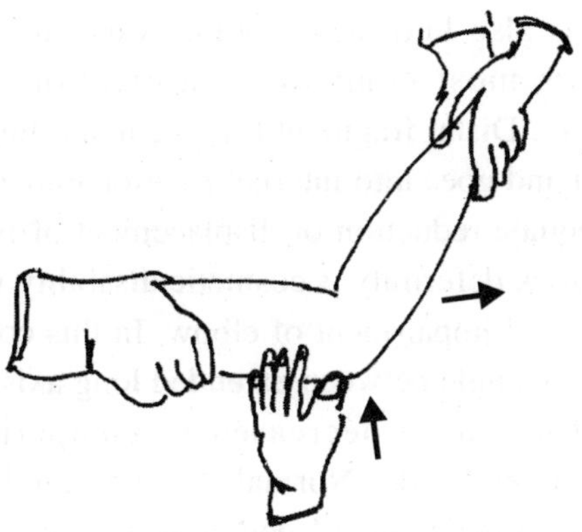

(*b*) Flexion during traction

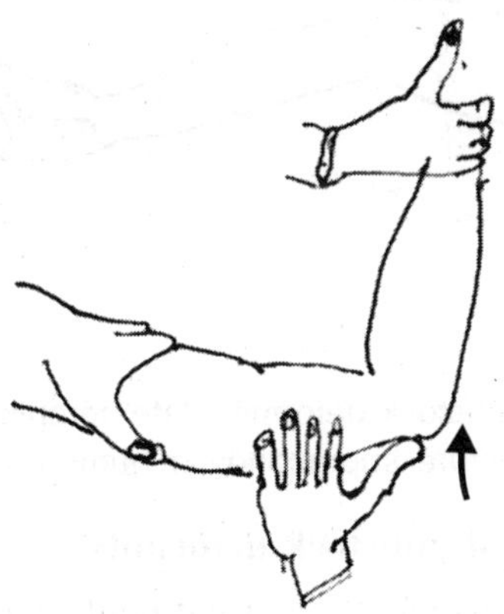

(*c*) Pushing the tip of elbow with thumb

Fig. 9.5 Technique of closed reduction of supracondylar fracture humerus

Indication of Smith Traction

This is an olecranon traction which can be applied by K wires inserted through olecranon. It can be maintained either over head or in side arm position. This traction is applied in fracture supracondylar humerus in following conditions:

a. Failure of closed reduction.

b. If reduction is achieved but inability to maintain it.

c. Threatened Volkman's ischaemia.

d. Grossly contaminated lesion where external fixation can not be done.

Dunlop Traction

This is a below elbow skin traction which is applied in supracondylar fracture of humerus. Drawback of this traction is that it can slip through skin, if not applied properly. It is rarely used now.

Role of Surgical Treatment

If methods of closed reduction fail, open reduction and internal fixation is the treatment of choice. It can be done by following two methods:

1. **Miller's method** of percutaneous K wire fixation. In this method distal fragment can be fixed with two K-wires. It should be only done when open reduction with internal fixation is preluded.
2. **ORIF:** This is indicated in failed closed reduction, vascular injury and associated fracture of humerus or forearm. Open reduction and internal fixation can be done by either Y plate or 2 plates fixed at right angle or by bicondylar screws.

COMPLICATIONS

Complications are divided into immediate, early and late types.

Immediate

a. Vascular injury

Brachial artery is most commonly injured in displaced fracture. Sharp edge of proximal fragment impinges the brachial artery, leading to vascular compromise of flexor group of muscle of forearm.

b. Nerve injury

Radial nerve is commonest nerve to be injured in this fracture. Other nerves to be injured are median and ulnar nerve in that order.

Early Complications

Volkman's Ischaemia

This is ischaemia of muscles and nerves of forearm (flexor compartment). Ischaemia occurs due to occlusion of brachial artery that causes reduced blood supply to flexor group of muscles of forearm. Flexor pollicis longus and Flexor digitorum profundus (medial half) are the commonly affected muscles in Volkman's ischaemia. It happens because these are supplied by an end artery; anterior interoseous artery. Ischaemia of these muscles causes **Compartment syndrome.**

Clinical features of Volkman's ischaemia

Volkman's ischaemia has classical features, known by 5 "P" as follows:

1. Pain in forearm. (pain on passive stretching of fingers)
2. Pallor (due to reduced capillary filling time).
3. Paresthesia.
4. Paralysis.
5. Pulselessness.
6. Swelling and tenderness over forearm.

Treatment of Volkman's ischaemia

Volkman's ischaemia should be treated on the following line of action:

1. Remove all the splint, bandage or slab/plaster.
2. Elevate the forearm and advice to do active and passive movement of fingers.
3. Urgent fasciotomy should be done if no improvement occurs in response to above mentioned treatment. Fasciotomy is recommended when compartment pressure is more than 30 mm Hg. In this method deep fascia is split longitudinally along its entire length.

Late Complications

a. Malunion (Gunstock deformity)

This is also known as cubitus varus deformity. This is most common complication of this fracture. Distal fragment tilts medially during the union and goes into internal rotation either due to inadequate reduction or displacement of fracture. Gunstock deformity is cosmetic disability without functional impairment of elbow. In this condition carrying angle between extended long axis of arm and forearm is decreased in comparison to contralateral side. Normal carrying angle is 11 degree in male and 14 degree in female.

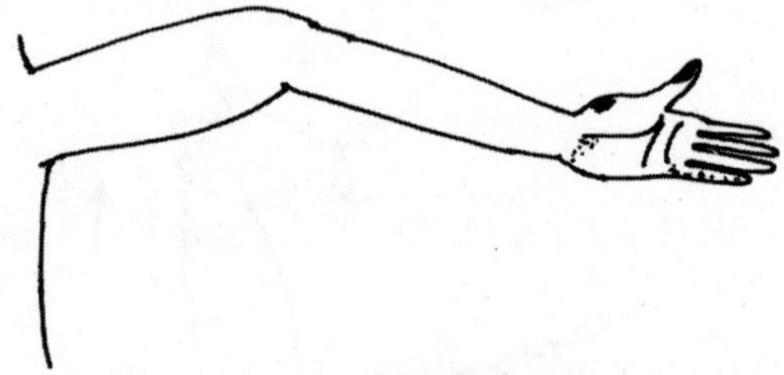

Fig. 9.6 Gunstock deformity; late complication of fracture supracondylar humerus

Treatment of gunstock deformity

Corrective osteotomy is treatment of choice. It should be done after the skeletal maturity, otherwise deformity can recur.

French osteotomy

This is lateral closed wedge osteotomy of lower end of humerus. This procedure involves removal of lateral wedge of bone from supracondylar area and closing the osteotomy. In this osteotomy one screw is placed anteriorly in distal fragment and second screw is placed slightly posterior in proximal fragment. Now osteotomy is done in between these screws. Distal fragment is rotated in such a manner that both screws become parallel to each other. Both screws are tied by a stainless steel wire in figure of eight manner. This method fills the gap in between proximal and distal fragment. Drawbacks of this osteotomy are chances of nonunion and lengthening of arm.

King's osteotomy

This is a medial open wedge osteotomy of lower end of humerus. A wedge of bone is removed from medial side of lower end of humerus.

Derotation osteotomy

This is not performed routinely.

b. Myositis ossificans

Frequent and prolonged massage around a post traumatic elbow gives rise to ectopic new bone formation around it, thus leading to stiff elbow. This is treated by immobilization in above elbow POP slab for three weeks. Later gentle mobilization exercises can be started.

c. Volkman's ischaemic contracture

This is deformity of hand, wrist and forearm developing as a sequel to Volkman's ischaemia in which wrist and fingers go into flexion contracture.

Clinical features of VIC

VIC can be diagnosed by following clinical features:

1. Flexion contracture of forearm due to involvement of flexor digitorum profundus and flexor pollicis longus.

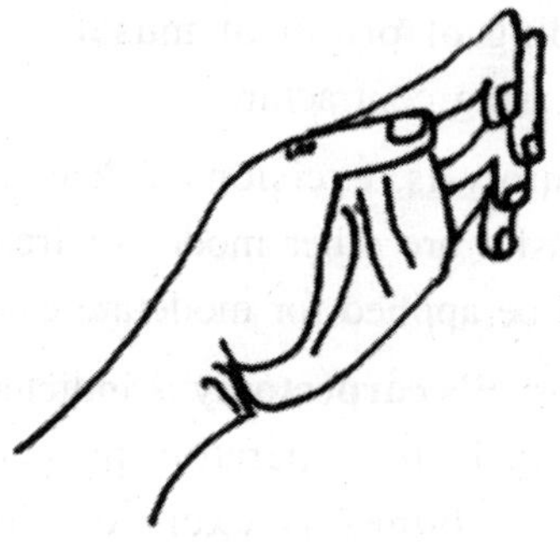

Fig. 9.7 (*a*) Volkman's ischaemic contracture

2. Claw hand deformity may be present.
3. **Volkman's sign** is positive. i.e. extension of wrist exaggerate the deformity while flexion causes opposite to it. In other words fingers can be extended at interphalangeal joint only when wrist is flexed.

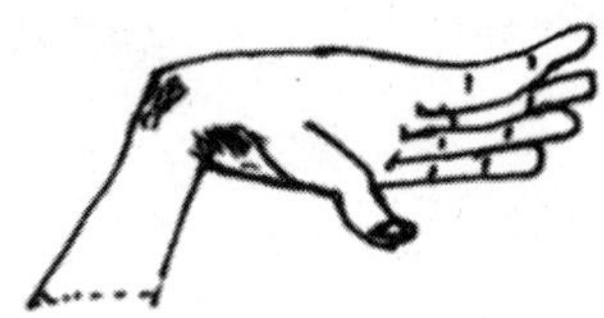

Fig. 9.7 (*b*) Fingers can be extended at I.P. joint while wrist is flexed. If we extend the wrist (*a*) finger become flexed at I.P. joint (Volkman's sign).

4. Contracture of joint and soft tissue with scarring of skin is also seen.
5. Bones are also deformed.
6. Sensory and motor loss may occur in forearm and hand due to peripheral nerve involvement.

Treatment of VIC

Volkman's ischaemic contracture can be managed by following methods:

1. Volkman's splint is applied in mild case.
2. **Maxpage operation** is indicated in moderate cases. In this operation muscles of common flexor origin are released from medial epicondyle and ulna. This makes

CHAPTER 9

sliding of origin of muscles down thus releasing contracture.

3. Neurolysis, excision of scar and tendon transfer are other modes of treatment that can be applied for moderate cases.
4. **Seddon's carpectomy** is indicted in severe cases. In this operation proximal row of carpal bones is excised. This causes shortening of forearm thus masking the effect of contracture.
5. **Arthrodesis** of wrist joint in functional position can also be done in severe cases.
6. Amputation is done in very severe cases where wrist and hand show gangrenous changes.

FLEXION TYPE OF SUPRACONDYLAR FRACTURE

Impaction of force against the posterior aspect of flexed elbow, leads to flexion type of supracondylar fracture.

Distal fragment is displaced anteriorly with the elbow joint. Posterior periosteum is torn. This type of fracture is usually compound but vascular injuries are rare. Patient presents with flexed elbow. Normal prominence of posterior aspect of elbow is lost. This fracture is difficult to manage. It can be reduced by Sultanpur technique of closed reduction followed by AEPOP slab for 6 weeks. Failure of conservative treatment requires ORIF by double plate.

CHAPTER

10 Fracture Lateral Condyle Humerus

- Classification
- Clinical features
- Complications
- Fracture intercondylar humerus
  - Clinical features
  - Complicatiions

This fracture is commonly seen in children. It is prone for nonunion due to rotation of distal fragment. Rotation occurs due to pull of extensor muscles. This is a Salter Harris type four fracture.

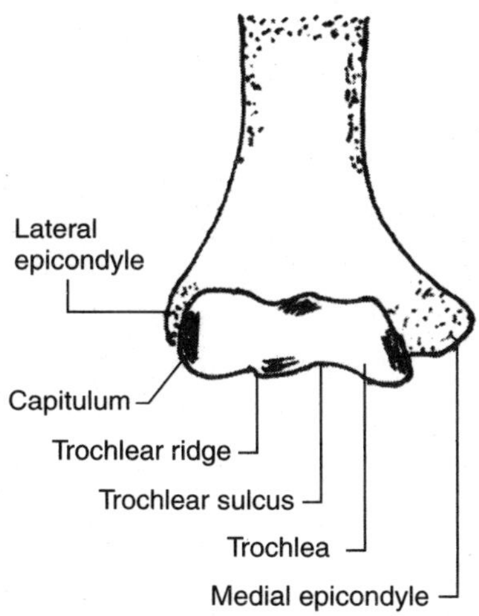

Fig. 10.1 Anatomical landmark of lower end humerus

CLASSIFICATION

This fracture has been classified into two types as follows:

Type I: In this type lateral trochlear ridge remains intact thus preventing dislocation of radius and ulna.

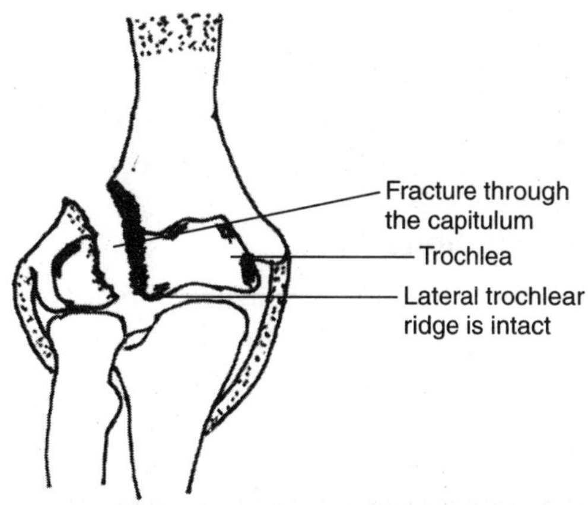

Fig. 10.2 Fracture lateral condyle humerus (Type !) (Lateral trochlear ridge is intact, thus preventing dislocation of radius and ulna.)

Type II: Lateral trochlear ridge is a part of fractured lateral condyle. Capsuloligamentous disruption may dislocate radius and ulna.

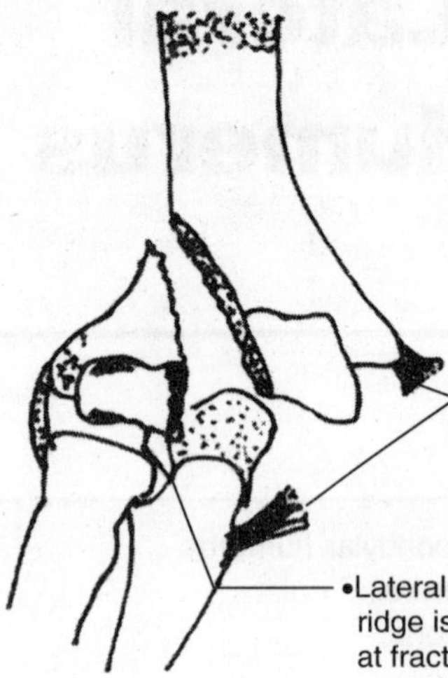

Fig. 10.3 Fracture lateral condyle humerus (Type II)

CLINICAL FEATURES

Patient may present with following clinical features:

1. Child presents with pain and swelling at lateral condyle of humerus.
2. Bony tenderness, crepitus and abnormal mobility is present at lateral condyle.

X-ray Findings

X-ray shows fracture line passing obliquely either from capitulotrochlear sulcus or from lateral border of trochlear groove upto supracondylar ridge.

TREATMENT

Undisplaced fractures can be treated conservatively by AEPOP cast. Displaced fractures can be treated by open reduction and internal fixation by screw.

COMPLICATIONS

Lateral condyle humerus is known for it's complications. This fracture may develop following complications:

1. Nonunion
2. Cubitus valgus
3. Tardy ulnar nerve palsy
4. Osteoarthritis.

Nonunion

This fracture is prone to undergo nonunion due to pulling action of extensor muscle attached to it. So this fragment rotates and gets displaced leading to nonunion. This is treated by open reduction and internal fixation by screws. Very old cases (>2-3 months) are very difficult to manage. Such cases can be treated conservatively.

Cubitus Valgus

Growth of lateral aspect of lower end of humerus epiphysis is retarded that causes cubitus valgus deformity. This is treated by corrective supracondylar osteotomy.

Tardy Ulnar Nerve Palsy

Development of cubitus valgus deformity stretches ulnar nerve while it passes across medial epicondyle (during flexion and extension of elbow). This causes friction neuritis of ulnar nerve leading to late (tardy) ulnar nerve palsy. This is treated by anterior transposition of ulnar nerve.

Osteoarthritis

Inaccurate reduction of articular surface leads to development of osteoarthritic changes in elbow later in life.

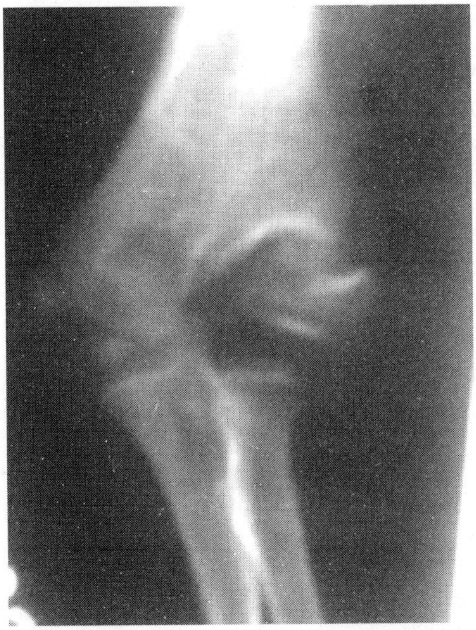

Fig. 10.4 Fracture lateral condyle humerus

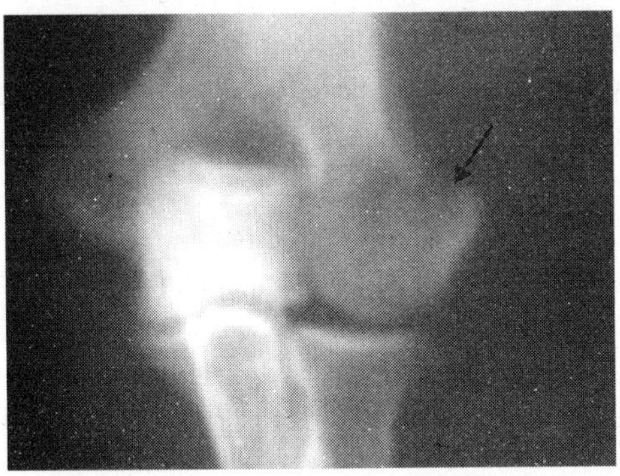

Fig. 10.5 Fracture lateral condyle humerus

FRACTURE INTERCONDYLAR HUMERUS

Intercondylar fracture humerus is most complicated fracture of upper extremity. Most of the cases require open reduction and internal fixation to establish the articular congruity.

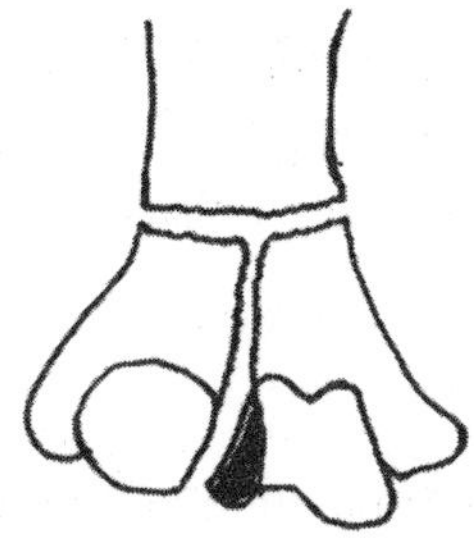

Fig. 10.6 Fracture intercondylar humerus (T-shaped)

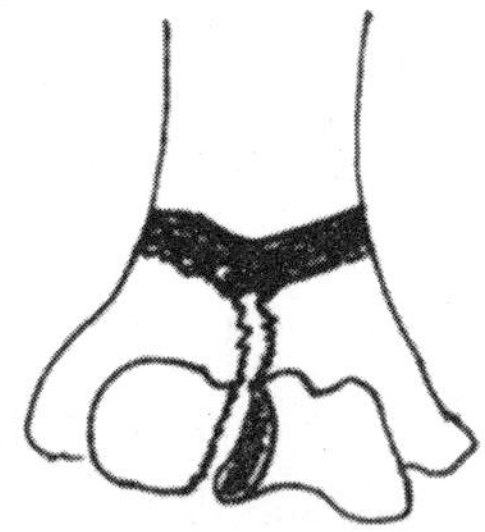

Fig. 10.7 Y-shaped intercondylar fracture humerus

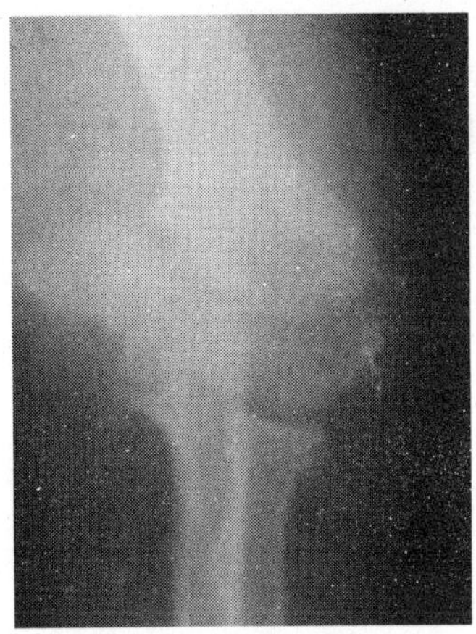

Fig. 10.8 Fracture supracondylar humerus with intercondylar extension

Mechanism of Injury

Impact of ulna in trochlear groove forces the condyle of humerus wide apart. It can occur both in flexion and extension.

Riseborough and Radin Classification

Riseborough and Radin have classified this fracture into four types as follows:

Type 1: Undisplaced fracture between capitulum and trochlea.

Type 2: Capitulum and trochlea are separated apart without rotation of fragment.

Type 3: Fragments are rotated and separated.

Type 4: Gross comminution of articular surface. Condyles are separated.

Clinical Features

Patient may present with the following clinical features:

1. Pain, swelling and deformity at elbow are common presentation. Swelling is usually gross.
2. Relationship of 3 bony landmarks is disturbed.

Treatment

Closed reduction can be done by bag of bone technique. Open reduction and internal fixation can be done by dual plate fixation. A semitubular plate on medial aspect and 3.5 mm reconstruction plate on posterolateral aspect can be fixed.

Complications

1. *Stiff Elbow*

This is most common complication following intercondylar fracture humerus. Elbow mobilization exercises and hot saline fomentation are mainstay of treatment.

2. *Malunion*

Malunited fracture can cause cubitus varus or valgus deformity.

3. *Osteoarthritis of elbow*

If articular congruity is not maintained after reduction, it can lead to osteoarthritic changes later in life.

CHAPTER

11 Injuries Around Elbow

- Pulled elbow
- Dislocation of elbow
- Unreduced dislocation of elbow
- Fracture medial condyle of humerus
- Fracture of olecranon
- Fracture of medial epicondyle
- Fracture head radius

PULLED ELBOW

If we lift a child by holding his wrist, head of radius may come out of annular ligament. This condition is known as *pulled elbow*.

Clinical Features

Child will present with the following clinical features:

1. This is commonly seen in between the age of 2–6 years.
2. Child presents with forearm in pronation with lot of pain almost crying.
3. Mild swelling may be seen at elbow.

X-ray Findings

Subluxated head of radius can not be seen in X-ray as it is cartilaginous.

Treatment

Closed reduction is done by full supination of forearm and pressing the head of radius directly with thumb. Reduction is confirmed by a sound of click, followed by normal range of motion at elbow.

DISLOCATION OF ELBOW

This is commonly seen after 10 years of age. Males are predominantly affected.

Mechanism of Injury

Dislocation of elbow is caused by fall on outstretched hand or wrist with elbow in slight hyperextension or at least full extension.

Clinical Features

Dislocation of elbow will present with the following features:

1. Pain, swelling and deformity at elbow are common symptoms in dislocated elbow.
2. Tip of the elbow is unduly prominent and goes posteriorly.
3. Relationship of three bony landmarks is disrupted.
4. Bony crepitus is absent.

5. Movements at elbow are grossly restricted.
6. Nerve injuries may be present. It happens because valgus displacement put the ulnar nerve under stretch. Median nerve can be injured either at the time of dislocation or during reduction.
7. Patient may have associated fracture of medial epicondylar epiphysis, proximal radius, olecranon, trochlea and coronoid process.

Stimson's Classification

Most of the dislocations are posterior type. Anterior dislocations are rare. Stimson has classified 4 types of elbow dislocation as follows:

1. Posterior(Posterolateral and Posteromedial).
2. Anterior dislocation.
3. Medial dislocation.
4. Lateral dislocation.

Stimson has also classified divergent type of dislocation which is also rare. In this type proximal radioulnar joint is disrupted.

X-ray Findings

X-ray shows dislocation of elbow mostly at ulnohumeral joint. Coronoid process comes to lie posterior to humeral condyle.

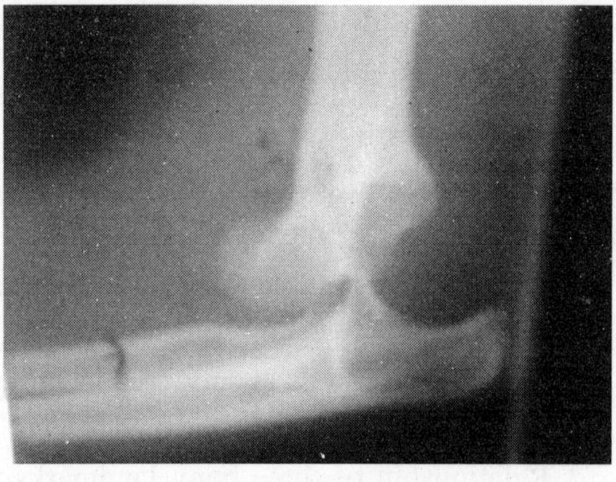

Fig. 11.1 Posterior dislocation of elbow

Treatment

Closed reduction done under general anaesthesia is usually successful. AEPOP slab is applied after reduction for a period of 3 weeks. Traction is applied at forearm with elbow flexed at 70 degree. Countertraction is applied at arm. This technique is called **Puller's technique** and applied in adults. To reduce dislocation, child should lie in prone position. Olecranon is pushed with thumb in the direction of forearm, till reduction is achieved.

If closed reduction fails, open reduction should be done.

Complications

1. Nerve injuries

Ulnar nerve is more commonly injured. Median and radial nerves can also be injured in this decreasing order of frequency.

2. Vascular injuries

Arterial injuries are very uncommon in dislocation of elbow.

3. Myositis ossificans

Excess of physiotherapy and massage of elbow give rise to this condition.

4. Recurrent dislocation

It is very uncommon to see recurrent dislocation of elbow.

5. Osteochondral fracture

6. Irreducible dislocation

UNREDUCED DISLOCATION OF ELBOW

If reduction is not done within a week, chances of closed reduction fade. In this condition open reduction should be done and incipient contracture is released to restore function. If dislocation is less than 3 weeks old, open reduction along with arthroplasty should be done. Following three types of arthroplasty can be used in dislocated elbow:

1. Fascial (Interpositional) arthroplasty.
2. Implant arthroplasty.
3. Resection arthroplasty.

FRACTURE MEDIAL CONDYLE HUMERUS

This fracture is not as common as lateral condyle. This fracture has certain features as follows:

1. This is caused by fall on outstretched hand.
2. Patient presents with pain, swelling and tenderness at medial condyle.
3. Ulnar nerve injury may be associated with it.

Classification

Type 1: Lateral trochlear ridge is intact thus providing stability to radius and ulna.

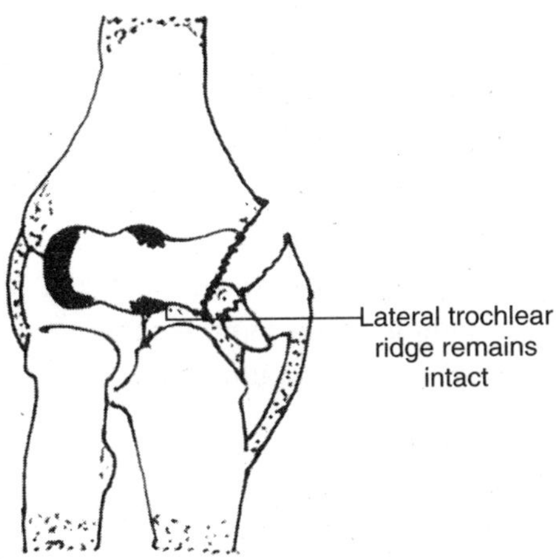

Fig. 11.2 (*a*) Fracture of medial condyle humerus (Type I)

Type 2: Lateral trochlear ridge is apart of fractured medial condyle. Radius and ulna may dislocate due to capsuloligamentous disruption.

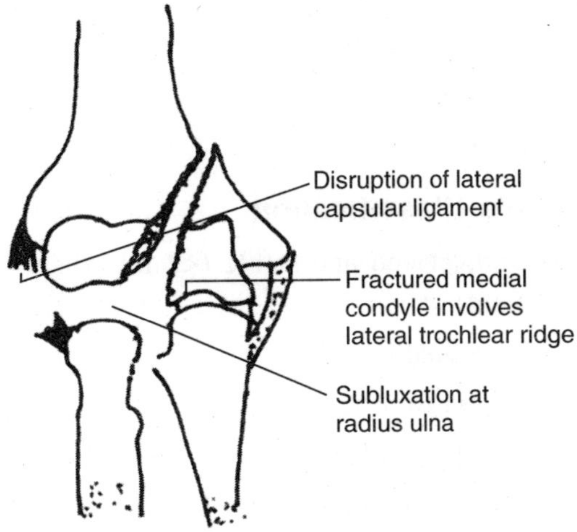

Fig. 11.2 (*b*) Fracture of medial condyle humerus (Type II)

Treatment

Closed reduction is difficult to achieve as well as to maintain. Open reduction and internal fixation is main stay of treatment as it may restore the joint congruity. If the ulnar groove is also fractured, anterior transposition of nerve can be done. Joint stability can be restored by repair of lateral collateral ligament. AEPOP slab is applied with elbow and wrist in flexed position while forearm in pronation.

FRACTURE OF OLECRANON

Olecranon fracture is commonly seen in adults. It is uncommon in children. Fracture of olecranon causes triceps insufficiency.

Mechanism of Injury

Direct impact at the posterior aspect of ulna and to fall on upper limb causes fracture olecranon. It can also happen as a result of side swipe injury.

Clinical Features

1. Pain, swelling and a palpable gap at the fracture site.

CHAPTER 11

2. Active extension of elbow against gravity is restricted.
3. Uncommonly ulnar nerve can also be injured.

Colton's Classification

1. Undisplaced and stable (<2 mm displacement).
2. Displaced
   — Avulsion fracture
   — Oblique/Transverse
   — Comminuted
   — Fracture/Dislocation

Displaced fractures show more than 2 mm displacement.

Avulsion fracture

In this type a small fragment of olecranon is separated from rest of ulna. It is common in elder patient.

Oblique/transverse fracture

Fracture line is oblique and begins near the deepest part of semilunar notch, extending dorsally and distally to emerge on subcutaneous surface of ulna.

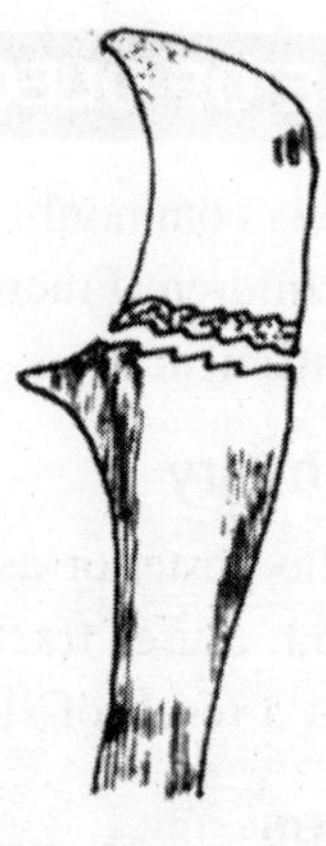

Fig. 11.3 (*a*) Transverse fracture of olecranon

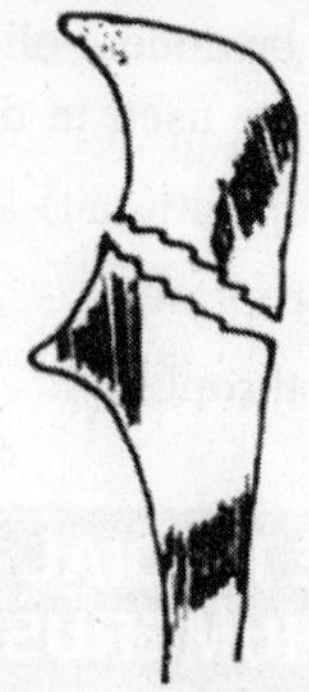

Fig. 11.3 (*b*) Oblique fracture of olecranon

Comminuted fracture

This fracture is grossly comminuted.This type of fracture may be associated with other fracture.

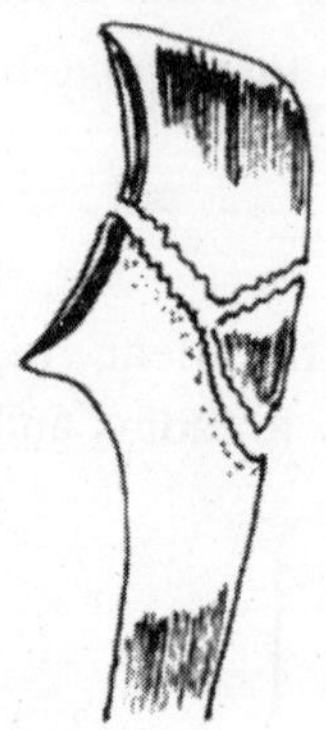

Fig. 11.3 (*c*) Comminuted fracture of olecranon

Fracture/dislocation

This fracture has a plane of instability at facture site and at radiohumeral joint, leading to anterior dislocation of radius and ulna.

X-Ray Findings

To detect fracture of olecranon always go for true lateral view of elbow.

Advantages of true lateral view

1. Extent of fracture can be detected.
2. Degree of comminution of olecranon can be visualized.

3. Disruption of articular surface can be seen.
4. Displacement of head of radius can seen.

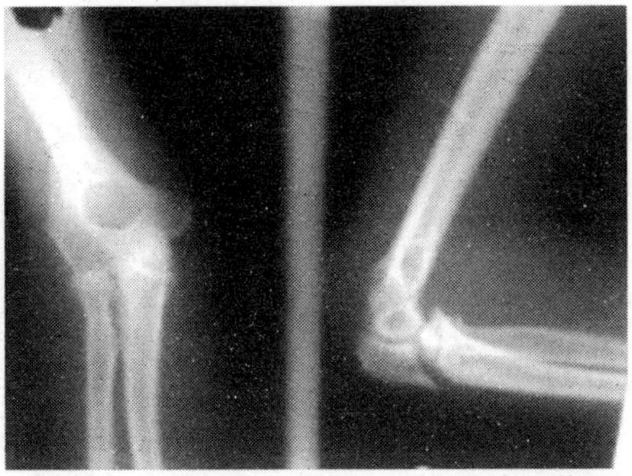

Fig. 11.4 Fracture olecranon (oblique type)

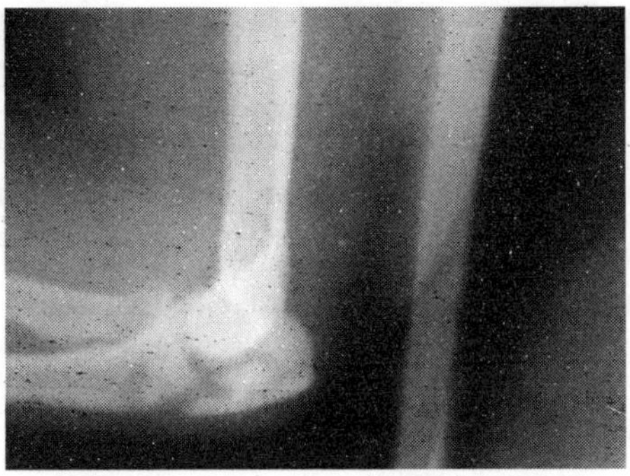

Fig. 11.5 Fracture olecranon

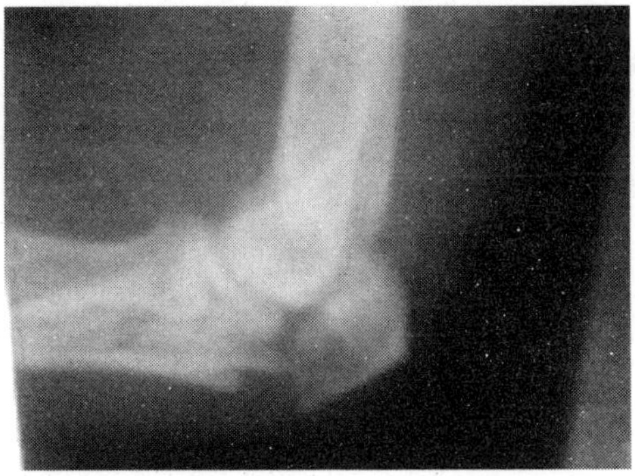

Fig. 11.6 Fracture olecranon (transverse type)

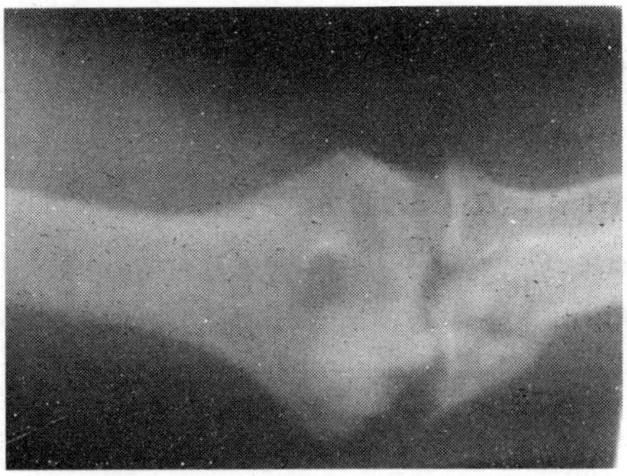

Fig. 11.7 Fracture olecranon (comminuted type)

Treatment (Undisplaced Fracture)

Undisplaced fracture should be immobilized in AEPOP cast in 45–90 degree flexion. Full extension is not recommended as it may cause stiffness of elbow. After 7 days a follow up X-ray should be done to rule out redisplacement.

Treatment (Displaced Fracture)

Displaced fracture should be treated by open reduction and internal fixation by following methods:

1. ORIF by TBW (Tension band wiring).
2. ORIF by Leinbach screw.
3. Bicortical screw fixation.
4. ORIF by A.O. plate.
5. ORIF by Zuelzer plate.

Tension band wiring

This is indicated in avulsion fracture. Basic principle of tension band wiring is that it converts shearing forces into compressive forces.

Leinbach/intramedullary screw

Leinbach screw can gain enough purchase in the distal fragment, but it can break at shank screw junction. So an intramedullary screw is better as it can get purchase in medullary cavity of distal ulna. Chances of breakage of intramedullary screw are less. A 6.5 mm cancellous intramedullary screw can be used.

Bicortical screw fixation

A cortical screw is inserted through the tip of olecranon till it engages the anterior cortex of coronoid process near sublime tubercle.

A.O. plate

This is indicated in oblique or comminuted fracture. 3.5 mm reconstruction plate is better option for this.

Zuelzer plate

This is indicated when a small fragment of bone is fractured from principal part of bone. This is a hook type of plate. Advantage of this plate over TBW is that it does not require any supplement fixation.

Indications of excision of proximal fragment of olecranon

1. Old ununited fracture.
2. Extensively comminuted fracture.
3. Fracture in elderly person.
4. Any fracture not involving trochlear notch.

Laugier Fracture

Fracture of trochlea is known as Laugier fracture. It is very rare.

Kocher Fracture

This is a fracture of capitullum and has following features:

1. This is of two types Type-1 **(Hahn-steinthal)** and Type-2 **(Kocher-Lorenz).**
2. Type 2 fracture is also known as Un capping of condyle.
3. Open reduction and internal fixation is very difficult. Excision of capitullum can be done.

FRACTURE OF MEDIAL EPICONDYLE

This fracture is more common than lateral epicondyle fracture. (Medial epicondyle fuses with distal humerus at 20th year). This fracture has few peculiar features:

1. Ulnar nerve may be involved.
2. Mode of trauma is commonly a direct blow to epicondyle.
3. AEPOP cast should be applied with forearm in pronation while wrist and elbow in flexion.

FRACTURE HEAD RADIUS

This is an intraarticular fracture and commonly seen in adults. It is rare in children. Head of radius remain in contact with ulna in lesser sigmoid notch throughout the movement of pronation and supination.

Mechanism of Injury

This type of injury is sustained as a result of fall on outstretched hand. Fracture head of radius can also be associated with dislocation of elbow.

Mason's Classification

Mason has classified fracture head radius into 3 types as follows:

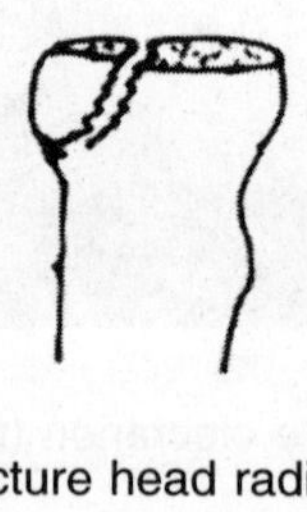

Fig. 11.8 (*a*) Fracture head radius fragment <1/3 the size of head of radius

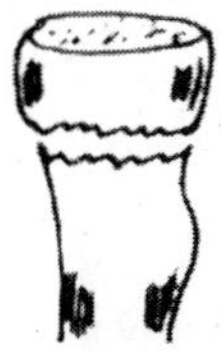

Fig. 11.8 (*b*) Complete fracture of head radius

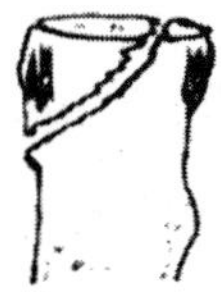

Fig. 11.8 (*c*) Fragment >1/3 the size of head of radius

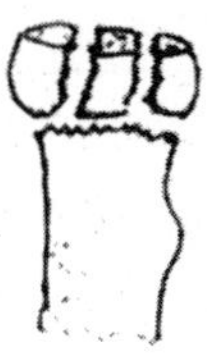

Fig. 11.8 (*d*) Comminuted fracture head radius

Type 1:

1. Undisplaced or minimally displaced fracture of head or neck.
2. Restriction of forearm supination and pronation due to pain and swelling.
3. Intraarticular displacement is less than 2 mm.

Type 2:

1. Intraarticular displacement is more than 2 mm.
2. Forearm rotation is restricted.
3. Marginal tip of radial head is fractured.

Type 3:

1. Severly comminuted fracture of head and neck radius.
2. It can not be reconstructed.
3. Excision is required to gain movement.

Clinical Features

1. Pain at lateral aspect of elbow that aggravates on forearm rotation.
2. **Terrible triad** may be present that includes fracture coronoid, fracture head radius and gross instability of elbow.

X-Ray Findings

X-ray elbow A.P. and lateral view shows fracture of head radius. If fracture is not visualized and a pad of fat is present a radiocapitellar view can be done.

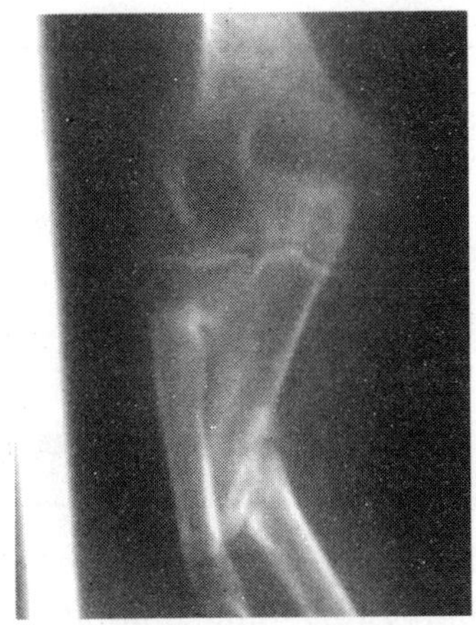

Fig. 11.9 Fracture head radius with fracture shaft of ulna

Role of CT Scan

Axial, sagittal and coronal section in CT scan of radial head can asses the size of head, degree of fragmentation and displacement.

Management

Type 1 fracture usually does not require surgical intervention. It can be managed in AEPOP cast. Haemorrhagic effusion can be aspirated.

Type 2 fracture is managed by surgical excision of head radius meeting the **Maclaughlin's criteria i.e. angulation > 30 degree, displacement >3 mm and >1/3rd head is involved).**

Type 3 fracture is strongly considered for surgical excision of head radius. Excised head of radius can be replaced by **Silicon prosthesis.**

CHAPTER

12 Fractures of Forearm

- Applied anatomy
- Fracture both bones forearm
- Monteggia fracture
- Galeazzi's fracture

APPLIED ANATOMY

Three muscles that play an important role in fracture shaft radius and ulna are Supinator, Pronator teres and Pronatus quadratus. These muscles keep the radius and ulna in approximation thus reducing interosseous space.

Other important muscles are flexor carpi radialis that pronate the forearm; abductor pollicis longus and brevis and extensor pollicis longus exert a supinating force.

Fracture of shaft radius between insertion of supinator and pronator teres causes proximal fragment in supination and distal fragment in pronation.

Fracture of shaft radius between pronator teres and pronator quadratus causes proximal fragment in neutral rotation while distal fragment in pronation.

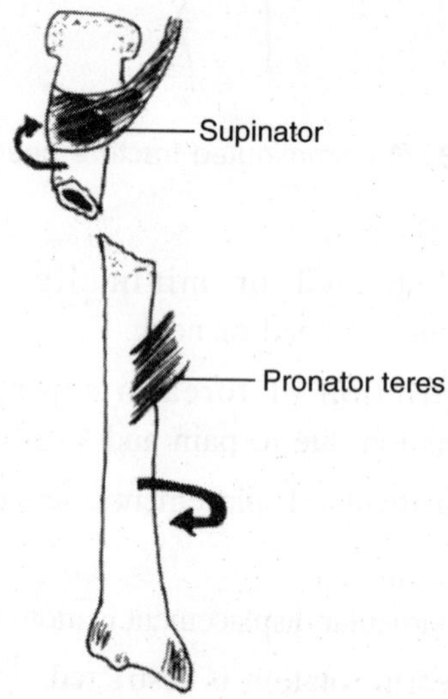

Fig. 12.1 Fracture between supinator and pronator teres. Proximal fragment is supinated while distal fragment is pronated

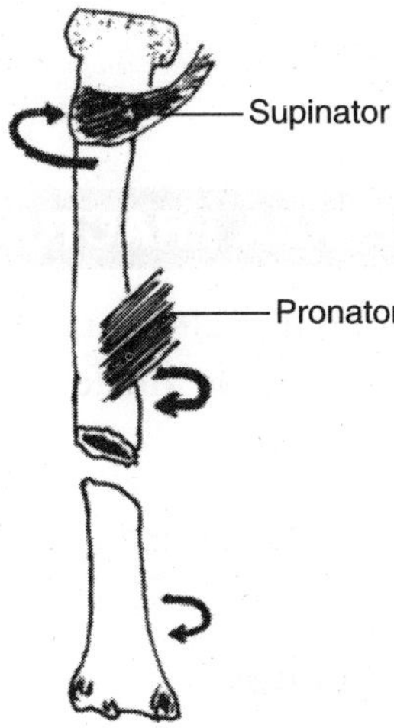

Fig. 12.2 Fracture distal to pronator teres keeps the proximal fragment in midprone position

FRACTURE BOTH BONES FOREARM

Children may present as green stick fracture. Displacement is unusual in children while an adult can have angulation, shift or rotation of fragment. Fractured fragment angulates anterior or ulnarward.

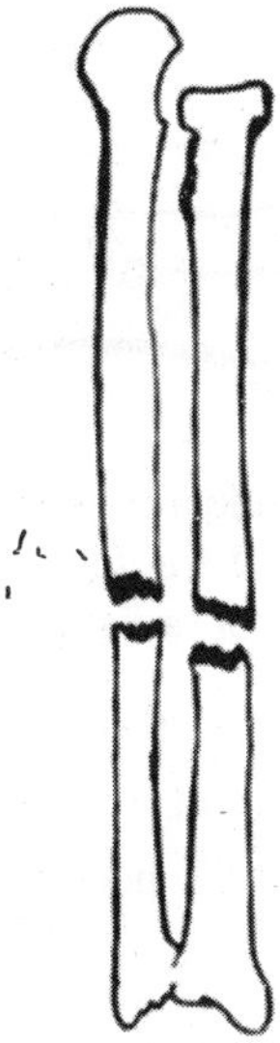

Fig. 12.3 Fracture both bones forearm

Clinical Features

1. Pain, swelling and deformity at the fracture site and inability to use forearm.
2. Bony tenderness, crepitus and abnormal mobility at the fracture site are clinical findings.

X-Ray Findings

X-ray forearm full length A.P. and Lateral view will show the fracture of shaft of radius or ulna (with angulation shift or rotation if present).

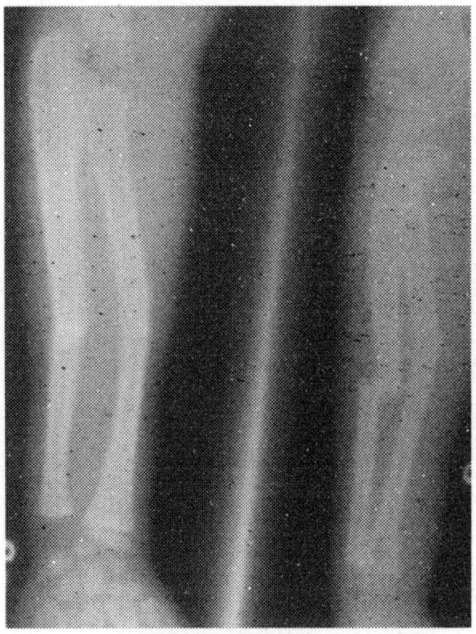

Fig. 12.4 Fracture both bones forearm

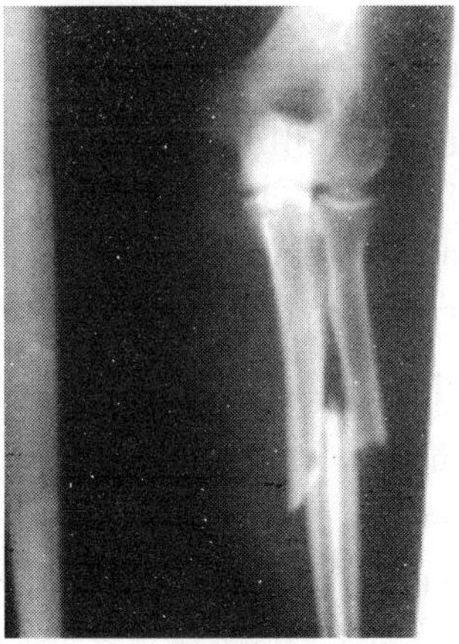

Fig. 12.5 Fracture both bones forearm

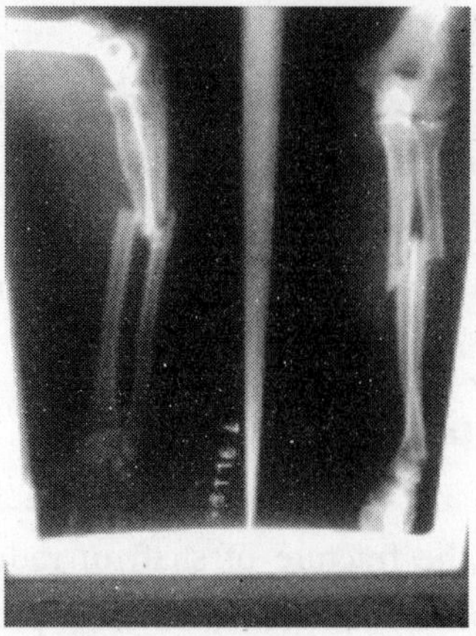

Fig. 12.6 Fracture both bones forearm

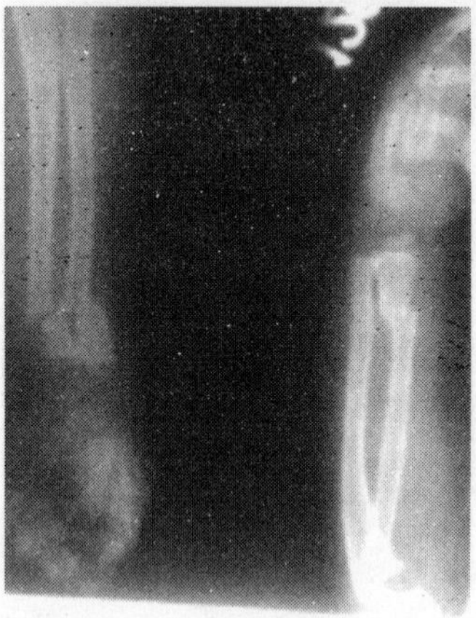

Fig. 12.7 Fracture lower end of both bones forearm

Treatment

Closed reduction followed by AEPOP cast is successful. If it fails ORIF of radius and ulna is done by dynamic compression plate (DCP/LCP) or by square nail.

Complications

Fracture both bones forearm can have following complications:

1. Volkman's ischaemia.
2. Delayed and nonunion.
3. Malunion.
4. Synostosis.

MONTEGGIA FRACTURE

Fracture of upper third of ulna with dislocation of head of radius is known as Monteggia fracture.

Aetiology

It is caused by forceful pronation of forearm or by a direct blow.

Bado's Classification

Bado has described four types of Monteggia fracture as follows:

Type 1: This is also known as extension or anterior type. It comprises of fracture of ulnar diaphysis with it's anterior angulation, associated with anterior dislocation of head radius. This is commonest type.

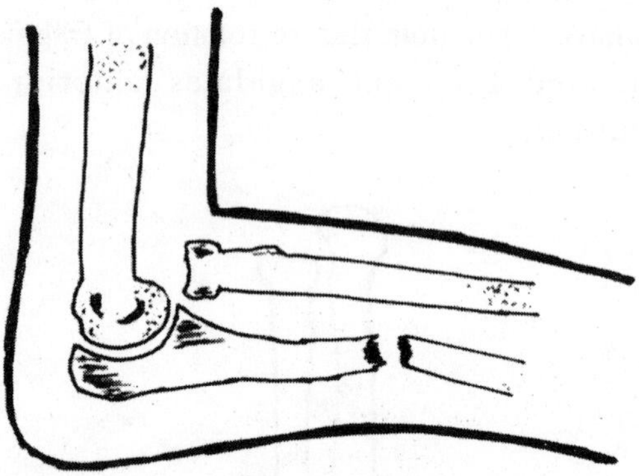

Fig. 12.8 (*a*) Monteggia fracture Type I shows anteriorly angulated fracture shaft ulna with anterior dislocation of radial head

Type 2: This is known as posterior or flexion type. It comprises of fracture of ulnar diaphysis with it's posterior angulation and posterior dislocation of head radius.

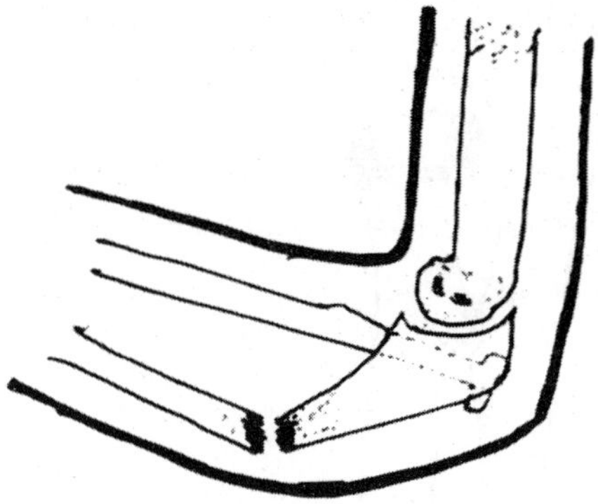

Fig. 12.8 (*b*) Monteggia fracture Type II shows posteriorly angulated fracture shaft ulna with posterior dislocation of head

Type 2A: Fracture of ulna occurs at olecranon and coronoid process.

Type 2B: Ulnar fracture is at the diaphyseal and metaphyseal junction.

Type 2C: It has diaphyseal fracture of ulna.

Type 2D: Fracture of ulna extends from proximal 1/3 to 1/2 of ulna.

Type 3: It has got lateral or anterolateral dislocation of head radius with fracture of ulnar metaphysis.

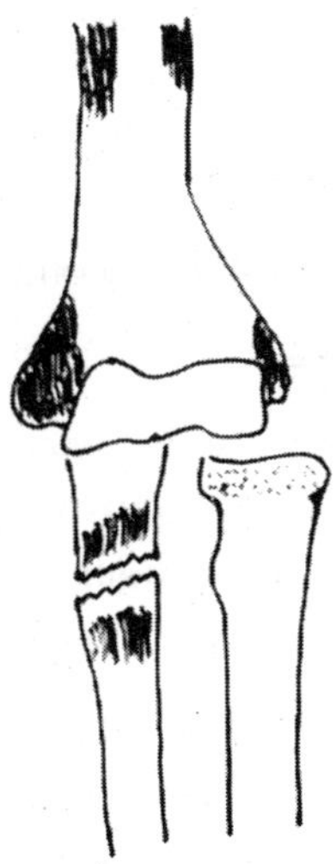

Fig. 12.8 (*c*) Monteggia fracture Type III shows fracture of ulnar metaphysis. It may be associated with anterior or anterolateral dislocation of head radius

Type 4: This type has fracture of radius and ulna wih anterior dislocation of head radius.

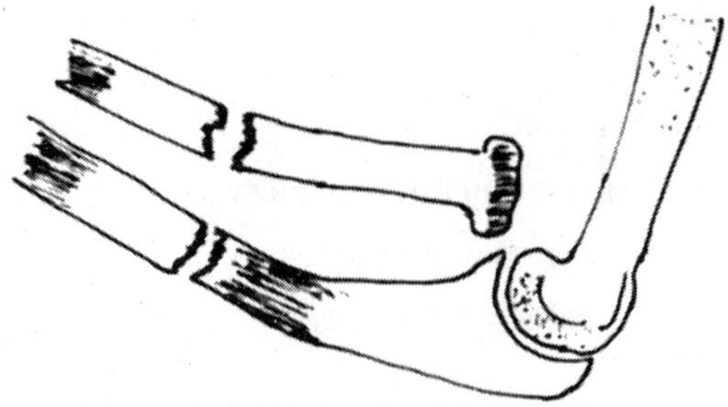

Fig. 12.8 (*d*) Monteggia fracture Type IV shows fracture of radius and ulna. With anterior dislocation of radial head

Clinical Features

1. Pain, swelling and deformity at upper end of ulna.
2. Dislocated head of radius can be palpated.
3. Bony tenderness, crepitus and abnormal mobility is present at the upper end of ulna.
4. Posterior type 2 fracture may be associated with posterior intersseous nerve injury.

X-ray Finding

X-ray will show fracture of upper third of ulna with dislocation of head radius.

Treatment

Closed reduction may be successful in children only. In adults it requires open reduction and internal fixation of ulna dynamic compression plate and closed reduction of head radius. Postoperatively AEPOP cast is applied in full flexion because it is an extension injury. Repeat X-ray is taken after 2nd, 4th and 6th week. After 6 weeks if X-ray shows adequate callus formation, cast can be removed, but sling is continued. Unreduced head radius in adults can be excised.

Complications

1. Post operative infection.
2. Implant failure.
3. Nonunion.
4. Malunion.
5. Posterior interosseous nerve injury.
6. Unstable radial head.
7. Radioulnar synostosis.

GALEAZZI'S FRACTURE

This is a fracture of shaft radius at the junction of middle and distal third, associated with subluxation or dislocation of distal radioulnar joint. This is also known as fracture of necessity i.e. open reduction and internal fixation is necessary if good result is to be achieved. This is also known as reverse of monteggia fracture.

If this fracture is reduced by closed method, it usually slips within 1-2 weeks because of following reasons:

1. Even in a cast, gravity acts through weight of hand that cause subluxation of inferior radioulnar joint. Along with that it causes dorsal angulation of fractured fragment.
2. Pronator quadratus rotates the distal fragment toward ulna and pulling it in proximal and volar direction. This makes reduction difficult.
3. Brachioradialis, abductors and extensor of thumb also make the reduction difficult.

Aetiology

It is caused by fall on outstretched hand combined with marked pronation of forearm.

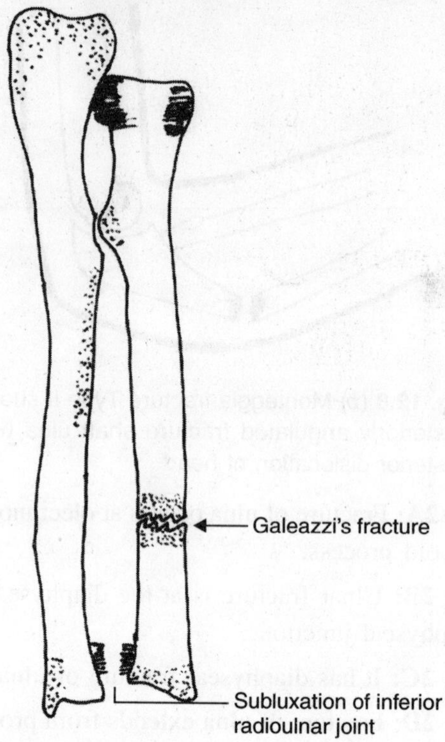

Fig. 12.9 Galeazzi's fracture

Clinical Features

1. Pain, swelling and deformity at the junction of middle third and lower third of shaft of radius. Bony tenderness, crepitus and abnormal mobility is present at the same site.
2. Head of ulna may become prominent.

X-Ray Findings

X-ray shows fracture at the junction of middle and distal third of shaft of radius with subluxation or dislocation of inferior radioulnar joint. Fracture is either transverse or short oblique.

Lateral view can show dorsal angulation of shaft of radius and prominence of head of ulna.

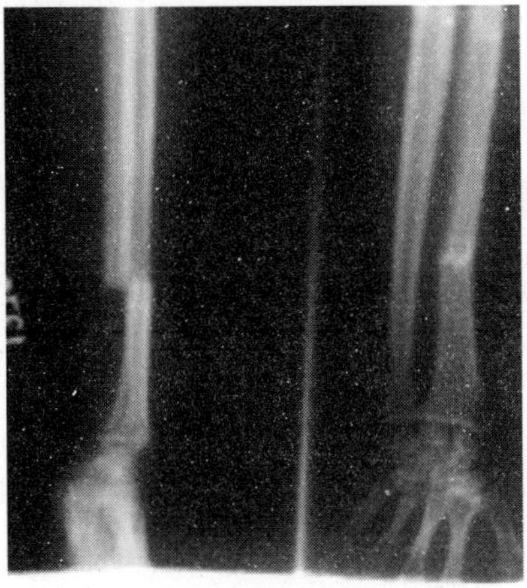

Fig. 12.10 Galeazzi's fracture

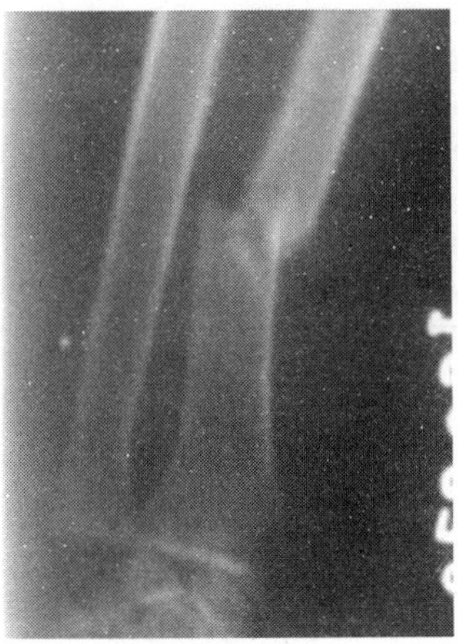

Fig. 12.11 Galeazzi's fracture

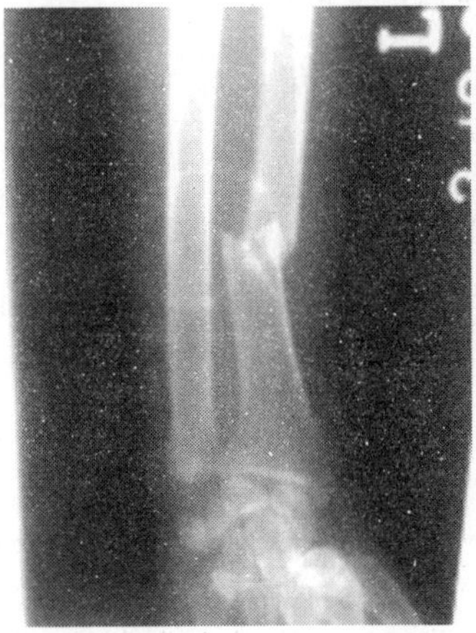

Fig. 12.12 Galeazzi's fracture

Treatment

Closed reduction usually fails. So it must be treated by open reduction and internal fixation by dynamic compression plate or locking compression plate (L.C.P.) followed by AEPOP cast in full supination. (supination is most stable position)

CHAPTER

13 Injuries Around Wrist

- Colles's fracture
- Smith fracture
- Scaphoid fracture
- Dislocation of lunate
- Bennett's fracture
- Rolando fracture
- Barton's fracture
- Chauffer's fracture
- Essex-Lopresti fracture
- Keinbock's disease
- Mallet finger
- Metacarpal fracture
- Boxer's fracture
- Dislocation of MP joint
- Kaplan's lesion
- Jersy finger

COLLES'S FRACTURE

Definition: This is a transverse fracture of lower end of radius within 3/4th of an inch from its distal articular margin at the corticocancellous junction occurring as a result of fall on outstretched hand leading to dinner fork deformity, commonly seen in post menopausal elderly females.

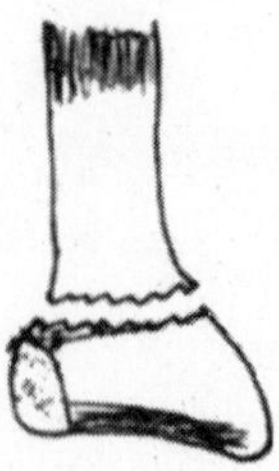

Fig. 13.1 (*a*) Colles's fracture

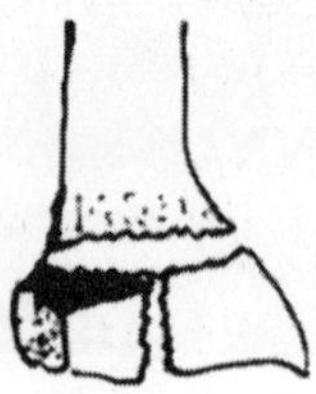

Fig. 13.1 (*b*) Intraarticular Colles's fracture

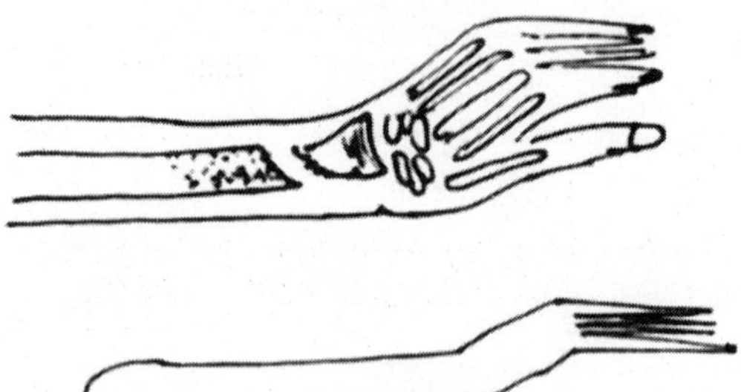

Fig. 13.2 Dinner fork deformity

Deformities of Colles's Fracture

Six deformities can be seen in this fracture.

1. Impaction

2. Dorsal displacement
3. Dorsal tilt
4. Lateral displacement
5. Lateral tilt
6. Supination.

Associated Injuries of Colles's Fracture

Colles's fracture has chances of having certain associated injuries as follows:

1. Ulnar styloid fracture.
2. Triangular cartilage of ulna may be ruptured.
3. Rupture of ulnar collateral ligament usually occurs after 4 weeks of injury.
4. Radioulnar subluxation can occur due to rupture of radioulnar interosseous ligament.

Clinical Features

Patient presents with pain, swelling and dinner fork deformity at wrist. Bony tenderness is present at lower end of radius. Radial styloid process lies at the same or little higher level of ulnar styloid process.

Frykman Classification

Frykman has classified this fracture into six types, as mentioned below in table.

Fracture	Distal ulnar fracture Absent	Distal ulnar fracture Present
Extraarticular	1	2
Intraarticular involving radiocarpal joint	3	4
Intraarticular involving lower radioulnar joint	5	6
Intraarticular involving both radiocarpal and distal radioulnar joint	7	8

X-ray Findings

Dorsal tilt should be looked for, in X-ray of wrist A.P. and Lateral view. If distal articular surface faces dorsally or in neutral position a dorsal tilt is present. Normally distal articular surface faces ventrally toward the side of thumb. We should also look for Smith or Barton's fracture. Intraarticular extension of fracture line should be looked for. A.P. view of wrist normally shows distal articular surface facing medially. In Colles's fracture if it faces laterally it means a lateral tilt is present. Supination of distal fragment can not be detected in X-ray. Associated fracture of ulnar styloid should be looked for.

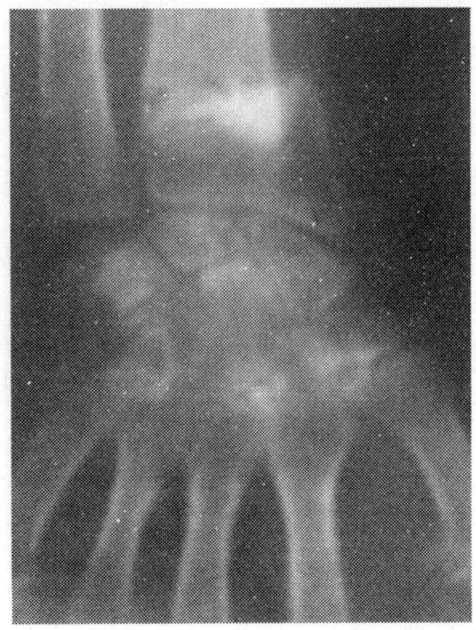

Fig. 13.3 Colles's fracture (extraarticular type 1)

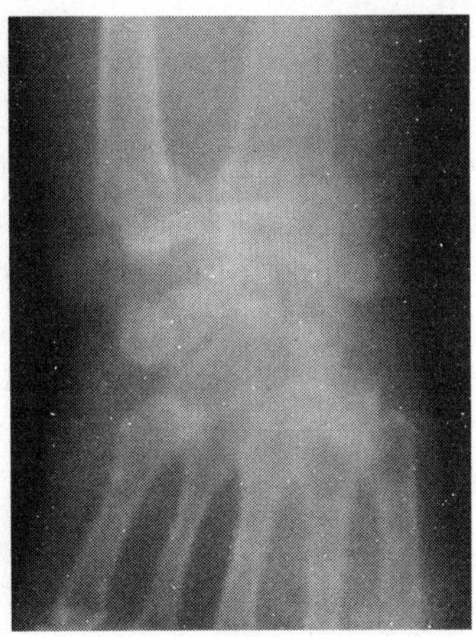

Fig. 13.4 Colles's fracture (extraarticular type 2)

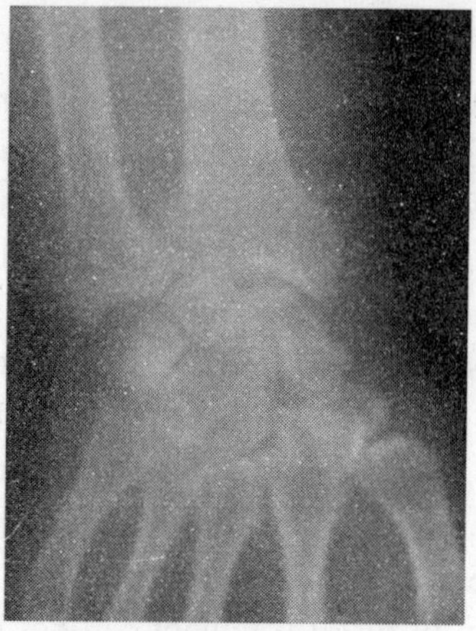

Fig. 13.5 Colles's fracture (intraarticular type)

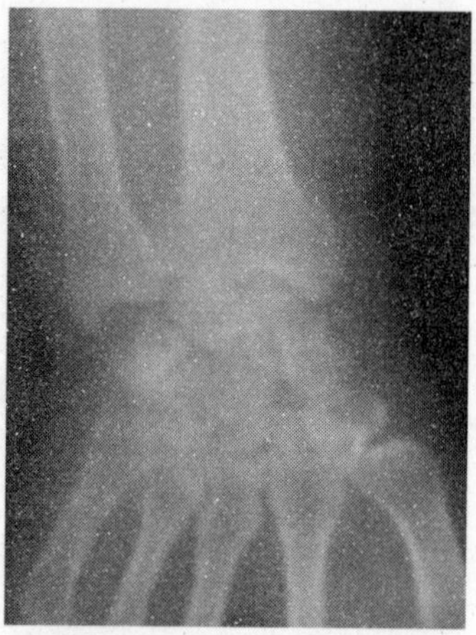

Fig. 13.6 Colles's fracture

Treatment

Colles's fracture can be reduced by shaking hand technique. It is maintained by BEPOP cast in palmar flexion and ulnar deviation, with forearm in pronation. BEPOP cast is applied for 6 weeks. AEPOP cast is applied if fracture is intraarticular/ comminuted or associated with ulnar styloid fracture. AEPOP cast is converted into BEPOP cast after 3 weeks for the purpose of physiotherapy.

Intraarticular fracture lower end radius can be treated by open reduction and internal fixation by volar buttress plate or LCP (Locking compression plate).

If subluxation of inferior radioulnar joint occurs, head of ulna becomes unduly prominent. This can be treated by **Darrach's procedure** in which lower end of ulna is excised.

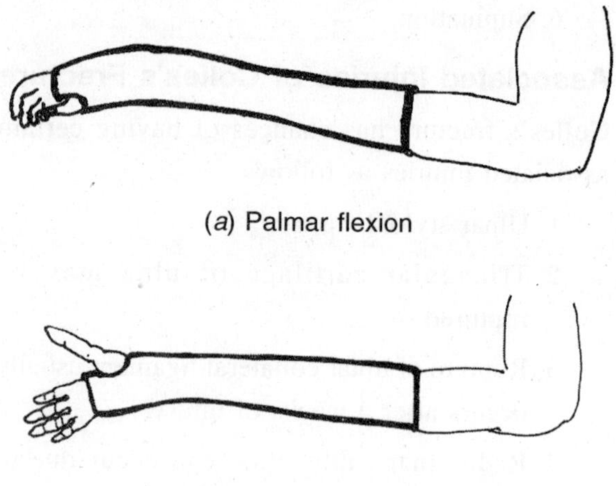

(*a*) Palmar flexion

(*b*) Ulnar deviation

Fig. 13.7 Colles' cast in palmar flexion and ulnar deviation

Complications

1. Stiffness of wrist joint
2. Malunion
3. Painful wrist joint
4. Sudeck's osteodystrophy
5. Subluxation of inferior radioulnar joint
6. Rupture of extensor pollicis longus
7. Carpal tunnel syndrome
8. Frozen shoulder hand syndrome.

Stiffness of Wrist Joint

This is most common complication of Colles's fracture. It is managed by physiotherapy. Stiffness can occur in fingers, wrist, shoulder and elbow joint.

Malunion

Malunion is second most common complication of this fracture. Malunion occurs because it has tendency to displace again within the plaster.

Painful Wrist Joint

Wrist joint may become painful due to post-traumatic stiffness, arthritis, intraarticular fracture of lower end radius, associated fracture of ulnar styloid process, fracture scaphoid, subluxation of inferior radioulnar joint, carpal tunnel syndrome and sudeck's atrophy.

Sudeck's Osteodystrophy

Patient presents with pain, swelling and stiffness in hand after removal of plaster. Overlying skin becomes shiny and stretched.

Rupture of Extensor Pollicis Longus

It can happen due to two reasons either hampered blood supply of tendon at the time of fracture or due to friction of tendon over fracture site.

Carpal Tunnel Syndrome

It may occur due to compression of median nerve in carpal tunnel by callus formation. It can be treated by decompression of nerve.

Frozen Hand Shoulder Syndrome

In this condition patient keeps his shoulder in immobilized condition to avoid pain at fracture site. This makes shoulder stiff.

Nonunion

It is very rare complication of Colles's fracture.

Universal Classification of Fracture Lower End Radius

Fractures of lower end radius are classified as Extraarticular and Intraarticular. Extraarticular fracture of lower end radius is known as Colles's fracture. These are of two types as follows:

Type 1: Stable and undisplaced

Type 2: Displaced and unstable

Intraarticular fractures are also of two types as follows:

Type 3: Undisplaced

Type 4: Displaced

Treatment of Malunited Fracture

In this condition patient presents with either of these problem:

1. Impaired function
2. Cosmetic deformity
3. Both of above

Impaired function is treated by **Darrach's operation.** In this operation lower end of ulna about 2.5 cm is excised including the head. Periosteum is left behind.

Cosmetic deformity can be corrected by **Fernandes and Campbell osteotomy** of radial fracture site. Fernandes osteotomy is dorsal wedge osteotomy while Campbell osteotomy is lateral wedge osteotomy.

Osteotomy and Darrach's operation can be done together if patient needs cosmetic correction as well as improved function.

If patient develops post-traumatic osteoarthritis following an intraarticular fracture; arthrodesis of wrist joint can be done in functional position.

SMITH FRACTURE

1. This fracture is reverse of Colles's fracture.
2. In this fracture distal fragment presents with ventral displacement and ventral tilt opposite to Colles's fracture.
3. This is volar angulated fracture of distal radius leading to garden spade deformity.
4. It can be treated by closed reduction followed POP cast for 6 weeks.
5. ORIF is treatment of choice for palmar displaced fracture, particularly intraarticular type 2 and type 3.

SCAPHOID FRACTURE

This is most common fracture among carpal bones and second most common fracture of wrist. 65%

of scaphoid fractures occur through its waist; 15% through proximal pole; 10% through distal body; 8% through tuberosity and rest at distal articular surface. It is caused by fall on outstretched hand with hyperextension.

Clinical Features

1. Pain and swelling at the wrist.
2. Bony tenderness at anatomical snuff box.

X-ray Findings

1. Initial X-ray may not show a fracture line in scaphoid. Fracture becomes visible 2-3 weeks later.
2. Following views of X-ray can be done e.g. A.P./Lateral, scaphoid view, motion view of wrist (flexion/extension and radioulnar deviation).
3. If diagnosis is still in doubt, technectium bone scan can be done.
4. If diagnosis is still not confirmed polytomography or MRI can be done in this order of preference.

Classification

Classification is of two types based on location of fracture within the scaphoid described above (65% occurring at waist of scaphoid) and displacement or stability of fracture as described below:

Stable scaphoid fracture. It is the fracture that is undisplaced and may have intact cartilage envelope.

Unstable scaphoid fracture. Displacement of more than 1 mm is defined as unstable scaphoid fracture.

Treatment

1. Stable fracture is treated by scaphoid cast for 8–10 weeks.
2. Unstable fracture should be treated by open reduction and compression screw fixation.
3. Scaphoid is notorious not to heal well. Treatment of choice for nonunion of scphoid is bone grafting i.e. cortico-cancellous graft. PEMS (Pulsed electromagnetic stimulation) is supposed to be good treatment option for undisplaced scaphoid nonunion.
4. **Vascularised bone graft** is used in AVN scaphoid, failure of bone grafting, **Preiser disease** (AVN of entire scaphoid bone).

Complications

1. Nonunion is the most common complication.
2. It may remain undiagnosed.
3. Preiser disease (avascular necrosis of entire scaphoid bone).

DISLOCATION OF LUNATE

Lunate dislocations are uncommon and are of two types as follows:

Anterior dislocation of lunate

This is common type of dislocation in which lunate dislocates anteriorly while other carpal bones remain stationary.

Perilunate dislocation

This is not so common. In this type lunate remains stationary at its position but other carpal bones around it dislocate. This is managed by open reduction.

BENNETT'S FRACTURE

Edward Bennett was the first person to describe this fracture. This is an intraarticular fracture of base of first metacarpal of thumb. It may be associated with subluxation or dislocation of first metacarpophalangeal joint.

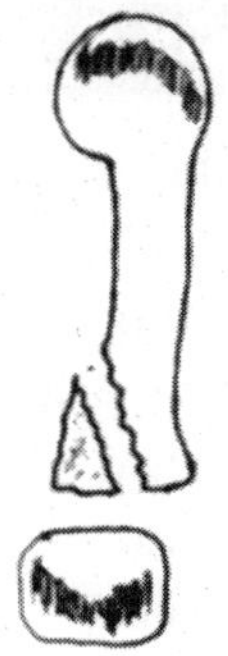

Fig. 13.8 Bennett's fracture
(Intraarticular fracture of base of first metcarpal)

Mechanism of Injury

It is caused by blow on partially flexed metacarpal.

Clinical Features

Patient presents with pain swelling and deformity at the base of first metacarpal. On examination we can get bony tenderness, crepitus and abnormal mobility at the base of first metacarpal.

Treatment

If closed reduction fails we should try to fix it by K wire (percutaneously). If this method fails; open reduction and internal fixation should be done with small screw or K wire.

Complications

1. Osteoarthritis of metacarpophalangeal joint can occur due to inaccurate reduction leading to irregular articular surface.
2. Pain and stiffness at metacarpophalangeal joint.

ROLANDO FRACTURE

Extraarticular fracture of base of first metacarpal is known as Rolando fracture. It can be managed by closed reduction followed by thumb spica for three weeks.

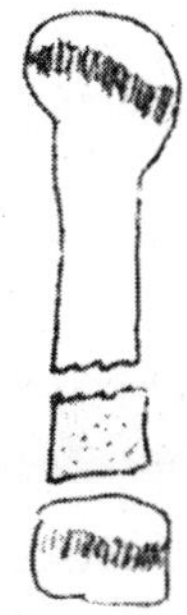

Fig. 13.9 Rolando fracture
(Extraarticular fracture of base of first metacarpal)

BARTON'S FRACTURE

This is fracture of distal articulating surface of radius. Barton's fracture is treated by closed reduction followed by cast immobilization. If closed reduction fails open reduction and internal fixation is done by buttress plate. Barton fracture is of two types as follows:

Volar Barton Fracture

If fracture line passes through volar margin of distal articulating surface of radius, it is called as Volar Barton fracture.

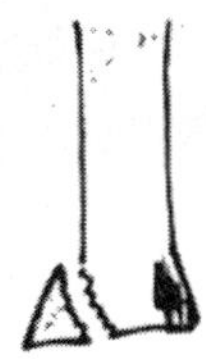

Fig. 13.10 Volar Barton fracture

Dorsal Barton Fracture

If fracture line passes through dorsal margin of distal articulating surface of radius, it is known as Dorsal Barton fracture.

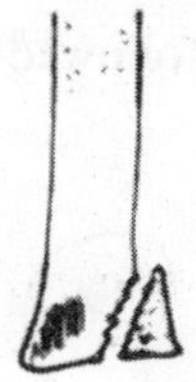

Fig. 13.11 Dorsal Barton fracture

CHAUFFER'S FRACTURE

This is the fracture of radial styloid process and usually associated with scapholunate ligament tear, radial shortening and significant dorsal angulation. It is treated by closed reduction and percutaneous pin fixation. Open reduction is done when more than 3 mm displacement is present or scapholunate dissociation is seen. Trabecular screw provides better fixation.

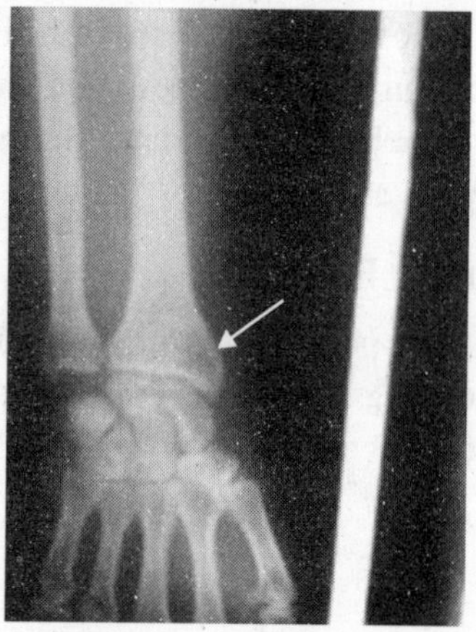

Fig. 13.12 Chauffer's fracture

ESSEX-LOPRESTI FRACTURE

Combination of fracture head radius with subluxation of inferior radioulnar joint is known as Essex-Lopresti fracture. It should be treated by excision of head radius which can be replaced by radial head sialistic prosthesis. If we do not put sialistic prosthesis there will be chances of proximal migration of radius.

KIENBOCK'S DISEASE

Fracture of lunate bone, progresses to osteochondrosis later. By the time it becomes symptomatic it is diagnosed as Kienbock's disease. It is caused by a hyperextension injury like a fall on outstretched hand. It is also known as **Leunatomalacia** or osteonecrosis/osteochondritis of lunate.

Stahl and Lichman Classification

Stahl and Lichman have classified Kienbock's disease into four stages as follows:

Stage 1. Normal appearance or linear fracture on tomogram.

Stage 2. Sclerosis and slight collapse of radial border.

Stage 3. Fragmentation and collapsed lunate with scaphoid rotation.

Stage 4. Advanced collapse of lunate with scaphoid rotation. Sclerosis and osteophytes at radiocarpal joint.

Treatment of Kienbock's Disease

Lunate fracture can lead to carpal instability, nonunion or avascular necrosis so CT scan should be done. Some times a MRI may be required. A long arm cast or Monster type cast, well moulded over wrist (to compress the lunate area) should be applied.

MALLET FINGER

This is also known as Baseball finger or Drop finger. This is an avulsion injury of extensor tendon slip attached to the terminal phalanx of a finger caused by forced flexion of distal phalanx while extensor tendons are trying to extend the fingers. Two types of injuries are seen in mallet finger:

1. Extensor tendon is torn at its origin.

2. Extensor tendon tear involves a piece of bone.

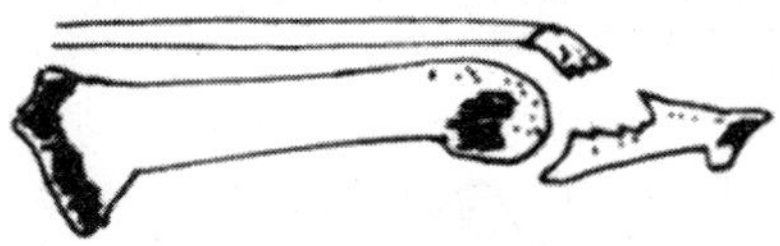

Fig. 13.13 Mallet finger resulting due to bony injury

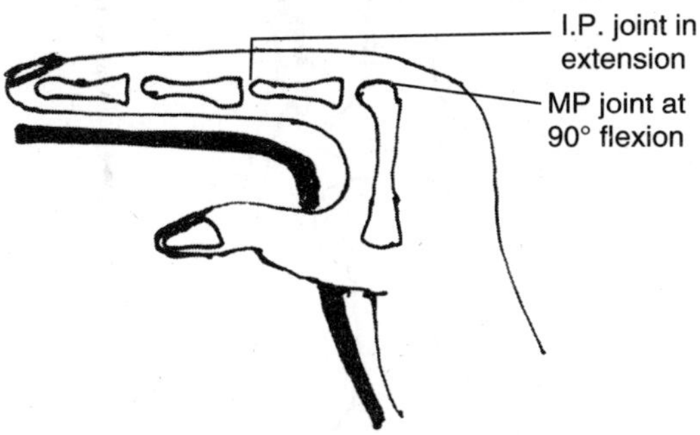

Fig. 13.14 Position of plaster (James position) in crush injury of hand. Collateral ligaments are relaxed in this position

Clinical Features

1. Patient presents with pain and inability to extend the terminal phalanx of finger or thumb.
2. Mild cases may show loss of 10–20 degree active extension while moderate and severe cases may show loss of 35–45 degree or active extension or no active extension.

Treatment

This is treated by continuous immobilization of distal joint for 6–10 weeks by mallet finger splint. Patient can also be immobilized by Smellie' cast. Mallet finger of bony origin can be fixed by K wire.

METACARPAL FRACTURE

Undisplaced metacarpal fractures can be managed by below elbow POP volar slab which is applied in cobrahood position. Displaced fracture can be fixed with K-wires. Boxer's fracture is one of the common fractures among metacarpal fractures.

BOXER'S FRACTURE

This is a fracture of neck of fifth metacarpal. This is sustained when a closed fist hits to a hard object as in boxers. This is treated by BEPOP slab applied dorsally on hand for three weeks. Displaced fractures can be fixed with K wire.

DISLOCATION OF MP JOINT

Dislocation of MP joint is caused by hyperextension, leading to tear of volar plate at its proximal insertion at metacarpal neck. It is of two types Simple and Complex.

Simple dislocations are those that can be reduced by closed method, while Complex dislocations are those that cannot be reduced by closed method.

Complex dislocation of MP joint is known as **Kaplan's Lesion.**

KAPLAN'S LESION

This is a complex dislocation of 2nd metacarpophalangeal joint that cannot be reduced because a volar plate is interposed in between. It is also known as **Button holing** of metacarpal head into palm.

Index finger is most common to be involved. Thumb and little finger can also be involved in decreasing order of frequency.

Clinical Features

1. Patient presents with flexed interphalangeal joint and mildly hyperextended metacarpophalangeal joint.
2. Examination shows puckered skin on volar aspect.

X-ray Finding

X-ray shows dislocated joint. Sometimes a sesamoid bone can be seen in widened joint space.

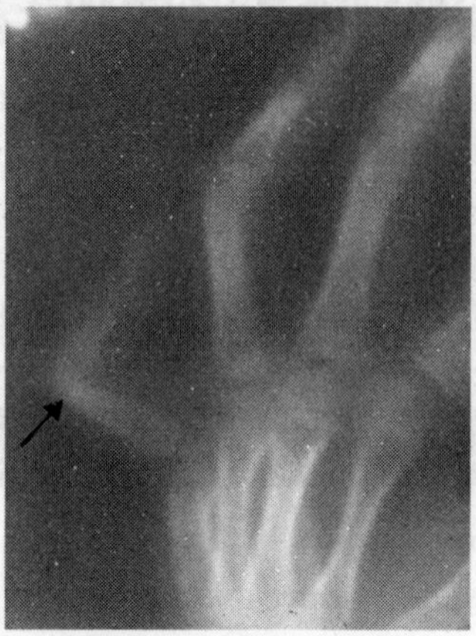

Fig. 13.15 Kaplan's lesion

Treatment

If closed reduction fails it should be managed by open reduction, known as **Kaplan's operation.**

JERSY FINGER

This is an avulsion fracture of flexor digitorum longus tendon from volar aspect of distal phalanx. This avulsion may accompany a metaphyseal fragment and a variable amount of physis.

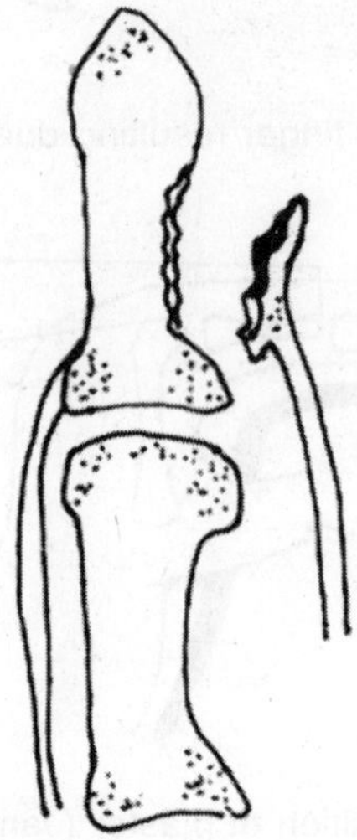

Fig. 13.16 Jersy finger (Instead of common avulsion of flexor digitorium profundus from its metaphysis on volar terminal phalanx, a metaphyseal fragment involving part of physis can accompany tendon

CHAPTER

14 Fracture Pelvis

- Tile's classification
- Straddle fracture
- Malgaigne's fracture
- Open book fracture
- Central fracture dislocation of hip

Fracture pelvis is an emergency, commonly seen in road traffic accidents. Patient may present with hypovolemic shock, rupture of bladder or urethra. Pain and swelling at pelvic area, inability to stand or walk are main clinical features of fracture of pelvis.

TILE'S CLASSIFICATION

This fracture has been classified into three types as follows:

Stable

a. Fracture of pelvis not involving ring.

b. Stable and minimally displaced fracture of ring.

Vertically Stable and Rotationally Unstable

a. Open book type fracture

b. Ipsilateral with lateral compression

c. Contralateral (Bucket handle type)

Rotationally and Vertically Unstable

a. Rotationally and vertically unstable

b. Bilateral

c. Associated with acetabular fracture

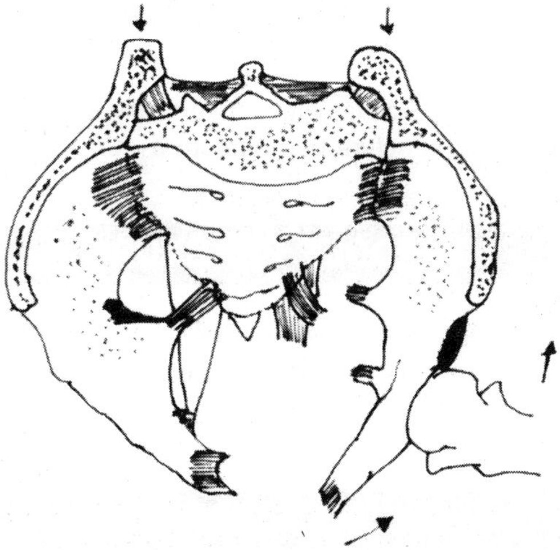

Fig. 14.1 (*a*) Open book type fracture

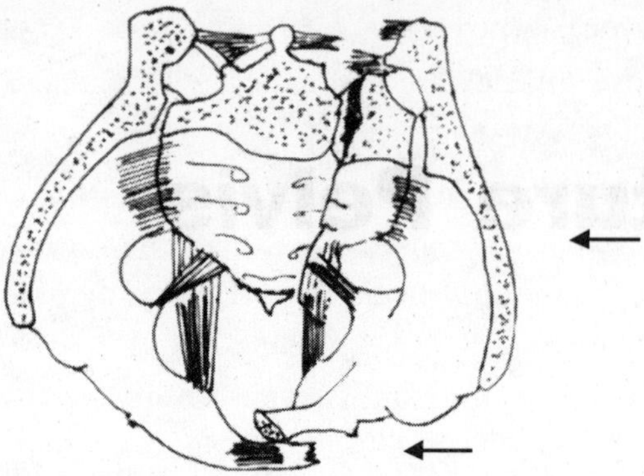

Fig. 14.1 (*b*) Lateral compression fracture

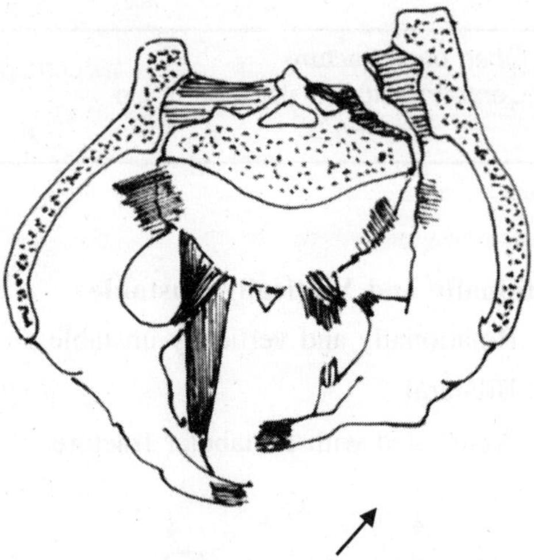

Fig. 14.1 (*c*) Rotationaly and vertically unstable fracture pelvis fracture

STRADDLE FRACTURE

This is type 3a fracture of Key and Canwell's classification involving double vertical fracture of pubis.

MALGAIGNE'S FRACTURE

This is a type 3b fracture of Key and Canwell's classification involving ipsilateral pubic rami fracture with ipsilateral sacroiliac joint dissociation.

OPEN BOOK FRACTURE

In this fracture pelvic ring opens up from the front like a book. It may be associated with **pubic diastasis** (disruption of pubic symphysis) or pubic rami fracture. In this type, one half of pelvis is externally rotated.

Clinical Features

Patient may present with the following features:

1. Pain at pelvic area.
2. Inability to stand or walk.
3. Haematoma at symphysis pubis.
4. Shortening of one of lower limb in case of displaced fracture.
5. Pelvic compression and distraction test is positive. This test is done in supine position. Both iliac crest are compressed toward each other (compression test) and distracted away from each other (distraction test). During this procedure patient will feel pain. Examiner will get springy feel.
6. Bony tenderness and crepitus can be felt at fracture site.
7. Hypovolemic shock.
8. Patient may also present with the following injuries, e.g., urethral injury, rupture of bladder, injury to common iliac artery or it's branches, perineal injuries with damage to rectum or vagina and lumbosacral injury.

Investigations

X-ray pelvis with both hip-AP view will show the fracture. CT scan can be helpful in planning of management.

Treatment

Pelvis fracture should be treated on following line of action:

1. We should correct hypovolemic shock by giving intravenous fluid/plasma expander/ blood.

2. Vital monitoring should be done at regular interval. Always keep a watch on blood pressure.
3. Undisplaced fracture can be treated by absolute bed rest for 3-4 weeks.
4. Open book type fracture (displacement > 2.5 cm) can be treated by hammock sling traction/external fixator applied through schanz pins. Internal fixation is treatment of choice for pubic diastasis. It can be done by single plate fixation or screws.
5. Percutaneous fixation is used for complete disruption of sacroiliac joint.
6. Posterior iliac ring fracture can be fixed with 6.5 mm screw.

Complications

Fracture pelvis may have following complications:

Urethral injury

It is more commonly seen in male patient and membranous urethra is commonest to be injured. Patient will present with blood per urethra, perineal haematoma and distension of bladder. This injury is associated with pubic diastasis and pubic rami fracture. It can be managed by suprapubic cystotomy.

Bladder rupture

Bladder rupture is usually extraperitoneal, where urine extravasates into perivesical space. In this condition patient dose not pass urine. It can be managed by repair of bladder.

Injury to common iliac artery or it's branches

This injury is not so common and to be managed by a vascular surgeon.

Perineal injuries

These injuries are associated with damage to vagina or rectum.

Lumbosacral injury

These types of injuries are treated conservatively and commonly seen in vertically displaced fracture.

Thromboembolism and malunion are other complications.

CENTRAL FRACTURE DISLOCATION OF HIP

Central fracture dislocation of hip (acetabulum) occurs due to direct blow at lateral aspect of trochanter thus transmitting the force through femoral head into acetabulum.

Following three types of acetabular fractures are seen:

1. Transverse fracture of anterior column.
2. Transverse fracture of posterior column.
3. Transverse fracture of anterior and posterior column.

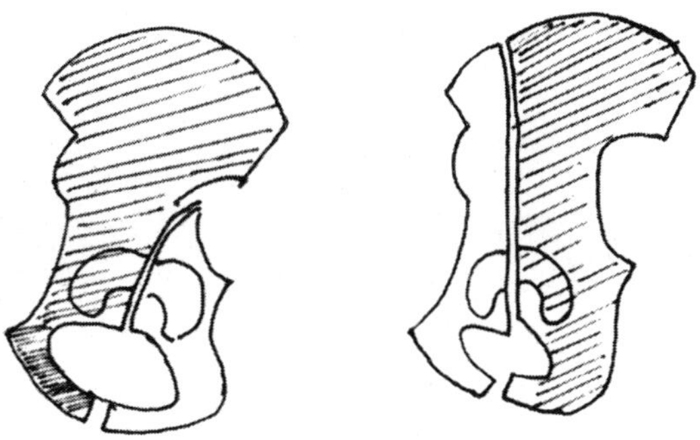

Fig. 14.2 (*a*) Universal classification of acetabular fracture (Type A)

CHAPTER 14

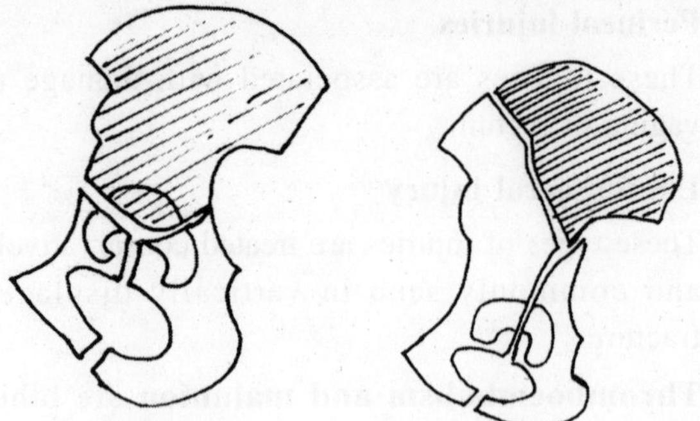

Fig. 14.2 (*b*) Universal classification of acetabular fracture (Type B and C)

Clinical Features

1. Pain, swelling and bruises around the hip joint are common features.
2. Limb shortening is seen.
3. Sciatic nerve injury may be present.
4. It may be associated with injury to chest, abdomen, head and other part of body.

Investigations

1. X-ray of hip (internal and external oblique views) should be done to see the fracture and displacement.
2. 3-D CT scan of hip joint can show 3 dimensional image of hip joint.
3. MRI can asses vascularity of femoral head and associated cartilaginous injury.

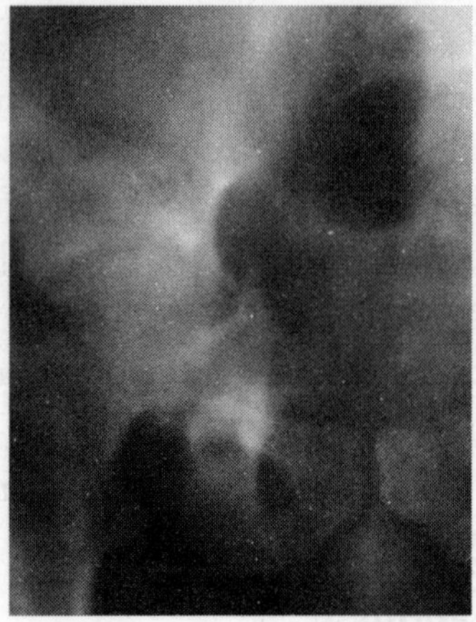

Fig. 14.3 Central fracture dislocation of hip

Treatment

Treatment should be done in a manner so that following aims are achieved:

1. Relationship of acetabulum and femoral head to be re-established.
2. Restore the congruity of articular surface.

CHAPTER

15 Dislocation of Hip

- Posterior dislocation of hip
- Recurrent dislocation of hip
- Anterior dislocation of hip

Dislocation of hip is an orthopaedic emergency. It should be reduced as soon as possible. Commonest dislocation of hip is posterior type (85–90%). Anterior dislocation is uncommon and seen in 10–15% cases.

POSTERIOR DISLOCATION OF HIP

This is a dash board injury sustained as a result dash board impacting at knee. In this fracture; head of femur rests posterior to coronal plane of acetabulum.

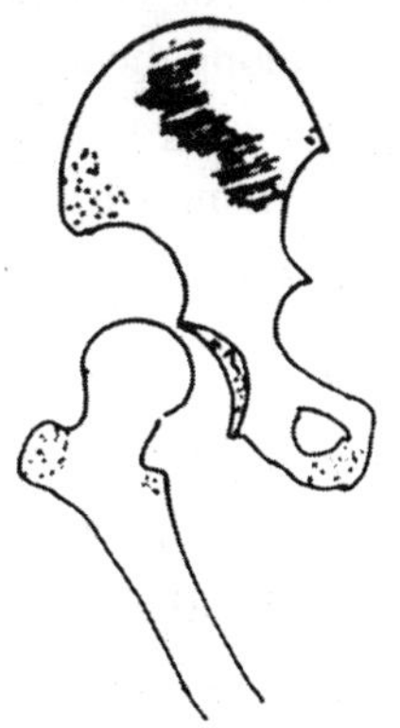

Fig. 15.1 Dislocation of hip joint

Thompson and Epstein Classification

Thompson and Epstein have classified posterior dislocation of hip into 5 types as follows:

Type 1: Posterior dislocation is associated with or without minor fracture.

Type 2: Posterior dislocation is associated with large single fracture of acetabulum.

Type 3: Comminuted fracture of acetabular rim is with or without a major fragment.

Type 4: Dislocation is associated with fracture of floor of acetabulum.

Type 5: Dislocation is associated with femoral head fracture.

Pipkin's Classification

Pipkin's has classified Type 5 fracture (Thompson classification) further into 4 subtypes as follows:

Type 5A: Fracture of femoral head is cauded to fovea centralis.

Type 5B: Fracture of femoral head is cephalic to fovea cenntralis.

Type 5C: It includes Type A + B + Fracture neck of femur.

Type 5D: It includes Type A + B + C + Fracture of acetabulum.

Clinical Features

Patient presents with the deformity of flexion, adduction and internal rotation at hip joint. Along with this; patient has severe pain and swelling at hip. Examination shows shortening of lower limb. Head can be palpated in gluteal region.

X-ray Findings

1. X-ray pelvis with both hip A.P. and Lateral views will show head lying out of acetabulum.
2. Shenton line is broken.
3. Lesser trochanter is less prominent due to internal rotation of femur.
4. Associated fracture of acetabulum/femoral head can be seen if present.

Role of CT Scan

1. It can asses anatomy and congruity of acetabulum and femoral head.
2. It can show intraarticular fragment.
3. CT scan should be done after closed reduction of hip in all cases to rule out osteochondral fragment and acetabular fracture.
4. It is also indicated when open reduction is planned.
5. It is also indicated in cases where patient has widened joint space in which no osteochondral lesion is seen in CT scan.

Role of MRI

1. MRI can show degree of comminution in a better way than CT scan.
2. It can evaluate integrity of labrum.
3. It can asses vascularity of head.
4. This is primarily indicated in hip that becomes unstable after reduction.

Treatment

Most common method of closed reduction is Biglow's 90-90 method. Other methods of closed reduction are, Gravity method of stimson and Allis maneuver. Dislocation of hip is an emergency and should be reduced as soon as possible.

Biglow's 90-90 Method

Reduction is done under general anesthesia. Patient lies supine on floor. Hip and knees are flexed up to 90 degree. Hold the knee with hands or flexed elbow, meanwhile assistant surgeon holds the pelvis firmly with both hands. Now a upward pull is applied along the axis of femur till a sound of click is heard. This sound of click confirms the reduction. It can also be confirmed by testing range of movements at hip. Now limb is kept in Thomas knee splint with light traction. Hip is kept in slight abduction. Traction is applied for 3–6 weeks and later hip mobilization exercises are started.

Gravity Method of Stimson

In this method patient is asked to lie in prone position with the hip flexed over the edge of table. Assistant surgeon holds the sacrum. Hip and knee are kept at 90 degree of flexion. Now apply a downward pressure along the axis of femur. When a sound of click is heard, reduction is achieved. It can also be confirmed by testing range of movements at hip joint.

Alli's Maneuver

This is also known as flexion adduction method of reduction of posterior dislocation of hip. In this method traction is applied in the line of deformity then we flex the hip up to 90 degree. Meanwhile longitudinal traction is continued. Now hip joint is internally and externally rotated until reduction is achieved.

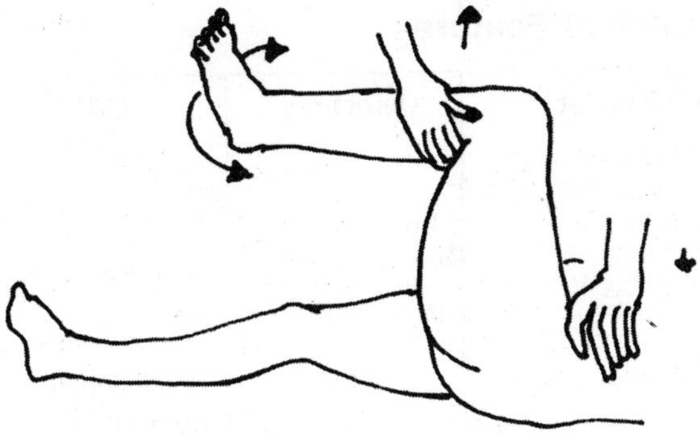

Fig. 15.2 Alli's reduction method for posterior dislocation of hip

Indications of Surgery

Open reduction is required in following conditions:

1. Unstable reduction (due to large posterior lip fragment).
2. Bony fragment is present in acetabular cavity.
3. Dislocation is associated with fracture of femoral head.

Complications

These are classified in early and late types as follows:

Early Complications

1. Sciatic nerve paresis
2. Irreducible posterior dislocation
3. Missed ligament injuries of knee
4. Recurrent dislocation in traction.

Late Complications

1. Myositis ossificans
2. Aseptic necrosis
3. Post traumatic arthritis.

Sciatic Nerve Paresis: Sciatic nerve is widened and stretched due to dislocated femoral head. Nerve cannot bear pressure changes, and likely to undergo ischaemic changes, if not treated early. Peroneal component of sciatic nerve is most commonly injured. This nerve injury is neuropraxia type of injury. Sometimes it may be an axonotmesis type of injury. Rarely ectopic bone formation around hip joint can cause sciatic nerve paresis. Nerve is decompressed during ORIF of displaced fragment of acetabbulum.

Irreducible Dislocation: Most common cause of irreducible dislocation is buttonholing of femoral head through hip capsule. Second most common cause is interposition of piriformis muscle between femoral head and acetabulum. If closed reduction is not achieved under general anesthesia, one more attempt can be taken. If still it is not reduced, open reduction is recommended to remove obstruction in the path of reduction.

Missed Ligament Injuries of Knee: Collateral and cruciate ligaments are likely to undergo injuries due to varus or valgus rotation of knee.

Recurrent Dislocation in Traction: This is seen in those patients who are in coma or have associated injuries.

RECURRENT DISLOCATION OF HIP

It may be due to following reasons:

1. Shallow acetabulum.
2. Deficient posterior rim of acetabulum.
3. Inadequate immobilization.
4. Gross soft tissue injuries.

This can be treated by resecting the pseudocavity and putting a bone block at posterior margin of acetabular rim, which acts as a support.

Capsular plication with or without muscle plication is another mode of treatment for recurrent dislocation of hip.

Myositis Ossificans

Incidence of myositis ossificans depends on muscle damage and haematoma at the time of injury. Delayed ORIF is another cause for development of myositis ossificans. It can be treated by giving rest to joint. Analgesics can be given for pain relief.

Aseptic Necrosis of Head of Femur

This is also known as avascular necrosis of head femur. Chances of necrosis depend on duration for which hip remains dislocated. If closed reduction is done within 6 hours of injury, chances of necrosis are less. Open reduction specially done from anterior approach has more chances of developing aseptic necrosis of femoral head.

Earlier diagnosis of AVN could be made by using technectium99m-sulfur colloid bone scaning. But now MRI has become a investigation of choice to detect avascular necrosis of femoral head.

Post Trumatic Arthritis

This is commonly seen in dislocation of hip associated with fracture of acetabulum or femoral head. Severity of trauma also plays a role in development of post traumatic arthritis. Articular cartilage is damaged leading to death of chondrocytes that causes post traumatic arthritis.

ANTERIOR DISLOCATION OF HIP

Only 10–15% of all dislocations constitute anterior dislocation. It is of two types as follows:

1. Superior Type
   a. Iliac type
   b. Pubic type
2. Inferior Type
   a. Obturator type
   b. Thyroid type
   c. Perineal type

Clinical Features

Superior type	**Deformity**	**C/F**
Iliac	Hip is extended and externally rotated	Head is palpable near ASIS
Pubic	Do	Head is palpable in groin. True lengthening of leg
Inferior type		
Obturator	Hip is in abduction and external rotation	Fullness is palpable in obturator foramen
Thyroid	Do	
Perineal	Do	Fullness in perineal region

Treatment

This should be treated under general anesthesia by closed methods as mentioned below:

1. Gravity method of Stimson
2. Alli's method
3. Reverse Biglow method

If closed methods of reduction fail, we should opt for open reduction.

Complications

Complications of anterior dislocations are same as seen in posterior type.

CHAPTER

16 Fracture Neck Femur

- Applied anatomy
- Classification
- Classification of fracture neck femur in children
- Hemireplacement arthroplasty of hip
  - Complications

APPLIED ANATOMY

Most valuable anatomy of neck of femur is it's vascular anatomy as fracture neck femur is more prone for nonunion due to disruption of its blood supply. Head of femur is supplied by 3 main sources as follows:

1. Retinacular vessels
2. Artery of ligamentous teres (branch of obturator or medial circumflex femoral artery)
3. Intraosseous cervical vessels.

Retinacular vessel is the major source of blood supply to head of femur. If it is damaged in fracture neck femur, avascular necrosis of femoral head will develop. Artey of ligamentum teres supplies a small portion of head of femur. Intraosseous cervical vessels are also damaged in fracture neck femur. Intracapsular area of neck of femur heals only by endosteal callus because cambium layer is not found in this area. Periosteal callus is not formed. Synovial fluid dissolves blood clot at fracture site, so delaying fracture healing.

Calcar femorale is another important anatomical landmark as far as surgical treatment of fracture neck femur is concern. This is a thick dense vertical plate of bone that extends from posteromedial part of shaft femur under lesser trochanter to greater trochanter. Calcar femorale strengthen the femoral neck posteromedially. This is thickest on medial side.

Mechanism of Injury

Most of the fractures neck femur are caused by trivial trauma. According to Kocher, two mechanisms of injuries are responsible for fracture neck femur.

1. Direct blow over greater trochanter can occur if patient fell down due to a trivial trauma.
2. Lateral rotation of extremity.

Aetiology

This is commonly seen in older patients who have marked osteoporosis or osteomalacia.

CLASSIFICATION

Fracture neck femur has been classified under three categories as follows:

1. Anatomical classification
2. Classification based on direction of angle
3. Classification based on displacement of fractured fragment

Anatomical Classification

Subcapital

Fracture occurs just beneath the articular surface of femoral head. [See Fig. 16.2 (*b*)]

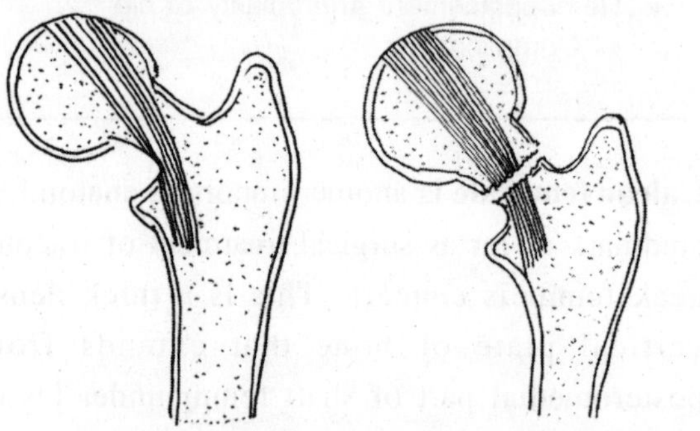

(*a*) Trabecular pattern deformed but not broken (*b*) Broken trabecular pattern without displacement

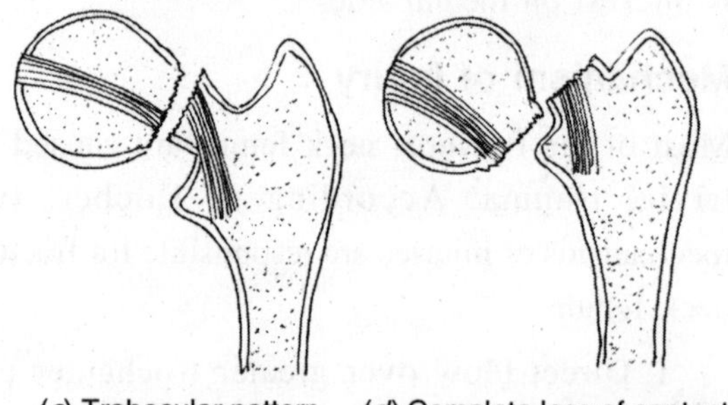

(*c*) Trabecular pattern is malaligned (*d*) Complete loss of contact between trabecular pattern at head neck

Fig. 16.1 Trabecular pattern of bone, during fracture neck femur

Transcervical

Fracture line passes through femoral neck. [See Fig. 16.2 (*c*)]

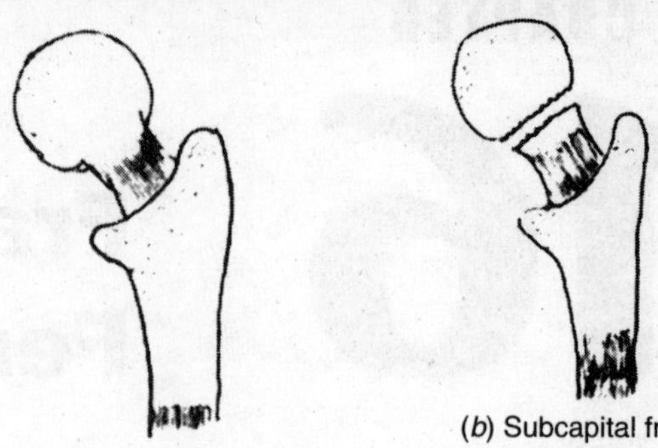

(*a*) (*b*) Subcapital fracture neck femur

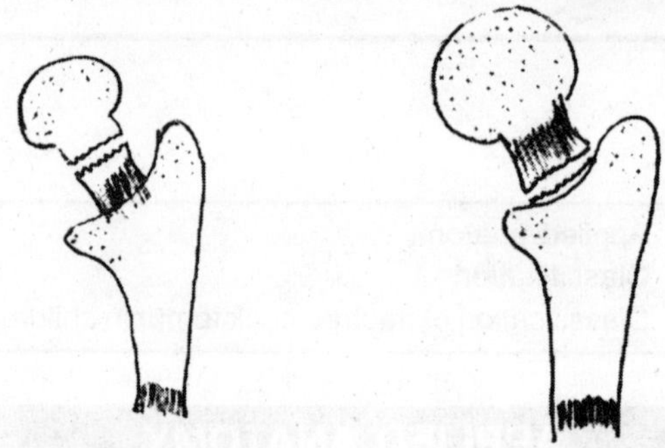

(*c*) Transcervical fracture neck femur (*d*) Basal fracture of neck femur

Fig. 16.2 Anatomical classification of fracture neck femur

Basal

Fracture line is present at the base of neck. [See Fig. 16.2 (*d*)]

Classification Based on Fracture Angle

Pauwel's Angle

Angle is formed by fracture line with respect to horizontal line.

Type 1: 30 degree [See Fig. 16.3 (*a*)]

Type 2: 50 degree [See Fig. 16.3 (*b*)]

Type 3: 70 degree [See Fig. 16.3 (*c*)]

Type 3 is most unstable fracture.

Perlington's classification

Angle is formed by a fracture line with respect to vertical plane. It is of three types as follows:

Type 1: 70 degree

Type 2: 50 degree

Type 3: 30 degree

Garden Classification

This is based on displacement of fracture. It is of four types as follows:

Type 1: Incomplete fracture

Type 2: Complete fracture, undisplaced

Type 3: Complete fracture, partially displaced

Type 4: Complete fracture with total displacement

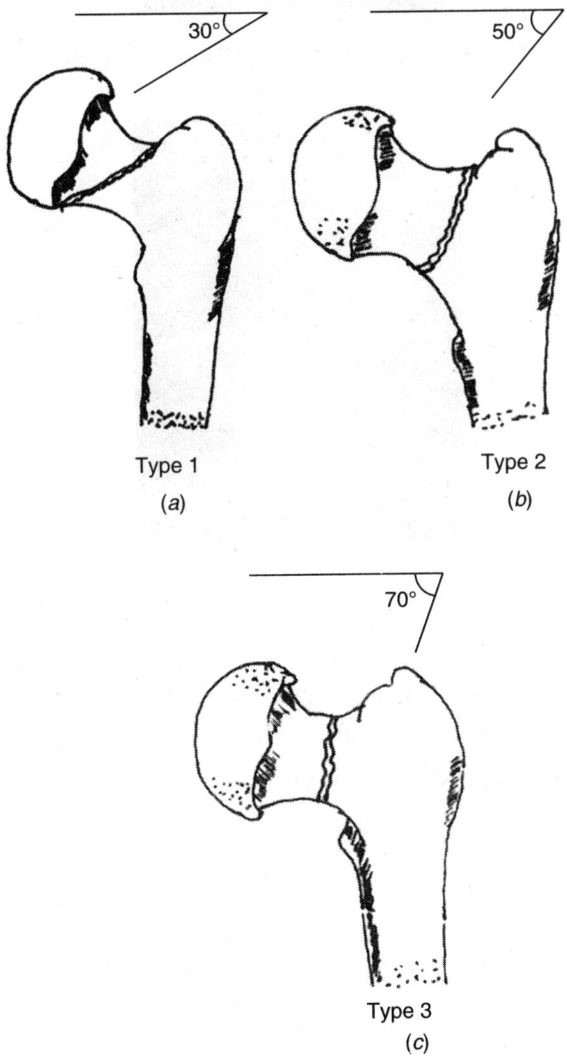

Fig. 16.3 Pauwel's angle

CLASSIFICATION OF FRACTURE; NECK FEMUR IN CHILDREN

Delbet has classified this fracture into five types as follows:

Peritrochanteric

Fracture line is present at trochanteric area.

Intertrochanteric

Fracture line is present in between greater and lesser trochanter.

Cervicotrochanteric

Fracture line is present in between neck and shaft.

Transcervical

Fracture line runs across the femoral neck.

Transepiphyseal

Fracture line is in between head and neck.

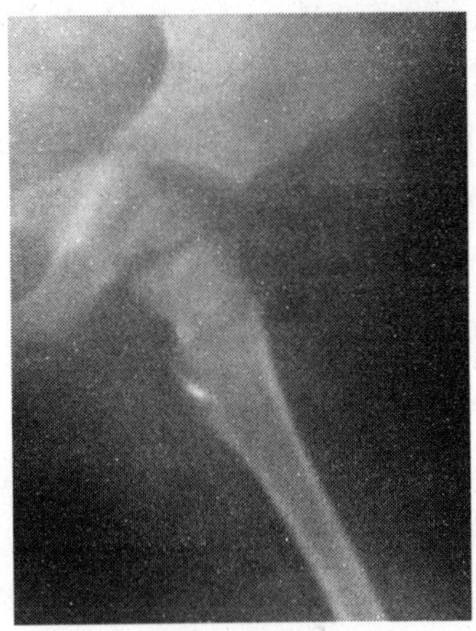

Fig. 16.4 Fracture neck femur in children (lateral view)

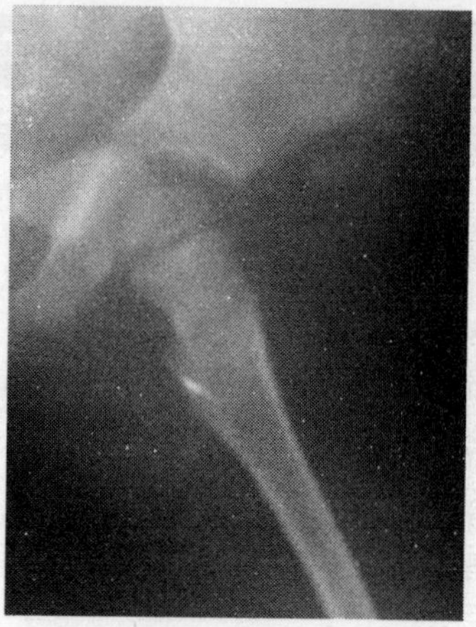

Fig. 16.5 Fracture neck femur in children (A.P. view)

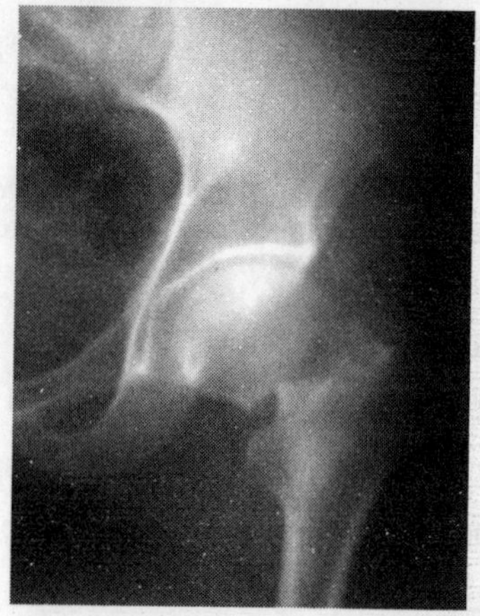

Fig. 16.6 Fracture neck femur (basal type)

Clinical Features

This fracture is most common in old age and very commonly kept in examination. This fracture has following clinical features:

1. History of fall on ground due to trivial trauma is usual presentation.
2. Pain and tenderness at the scarpa's triangle
3. Limb is externally rotated.
4. Minimal shortening of limb is present.
5. Movements at hip are restricted.

X-ray Findings

Fracture neck femur has following classical radiological features:

1. Breech in lamellar pattern of cortex of neck femur.
2. Shenton line is broken.
3. Greater trochanter is shifted upward
4. Lesser trochanter becomes more prominent.
5. ASIS is shifted upward on same side.

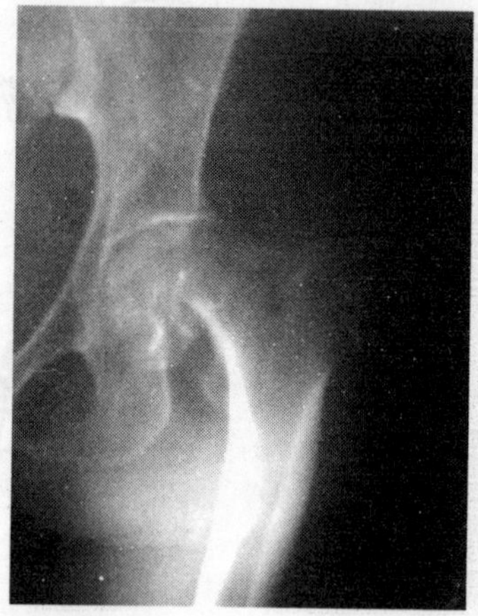

Fig. 16.7 Fracture neck femur (capital type)

Treatment

Treatment of fracture neck femur is decided on the basis of age of patient and duration of fracture.

CHILDREN < 16 YEARS

< 3 weeks old fracture

Undisplaced fracture can be treated by internal fixation by Austin moore pins or POP hip spica.

Displaced fracture can be treated by closed reduction and internal fixation by Austin moore pins.

> 3 weeks old fracture

This can be treated by McMurray's osteotomy. In this method osteotomy is done at the intertrochanteric region directed upward and medially, starting at the base of greater trochanter and finishing just above the lesser trochanter. This is a displacement abduction osteotomy. Advantage of this osteotomy is that it increases osteogenesis and blood supply at the local area. Most important advantage of this osteotomy is that it converts shearing forces into compressing forces.

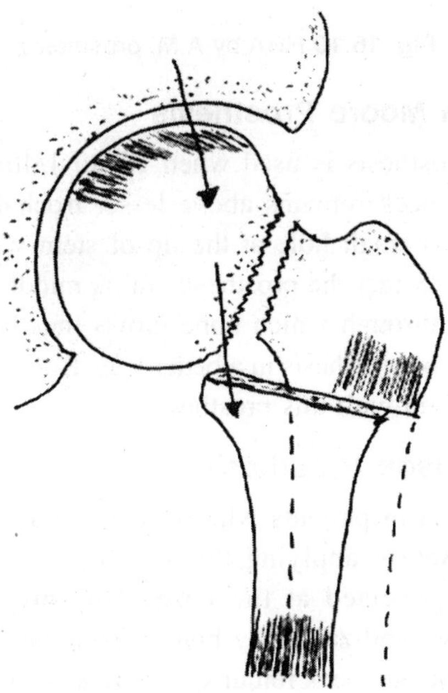

Fig. 16.8 McMurray's Osteotomy. Line of weight bearing (bypasses the fracture site) passes from head to distal fragment

YOUNG ADULTS 16–60 YEARS

< 3 weeks old

Undisplaced fracture can be fixed by **Cancellous screws**, SP nail, Dynamic hip screws, Knowle's pins, Canulated bolt or Asnis screw.

Displaced fracture can be treated by closed/open reduction and internal fixation by above mentioned methods.

> 3 weeks old

If neck is not absorbed it can be managed by internal fixation with bone graft like vascularised muscle pedicle graft. This graft is taken from quadratus femoris. This is known as **Meyer's procedure.**

If neck is absorbed, it can be managed by **McMurray's displacement osteotomy.**

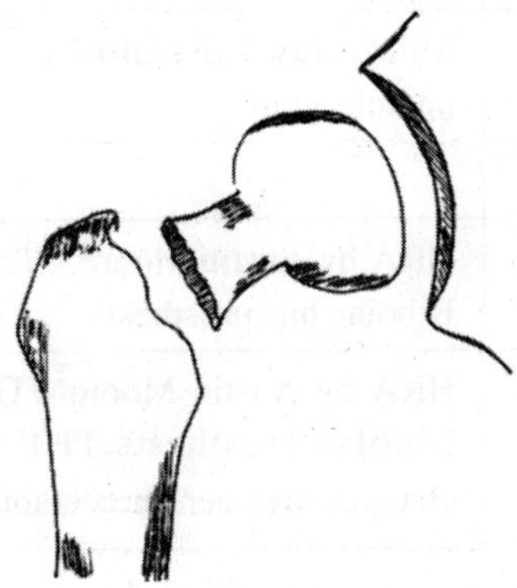

(*a*)

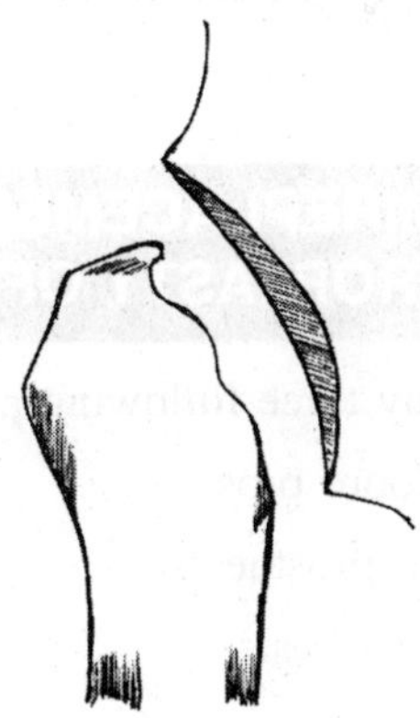

(*b*) Girdlestone arthroplasty of hip (Head and neck of femur are excised)

Fig. 16.9

ELDER PATIENT > 60 YEARS

< 3 weeks old

It can be treated by hemireplacement arthroplasty.

> 3 weeks old

It can also be managed by hemireplacement arthroplasty. If osteoartritic changes are seen in acetabulum, total hip replacement is the treatment of choice.

< 16 years	
< 3 weeks	CR and IF by A.M. pins
> 3 weeks	McMurray's osteotomy
16–60 years	
< 3 weeks	IF by 3 cancellous screws
> 3 weeks	McMurray's osteotomy or Muscle pedicle graft
> 60 years	
< 3 weeks	HRA by Austin Moore's/Thompson / Bipolar hip prosthesis.
> 3 weeks	HRA by Austin Moore's/Thompson/ Bipolar prosthesis.THR (if O.A. changes are seen in acetabulum)

Now hemireplacement arthroplasty of hip has become treatment of choice, if patient is more than 50 years of age.

HEMIREPLACEMENT ARTHROPLASTY OF HIP

It can be done by three following prosthesis:

1. Austin Moore prosthesis
2. Thompson prosthesis
3. Bipolar prosthesis
4. Proxima hip (discussed in implants section)

Prosthesis should be inserted in such a way that the distance between superior aspect of lesser trochanter and acetabulum is anatomically restored.

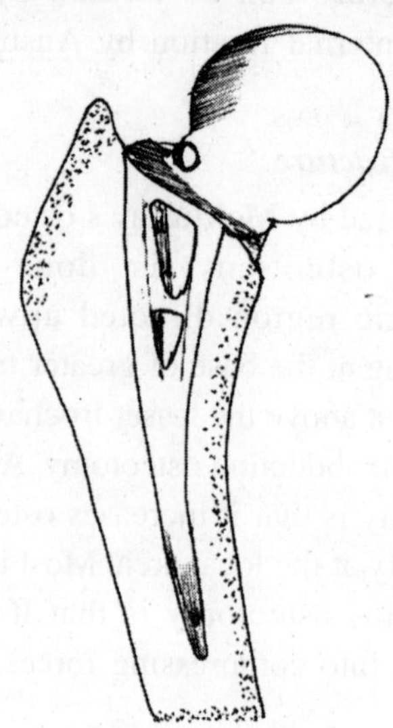

Fig. 16.10 HRA by A.M. prosthesis

Austin Moore Prosthesis

This prosthesis is used when 1/2 to 1/4th of an inch of neck remains above lesser trochanter. It has got a small hole at the tip of stem which is used to extract the prosthesis. In its middle it has 2 holes through which bone grows thus helps in fixation of prosthesis in a better way. Bone cement is not used with this prosthesis

Thompson Prosthesis

It is used in patients who have limited femoral neck. Before applying this prosthesis, femoral neck is excised at the base. This prosthesis requires stabilization by bone cement. It is used in old fracture neck femur where neck is absorbed.

Bipolar Prosthesis

This is indicated when chances of acetabular erosion and protrusion are high (by a prosthesis). Advantage of bipolar prosthesis is that this can be easily converted into total hip arthroplasty.

COMPLICATIONS

Fracture neck femur has risk of developing certain complications as follows:

1. Most common complication is nonunion.
2. Avascular necrosis of head femur
3. Limb shortening
4. Osteoarthritis

Nonunion

Cause of nonunion is inadequate immobilization and poor blood supply to head of femur. Patient comes with complaints of pain and inability to bear weight on affected limb. Telescopy test and Trendlenberg test become positive. Absence of cambium layer in periosteum of femoral neck makes it prone to undergo nonunion.

Following three factors should be decided to treat nonunion:

a. Viability of head
b. Degree of absorption of neck
c. Degree of osteoporosis

If patient has viable femoral head and adequate neck, it can be treated by McMurray's or Dickson's geometric osteotomy in young adults. Elderly patients of more than 60 years of age can be treated by replacement arthroplasty. Other methods of treatment of nonunion are as follows:

1. Muscle pedicle bone grafting
2. Cortical bone grafting
3. Cancellous bone grafting
4. Osteotomy with bone grafting.

Avascular Necrosis of Femoral Head

It is caused by disruption of retinacular vessels and vessels within the femoral neck in widely displaced fractures.

Young patient can be treated by Meyer's procedure, bipolar arthroplasty or arthrodesis of hip. Replacement arthroplasty is reserved for older patients.

Avascular Necrosis of Femoral Head in Children

This is most common complication after fracture neck femur in children. Avascular necrosis depends on following three factors:

1. Initial displacement of fracture.
2. Compromise of blood supply at the time of fracture.
3. Type of treatment. Single attempt of closed reduction does not affect rate of avascular necrosis.

Types of avascular necrosis in children

Type 1: This shows complete collapse of femoral head. Diffuse increased density is seen in whole of head.

Type 2: This shows minimum collapse of femoral head. Increased density is confined to a part of epiphysis.

Type 3: Femoral head is spared in this type. Increased sclerosis is seen in femoral neck from fracture line to physis. [See Fig. 4.11 (*a*), (*b*) (*c*)]

Osteoarthritis

Cause of arthritis is either faulty union or avascularity of femoral head. It can be managed by osteotomy in young patients or by THR in older patients.

Limb Shortening

Limb becomes short due to absorption of neck and mismatch of size of prosthesis.

CHAPTER

17 Trochanteric Fractures

- Fracture of intertrochanteric femur
- Fracture subtrochanteric femur
- Fracture of greater trochanter
- Isolated avulsion fracture of lesser trochanter

FRACTURE OF INTERTROCHANTERIC FEMUR

Applied Anatomy

Intertrochanteric fracture is purely extracapsular in nature. This fracture occurs through the cancellous bone, which has rich blood supply. That is why this fracture heals well. Neck shaft angle is crucial in planning of open reduction and internal fixation of fracture. Normal neck shaft angle is 135 degree which decreases with age.

Mechanism of Injury

This fracture is caused by a fall or impaction of direct or indirect forces.

Boyd's Classification

Boyd has classified this fracture in four types as follows:

Type 1: Undisplaced and stable fracture.

Type 2: Stable, displaced with minimum comminution.

Type 3: Unstable with large posteromedial comminuted area.

Type 4: Intertrochanteric fracture has subtrochanteric component.

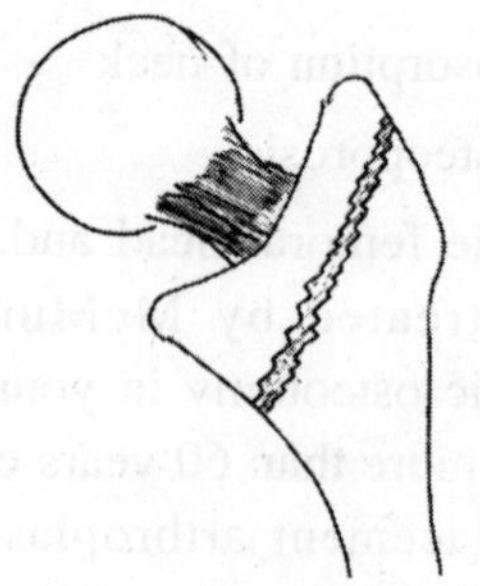

Fracture intertrochanteric femur
Type I : Undisplaced and stable

Fig. 17.1 (*a*)

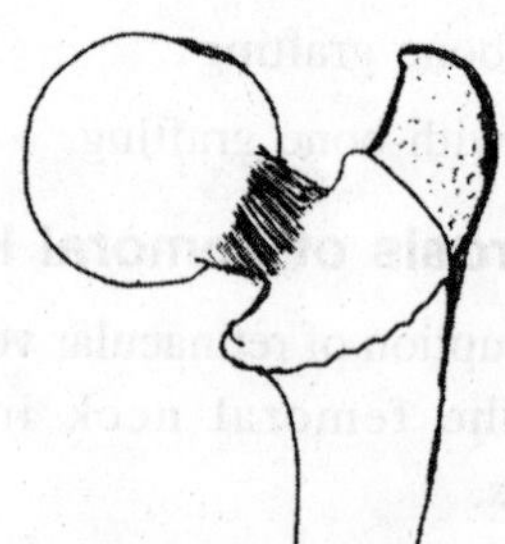

Type II : Stable and displaced intertrochanteric fracture femur

Fig. 17.1 (*b*)

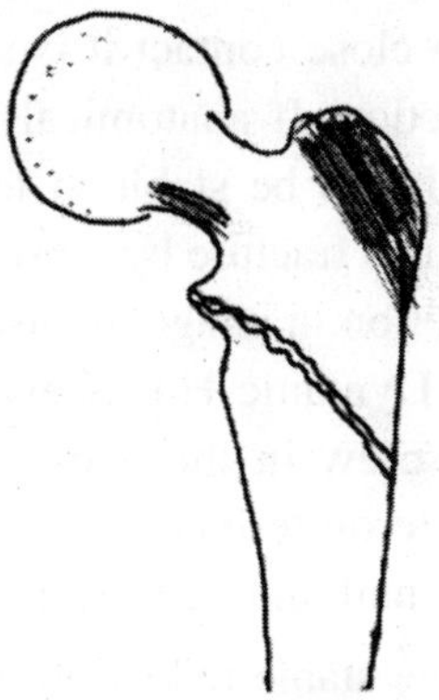

Type III : Posteromedial comminuted area (unstable)

Fig. 17.1 (*c*)

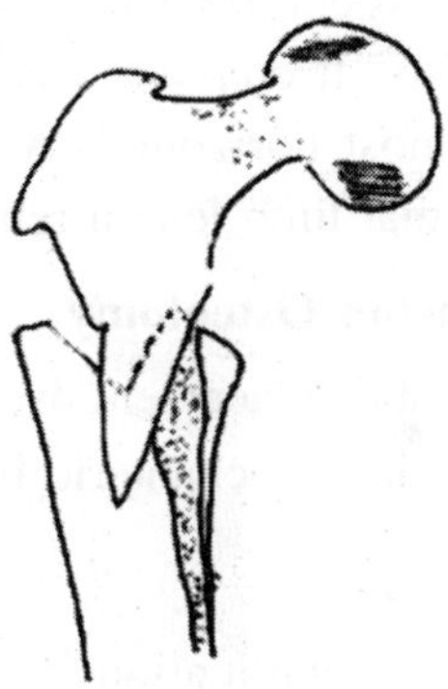

Type IV : Intertrochanteric fracture with subtrochanteric extension

Fig. 17.1 (*d*)

Clinical Features

Patient of intertrochanteric fracture can be diagnosed by following clinical features:

1. Pain, swelling and echymosis at greater trochanter.
2. Marked shortening of lower limb.
3. Limb is in complete external rotation.
4. Anteroposterior tenderness is present at greater trochanter.
5. Greater trochanter is markedly broadened.
6. Marked tenderness is present at trochanteric area.

X-ray Findings

Fracture line is seen in between greater and lesser trochanter. A.P. view of hip in internal rotation can show fracture obliquity and quality of bone. Stability of fracture can be determined in lateral view of hip.

Stable fracture is that in which medial cortices of proximal and distal fragment are not comminuted. Along with this; it does not have displaced fracture of lesser trochanter.

Unstable fracture is reverse of stable type. It has reverse obliquity of fracture. In this type, adductor muscles try to displace the shaft medially.

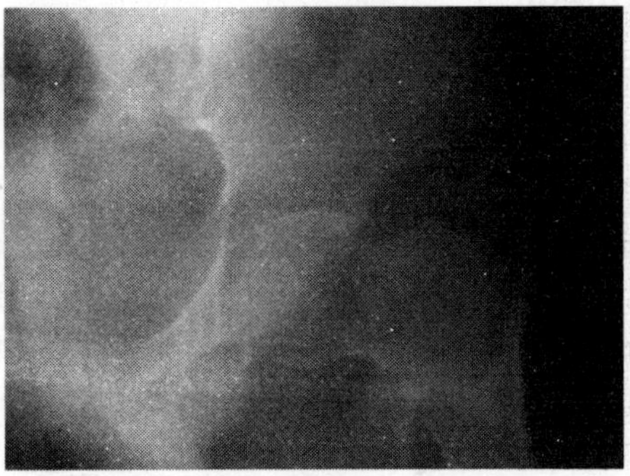

Fig. 17.2 Fracture intertrochanteric femur

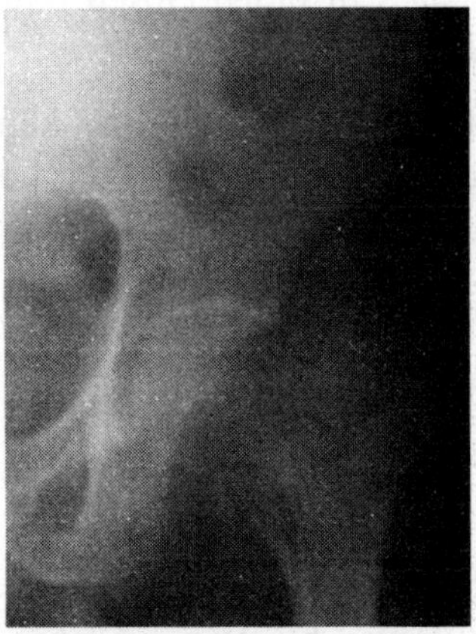

Fig. 17.3 Fracture intertrochanteric femur

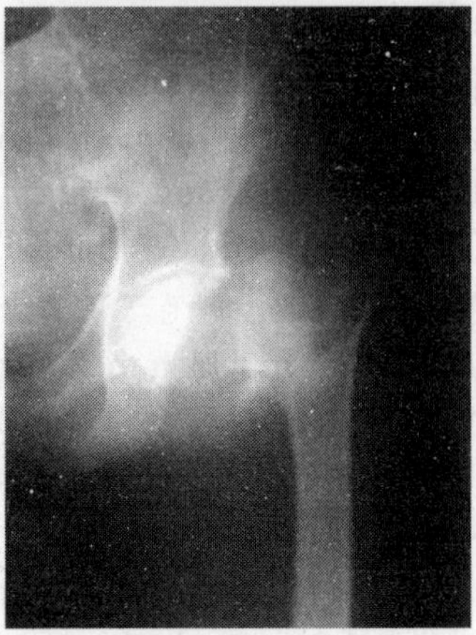

Fig. 17.4 Fracture intertrochanteric femur

Treatment

This fracture can be managed by closed reduction as well as by open reduction.

Closed Reduction

Traction is applied along the axis of femur. Counter traction is applied at pelvis. Now thigh is abducted and externally rotated. Reduced fracture is immobilized in Thomas knee splint, which can be incorporated with POP bandage, known as Tobreak application.

Open Reduction

This is indicated in failed closed reduction and unstable fractures.

Following five factors should be kept in mind before surgeries:

1. Bone quality
2. Geometry of fragment
3. Reduction
4. Design of implant
5. Placement of implant

Aim of surgical treatment is to achieve stable reduction followed by its good fixation. When posteromedial cortices of proximal and distal fragment come into close contact it is said to be an anatomical reduction. If anatomical reduction is not achieved it should be stable at least. First we should try to reduce fracture by closed method then check the reduction in image intensifier, then we can fix it with Dynamic Hip Scews (DHS). Insertion of DHS screw in the neck should be either central or posteroinferior. This fracture can also be fixed by SP nail and Ender's nail.

Sometimes to achieve stable reduction osteotomy is required e.g., **Sarmiento Osteotomy** and **Dimon Hughston Osteotomy**.

Sarmiento Osteotomy

This is valgus osteotomy which is done to obtain cortical stability. It converts fracture plane from vertical to almost horizontal. Advantage of this osteotomy is that limb length remains equal.

Dimon Hughston Osteotomy

This is a medial displacement osteotomy which is done in 4 part intertrochanteric fracture.

Complications

Most common complication is malunion, other complications are limb shortening and osteoarthritis.

FRACTURE SUBTROCHANTERIC FEMUR

Fracture occurring between lesser trochanter and a point 5 cm distally is known as fracture subtrochanteric femur. This fracture is likely to undergo malunion or nonunion because cortical bone present at subtrochanteric area is less vascular and more comminuted. Large biomechanical stress also plays an important role in malunion and nonunion.

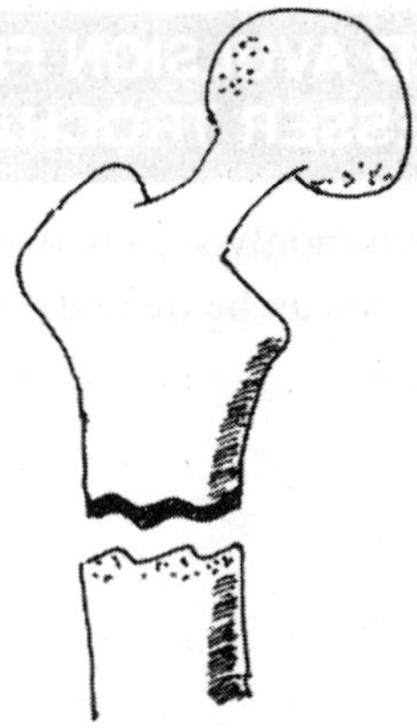

Fig. 17.5

Seinshemer's Classification

Seinshemer has classified this fracture into five types as follows:

Type 1: This is undisplaced fracture with < 2 mm displacement.

Type 2:

a. Two part transverse fracture

b. Two part spiral fracture with lesser trochanter attached to proximal fragment.

c. Two part spiral fracture with lesser trochanter attached to distal fragment.

Type 3:

a. Three part spiral fracture, lesser trochanter is a part of third fragment.

b. Three part spiral fracture with third part being a butterfly fragment.

Type 4: Comminuted four part fracture.

Type 5: Subtrochanteric fracture has intertrochanteric extension. (See Fig. 17.6)

Treatment

Conservative treatment is indicated in severely comminuted fractures in young patient in whom stable internal fixation cannot be done and in compound fractures.

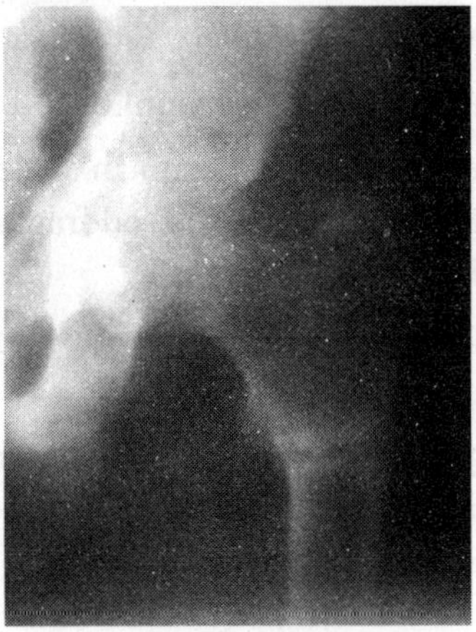

Fig. 17.6 Fracture subtrochanteric femur

Open reduction and internal fixation can be done by proximal femoral nail (PFN), long tail DHS, Ender's nail and external fixator.

Proximal Femoral Nail

This is an implant that is indicated in high subtrochanteric fracture femur and in pertrochanteric fracture. This is contraindicated in fracture shaft femur, gross abnormality of intramedullary canal and infection.

FRACTURE OF GREATER TROCHANTER

This uncommon fracture results in the form of isolated avulsion or comminuted fracture of greater trochanter. In children mechanism of injury is strong muscle contraction, while in adults it is caused by a direct blow to greater trochanter resulting into comminuted fracture.

Clinical Features

Patient presents with pain, swelling and echymosis at greater trochanter. Due to severe pain and spasm patient keeps his hip in flexed position. (Flexion deformity of hip)

Treatment

1. This fracture always unites.
2. Keep the affected limb in wide abduction to counteract the displaced fragment with its bed.
3. Full weight bearing is allowed after 4–6 weeks.
4. In young patients displacement of more than 1 cm can be fixed with 2 cancellous screws or by a wire loop.

ISOLATED AVULSION FRACTURE OF LESSER TROCHANTER

This is most commonly seen between 12–16 years age. This fracture can be treated conservatively by bed rest.

CHAPTER

18 Fracture Shaft Femur

- Fracture shaft femur
- Supracondylar and intercondylar fracture of femur

FRACTURE SHAFT FEMUR

Clinical Features

Patient presents with pain, swelling, deformity and inability to use affected limb. It is associated with history of severe trauma. Examination findings show bony tenderness, crepitus and bony abnormal mobility at the fracture site. Patient may also present with associated features of shock due to intramedullary bleeding.

X-ray Findings

Fracture line will be seen in shaft of femur according to anatomical or radiological type of fracture.

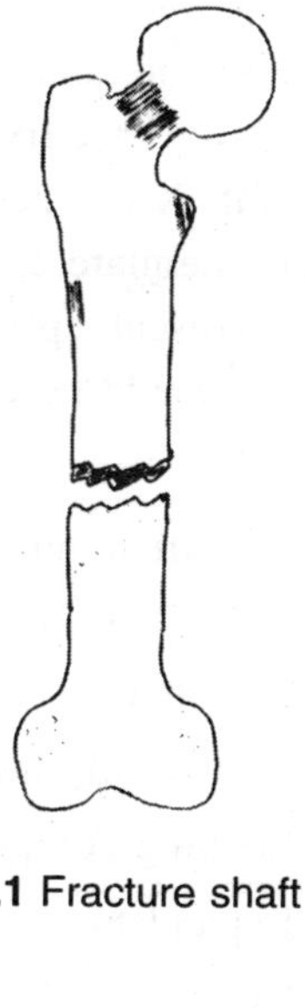

Fig. 18.1 Fracture shaft femur

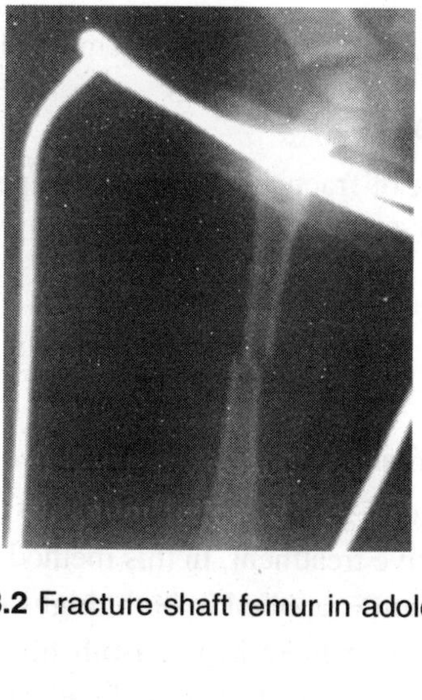

Fig. 18.2 Fracture shaft femur in adolescent

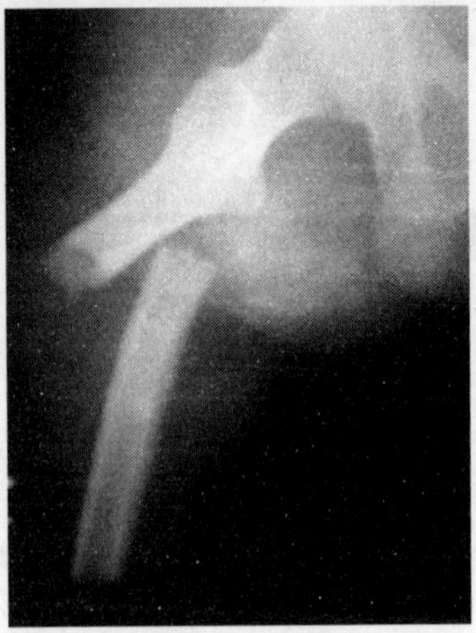

Fig. 18.3 Fracture shaft femur in adult

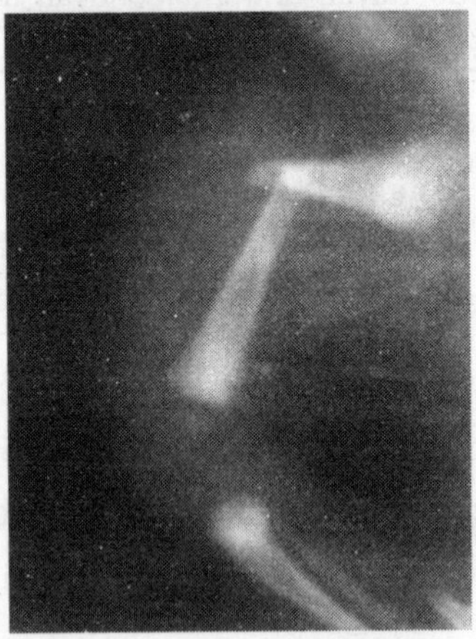

Fig. 18.4 Fracture shaft femur in infant

Treatment

Treatment of fracture shaft femur depends on age of patient as follows:

Neonate

Thigh to abdomen strapping is sufficient in this age group.

Upto 2 Years

In this age group Gallow's traction is best conservative treatment. In this method above knee skin traction is applied in both thighs and legs are tied to a over head beam. Both hips should be lifted above the bed to provide adequate counter traction. Fracture unites within 4–6 weeks.

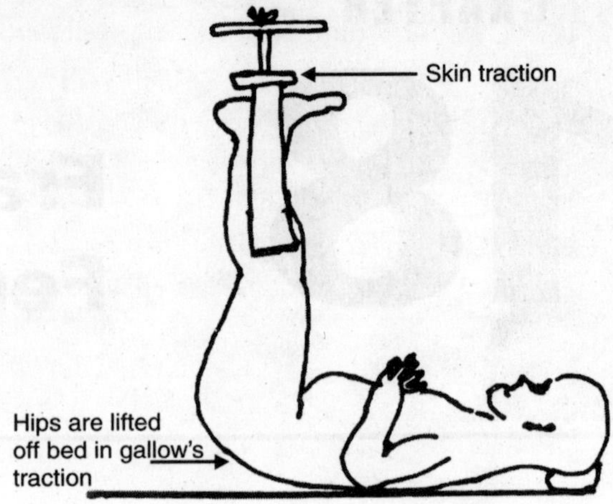

Fig. 18.5 Gallow's traction

2–6 Years

In this age group closed reduction is done which is maintained on POP hip spica.

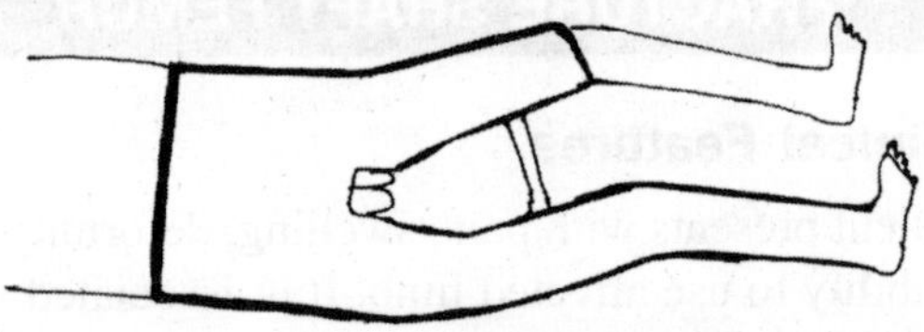

Fig. 18.6 1½ POP hip spica

6–16 Years

Closed reduction is done under anesthesia which is maintained by above knee fixed skin traction on Thomas knee splint. X-ray is repeated after 3-4 weeks to see the adequate callus formation. If adequate callus is present, splint can be removed and POP hip spica should be applied.

Adults

In adults fracture shaft femur can be treated by following surgical methods:

1. ORIF by KIM nail
2. CRIF by Interlocking nail
3. ORIF by Locking compression plate
4. ORIF by Expandable nail
5. ORIF by DCP.

ORIF by KIM nail: This is the treatment of choice. This is indicated in fracture mid shaft femur or fracture at the junction of upper and middle third of shaft femur. Fracture should be transverse or short oblique.

CRIF by Interlocking nail: This is done under image intensifier. First closed reduction is done then an interlocking nail is inserted into shaft of femur from the tip of greater trochanter till it reaches at the end of medullary canal. Now proximal and distal locking is done under image intensifier. This is indicated in fracture of distal third or proximal third of shaft femur.

CRIF by Expandable nail: This nail is also known as Israel nail. (discussed later). In this method, nail is inserted into medullary canal and later expanded by infusion of saline.

ORIF by DCP: This method is not performed in these days. This is done when other options are not available. This is done in comminuted fractures.

Acceptable Position in Fracture Shaft Femur

Age	*Birth–2 years*	*2–5 yrs*	*6–10 yrs*	*>10 yrs*
Varus/Valgus	30 deg	15 deg	10 deg	5 deg
Ant./Post.	30 deg	20 deg	15 deg	10 deg
Shortening	1.5 cm	2 cm	1.5 cm	1 cm

Complications

Early

1. Shock
2. Fat embolism
3. Neurovascular injuries.

Late

1. Delayed union
2. Malunion
3. Non union
4. Post traumatic stiff knee.

Shock

Fracture shaft femur can cause 1–1.5 liter of blood loss internally. It will present as hypovolemic shock.

Fat Embolism

Manifestation of fat embolism starts after 24–48 hours of trauma. Fat globules block the passage of small vessels of brain (cerebral type) or of lung (pulmonary type). Patient presents with tachypnoea, tachycardia, drowsiness, restlessness, petechial rash at lower conjuctiva, neck and at axillary fold. Patient may die due to respiratory failure.

Neurovascular Injuries

Sciatic nerve or femoral artery can be damaged due to penetration of sharp edge of bone.

SUPRACONDYLAR AND INTERCONDYLAR FRACTURE OF FEMUR

Fracture occurring between femoral condyles and metaphyseal junction with femoral shaft is known as supracondylar femur fracture.

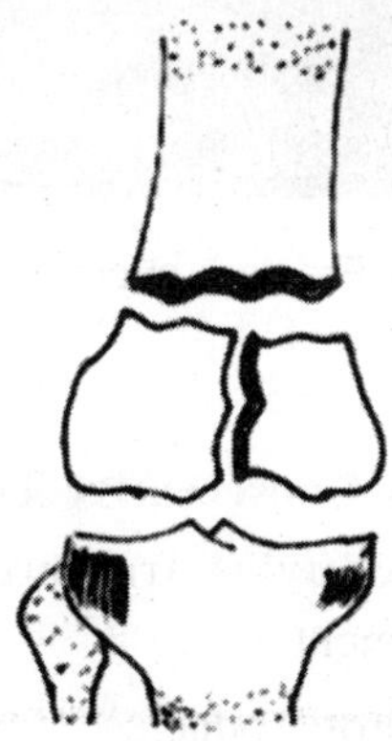

Fig. 18.7 T-shaped fracture intercondylar femur

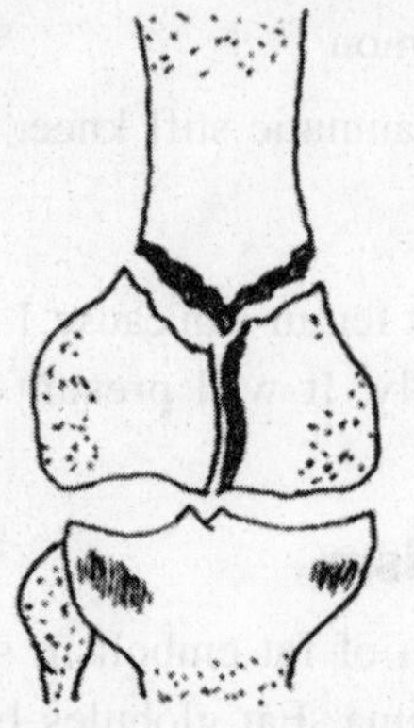

Fig. 18.8 Y-shaped fracture intercondylar femur

Mechanism of Injury

This fracture occurs due to axial loading with varus or valgus rotation force.

Clinical Features

Pain, swelling and deformity at supracondylar area are main clinical features. Bony tenderness and crepitus are present at fracture site.

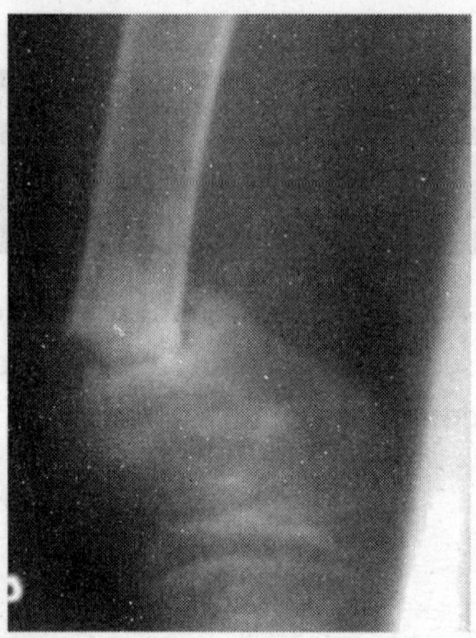

Fig. 18.9 Fracture supracondylar femur

Treatment

Indications of Conservative Treatment

1. Supracondylar fracture without joint involvement.
2. Osteoporotic bone
3. Undisplaced fracture
4. Associated illness (cardiopulmonary or neurological disease)
5. Contaminated compound fracture.

These fractures can be managed by upper tibial skeletal traction (30 pounds). Once the limb length and alignment is maintained, weight of traction can be reduced. In mediolateral (frontal) plane malalignment should not be more than 7 degree. In sagittal plane it should not exceed 7–10 degree. 1–1.5 cm of limb shortening can be accepted.

Surgical Treatment

ORIF can be done in displaced intraarticular and extraarticular fracture. ORIF can be done by following methods:

- Dynamic condylar screws
- 95 degree condylar blade plate
- Condylar buttress plate
- Reamed intramedullary nail
- Intramedullary supracondylar (IMSC) femoral nail
- Flexible and semirigid nail.

IMSC femoral nail is indicated for comminuted fracture extending up to articular margin. Nail is inserted in retrograde fashion from knee, through intercondylar notch thus stabilizing the fracture below isthmus. Nail is fixed with 2 proximal and 2 distal screws. This is contraindicated in active infection and where epiphyseal plates are open.

Complications

1. Post traumatic stiffness of knee
2. Inaccurate reduction
3. Infection
4. Post traumatic arthritis
5. Non union

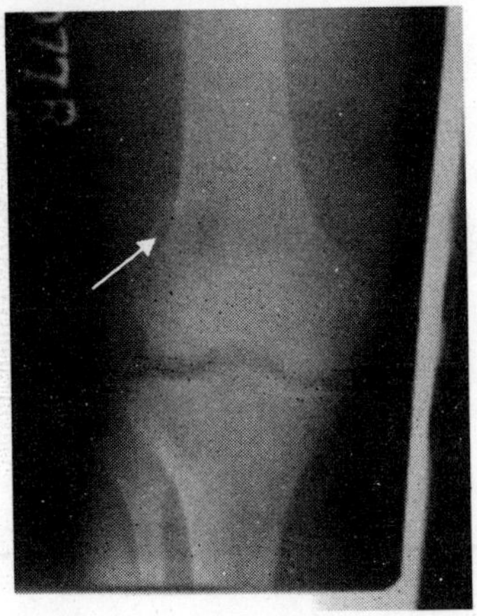

Fig. 18.10 (*a*) Fracture lateral condyle femur. AP view

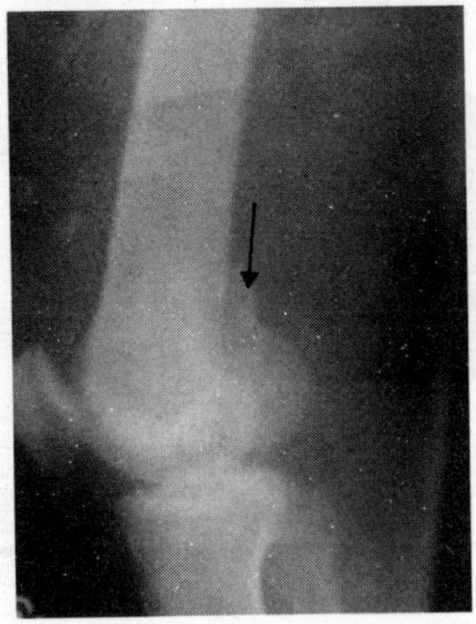

Fig. 18.10 (*b*) Fracture lateral condyle femur. Lateral view

CHAPTER

19 Injuries Around Knee

- Fracture of proximal tibia
- Fracture of patella
- Classification of knee ligament injuries
- Anterior cruciate ligament injury
- Arthroscopic reconstruction of ACL
- Posterior cruciate ligament injury
- Meniscus injury
- Other ligaments of knee
    - Collateral ligament injury
- Dislocation of knee

FRACTURE OF PROXIMAL TIBIA

This is also known as tibial plateau fracture. Lateral tibial plateau is more commonly fractured (60–70%) than medial plateau. Bicondylar fracture is seen in 15–25% cases. Lateral condyle fracture is also known as **Bumper fracture.**

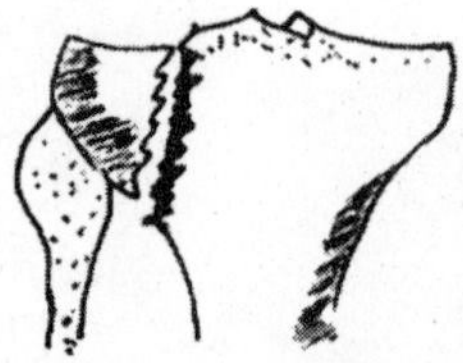

Fig. 19.1 Lateral tibial plateau fracture

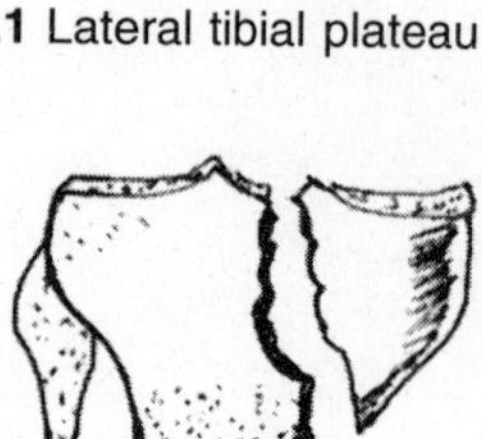

Fig. 19.2 Medial tibial plateau fracture

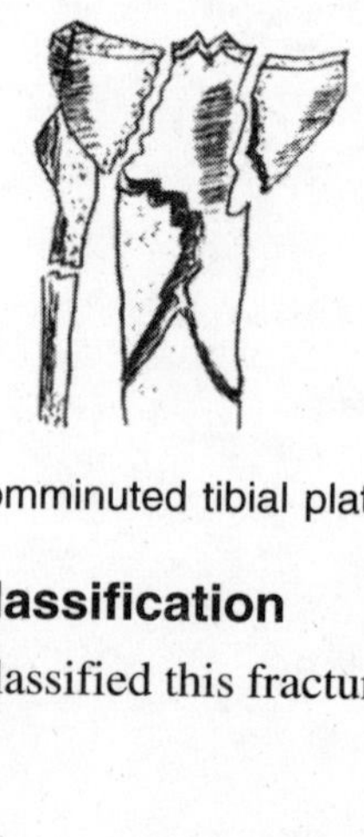

Fig. 19.3 Comminuted tibial plateau fracture

Schatzkar Classification

Schatzkar has classified this fracture into six types as follows:

Type 1:

1. Split fracture of lateral tibial plateau.
2. No articular depression.

Type 2:

1. Split fracture of lateral tibial plateau.
2. Articular area is depressed.

Type 3:

1. Isolated depression of lateral tibial plateau.
2. Joint becomes unstable.

Type 4:

1. Medial tibial plateau fracture.
2. It may be associated with cruciate and collateral ligament injury.

Type 5:

1. Bicondylar plateau fracture.
2. Articular area is depressed.
3. Condyles are displaced.

Type 6:

This is bicondylar tibial plateau fracture with diaphyseal and metaphyseal dissociation.

Mechanism of Injury

This type of fracture is caused by a valgus force.

Clinical Features

Patient may present with the following clinical features:

1. Pain, swelling and deformity at knee.
2. Bony tenderness and crepitus is present at upper end of tibia.
3. Associated ligament injuries will show corresponding sign.

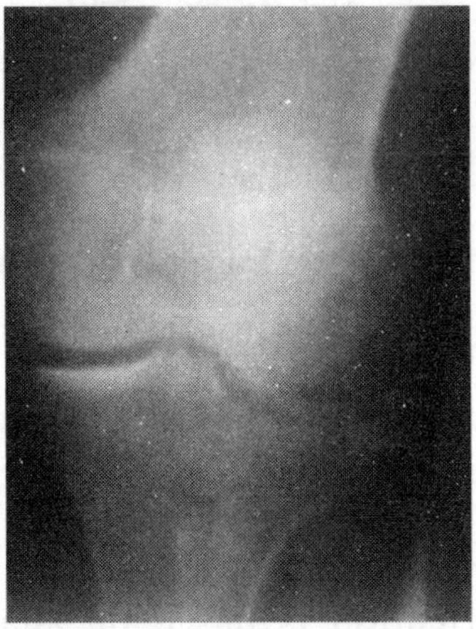

Fig. 19.4 Fracture proximal tibia (Type 2)

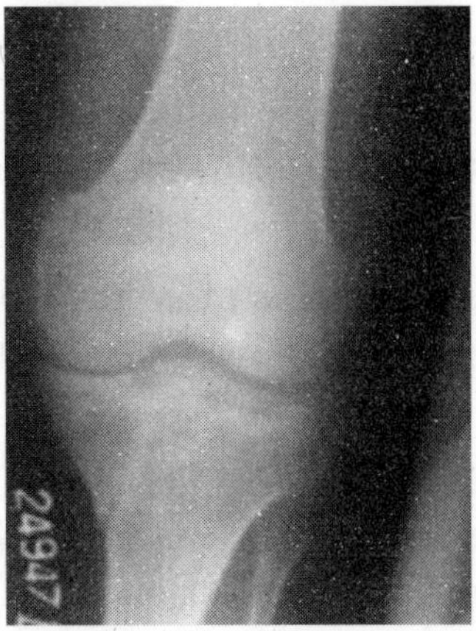

Fig. 19.5 Fracture proximal tibia (Type 4)

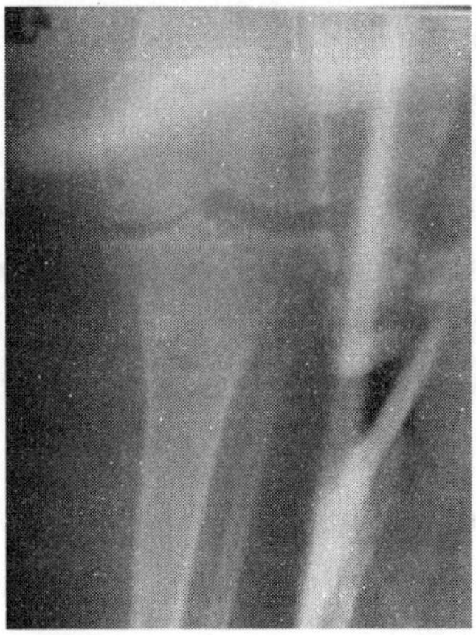

Fig. 19.6 Fracture proximal tibia (Type 6)

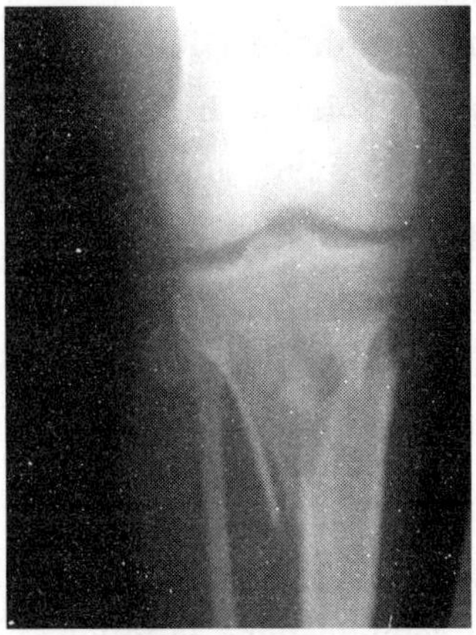

Fig. 19.7 Fracture upper end of tibia and neck of fibula

Treatment

Undisplaced fracture can be treated by AKPOP cast for 3-4 weeks, followed by early knee mobilization.

Displaced fracture can be treated by lower tibial skeletal traction followed by early knee mobilization.

Depressed fracture of lateral tibial plateau should undergo MRI-scan to see injury/compression of meniscus. If meniscus is compressed, fracture should be opened and meniscus should be repositioned, by lifting it with a suture. Depressed fracture should be lifted up, to make articular congruity of joint. Raw area (left beneath articular area) should be filled with bone graft in such a way that articular cartilage does not collapse. If meniscus is torn, it should be excised or repaired. Post operatively knee should be mobilized early, at 3-4 weeks. Full weight bearing can be allowed after 3 months.

Absolute indications of ORIF

1. Compound tibial plateau fracture.
2. Associated compartment syndrome or vascular injury.

Relative indications of ORIF

1. Unstable joint with lateral tibial plateau fracture.
2. Widely displaced medial tibial plateau fracture.
3. Widely displaced bicondylar tibial plateau fracture.

Complications

Fracture of proximal tibia has higher chances of developing complications as follows:

1. Stiff knee
2. Osteoarthritis of knee
3. Nonunion (rare)

FRACTURE OF PATELLA

Main function of patella is to improve leverage of quadriceps femoris muscle. It also protects femoral condyles from injury.

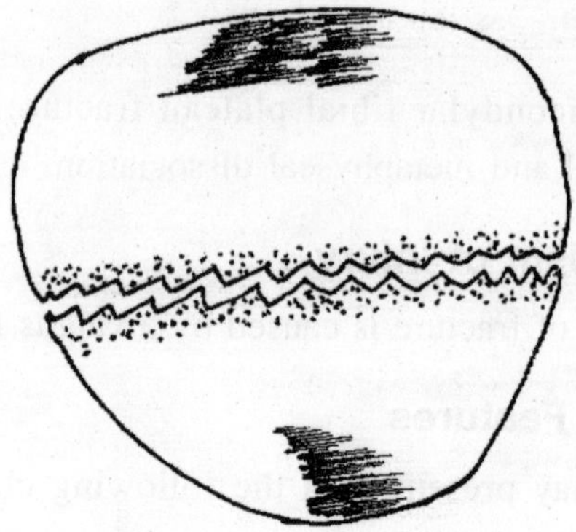

Fig. 19.8 Transverse fracture of patella

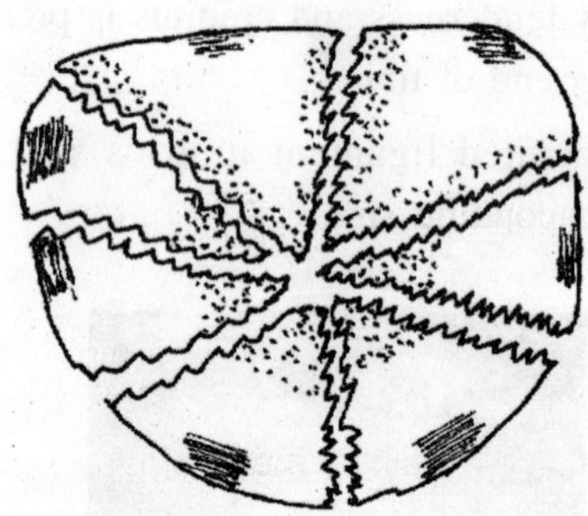

Fig. 19.9 Stellate fracture of patella

Mechanism of Injury

This is commonly caused by a dashboard injury or a direct fall over patella.

Radiological Classification

This classification is based on anatomical displacement of patella.

1. Undisplaced.
2. Displaced
   a. Transverse fracture (50–80%)
   b. Stellate fracture (30–35%)
   c. Comminuted fracture
   d. Proximal or distal pole fracture
   e. Osteochondral fracture
   f. Vertical fracture (12–17%).

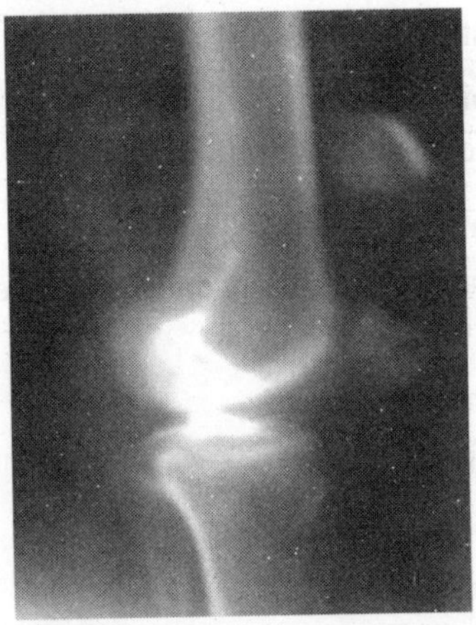

Fig. 19.10 Fracture patella (transverse type)

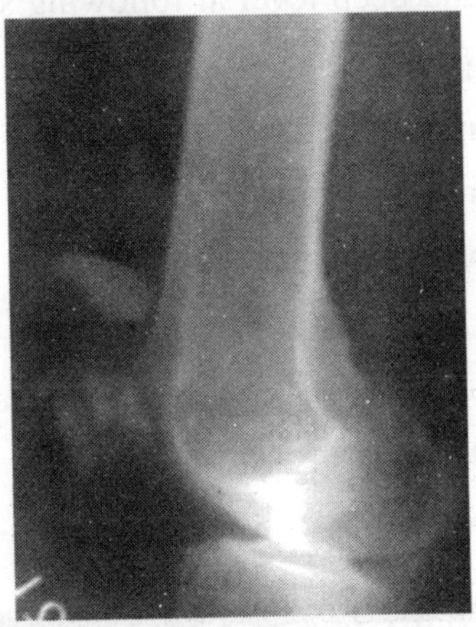

Fig. 19.11 Fracture patella (comminuted)

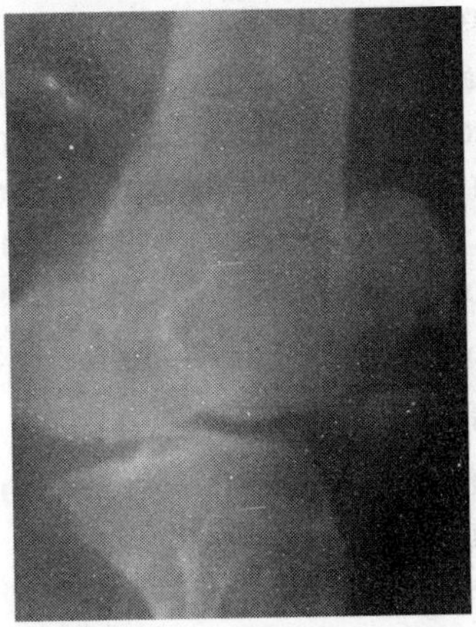

Fig. 19.12 Fracture patella (distal pole)

Clinical Features

Fracture patella can be diagnosed by following clinical features:

1. Pain and swelling (due to haemarthrosis) at knee joint.
2. Patient cannot extend knee.
3. Patellar gap and patellar tap are present.
4. Bony tenderness and crepitus is felt at fracture site.

X-ray Finding

X-ray can be taken in three views, A.P., Lateral and Skyline view. X-ray shows fracture line.

Treatment

Aspiration should be done if haemarthrosis is present. Undisplaced fractures can be managed conservatively by AKPOP cylinder cast. Quadriceps exercises are adviced to patient. Weight bearing can be allowed after 4–6 weeks.

Surgical Treatment

Surgical treatment is opted for displaced fracture with patellar gap more than 2-3 mm. Transverse fracture can be treated by **Tension band wiring** (TBW). It can also be fixed by circumferential wiring around patella, known as **Martin's wiring.**

Other methods of ORIF are as follows:

1. Modified TBW
2. Interfragmentary wiring **(Manuson's method)**
3. ORIF by Shaeuwacker method. In this method along with figure of eight wiring, interfragmentary screws are also fixed into patella.

Complications

Fracture of patella may develop following complications:

1. Post operative fracture dehiscence.
2. Infection
3. Avascular necrosis
4. Refracture.
5. Extensor lag (patient cannot perform terminal extension of leg).
6. Osteoarthritis of patellofemoral joint may develop later in life.

CLASSIFICATION OF KNEE LIGAMENT INJURIES

Injuries of knee ligaments have been classified on the basis of numbers of fibre torn and on the basis of their anatomy.

First degree sprain

Minimum fibres are torn. Localized tenderness is present. Joint is stable.

Second degree sprain

Significant numbers of ligament fibres are torn. Loss of function is seen but instability is not significant.

Third degree sprain

Complete disruption of ligament causes joint instability. Instability may present in one or more than one plane.

Anatomical Classification

ACL and PCL Injury

ACL and PCL can be injured at the following sites:

1. At femoral origin
2. Interstitial
3. At tibial insertion: with or without avulsion of intercondylar eminence.

LCL Injury

Lateral collateral ligament can be injured at the following sites:

1. At femoral origin
2. At middle portion
3. At fibular insertion.

MCL Injury

Medial collateral ligament can be injured at superficial and deep level at following sites:

Superficial:

1. At femoral origin
2. At middle portion
3. At tibial insertion.

Deep:

1. Meniscofemoral
2. Middle portion
3. Meniscotibial.

ANTERIOR CRUCIATE LIGAMENT INJURY

Applied Anatomy

Anterior cruciate ligament starts from anterior aspect of intercondylar notch of tibia and runs upward, backward and laterally and attaches to medial surface of lateral condyle of femur.

Posterior cruciate ligament starts from posterior aspect of intercondylar notch of tibia and runs upward, forward and medially and attaches to lateral surface of medial condyle of femur.

Anterior cruciate ligament becomes taut during extension while posterior cruciate ligament does so during flexion. Cruciate ligaments maintain anteroposterior stability of knee joint.

Anterior cruciate ligament is most commonly injured than any other ligament. Most common injury is hyperextension of knee with internal rotation of femur or external rotation of femur with abduction of flexed knee. Isolated injury of anterior cruciate ligament is uncommon. It may be associated with injury to medial or lateral collateral ligament. Avulsion fracture of tibial spine confirms injury to anterior cruciate ligament.

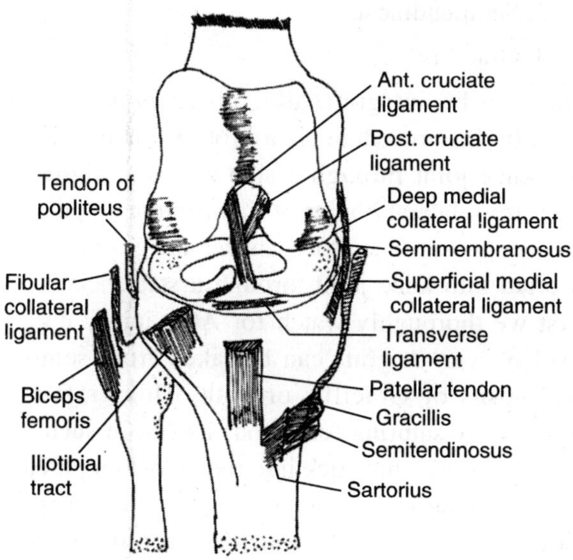

Fig. 19.13 Relationship of intercondylar structures

Clinical Features

Patient of ACL injury may present with the following clinical features:

1. Pain and swelling around knee joint.
2. This swelling is caused by haemarthrosis.
3. Tenderness is vague at knee joint.
4. Anterior Drawer test is positive.
5. Lachman test is positive.

Anterior Drawer Test

In this test patient lies supine on bed. Knee is kept in 90 degree flexion. Clinician sits on foot of patient. Now upper end of tibia is brought forward with both hands. Anterior translation of tibia between 5–10 mm confirms ACL ligament injury.

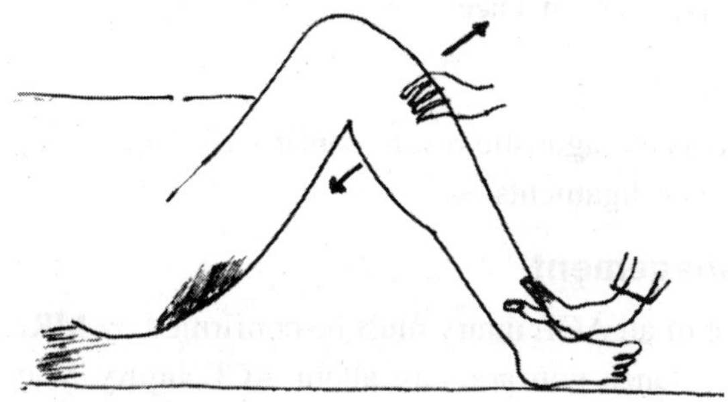

Fig. 19.14 Test for anterior and posterior cruciate ligaments injury

Lachman Test

This test is done in 20–30 degree flexed knee. It can also be done in effusion of knee. It is less painful.

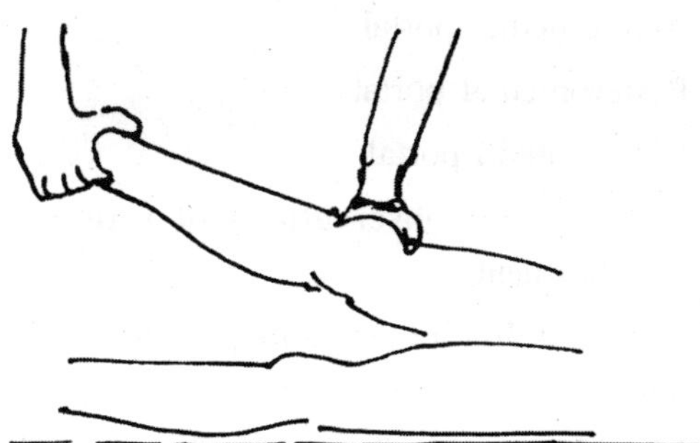

Fig. 19.15 Abduction and adduction test to check the integrity of cruciate ligament

This test has been graded into 3 types as follows:

Grade 1: If anterior translation of tibia is 0–5 mm it is called as Grade 1.

Grade 2: 5–10 Degree anterior translation is called Grade 2.

Grade 3: > 10 mm anterior translation is called Grade 3.

X-ray Findings

ACL tear is not visible in X-ray. Associated fractures may be visible in Tunnel's view and sunrise view of knee.

MRI

MRI is a diagnostic test to confirm the injuries of cruciate ligaments.

Management

First of all ACL injury must be confirmed by MRI scan. Once you are sure about ACL injury, you can go ahead with diagnostic/therapeutic arthroscopy of knee. Arthoscopy should be done 3-4 weeks after the injury.

Arthroscopy of Knee

Diagnostic arthroscopy of knee can be done through four standard portals as follows:

1. Anterolateral portal
2. Anteromedial portal
3. Posteromedial portal
4. Superolateral portal.

Arthroscopy needs observations of following seven compartments:

1. Suprapatellar pouch and patellofemoral joint
2. Medial compartment
3. Medial gutter
4. Lateral compartment
5. Lateral gutter
6. Poseromedial compartment
7. Intercondylar notch.

Complications of Arthroscopy

Arthroscopy of knee can develop following complications:

1. Haemarthrosis is commonest complication
2. Infection
3. Thromboembolism
4. Anaesthetic complication
5. Failure of instruments
6. Reflex sympathetic dystrophy
7. Injury to other ligament.

ARTHROSCOPIC RECONSTRUCTION OF ACL

Arthroscopic reconstruction of anterior cruciate ligament can be done by taking following graft:

1. Patellar tendon bone graft
2. Semitendinosus
3. Gracillis.

Graft can be autograft, allograft or an artificial graft. In this procedure an arthroscope is inserted into knee joint through a stab incision slightly away from lateral border of ligamentum patellae. On the opposite side probe, shaver and grasper are inserted into knee joint through a stab incision. First we thoroughly watch for ACL injury e.g., level of tear. A graft can be taken from semi-tendinosus or Gracillis or both. This graft is prepared by suturing (ethibond) its end in such a way that it does not stick into the tunnel prepared in lateral condyle of femur. Length of this graft should be 8–10 cm. A tunnel is made in lateral condyle of femur. Prepared graft is taken into this tunnel. Proximal end of suture of graft is pulled out through shaft of femur on lateral side. Now this end of graft is fixed with screw/endo button into tunnel made into medial surface of later-al condyle. Fixation of graft can be checked by pulling it's distal end.

Distal end of graft is fixed at upper end of tibia either by a screw or a metallic staple or button. Stability of knee is checked by anterior drawer test and Lachman test.

POSTERIOR CRUCIATE LIGAMENT INJURY

PCL injury is less common. Mechanism of injury may be a backward push on upper end of tibia or complete dislocation of knee or a severe rotational injury of knee. It is also associated with other ligamentous injuries.

Clinical Features

1. Pain and diffuse swelling (due to haemarthrosis) in knee.
2. Knee joint becomes tender.
3. Posterior drawer test is positive.

X-ray Finding

X-ray will not show any ligamentous injury.

MRI

MRI is a diagnostic tool to confirm ligamentous injury.

Treatment

It can also be repaired arthroscopically by using same graft which are used for ACL reconstruction.

Triad of Donoghue

This triad includes following three injuries:

1. Injury to medial structures
2. ACL injury
3. Medial meniscus injury.

Mechanism of injury in this triad is internal rotation with abduction of femur on flexed knee.

MENISCUS INJURY

Applied Anatomy

Meniscus is also called as Semilunar cartilage. Menisci are disc shaped and fibrocartilaginous in nature. Menisci are two in number; medial and lateral. Medial meniscus is semicircular while lateral meniscus is circular. These two menisci divide knee joint into upper and lower compartment. Upper compartment provides space for flexion and extension of knee while rotation takes place in lower compartment. Both the ends of menisci are attached to tibia. Thick and convex outer border of meniscus are vascular and fixed to fibrous capsule. Inner border of menisci are avascular, concave and thin. Tendon of popliteus and capsule separate the lateral meniscus from fibular collateral ligament. Medial meniscus is adherent to deep part of tibial collateral ligament at its peripheral margin.

Functions of Menisci

Menisci have a lot of functions to perform:

1. Menisci make the knee joint more congruent.
2. They act as a shock absorber for knee joint.
3. Menisci provide lubrication to joint.
4. Menisci also provide proprioceptive impulses.
5. They provide stability to joint.
6. Menisci also help in locking of knee joint.

Mechanism of Injury

Menisci are injured when femur rotates on partially flexed knee. (Twisting strain) Medial meniscus is more commonly injured than lateral, as previous one is fixed to tibial collateral ligament and is less mobile.

Classification

1. Bucket handle tear is commonest injury.
2. Longitudinal tear.
3. Radial tear.
4. Anterior horn tear.
5. Posterior horn tear.
6. Discoid meniscus.
7. Meniscal cyst.

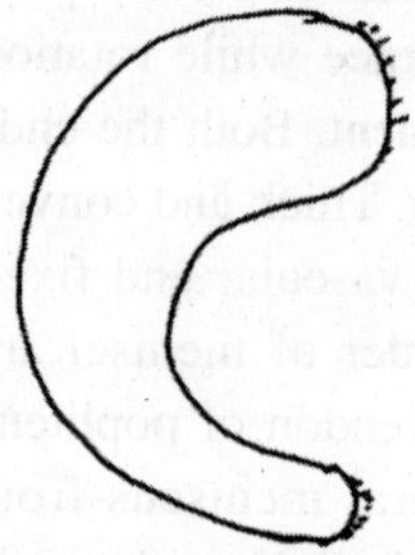

Fig. 19.16 Normal meniscus

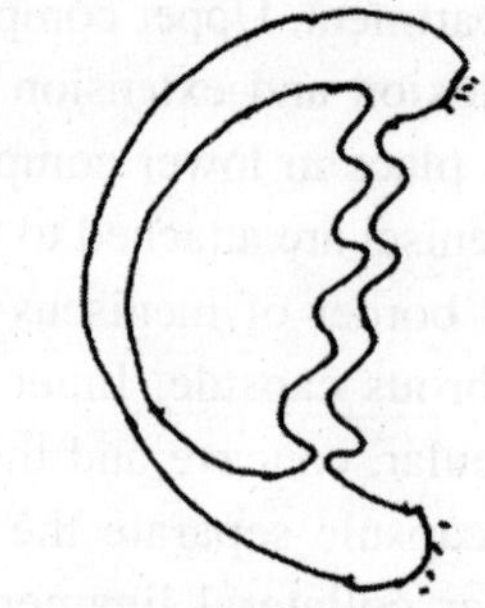

Fig. 19.17 Bucket-Handle tear

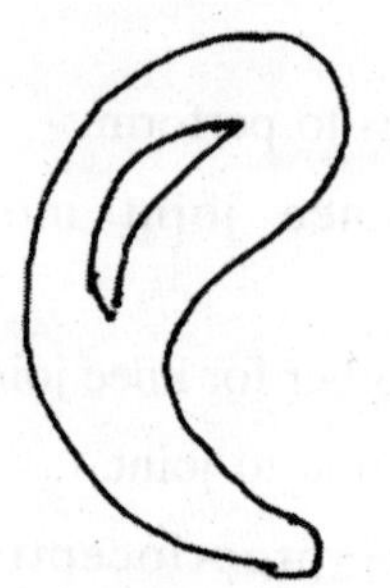

Fig. 19.18 Longitudinal tear

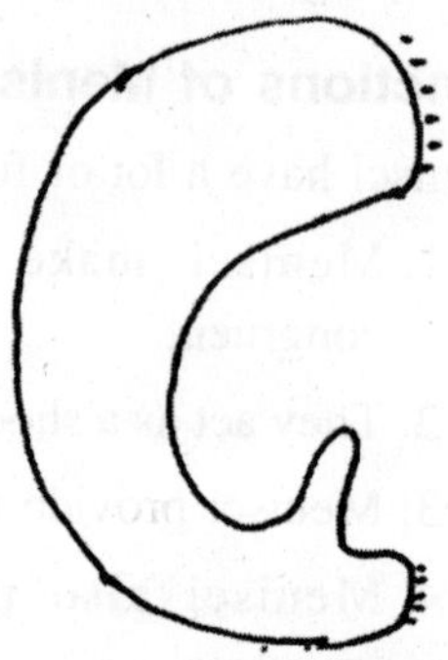

Fig. 19.19 Anterior horn tear

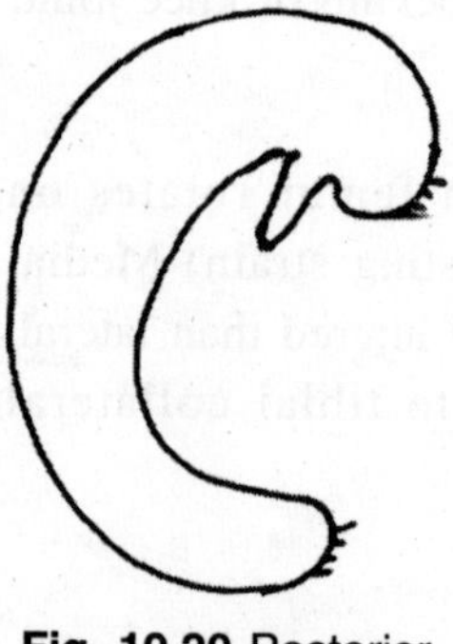

Fig. 19.20 Posterior horn tear

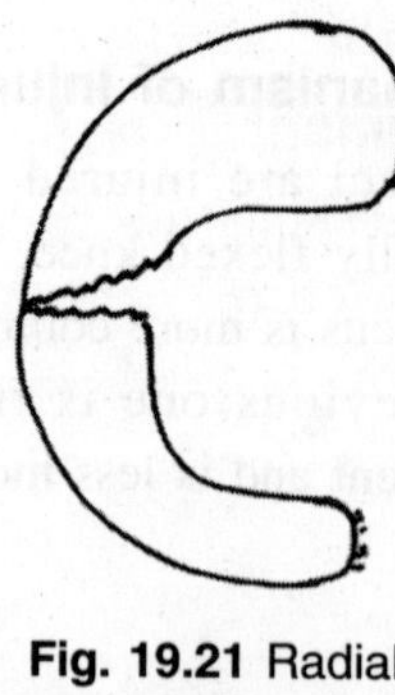

Fig. 19.21 Radial tear

Clinical Features

Meniscus injury has classical clinical features as follows:

1. Pain in affected knee
2. Swelling usually occurs 2 hours after injury
3. History of locking of knee is present. Locking occurs due to interposition of torn meniscus in between tibial and femoral condyle
4. Patient may also present with history of sudden unlocking
5. Medial joint line tenderness is present
6. **McMurray's test** is positive
7. **Apley's grinding test** is positive.

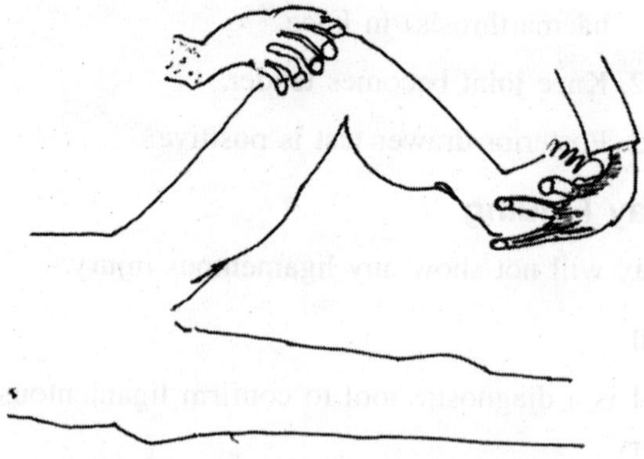

Fig. 19.22 Testing for meniscus injury

McMurray's test

In this test patient lies supine on a couch. Hip is flexed upto 90 degree. Now knee is flexed till heel touches thigh. Now limb is slowly extended by holding ankle in external rotation. Meanwhile valgus stress is given at knee during extension. Pain at medial aspect of knee during valgus stress indicates medial meniscus injury. This test can be repeated by holding ankle in internal rotation and giving varus stress at knee. If patient complaints of pain at lateral aspect of knee, it indicates lateral meniscus injury.

Apley's grinding test

This test is done in prone position. Examiner keeps his knee over patient's lower end of thigh. Knee is flexed up to 90 degree. Now distract leg upward and rotate it internally and externally. If patient has collateral ligamentous injury, he will complaint of pain at corresponding site. Now leg is pushed downward and same rotatory movements are repeated. If meniscus is injured patient will complaint of pain at corresponding site.

Investigations

MRI

MRI is most useful investigation to confirm meniscus injury.

Arthroscopy

This can be used for diagnostic as well therapeutic purpose.

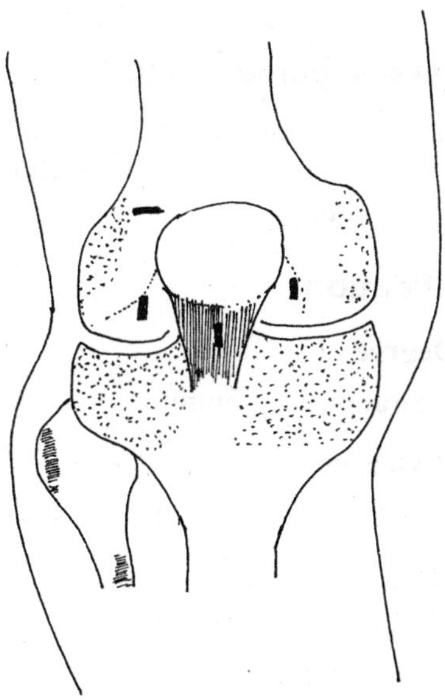

Fig. 19.23 Sites of arthroscopic incision

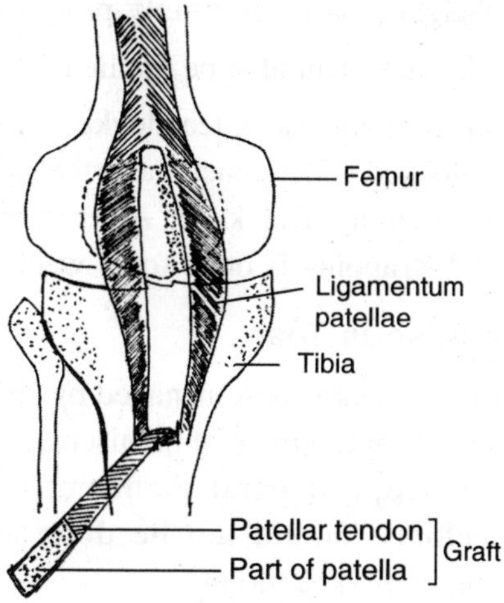

Fig. 19.24 Patellar tendon bone graft is taken for reconstruction of ACL

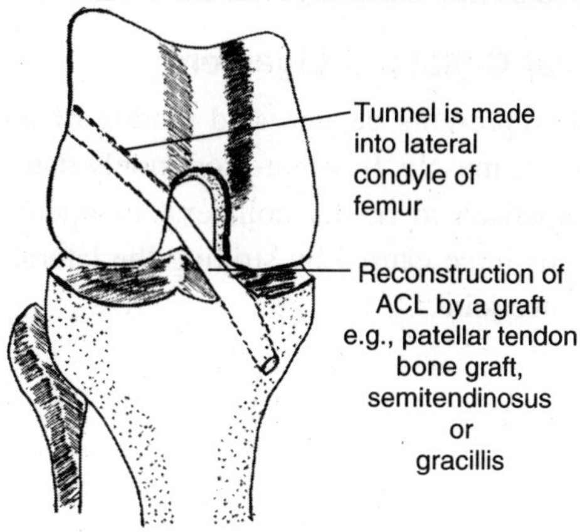

Fig. 19.25 Reconstruction of anterior cruciate ligament

Arthrography

In this method X-ray of knee is taken after injecting a radio opaque dye.

Treatment

1. Haemarthrosis should be aspirated and Roberts John strapping should be done.
2. AKPOP cylinder cast may be applied.

3. Weight bearing is strictly prohibited.
4. Ice packs can also be applied.
5. In fresh meniscus tear locked knee can be unlocked under general anesthesia by gentle manipulation of knee. After manipulation R-J strapping is done for 3 weeks.

Old Meniscus Tear

Old meniscus tear is best managed by arthroscopic removal of torn fragment of meniscus, also known as arthroscopic partial menisectomy. Total menisectomy should not be done as it may incapacitate the knee joint.

OTHER LIGAMENTS OF KNEE

Tibial Collateral Ligament

This represents degenerated tendon of adductor magnus muscle. It is more commonly damaged in comparison to fibular collateral ligament due to valgus force caused by striking the lateral aspect of knee joint.

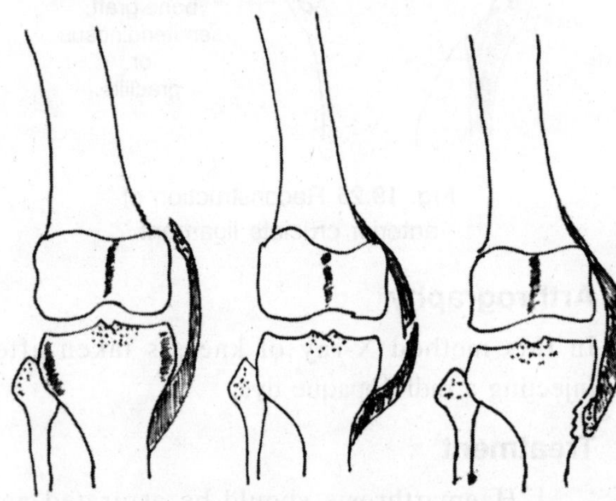

(*a*) Femoral origin (*b*) Middle portion (*c*) Tibial insertion

Fig. 19.26 Anatomical classification of medial collateral ligament injury

Fibular Collateral Ligament

This represents femoral attachment of peroneus longus.

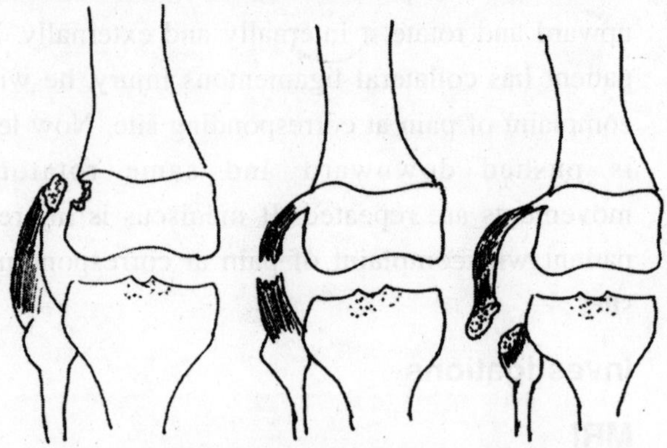

(*a*) Femoral origin (*b*) Middle portion (*c*) Fibular insertion

Fig. 19.27 Anatomical classification of lateral collateral ligament injury

Oblique Popliteal Ligament

This is an extended part of semimembranosus muscle.

Collateral Ligament Injury

This is more common in tibial collateral ligament due to valgus force caused by striking force to lateral part of knee.

Classification

First Degree

Joint separation is < 5mm

Second Degree

Joint separation is 5–10 mm.

Third Degree

Joint separation is >10 mm.

Clinical Features

Collateral ligament injuries may present with following clinical features:

1. This is commonly seen in football and rugby players.
2. Pain, swelling and haemarthrosis of knee is usual presentation.
3. Sometimes it is associated with ACL and medial meniscus injury which is known as Triad of Donoghue.
4. Tenderness is present at the insertion site of tibial collateral ligament.
5. Valgus stress test is positive.

Treatment

1. First and second degree of injury can be treated conservatively by analgesics and AKPOP slab for 6 weeks with knee in 30 degree of flexion.
2. Third degree tear should be repaired by surgery.
3. Old TCL and FCL should be transferred distally.
4. Old destroyed TCL can be reconstructed by semitendinosus or hamstring.
5. Old destroyed FCL can be reconstructed by fascia lata or biceps tendon.

DISLOCATION OF KNEE

Knee dislocations are usually seen in severe road traffic accidents. Most common type of dislocation is posterior one. Popliteal artery is most commonly injured in posterior dislocation. This is a dangerous injury and it should be managed immediately.

CHAPTER

20 Fracture Both Bones Leg

- Introduction
- Treatment
- Complications

INTRODUCTION

Tibia and fibula can be fractured by direct or indirect trauma.

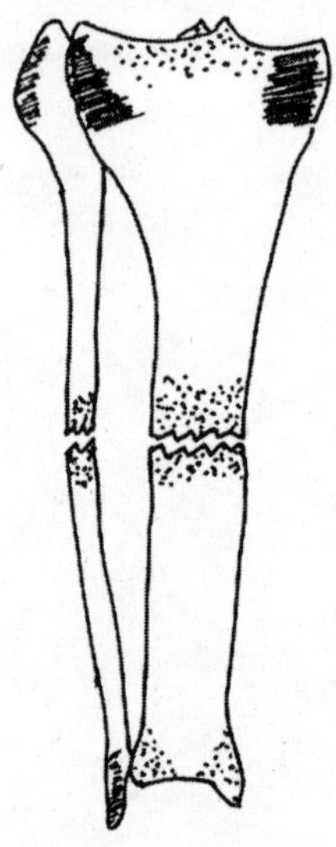

Fig. 20.1 (*a*) Fracture both bones leg

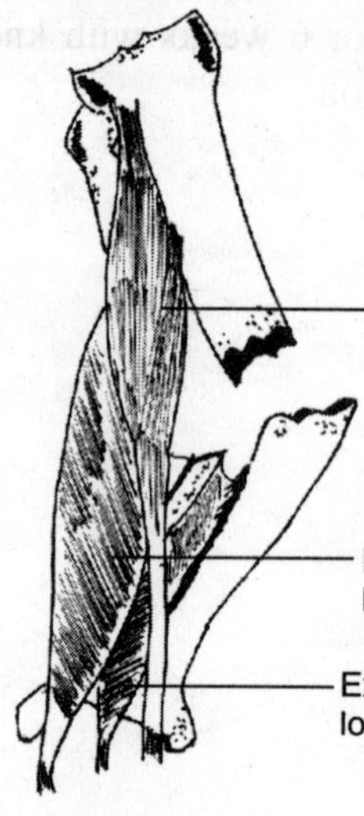

Fig. 20.1 (*b*) Fracture both bones leg

Clinical Features

1. Pain, swelling and deformity at the fracture site are usual presentation.
2. Bony tenderness, crepitus and abnormal mobility at the fracture site will be felt.

X-ray Findings

X-ray will show fracture at shaft of tibia and fibula.

Treatment

Children

Undisplaced fracture can be managed by AKPOP cast for 2-3 months. Displaced fracture can be managed by reduction setting followed by AKPOP cast for 2-3 months.

Adults

Displaced fracture can be managed by ORIF by DCP/Intramedullary V nail/Tibial interlocking nail/expandable nail.

Unstable fracture of shaft (e.g. spiral fracture or fracture of upper and lower end) tibia can be managed by closed reduction and internal fixation by tibial interlocking nail.

Wedging of cast

This procedure is required if angulation is seen in follow up X-ray of fracture of both bones leg. In this procedure plaster is cut circumferentially at the level of fracture. After correcting angulation, plaster is completed.

Complications

1. Delayed union
2. Nonunion
3. Malunion
4. Compartment syndrome
5. Injury to popliteal artery and common peroneal nerve (rare).

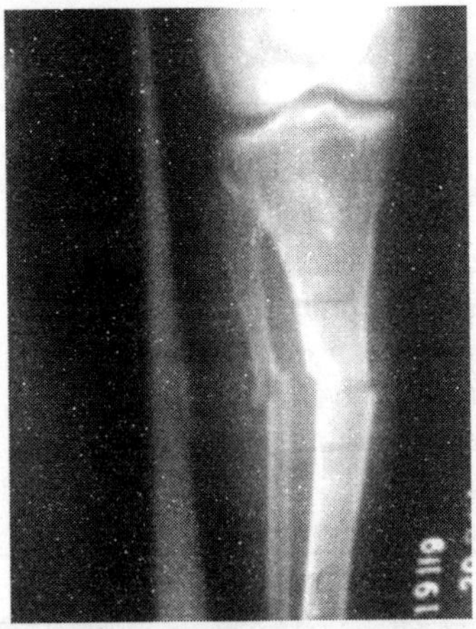

Fig. 20.2 Fracture both bones leg

CHAPTER

21 Injuries Around Ankle Joint

- Applied anatomy
- Lauge-Hansen classification
- Other classification of ankle injury
- Common fractures at ankle
- Pott's fracture
- Rupture of tendoachillis
- Ankle sprain
- Dislocation of ankle
- Fracture of calcaneum
- Fracture of talus
- Fracture of metatarsal

APPLIED ANATOMY

Ankle joint is formed by lower end of tibia, fibula and talus. Ankle joint is a synovial joint of hinge variety. This joint has main three ligaments as follows:

1. Deltoid Ligament
2. Lateral Ligament
3. Syndesmotic Ligament

Deltoid Ligament

This is also known as medial ligament of ankle. It has two parts Superficial and Deep.

Superficial part

This is further subdivided into three ligaments as follows:

a. Tibionavicular ligament (anterior fibres)
b. Tibiocalcaneal ligament (middle fibres)
c. Posterior tibiotalar ligament

Deep part

This is also known as anterior tibiotalar ligament.

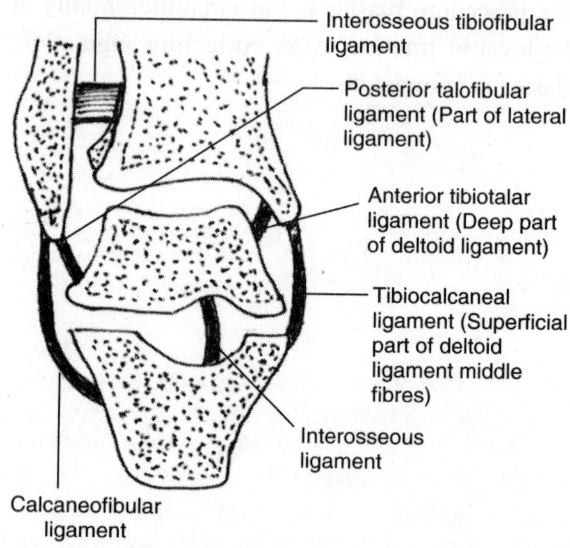

Fig. 21.1 Ankle joint (coronal section)

Lateral Ligament

This ligament is divided into three parts as follows:

a. Anterior talofibular (ATF) ligament (commonest to be injured)
b. Posterior talofibular (PTF) ligament
c. Calcaneofibular (CF) ligament

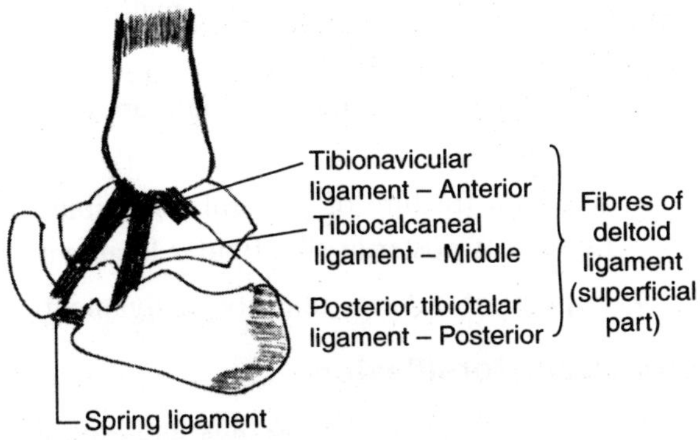

Fig. 21.2 Ankle joint showing parts of deltoid ligament [Medial collateral ligament (MCL)]. Medial collateral ligament injury can be diagnosed by doing eversion in neutral position of food. Patient feels severe pain.

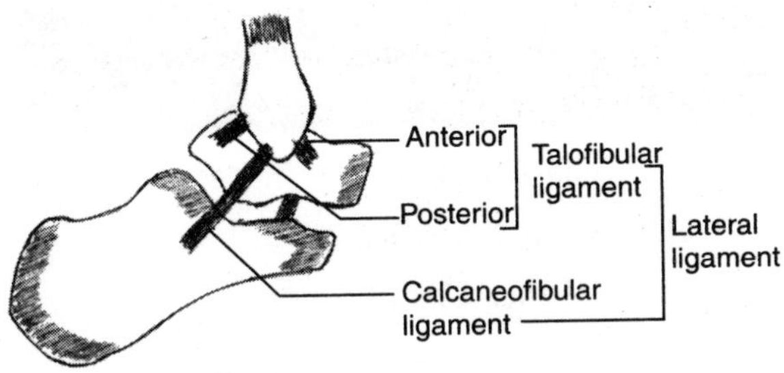

Fig. 21.3 Anatomy of lateral collateral ligament at ankle joint. Lateral collateral ligament injury can be diagnosed by doing inversion in neutral position. Patient feels severe pain.

Anterior talofibular injury (commonest) can be diagnosed by doing inversion in a plantar flexed position. Patient feels severe pain.

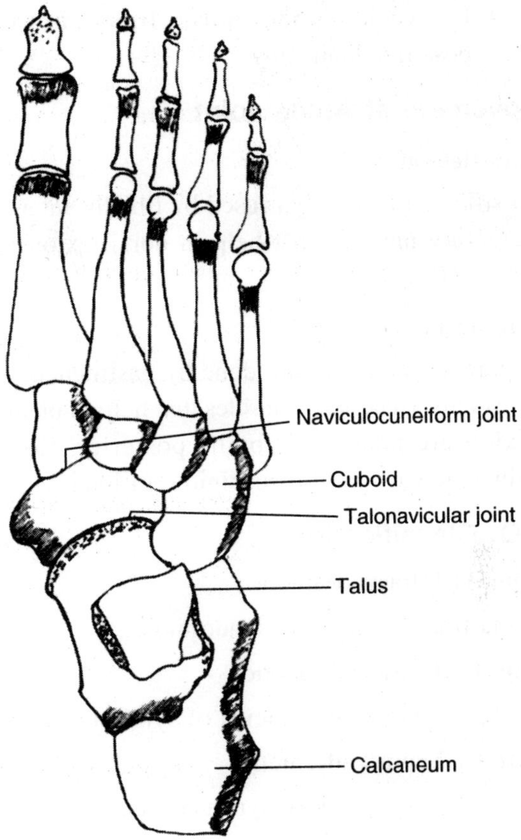

Fig. 21.4 Anatomy of foot

Syndesmotic Ligament

This is formed by tibiofibular ligament (anterior and posterior), interosseous ligament and inferior transverse ligament.

Stability of Ankle Joint

Stability of ankle joint depends on following structures:

1. Medial malleolus and medial collateral ligament.
2. Lateral malleolus and lateral collateral ligament.
3. Anterior syndesmotic ligament.

4. Posterior syndesmotic ligament and posterior malleolus.

Movement at Ankle Joint

Dorsiflexion

Dorsiflexion is mainly caused by tibialis anterior. Accessory muscles that help in dorsiflexion are EDL, EHL and PT.

Plantar Flexion

Plantar flexion is mainly done by gastrocnemius and soleus. Accessory muscles that help in plantar flexion are plantaris, tibialis posterior, flexor hallucis longus and flexor digitorum longus.

A.O. Classification

Type A: Infrasyndesmotic

Fibula fracture is below syndesmosis.

Type B: Transsyndesmotic

Fibula fracture is at the level of syndesmosis.

Type C: Suprasyndesmotic

Fibula fracture is above syndesmosis.

LAUGE-HANSEN CLASSIFICATION

Supination Adduction (SAD)

This type of injury causes:

1. Transverse fracture of fibula below ankle joint line or tear of lateral collateral ligament.
2. Vertical fracture of medial malleolus.

Supination Eversion (External Rotation) (SER)

This type of injury causes:

1. Spiral oblique fracture of distal fibula.
2. Fracture of posterior malleolus or tear of posterior tibiofibular ligament.
3. Fracture of medial malleolus or tear of deltoid ligament.
4. Disruption of anterior tibiofibular ligament.

Pronation Abduction (PAB)

1. Transverse fracture of medial malleolus or tear of deltoid ligament.
2. Short oblique fracture of fibula above the joint level.
3. Tear of syndesmotic ligament.

Pronation Eversion (External Rotation)

1. Transverse fracture of medial malleolus or tear of deltoid ligament.
2. Short oblique fracture of fibula above the joint level.
3. Avulsion fracture of posterolateral tibia or rupture of posterior tibiofibular ligament.
4. Rupture of anterior tibiofibular ligament.

Pronation Dorsiflexion

1. Fracture of medial malleolus and anterior margin of tibia.
2. Transverse fracture of posterior tibial surface.
3. Supramalleolar fracture of fibula.

OTHER CLASSIFICATION OF ANKLE INJURY

1. A.O. Classification
2. Henderson Classification
3. Denis Weber Classification

COMMON FRACTURES AT ANKLE

Maisonneuve Fracture

Maisonneuve was the first person to describe this fracture. According to him external rotation injury causes fracture of fibula at the joint level and at proximal end of fibula (If anterior tibiofibular ligament is ruptured first). This is known as Maisonneuve fracture.

Leforte-Wagstaffe Fracture

This is an avulsion fracture of anterior margin of fibula at the insertion site of anterior tibiofibular ligament.

Tillaux-chaput Fracture

This is a fracture at the lower end of tibia at posterolateral margin.

Boswarth Fracture

This is a fracture of lower end of fibula that is displaced behind tibia.

Pilon Fracture

Pilon was the first person to describe this fracture. This is a burst fracture of talus impacting against lower end of tibia as a hammer striking a nail.

Aviator's Fracture

This is fracture of neck of talus caused by forced dorsiflexion of ankle, sustained in aircraft crash. It may be associated with posterior dislocation of body of talus.

Cotton's Fracture

This was described by Cotton. This includes fracture of medial, lateral and posterior malleolus.

POTT'S FRACTURE

This was described by Sir Percivial Pott. This is bimalleolar fracture of ankle i.e. Fracture of medial and lateral malleolus.

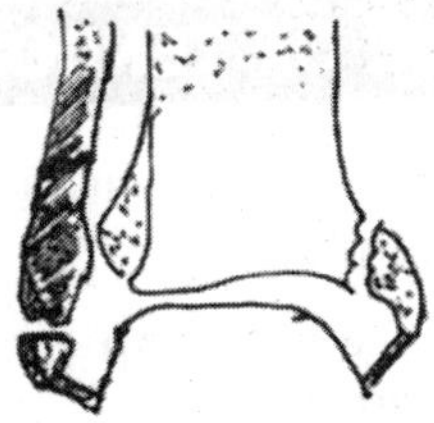

Fig. 21.5 Pott's fracture: Fracture medial malleolus and fracture lower end fibula (Adduction injury)

Clinical Features

1. Patient presents with pain, gross swelling and deformity at ankle.
2. Bony tenderness, crepitus are present at both malleoli.
3. Anterior Drawer test is positive.
4. Inversion and eversion stress tests are positive.

Anterior Drawer Test For Ankle

This test checks integrity of anterior talofibular ligament. Ankle is kept in neutral position. Now heal is pulled forward, while tibia is pushed backward. Anterior subluxation of 3 mm of talus is pathological.

X-ray Findings

Talocrural Angle

Normal range is 8–15 degree. Difference of 2–3 degree indicates fibular shortening. This angle is formed on X-ray of ankle in mortise view (X-ray beam is given perpendicular to intermalleolar line with leg internally rotated 15–20 degree) by making a line parallel to distal articular surface of tibia. Second line is drawn connecting two malleoli. Now angle formed between these 2 lines is called as Talocrural angle.

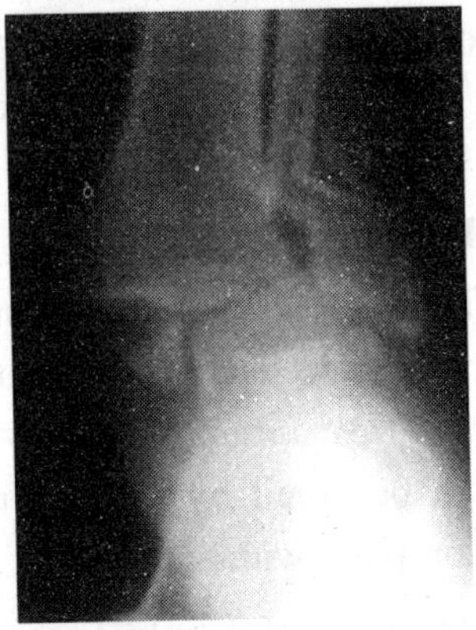

Fig. 21.6 Bimalleolar fracture (Pott's fracture)

CHAPTER 21

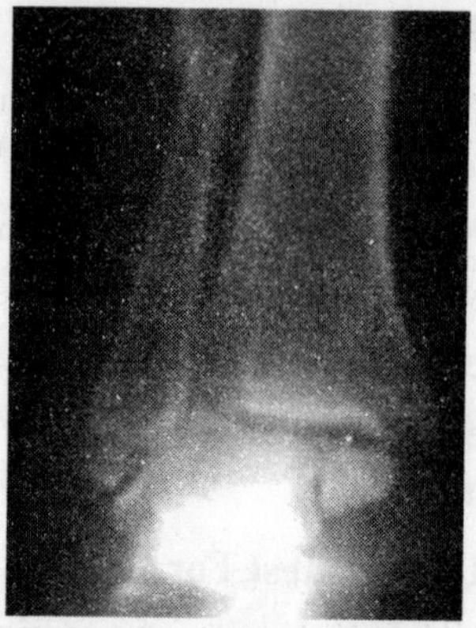

Fig. 21.7 Bimalleolar fracture with fracture shaft fibula

Talar Tilt

Normal talar tilt is less than 5 degree. 10–15 degree tilt indicates tear of anterior talofibular and calcaneofibular ligament.

Role of Arthroscopy

Arthroscope can be used to remove osteochondral lesion of talus. Any intraarticular pathology can also be dealt by arthroscopy.

Treatment

Undisplaced fracture (< 2 mm displacement) can be managed by BKPOP cast.

Displaced fracture should be tried first for closed reduction. If closed reduction fails, ORIF becomes treatment of choice. For all practical purposes any displaced fracture involving articular surface, should be managed by ORIF.

Lateral Malleolus

It can be fixed by tension band wiring, lag screw or 1/3rd tubular plate. Transverse fracture of fibula is fixed with 1/3rd tubular plate, while oblique fracture can be fixed by a lag screw or with neutralization plate with screw.

Avulsion fracture of fibula (associated with fracture of medial malleolus) can be managed by tension band wiring or lag screw.

Medial Malleolus

This can be fixed with either malleolar screw (if adequate bone is present in distal fragment to provide space for insertion of malleolar screw) or tension band wiring.

Posterior Malleolus

ORIF of posterior malleolus is indicated when more than 25% of posterior articular surface is involved and when more than 2 mm displacement is present.

Posterior malleolus can be approached from anterior to posterior (indirect) route or from posterior to anterior (direct) route. If we plan to choose a direct approach one should always reduce fibula first.

Anterior Malleolus

This should be fixed with a lag screw.

Complications

1. Post traumatic stiffness in ankle.
2. Malunion (fibula)
3. Nonunion is common in medial malleolus, uncommon in lateral and posterior malleolus.
4. If congruity of articular surface of ankle joint is not maintained it can lead to osteoarthritic changes later in life.
5. Synthesis of heterotrophic bone between lower end of tibia and fibula can form **Synostosis.**

RUPTURE OF TENDOACHILLIS

1. This is commonly seen among football and basketball players.
2. Common age group to be affected is between 30–35 years.
3. This is caused by sudden forceful dorsiflexion of ankle.

4. Common site of rupture is 2–6 cm proximal to its site of insertion on calcaneum.
5. Plantar flexion is absent.
6. **Thompson sign** is positive. In this test plantar flexion will be absent if we squeeze the calf muscle. This is also known as Calf squeeze test.
7. This rupture can be repaired by percutaneous technique of **Mac Griffith.**
8. Old rupture can be repaired by **Bosworth technique.**

ANKLE SPRAIN

It is anterior talofibular ligament (part of lateral ligament of ankle) which is commonly injured in ankle sprain. Sprain is caused by twisting of ankle due to inversion movement. Eversion force may cause sprain of medial collateral ligament of ankle.

Clinical Features

1. Pain, swelling and echymosis at ankle joint.
2. Patient experiences pain if stress is given to torn ligament.
3. If patient complaints of severe pain while doing inversion in neutral position of foot it means lateral collateral ligament is injured.
4. If inversion of a plantarflexed foot is painful it means anterior talofibular ligament is injured.
5. If eversion in nutral position is painful it means medial collateral ligament is injured.

Grades of Ankle Sprain

Grade 1: Only a few fibres of ligament are injured.

Grade 2: Most of the fibres of ligament are injured.

Grade 3: Ligament is completely torn.

Treatment

1. BKPOP slab can be applied for 3-4 weeks in grade 1 sprain.
2. BKPOP cast can be applied for 4 weeks in grade 2 sprain.
3. Grade 3 sprain is managed by surgical repair of ligament and BKPOP cast for 6 weeks.

DISLOCATION OF ANKLE

Pure ankle dislocations are uncommon. It usually occurs in association with fracture of ankle joint. It is caused by force directed against the plantigrade foot.

Types of Dislocations

1. Medial
2. Lateral
3. Posteromedial
4. Posterior
5. Rotatory

Clinical Features

1. Pain, swelling and deformity at ankle joint.
2. Compound dislocations may present with injury to dorsalis paedis artery/posterior tibial vessels.

Treatment

1. Ankle dislocation is an emergency and should be reduced as soon as possible.
2. Closed reduction is usually successful.
3. If fibula is also dislocated it may require open reduction.
4. After reducing the dislocation BKPOP cast is applied for 6 weeks.

FRACTURE OF CALCANEUM

70–75% Fractures of calcaneum are intraarticular type. Rests of them are extraarticular type.

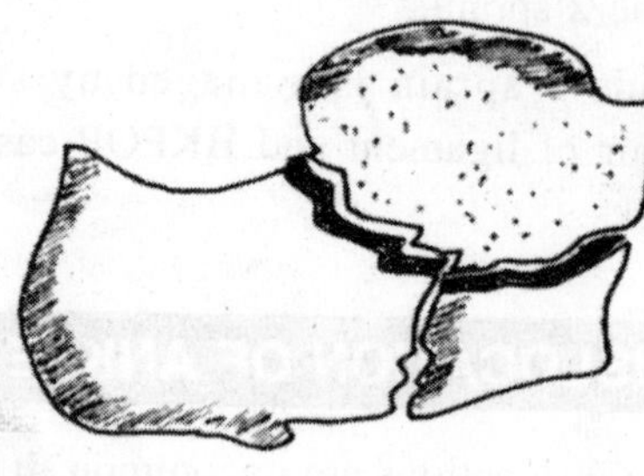

Fig. 21.8 Comminuted fracture calcaneum

Intraarticular fractures are subdivided into four types as follows:

Type 1: Undisplaced

Type 2: Two part fracture

Type 3: Three part fracture

Type 4: Comminuted fracture

Extraarticular type can be divided into five subtypes as follows:

1. Anterior process
2. Tuberosity
3. Medial process
4. Sustentaculum tali
5. Body

Mechanism of Injury

1. Intraarticular fractures are caused by axial loading and following a fall from a hight.
2. Extraarticular fractures are caused by a twisting force.

Clinical Features

1. Pain, swelling and echymosis at ankle.
2. Patient will not keep his ankle on ground due to pain.
3. Broadening of heel.

X-ray Findings

1. X-ray will show type of calcaneal fracture.
2. **Bohler's tuber joint angle** will be reduced. Normally it is 25–40 degree. It can be seen in lateral view. It is formed between two lines drawn at superior articulating surface and upper surface of tuberosity.

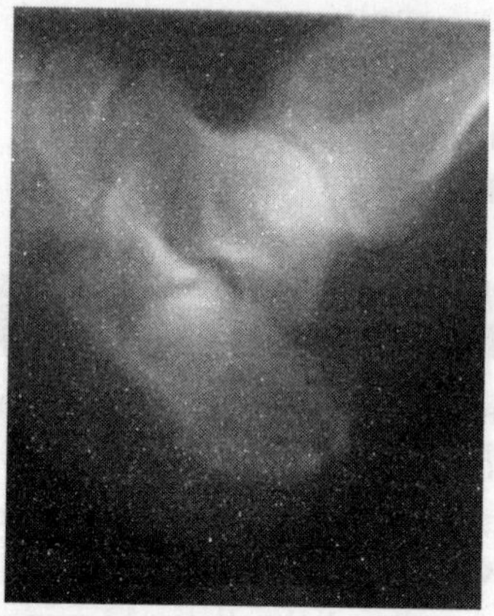

Fig. 21.9 Fracture calcaneum

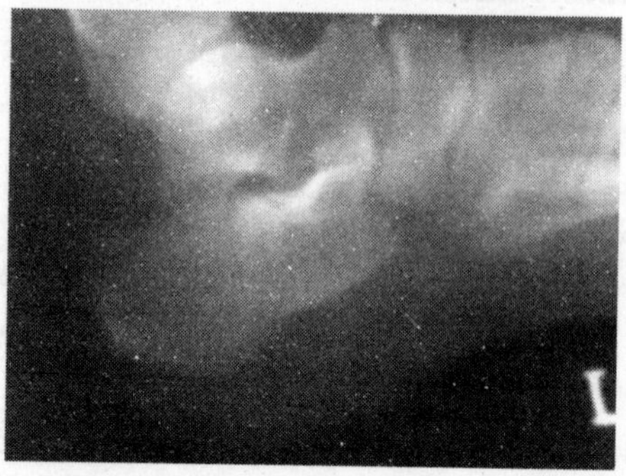

Fig. 21.10 Fracture calcaneum

Treatment

Displaced fractures should be reduced and BKPOP cast should be applied. Limb should be strictly elevated. Cast is applied for 3-4 weeks. Weight bearing is allowed after 4 weeks.

Undisplaced fractures are managed by BKPOP cast for 3-4 weeks.

Open Reduction

Open reduction of calcaneum can be done by following methods:

1. Essex-Lopresti method
2. Palmar method
3. McReynold method

Complications

1. Most common complication is stiffness at subtalar and midtarsal joint.
2. Patient with fracture calcaneum may present with osteoarthritic changes at subtalar joint later in life.

FRACTURE OF TALUS

This is second most common bone to be fractured among tarsal bone. Talus bone does not have any muscular or tendinous attachment. Fracture of lateral tubercle of posterior process of talus is known as **Shephard fracture.** It was described by Shephard in English literature.

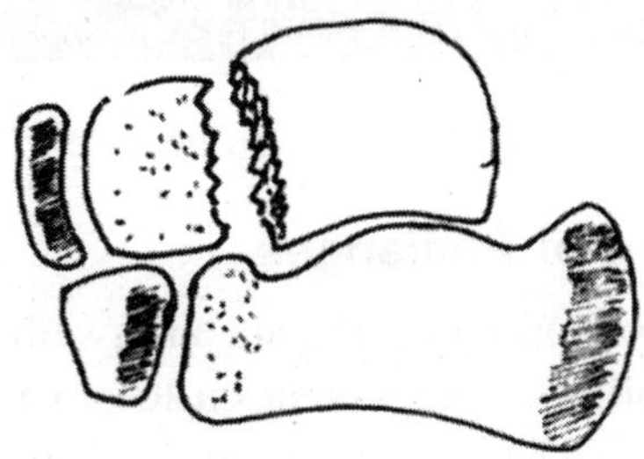

Fig. 21.11 Fracture talus (Aviator's fracture)

Blood Supply of Talus

Head of talus is supplied by branch pf dorsalis paedis artery and artery of sinus tarsi. Anastomosis ring is formed by artery to sinus tarsi, perforating branch of dorsalis paedis artery, branch of posterior tibial artery and artery of canal.

In fracture of talus, interosseous branch of arteries of tarsal sinus and tarsal canal are disrupted.

Mechanism of Injury

It is caused by forceful dorsiflexion of ankle, sustained as a result of air craft crash. It is also known as Aviator fracture. It may present with posterior dislocation of talus.

Clinical Features

1. Pain, swelling and deformity at ankle joint.
2. Difficulty to put weight on affected ankle.

Hawkins Classification

Type 1: Undisplaced vertical fracture of neck of talus.

Type 2: Displaced fracture with subluxation/ dislocation of subtalar joint.

Type 3: Displaced fracture of neck of talus and dislocation of body of talus from both ankle and subtalar joint.

X-ray Findings

This fracture can be missed on X-ray due to superimposition of tarsal bone. **Hawkin's sign** may be deteced on X-ray. This sign shows viability of head of talar body.

Treatment

Undisplaced fracture can be treated by BKPOP cast for 3-4 months. Displaced fracture may require ORIF by a screw.

Complications

Fracture talus can develop certain complications e.g. AVN, nonunion of talus and posttraumatic arthritis.

1. **Avascular necrosis and nonunion of talus** is most common complication of fracture of neck of talus because arterial supply is disrupted. This osteonecrosis can be treated by Blair's ankle fusion. In this procedure avascular part of talar body excised and replaced by sliding corticocancellous graft from anterior surface of lower end of tibia.

2. **Post traumatic arthritis** can occur due to osteonecrosis and immobilization of ankle.

FRACTURE OF METATARSAL

Patient will present with pain, swelling, deformity in foot and inability to walk. X-ray of foot A.P. and oblique will show fracture of metatarsal. Fracture may be displaced or undisplaced.

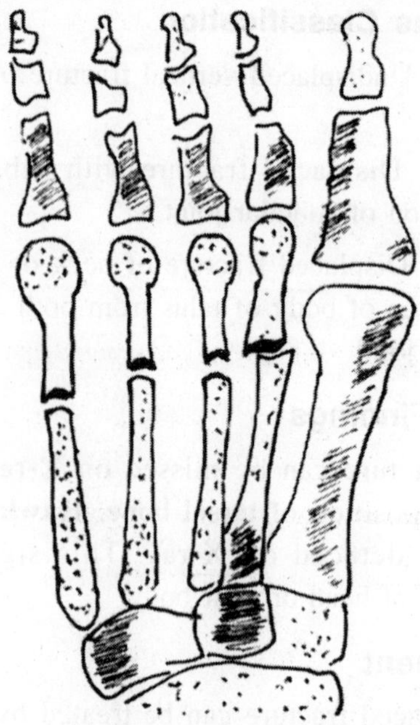

Fig. 21.12 Fracture metatarsals

Undisplaced fracture of metatarsal can be managed conservatively by below knee POP cast for 3–4 weeks. Displaced fractures can be fixed with Kwires or screws. Status of lisfrank joint should be looked for subluxation or dislocation. If found, it should be fixed with screws preferably.

March Fracture

This is fracture of second metatarsal (usually). It is caused by repeated stress in soldiers who perform march past phenomenon. This fracture heals spontaneously.

Jone's Fracture

This is fracture of base of 5th metatarsal. This is caused by pull of tendon of peroneus brevis muscle which is attached here. Patient may present with gross swelling in foot. Sumag (hygroscopic) dressing and limb elevation should be done. Below knee POP slab can be applied. If swelling subsides, below knee POP cast can be applied for 3-4 weeks.

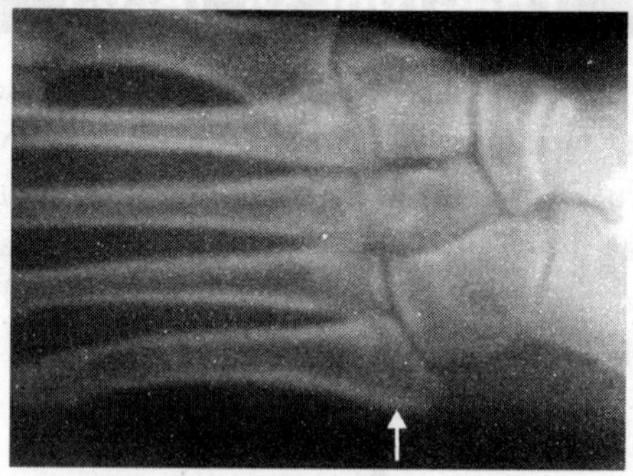

Fig. 21.13 Jone's fracture

Fracture of Phalanges

Patient will present with pain and swelling in toes and inability to put weight on toes. Undisplaced fractures can be managed by toe spica for 3 weeks. Displaced fractures can be fixed with Kwires.

CHAPTER

22 Fractures in Children

- Greenstick fracture
- Torus fracture
- Plastic bowing
- Epiphyseal injuries
- Complications

Following types of fractures are common in children:

1. Greenstick fracture
2. Torus fracture
3. Plastic bowing
4. Epiphyseal injury

GREENSTICK FRACTURE

When only one cortex is broken and other cortex remains intact, it is known as greenstick fracture. As this fracture pattern is similar to breakage of tender green stick of plant (it breaks on convex side only while concave side remains intact) it is termed as green stick fracture. This is common in both bones forearm. This type of fracture is managed by osteoclysis and reduction of fracture followed by AEPOP cast for 4–6 weeks. In osteoclysis, intact cortex is broken (because it may cause malunion) and plaster is applied.

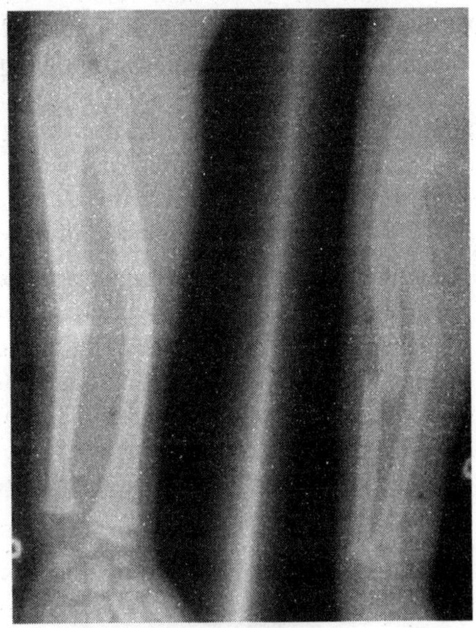

Fig. 22.1 Greenstick fracture of radius

TORUS FRACTURE

In this fracture, cortex of bone is buckled due to compressive forces. This fracture is common in metaphyseal region.

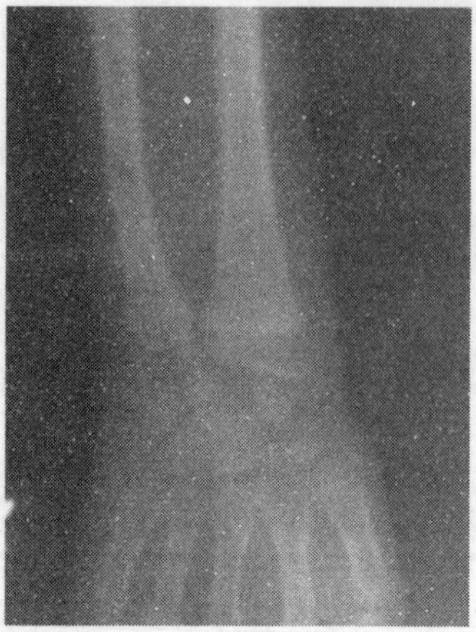

Fig. 22.2 Torus fracture of radius

PLASTIC BOWING

In this condition bone does not break but deforms. Microfractures are seen on concave side of bone. This bowing is common in paired bone e.g. both bones of forearm.

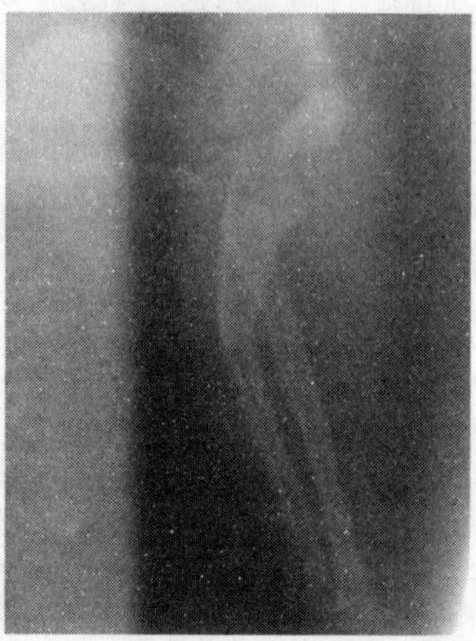

Fig. 22.3 Bowing of shaft ulna

EPIPHYSEAL INJURIES

Epiphyseal injuries are more common after the age of 10 years. Examples of such injuries are fracture lower end radius, fracture neck radius and fracture lower end tibia.

Salter-Harris Classification

Salter and Harris have classified epiphyseal injuries into six types as follows:

Type 1: Epiphysis is completely separated from metaphysis without fracture.

Type 2: This is most common type of epiphyseal injury. In this fracture physis and triangle of metaphysis bone is involved. This is known as **Thurston Holland sign.**

Type 3: This fracture occurs through physis and growth plate. This is an intraarticular fracture and should be managed by open reduction.

Type 4: Fracture line passes through epiphysis, physis and metaphysis and requires perfect reduction, because this is an intraartcular fracture. This is usually managed by open reduction to prevent growth arrest.

Type 5: In this type epiphysis is crushed, which later on causes growth arrest.

Type 6: This type involves peripheral physis injury.

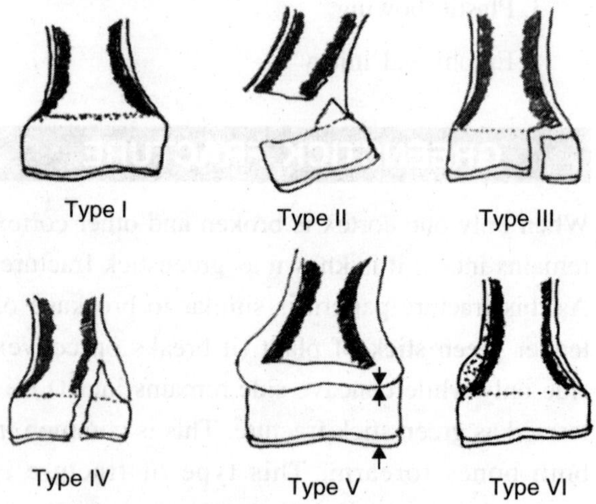

Fig. 22.4 Salter-Harris classification of epiphyseal injury

Treatment

While treating such injuries in children below mentioned principles should be kept in mind:

1. Rotation is not accepted in children.
2. Angulation should not be more than 10 degree.
3. Overlapping of fracture site can be accepted up to 1–1.5 cm.

Displaced fractures can be managed by closed reduction with manipulation or traction. ORIF is required in Type 3 and 4 injuries. Unstable fractures can also be fixed with pins and screw.

Table 22.1: Classification based treatment plan of epiphyseal injury

Type 1	Closed reduction followed by POP cast. Case should be followed up to 3 months.
Type 2	Closed reduction can be done under anesthesia or nerve block. Unstable fracture of distal end tibia can be fixed by pins and screws.
Type 3	Closed reduction and cast application.
Type 4	Open reduction (anatomical) and epiphysis to epiphysis internal fixation.
Type 5	Open reduction and internal fixation.
Type 6	These are compound injuries; so require debridement and secondary closure. Follow up should be done till maturity of bone.

COMPLICATIONS

(A) Growth disturbances

1. Over growth, due to increased vascularity and stimulation of epiphysis.
2. Growth arrest can occur due to injury to growth plate. (premature growth arrest is commonest complication)

(B) Angular Deformity of Limb

(C) Hypoplasia of Epiphysis

CHAPTER

23 Cervical Spine Injuries

- Atlas fractures
  - Fracture of odontoid process
- Atlanto-axial rotatory subluxation
- Clay shoveler's fracture
- Chance fracture
- Sentinel fracture
- Frankel classification
- Denis 3 column theory of spine
- Factors responsible for unstable fracture
- Clinical features of cervical spine injury
- Traumatic paraplegia
- Denis classification of spinal fractures

ATLAS FRACTURES

Atlas vertebra can show three types of fractures:

1. Jefferson fracture.
2. Fracture of its arch and lateral masses.
3. Fracture of posterior arch.

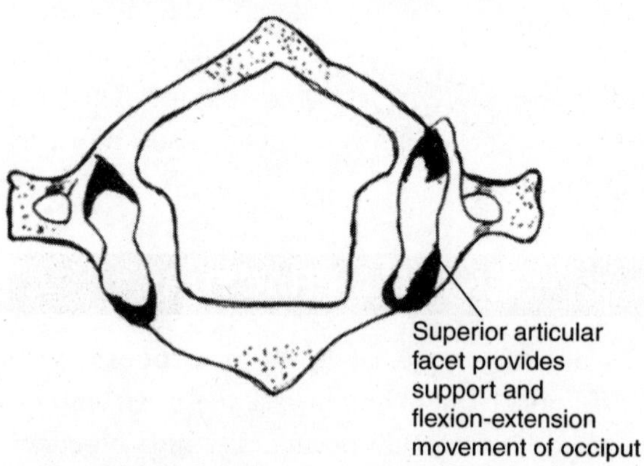

Fig. 23.1 Superior view of atlas vertebra (C_1)

Jefferson Fracture

Jefferson fracture is caused by direct, symmetrical and compression force that leads to fracture of ring at 3 or 4 sites thus separating the lateral masses. Jefferson fracture which has <7 mm of overlap on the open mouth odontoid view is treated by rigid halo immobilization. (If lateral overhang of C1 and C2 is >7 mm it means transverse ligament is

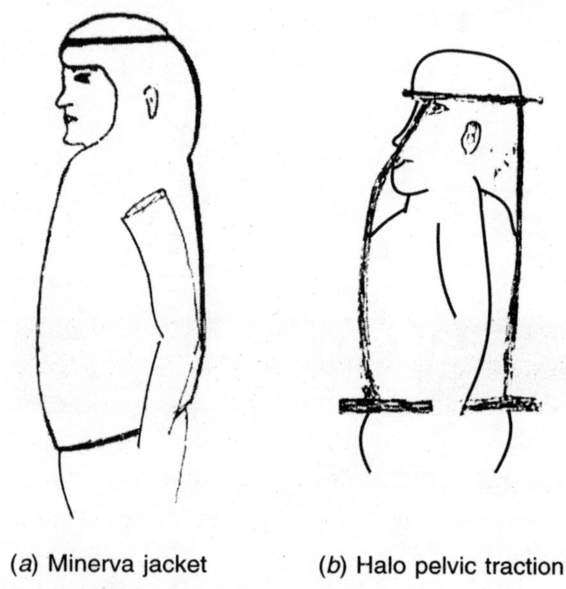

(*a*) Minerva jacket (*b*) Halo pelvic traction

Fig. 23.2

ruptured.) Minerva jacket is also useful in treatment of this fracture.

Fracture Axis Vertebra (Odontoid Process)

Anderson and D'Aonzo have classified this fracture into 3 types as follows:

Type 1: Oblique fracture of dens

Type 2: Fracture is at the junction of dens and central body of axis.

Type 3: Fracture mainly involves cancellous bone. Body of axis is separated.

Type 1 is treated by cervical orthosis as these are stable fracture. Type-2 fracture has high risk of non union and can be treated by halo immobilization, primary posterior C1-C2 fusion and anterior screw fixation of odontoid. Even with these options there are still chances of nonunion.

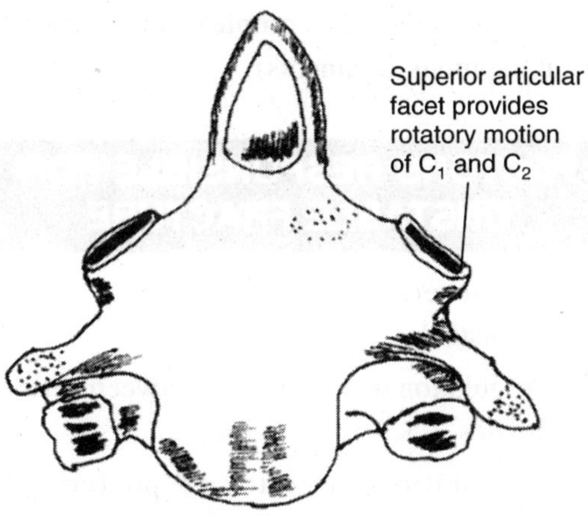

Fig. 23.3 Axis vertebra (C_2)

ATLANTOAXIAL ROTATORY SUBLUXATION

Patient presents with cervical pain and occipital neuralgia. Uncommonly patient may have symptoms of vertebrobasilar insufficiency. This is of four types as follows:

Type 1: This type has atlantodental interval <3 mm i.e. transverse ligament is intact.

Type 2: Atlantodental interval is 3–5 mm i.e. transverse ligament is inefficient.

Type 3: Atlantodental interval is >5 mm i.e. failure of alar ligaments.

Treatment

- Cervical head halter traction in supine position.
- Active ROM exercise for 24–48 hours.
- After 2 days ambulatory orthotic immobilization with active ROM exercises are adviced until free motion returns.

CLAY SHOVELER'S FRACTURE

This fracture occurs through spinous process of lower cervical and upper thoracic vertebrae. It is seen in clay shovelers; when shovel remains fixed in clay that causes muscular pull in spinous process leading to this fracture. Stable fractures are treated conservatively.

CHANCE FRACTURE

This is a fracture of vertebra that primarily involves bone and caused by failure of anterior, middle and posterior column of spine. This is a flexion distraction type of injury also known as **Seat belt injury.**

SENTINEL FRACTURE

Unstable fracture of spinous process with neurological involvement is known as sentinel fracture. This fracture occurs at lamina on either side of spinous process. Neurological involvement is caused by impingment of loose posterior element.

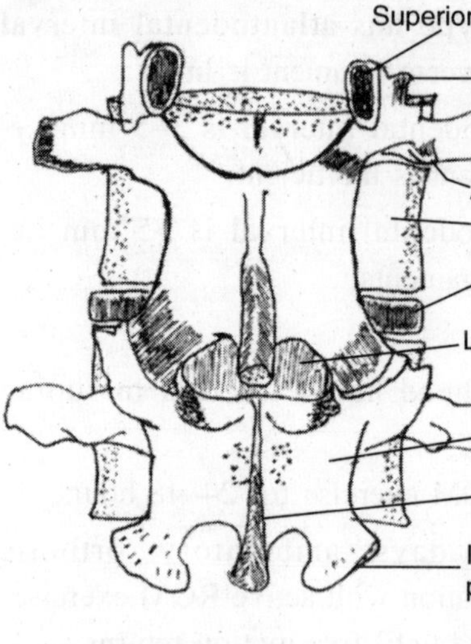

Fig. 23.4 Anatomy of vertebral column

FRANKEL CLASSIFICATION OF NEUROLOGICAL DEFICIT

Frankel has classified neurological deficit into five types as follows:

Type A: Sensorymotor functions are absent.

Type B: Sensation is present but motor functions are absent.

Type C: Sensation is present. Motor functions are active but not useful. (grade 2-3 power)

Type D: Sensation is present. Motor functions are active and useful.

Type E: Normal sensorymotor function

DENIS 3 COLUMN THEORY OF SPINE

Denis has divided spine into three columns anterior, middle and posterior.

Anterior column consists of:

1. Anterior longitudinal ligament
2. Anterior part of vertebral body
3. Anterior portion of annulus fibrosus

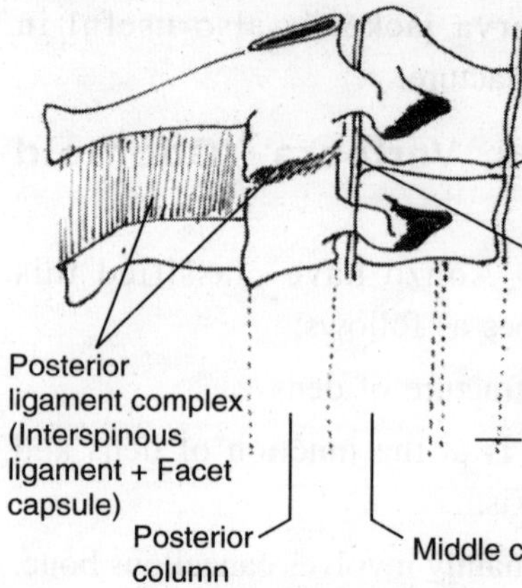

Fig. 23.5 Division of spine in 3 column

Middle column consists of:

1. Posterior longitudinal ligament
2. Posterior part of vertebral body
3. Posterior part of annulus fibrosus

Posterior column consists of:

Posterior ligamentous complex (Facet capsules and interspinous ligaments)

FACTORS RESPONSIBLE FOR UNSTABLE FRACTURE

There are several factors that make a vertebral fracture unstable:

1. Angulation of >11 degree between vertebral bodies.
2. Translation (anterior or posterior) of vertebral body >3.5 mm.
3. Loss of 25% posterior vertebral hight.
4. Loss of 20% anterior vertebral hight.
5. Intervertebral disc separation is more than 1.7mm.
6. Spinous process widening.
7. Widening of facet joint
8. Malaligned spinous process
9. Rotation of facet
10. Vertebral body is tilted laterally.

CLINICAL FEATURES OF CERVICAL SPINE INJURY

Patient with cervical spine injury may have following clinical features:

1. Pain, swelling and deformity at cervical spine.
2. Weakness or paralysis of upper and lower limb.
3. Sensory deficit corresponding to spinal injury.
4. Bladder and bowel is usually involved.
5. Bulbocaverous reflex is absent in phase of spinal shock.
6. Intact perianal sensation indicates, incomplete cord lesion.
7. Intact sharp-dull discrimination indicates preserved lateral spinal column.
8. If injury is proximal to C4 level (which is uncommon) patient will present with paralysis of all respiratory muscle. Prognosis is very poor in these cases. Patient may die instantly.

Depending upon level of spinal injury patient may present with either of the clinical entity:

1. Brown-Sequard syndrome
2. Central cord syndrome
3. Anterior cord syndrome
4. Posterior cord syndrome
5. Complete/incomplete spinal cord injury
6. Root injury

Brown-Sequard syndrome

This is also called as hemisection of spinal cord, as injury is limited to either side of spinal cord. Patient presents with ipsilateral muscle paralysis and loss of vibration, position sense on same side, while pain and temperature is lost on opposite side. Patient has good prognosis as most of them, regain bladder and bowel control and ability to walk.

Central cord syndrome

In this condition patient presents with complete flaccid quadriplegia, sevre flaccid lower motor neuron paralysis of arm, fingers and hand and upper motor neuron spastic paralysis of trunk and lower extremities. This is commonly seen in middle aged person with osteoarthritc changes in spine. This is an extension type of injury. Patient has good prognosis.

Anterior cord syndrome

This condition is characterized by sensory deficit with spared dorsal column of spine (deep pressure and proprioception are intact) and incomplete motor paralysis. Patient may recover from this condition within 24 hours.

Posterior cord syndrome

This condition is not common. Patient presents with loss of deep pressure, deep pain and proprioceptive sensation. Pain and temperature sensation are intact. Patient has full voluntary motor power.

Incomplete neurological deficit

This has following three distinctive features:

1. Preserved perianal sensation.
2. Voluntary rectal motor function.
3. Great toe flexor activity

Complete neurological deficit

This has following two features:

1. No sensorymotor function is seen distal to spinal cord injury.
2. Bulbocavernous reflex is present. (spinal shock is absent)

Root injury

Partial recovery is possible in this kind of peripheral nerve lesion. This type of injury may be seen in brachial plexus injury, otherwise it is uncommon.

X-ray Findings

X-ray will show type and stability of vertebral fracture, status of disc space and deformity of spine.

MRI Findings

MRI is done to rule out cord compression. However it can also show vertebral fracture.

Treatment

Transportation

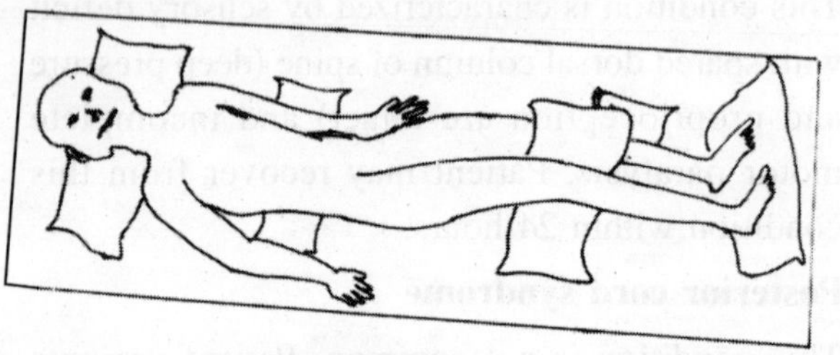

Fig. 23.6 (*a*)

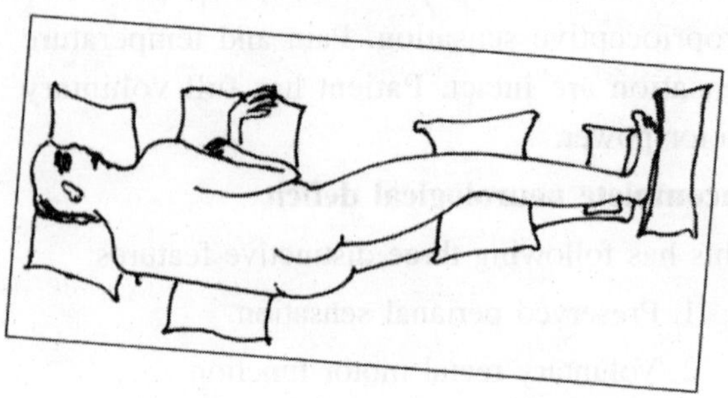

Fig. 23.6 (*b*) Proper positioning of paraplegic patient in bed

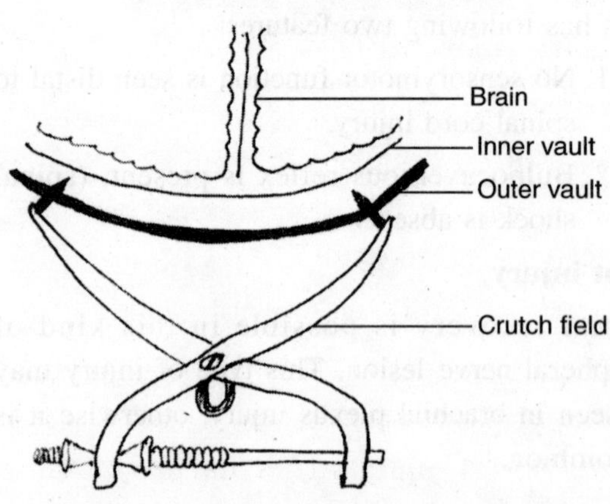

Fig. 23.6 (*c*) Crutchfield for skull fraction

Transportation of patient with spinal injury is most important step in management. Patient should be transported in such a way that his neck is held in traction by pulling the held in axis of cervical spine. Rest of body should be supported separately by 3 persons at shoulder, pelvis and legs. Other important step is that the trolly on which patient has come in emergency should not be changed until it is proved that spinal injury is stable.

Definitive Treatment

- Hard cervical collar should be applied as soon as possible.
- If bladder is involved, patient should be catherterized.
- X-ray of cervical spine (A.P., Lateral and swimmer's view) should be done.
- Undisplaced stable fracture without neurological deficit should be treated conservatively. Cervical collar is applied and patient is adviced bed rest for 6 weeks.
- Displaced unstable fracture is associated with neurological deficit. Fracture should be reduced by Crutch-Field skeletal traction applied in skull. Check X-ray should be done to see reduction. This reduction should be checked every 12 hourly by repeating X-ray. 10 pounds of weight is applied for head and 5 pounds for each additional vertebral injury.
- To see improvement; we should examine neurological status daily. Traction is continued for 6 weeks. After this period patient is adviced to wear cervical collar for 4 months.
- Care of bladder, bowel and back should be done.
- An air ring covered with a cotton cloth can be kept under hips to prevent bed sores.
- Patient should be turned side to side at the interval of two hours to prevent development of bed sore.

- Neurotropics should be given.
- Water bed can also be helpful in prevention of bed sores.

Indications of Surgery

If facture/dislocation is not reduced by crutch-field skull traction, it should be managed by open reduction and internal fixation. Cervical spine can be fixed by following surgical methods:

1. Lateral mass fixation
2. Bicortical screw fixation (anterior cervical decompression and fusion)
3. Midline wiring of lower cervical spine.
4. Facet wiring
5. Interlaminar clamps
6. Screw fixation of Dens.
7. Transarticular fixation (C1-C2 fixation)
8. Brook's fusion (C1-C2)

TRAUMATIC PARAPLEGIA

Injury to thoracolumbar spine may lead to traumatic paraplegia. Spinal cord injury can manifest in 3 ways as follows:

1. Cord concussion.
2. Cord transection
3. Root injury

Cord concussion

This type of spinal injury presents with transient functional loss that recovers within 12 hours of injury. There is no anatomical lesion in this type of injury.

Cord transection

This is a permanent spinal injury in which spinal cord is transected. Patient presents with total sensory loss and autonomic functions at the site of lesion.

Root injury

Neural foramen is the site where nerve root is damaged. Partial recovery can occur in root injury.

DENIS CLASSIFICATION OF SPINAL FRACTURES

This classification is based on analysis of CT-scan and X-ray.

1. Compression
   — Anterior flexion
   — Lateral flexion
2. Burst
3. Flexion distraction (seat belt type)
4. Fracture dislocation
   — Flexion rotation
   — Shear
   — Flexion distraction

Compression fracture

Compression fracture is caused by anterior or flexion injury leading to failure of anterior column. Anterior hight of vertebral body is reduced, whereas posterior hight of vertebral body is normal. Middle column is intact in this fracture. This is a stable injury.

Burst fracture

This fracture manifests in five following pattern:

Type A: Involves both end plate

Type B: Involves only superior end plate

Type C: Involves inferior end plate

Type D: Involves rotation of vertebra

Type E: Lateral wedging of vertebra.

Flexion distraction

(Seat belt type injury)

This is an unstable fracture and presents in following two patterns:

Chance fracture (occur through bone)

Dislocation occurs through soft tissue.

Fracture dislocation

1. In this injury all the three columns are disrupted.

2. This is a highly unstable injury.
3. Neurological deficit is usually present.
4. This fracture may be associated with dural tear or intraabdominal injury.

Clinical Features

1. Thoracolumbar spine injury may present with paresis/paralysis of trunk and both lower limbs.
2. Rest of the clinical features are same as in cervical spine injuries.
3. Patient may present with comlete/incomplete neurological deficit. Complete neurological deficit means sensorymotor functions are lost caudal to spinal cord injury. Bulbocavarnosus reflex is present i.e. S3-S4 area of conus medullaris is intact. Incomplete neurological deficit means some sensorymotor function persists below the level of spinal cord injury. Sacral sparing is an essential feature of incomplete deficit. Sacral sparing includes perianal sensation, voluntary motor function and great toe flexor activity.

Investigations

X-RAY can show type and stability of fracture.

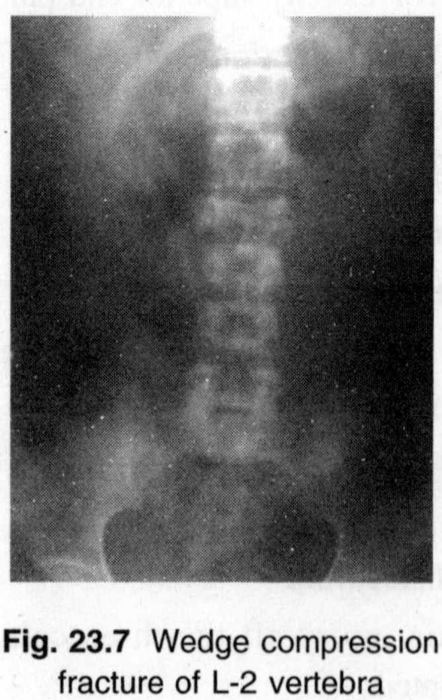

Fig. 23.7 Wedge compression fracture of L-2 vertebra

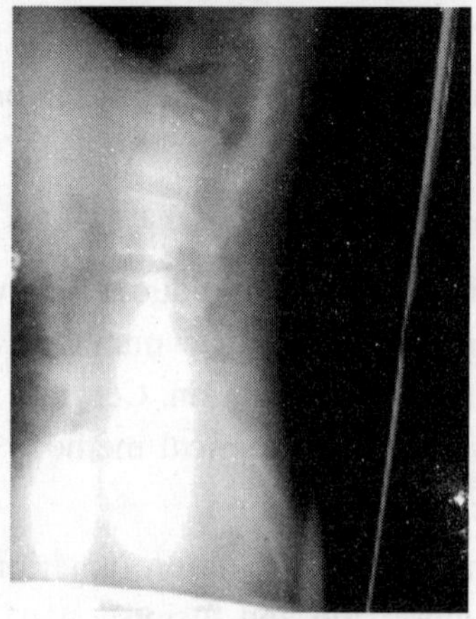

Fig. 23.8 Wedge compression fracture of L-2 vertebra (Lateral view)

CT-SCAN can show vertebral arches, facet joint and neural canal.

MRI can show the level of spinal cord compression.

Treatment

1. Hyperextension cast is applied in stable compression type of fracture. But upper thoracic compressive fractures should be stabilized by surgery if significant kyphosis is present.
2. Stable burst fractures can also be managed conservatively by a hyperextension cast. But unstable burst fracture is managed by posterior stabilization. Harrington system is contraindicated in lower lumbar spine injury.

Surgical Instrumentation In Spine

Today we have a lot of surgical implants to fix the spine. Commonly used implants are as follows:

1. Harrington's system
2. Kaneda fixation
3. Cotrel-Dubousset system
4. Pedicle screw fixation
5. Jacob rod

6. Cervical locking plate
7. Staffee plate.

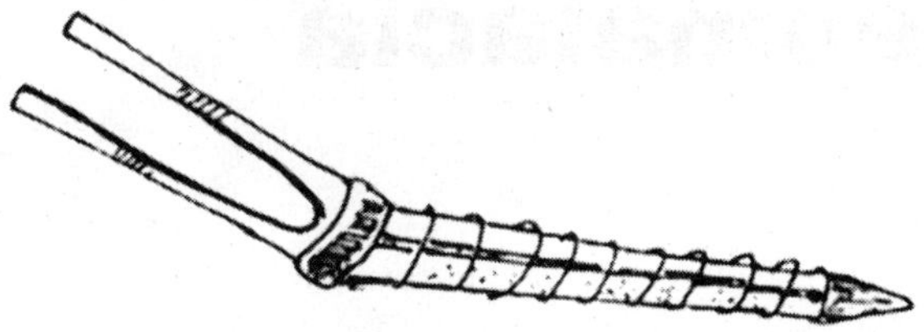

Fig. 23.9 Poly axial spine reduction screw

Indications of spine screw fixation

This implant can be used in following conditions:

1. Fracture spine
2. Pott's spine
3. Tumor of spine
4. Spinal deformity
5. Degenerated central disc prolapse with cauda equina syndrome.
6. Failed back syndrome
7. Degenerative and lytic lysthesis.

CHAPTER

24 Osteomalacia

- Calcium metabolism
- Rickets
- Coeliac rickets
- Osteomalacia

CALCIUM METABOLISM

Human body contains about 1100 gm (27.5 mmol) of calcium, about 99% of which exists in skeleton. Plasma calcium level is about 9–11 mg/dl or 5 meq/l or 2.5 mmol. Free ionized calcium acts as second messenger. Calcium is required for blood coagulation, muscle contraction and nerve function. Ionized calcium level can be measured by sensitive electrode. Reduced calcium level causes spasm of skeletal muscle, mainly of extremities and larynx, thus results in hypocalcemic tetany. Total diffusible calcium level is approximately 1.34 mmol/l of which 1.18 mmol is ionized.

About 0.92 mmol/l calcium bounds to albumin and 0.24 mmol/l bounds to globulin. Both of which makes total non diffusible (protein bound) calcium. (1.16 mmol/l)

Regulation of Plasma Calcium Level

Plasma calcium level is regulated by PTH, Vitamin D and calcitonin. Absorption of calcium takes place in upper small intestine. Phytates, citrate, oxlate and phosphates impair calcium absorption.

PTH

It increases calcium level by acting over bone, kidney and intestine.

- Most important action of PTH over bone is that it increases the resorption of calcium from bone by increasing number of **bone** remodelling units and inhibiting osteoclast.
- PTH increases calcium reabsorption in distal tubule and regulates the calcium excretion.
- In **intestine** PTH has no direct effect on calcium absorption but it increases it indirectly by enhancing the formation of calcitriol in kidney by activating 1 alpha hydroxylase.
- PTH decreases calcium level in milk, saliva and ocular lens. It may cause developmental cataract in hypoparathyroidism.
- Fall in plasma calcium level induces PTH release and increased calcium level does the

reverse probably by decreasing C-AMP. Prolonged hypocalcemia cause hypertrophy and hyperplasia of parathyroid, while sustained hypercalcemia has opposite effect.

Vitamin D

- Calcitriol (active form of vitamin D) increases resorption of calcium and phosphate from bone by promoting recruitment and differentiation of osteoclast precursors in bone remodelling unit.
- It increases absorption of calcium and phosphates from intestine by enhancing the synthesis of calcium binding protein (Calbindin).
- Calcitriol increases proximal tubular reabsorption of both calcium and phosphate in kidney. (In comparison to PTH, calcitriol action is less marked.
- Generally speaking vitamin D deficiency causes fall in plasma calcium level and vice versa.

Calcitonin

Calcitonin causes fall in plasma calcium level, opposite to that of PTH. High plasma calcium level causes calcitonin release while low plasma calcium causes decreased calcitonin release. Calcitonin acts through increase in c AMP formation. Calcitonin inhibits bone resorption by direct action on osteoclast. In proximal tubule it inhibits calcium and phosphate reabsorption by direct action on kidney.

Predisposing Factors for Hypercalcemia

1. Corticosteroid
2. PTH
3. Thyroxin
4. Excess hypervitaminosis D
5. PGE2
6. IL-1 and IL-6
7. Alcohol
8. Loop diuretics

Predisposing Factors for Hypocalcemia

1. Estrogen
2. Androgen
3. Calcitonin
4. Growth hormone
5. Biphosphonate
6. Fluoride
7. Gallium nitrate
8. Mithramycin
9. Thiazide diuretics

Physiological Role of Calcium in Human Body

1. It is essential element for excitation-contraction coupling.
2. It regulates excitation of nerves and muscles.
3. Calcium acts as intracellular messenger for hormone, autocoids and transmitter.
4. Calcium is required for blood coagulation.
5. Calcium generates impulse in heart and determines level of automaticity and A.V. conduction

RICKETS

Rickets is a metabolic bone disease of children in which osteoid fails to mineralize due to faulty calcium metabolism. It is characterized clinically by softening of bone and development of bony deformity, radiologically by delayed appearance of epiphysis and widened epiphyseal plate, cupping and slipping of metaphysis (champagne glass appearance).

Metabolic Changes

Due to deficiency of vitamin D intestinal absorption of calcium is reduced leading to hypocalcemia, which in turn stimulates PTH release. PTH increases calcium resorption from bone through action on osteocytes. PTH activates renal 1 alfa hydroxylase that increases the amount of vitamin D and calcium absorption. PTH also decreases the calcium excretion from kidney but it increases phosphate excretion. As a result serum calcium level comes to normal and serum phosphorus decreases. If treatment is not given to patient, PTH no more can sustain normal serum calcium level. So later serum calcium and phosphorus level both fall. Increased osteoblastic activity leads to rise in serum alkaline phosphatase level.

Clinical Features

Rickets is uncommon below 3 months of age. It presents in later half of first year or second year. Following clinical features can be seen in rickets:

1. Earliest clinical feature is **craniotabes**, usually seen in occipital or posterior part of parietal bone. Bone can be buckled inward by pressure but with release of pressure elastic recoil snaps the bone back into original position (ping pong ball like feeling). It is known as craniotabes.
2. Frontal bossing of skull is seen because of excess osteoid. Bossing is usually seen after 6 months of age and can also be present in parietal bone.
3. Over growth of cartilage or osteoid tissue at osteochondral junction leads to deformed chest known as **Rachitic rosary.**
4. **Pigeon chest deformity** is a common finding. Metaphyseal ends of ribs are weak in rickets. These are pulled inward by respiratory muscles creating anterior protrusion of sternum.
5. **Harrison groove** is a horizontal depression along the lower part of chest created by inward pull of lower part of chest.
6. **Pott-belly** appearance of abdomen is caused by muscular hypotonia. It leads to viscerptosis and lumbar lordosis that causes protruberant abdomen (pott-belly).
7. **Broadening of ends of long bones** occurs due to widening of epiphysis. Wrist and knee are common joint to be involved. It is seen around 6–9 months of age.
8. Delayed teeth appearance.
9. Deformity of legs is seen when child starts bearing weight on legs. Knock knee and coxa vara are common deformity.
10. Vitamin D deficiency in early infancy may result in bilateral lamellar cataract.

Investigations

1. Serum calcium is either normal or low.
2. Serum phosphorus is low.
3. Serum alkaline phosphatase is high.
4. Serum bicarbonate and serum chloride are decreased.

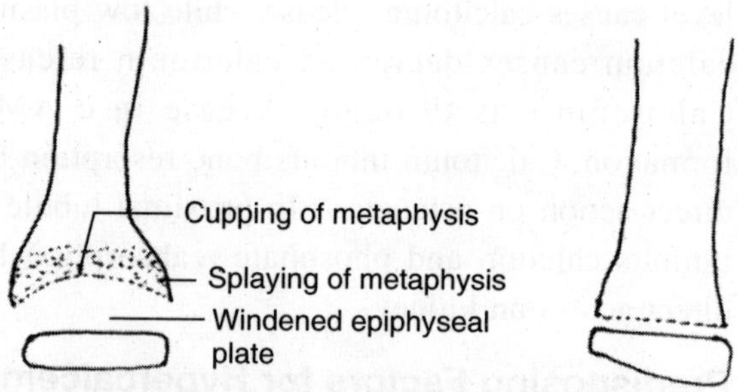

Fig 24.1 X-ray findings of rickets

Radiological findings

1. Early changes are seen in lower end of radius and ulna.
2. Epiphysis appears late. Epiphysis plate is widened due to uncalcified osteoid. (normal width is 2–4 mm)

3. Space between epiphysis and metaphysis is increased.
4. Widening and cupping of ends of long bones is known as **Champagne glass appearance** or trumpeting cortex.
5. Density of cortex is decreased which is known as rarefaction.

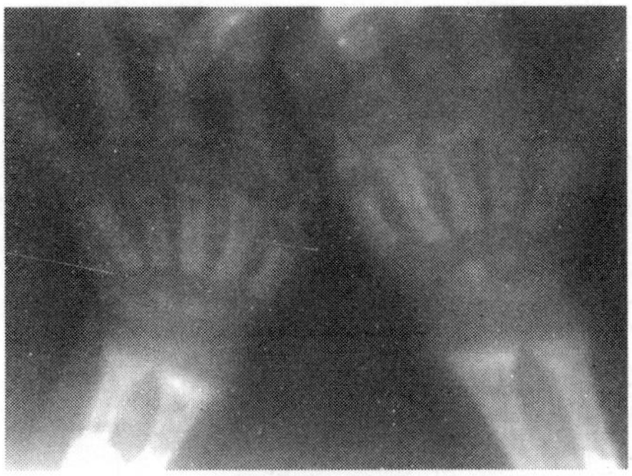

Fig. 24.2 Metaphyseal cupping and irregular epiphyseal plates in rickets

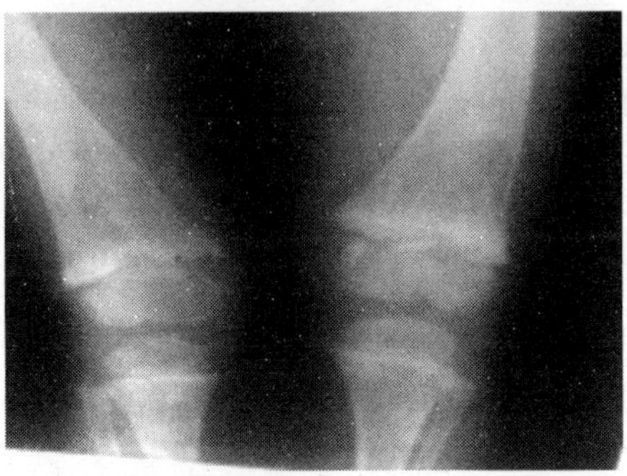

Fig. 24.3 Champagne glass appearance of distal ends of long bones in rickets

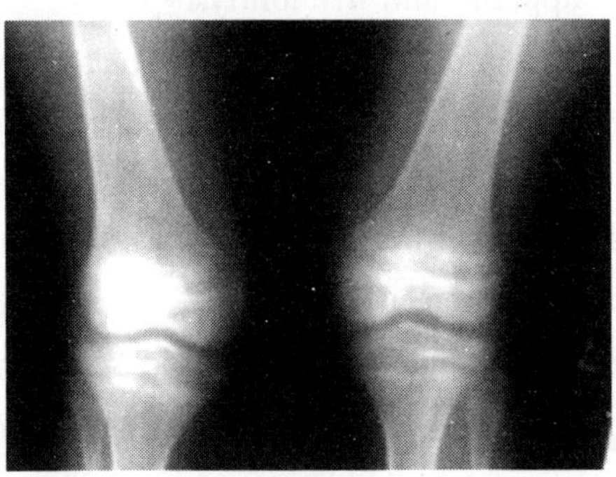

Fig. 24.4 Widening of epiphyseal plates in rickets

6. Bony deformity like genu valgum or genu varum can be seen on single large plate X-ray in standing position including both knees.

Treatment

Administration of 6 lac i.u. of vitamin D (oral or intramuscular) induces rapid healing. Follow up X-ray is done after 3–4 weeks of therapy. If healing line is not seen on X-ray, above mentioned dose can be repeated. Failure to respond to second dose of vitamin D is called **Refractory rickets.** If child responds to vitamin D therapy a maintenance dose of 400 units or 10 μg is given daily.

Prevention of Deformities

It can be prevented by absolute bed rest and application of mermaid splint. This splint is very effective in preventing the deformity of lower limb. It is helpful during active phase of disease. In requires regular supervision.

Surgical Treatment

When active rickets is brought under control and when growth stops, surgery is done in form of osteotomy; around the joint.

TYPES OF RICKETS

Before describing the types of rickets, it should be clear in mind that what is refractory rickets/ vitamin D resistant rickets/vitamin D dependent rickets?

Refractory Rickets

To treat rickets; first we give 6 lac I.U. of vitamin D. Then we do the X-ray of bone to see the line of healing. If we do not find this line a second dose of vitamin D (6Lac I.U.) is given. Failure to respond to second dose of vitamin D is diagnosed as refractory rickets.

Vitamin D Resistant Rickets

This is late onset rickets which is familial in pattern. It is also known as Late rickets or rachitis tarda. Patient presents with Tackle deformity i.e. genu valgum on one side and genu varum on other side. Patient suffers form excessive loss of faecal calcium and faulty synthesis of 1,25$(OH)_2$ vitamin D by kidney. It requires large dose of vitamin D (2000 U) and 0.5–1.5 gm phosphate (disodium hydrogen phosphate 13.6 gm/dl and phosphoric acid 5.9 gm/dl) given daily till bony maturity is achieved.

Vitamin D Dependent Rickets (Type-1)

It is an autosomal recessive disease. In this type due to deficiency of 1-alfa hydroxylase (in renal tubules) 25(OH) vitamin D can not be converted into 1,25$(OH)_2$ vitamin D3.

Vitamin D Dependent Rickets (Type-2)

In this type target cells do not respond to 1,25$(OH)_2$ vitamin D.

Type 1: Rickets

In this type patient has either vitamin D deficiency or its metabolic abnormality. Patient also develops secondary hyperparathyroidism.

CAUSES

Vitamin D deficiency

1. Reduced intake
2. Due to lack of exposure to sun light
3. Malabsorption

Vitamin D Metabolic Abnormality

Liver

1. Liver damage causes failure of synthesis of 25(OH) vitamin D3.
2. Long term anticonvulsant drug stimulate hepatic microsomal enzyme which convert vitamin D3 to 25(OH)D-26,23 lactone.

Kidney

1. Vitamin D dependent type-1 rickets.
2. Vitamin D dependent type-2 rickets.
3. Renal osteodystrophy in which kidney can not synthesize 1,25 $(OH)_2$ vitamin D3 due to damage of glomerulus and renal tubules.

Type 2: Rickets

Phosphate reabsorption defect in tubules.

1. Familial hypophosphatemic vitamin D refractory rickets (FHVRR). It has phosphate transportation defect across cell membrane of tubules and intestine. Synthesis of 1,25$(OH)_2$ vitamin D is reduced.
2. Fanconi Sydrome. Component of this syndrome includes cystinosis, tyrosinosis and lowe syndrome. In fanconi syndrome phosphate, amino acid and glucose are not reabsorbed through renal tubules.
3. Renal tubular acidosis
4. Isolated phosphaturia.
5. Oncogenic tumors

COELIAC RICKETS

This is also known as non tropical sprue, idiopathic steatorrhoea, Gee-Theyson disease or Gee disease. This is a gluten sensitive enteropathy which presents with malabsorption defect leading to loss of fat and fat soluble vitamin D in stool.

Clinical Features

1. It may cause rickets in growing child and osteomalacia in adult.
2. It starts in infant period or early childhood.
3. Infant presents with loose motion, loss of appetite and irritability.
4. Pale foul bulky stool and steatorrhoea.
5. Growth and development may undergo retardation.
6. Proximal muscle group may show wasting.
7. Abdomen is protruded.
8. Iron deficiency anemia.

Diagnostic Findings

1. Total loss of villi in duodenal biopsy.

2. Microscopic faecal smear shows fat.
3. X-ray may show intestinal dilatation.

Treatment

1. Gluten free diet. If we do not give gluten free diet, vitamin D given to patient will not be helpful in correction of intestinal malabsorption.
2. Parentral dose of high potency vitamin D.
3. Calcium lactate injection to be given by intramuscular route.
4. High protein diet.

OSTEOMALACIA

Osteomalacia is a clinical entitiy in which bones become soft due to excess of osteoid tissue and bone matrix fails to mineralize. It is adult counterpart of rickets.

Clinical Features

1. Generalized bony pain.
2. Typical muscle weakness. Patient feels himself so weak that he can not do his daily routine activity comfortably.
3. Patient has thin built contour.
4. Pathological fractures of bones are very common.
5. Bony deformities are commonly seen e.g. scoliosis, kyphosis, coxa vara, protrusion acetabuli and Regger's zersy spine.

Radiological Findings

X-ray shows following findings:

1. Persistent transverse looser's zone and demineralization are two diagnostic findings.
2. Skeletal bones show diffuse rarefaction and thinning of cortex.
3. **Looser's zone** (Milkman pseudofractures) is transverse bilateral symmetrical lines of rarefaction that do not cross the bone completely. These are commonly seen at neck femur, pubic rami, ischium, ribs, axillary border of scapula and immediately below glenoid.
4. Vertebral column gives **codfish spine** appearance because vertebral body develops biconcave shape.
5. **Compression fractures** can occur in vertebral body.
6. Females can have **triradiate pelvis.**
7. Some times **protrusion acetabuli** can also be seen.

Laboratory Findings

1. Serum calcium and phosphorus level is low.
2. Serum alkaline phosphatase is high (200–300 IU).
3. Faecal calcium is increased.
4. 24 hours urine calcium output is decreased. (80–150 mg)
5. Urine phosphorus level is also decresed.
6. Serum PTH level is increased.
7. Bone biopsy taken from iliac crest shows excess uncalcified osteoid that confirms the diagnosis.

Pathological Findings

Excess of osteoid is seen at the site of maximum stress. Compact bone is converted into cancellous bone. Fracture heals with abundant callus mainly of osteoid. So union is markedly delayed.

Treatment

Principal of treatment is that we should treat the cause of osteomalacia. Following are likey pathologies that cause development of osteomalacia:

Primary Vitamin D (nutritional) deficiency

It is not so common as vitamin D2 is supplied in fortified foods. Vitamin D given in the dose of 1000 IU–2000 IU responds well.

Vitamin D Dependent Osteomalacia

It is also known as pseudovitamin D deficiency. It has inborn error of vitamin D metabolism and inherited as recessive trait. It is most severe type of osteomalacia and requires large dose of vitamin D for treatment.

Vitamin D Resistant Familial (primary) Hypophosphatemia

In this category serum phosphorus level is low throught the life and it is sex linked dominant trait. 50,000–80,000 IU of vitamin D is required for treatment.

Phosphate Depletion (secondary) Hypophosphatemia

Some non absorbable antacids which bind to phosphate may cause phosphate depletion (on prolonged use) leading to osteomalacia. To treat this condition antacid should be stopped and phosphate supplementation should be started.

Drug Induced

Sedative, hypnotic, anticonvulsant, muscle relaxant and oral antidiabetic induce hepatic microsomal oxidase degradative enzyme, interfering in hydroxylation and conversion of vitamin D to more active metabolite. Thus it creates low level of 25(OH) calcitriol thus leading to osteomalacia. 50,000 IU of vitamin D once or twice in a week is required for treatment.

Post Gastrectomy

One gram calcium is sufficient in treatment and prophylaxis of this condition.

Renal Tubular Acidosis

In this condition hyperchloremic acidosis with hypokalemia is seen; while serum calcium level is normal. Impaired tubular transport of glucose, phosphate and amino acid is called Fanconi syndrome. Treatment includes $NaHCO_3$, K+ calcium and phosphate supplementation.

Celiac Disease

This is treated by gluten free diet and protein supplementation.

Hepatobiliary and Pancreatic disease

To treat this condition vitamin D is given through intravenous route because oral vitamin D is not effective.

Renal Osteodystrophy

This condition is treated by large doses of vitamin D (300,000 IU or 5 mg vitamin D)

Treatment of osteomalacia

Vitamin D is given in the dose of 10,000 IU. Alfacalcidol (1 alfa hydroxy vitamin D3) can be given in patient of renal disease. Hypercalcimia is it's side effect so serum calcium level should be watched during the therapy.

Calcium can be given in the dose of 0.5 gm–3 gm.

High protein diet is also required that helps in increasing the synthesis of organic matrix of bone (1 gm/kg for an adult).

Differential Diagnosis

Osteoporosis: In osteoporosis serum calcium, phosphorus and alkaline phosphatase are normal. Bone biopsy does not show osteoid tissue. In osteoporosis tissue metabolism is disturbed while calcium metabolism is normal.

Osteitis Fibrosa

It is commonly seen in hyperparathyroidism. Serum calcium and alkaline phosphatase levels are high. Serum phosphorus is low. Lamina dura is not present. Bone may show cyst or moath eaten appearance.

CHAPTER

25 Osteoporosis

- Aetiology
- Clinical features
- Treatment

When the rate of bone resorption (osteoclastic activity) exceeds the bone formation (osteoblastic activity) it results in deficiency of protein matrix in which calcium is laid down. This condition leads to diffuse reduction in bone density; known as osteoporosis. This is a metabolic bone disease commonly seen in old age people. Thickness of cortex is reduced and marrow space is widened. Cancellous trabeculae are thinned.

AETIOLOGY

(A) Postmenopausal Women

This is the most common cause of osteoporosis. In this age group sex hormones are not adequate so protein synthesis is decreased, while protein breakdown is continued.

(B) Senility

In senile age group rate of bone catabolism exceeds the bone anabolism that results in osteoporosis.

(C) Prolonged Immobilization

Bone production occurs in response to stress and strain. If patient is kept immobilized for a prolonged period he will not face major stress and strain which is essential stimuli for bone production. So bone production hampers while breakdown process exceeds the buildup rate. So patient suffers from osteoporosis.

(D) Protein Deficiency

Protien deficiency occurs in malabsorption, malnutrition, third degree burn, chronic draing sinus and nephrosis.

(E) Sudeck's Dystrophy

Traumatized areas stimulate sympathetics that causes local vasodilatation and sluggish blood flow and cause local osteoporosis. Other features of sudeck's dystrophy are pain, swelling, red shiny skin, raised temperature of skin and hyperhydrosis.

(F) Endocrinal Causes

1. Hypogonadism
2. Early menopause
3. Thyrotoxicosis
4. Hyperparathyroidism

(G) GIT Causes

1. Malabsorption

2. Inflammatory bowel disease
3. Chronic liver disease

(H) Inflammatory Causes

1. Ankylosing spondylitis
2. Rheumatoid arthritis

(I) Inherited Disease

1. Osteogenesis imperfecta
2. Gaucher disease
3. Homocystinuria

(J) Others

1. Corticosteroid intake
2. Alcohol and smoking
3. Low calcium intake
4. Highly trained atheletes
5. Neoplasia
6. Myeloma
7. Anorexia nervosa
8. Mastocytosis
9. Juvenile cause
10. Pregnancy associated

CLINICAL FEATURES

Patient often seeks medical advice with complaint of pain in thoracic region or lumbar region. Patient also presents with fracture (colles/vertebral/hip) as a result of trivial trauma. Pain of vertebral fracture often radiates anteriorly with a nerve root distribution. This acute backache is sometimes is so severe that it may mimic myocardial infarction. Kyphosis (Gibbus) may be seen due to anterior wedge compression fracture of vertebrae.

X-ray Findings

Osteoporosis has a list of radiological features as follows:

1. X-ray shows diffuse radiolucency in bone.
2. Transverse trabeculation cannot be seen.
3. Anterior cortices are not well defined.
4. Anterior wedge compression of thoracic vertebrae.
5. Lumbar vertebrae are biconcave and lumbar disc are ballooned.
6. Compression fractures of vertebrae are seen.
7. Loss of vertebral hight.
8. Codfish spine. Disc bulges into vertebral bodies and cause biconcave central compression.
9. Ground glass appearance.
10. Singh index: It is based on trabecular pattern of neck femur and has been graded from 1–6.
11. Metacarpal and vertebral index.
12. Pathological fractures.

Indications for Bone Densitometry

1. It should be reserved for those patients who have been diagnosed as osteoporosis on clinical ground and their plane X-ray is normal.
2. Elderly menopausal females.
3. All the causes of osteoporosis as mentioned above.

Technique for Bone Densitometry

Cortical bone minerals in appendicular skeleton can be assessed by a single photon absorptiometry, while dual photon absorptiometry and quantitative CT scan is helpful in assessment of mineral status of axial skeleton.

Total body neutron activation is helpful in determination of calcium content of whole body.

Lab Findings

Serum calcium, phosphorus and alkaline phosphatase are within normal limit. Level of 17 ketosteroid in urinary excretion is slightly on higher side. Urinary excretion of calcium and phosphorus is slightly higher than intake.

TREATMENT

1. **Estrogen and Androgen** produce protein anabolic effect. We should start with Premarin (1.25 mg) orally thrice in a day for one month. Skip this treatment for one week. After one week this treatment is repeated. Premarin is a conjugated estrogen. Major action of estrogen is to reduce maturation and activity of osteoclast by modifying regulatory cytokine signals from osteoblast. Estrogen directly accelerates their apoptosis of osteoclasts. Estrogen maintains the bone mass by retaining bone resorption. It inhibits osteoclasts formation and increases expression of bone matrix protein (osteonectin, osteocalcin, collagen and alkaline phosphatase. Estrogen induces the renal hydroxylating enzyme which generates active vitamin D3 which in turn promotes positive calcium balance. Estrogen must be continued for long duration even for years. Estrogen starts it's effect within 6 days. It reaches at maximum level in one month. Its effect is maintained for 30–50 days after the treatment is stopped. Androgen is given through buccal mucosa in the form of linguasorbs (6mg) thrice in a day.
2. **Calcium & Vitamin D** can only be given in presence of negative calcium balance. Otherwise excess of calcium may cause hypercalcimia and renal calculi. Calcium gluconate (10%) can be given by intravenous injection once in a day for two weeks (15 mg/kg body weight). This calcium suppresses parathyroid functions and stimulates the release of thyrocalcitonin which decreases the resorption of bone mineral. Vitamin D is given in the form of **calcirol D3 sachet** in ½ cup of milk twice in a week. It increases calcium absorption from gut. Calcirol D3 contains 60,000 IU in 1gm granule given at 3–4 weeks interval followed by every 2–6 months. Alfacalcidol is equally effective as calcirol D3. It can be started with the dose of 1–2 microgram/day. Repeated serum calcium level is essential for regulation of maintenance dose. Alfacalcidol should be stopped if serum calcium level rises.
3. **High protein diet and low fat diet** is required in case of gastrointestinal pathology. Vitamin B_{12}, Calcium lactate and liver extract can be given by intramuscular route.
4. **Calcitonin** inhibits bone resorption by direct action on osteoclast. It also inhibits proximal tubular reabsorption of calcium and phosphate by direct action on kidney thus producing hypocalcemia. This is usually given in postmenopausal osteoporosis. (100 IU s.c./i.m. route daily along with calcium and vitamin D. A nasal spray (MIACALCIN 200 IU) is also available in our country. Its effect is seen after 6 month therapy. One spray is given in each nostril at a time in a day. It increases bone mineral density in postmenopausal women. Calcitonin is given when estrogen can not be given and women are in menopause for at least 5 years.
5. **Biphosphonate** inhibits bone resorption. Alendronate (Osteophos 5–10 mg 1 OD) is most suitable drug in prevention and treatment of osteoporosis. This is given with empty stomach in morning with a glass of water. Patient is instructed neither to lie down nor to take food for 30 minutes to prevent oesophagitis. Tea, coffee, fruit juice,

calcium, iron, antacids and mineral water interfere its absorption. NSAID may precipitate gastric irritation.

Zolandronic acid is also being used for the treatment of postmenopausal osteoporosis. This is given by diluting it with 500 ml of normal saline and to be infused at least in one hour.

6. **Sodium fluoride** is effective in reducing the pain and tendency to fracture in osteoporosis. This is given in the form of gelatin capsule because it may cause gastric irritation. (0.5 mg/kg/day) Bone matrix is deposited around thin trabeculae by fluoride.
7. **Exercises** are also effective specially spinal extension exercises which provoke new bone formation and reduce compression forces on vertebral bodies.
8. **Bracing/Spinal orthosis** is also effective. ASHE brace or Taylor brace can also be prescribed prophylactically to prevent major pathological fractures.

Latest Treatment of Osteoporosis

Denosumab

(Ref: New England journal of medicine feb 2000). This is a fully human monoclonal antibody (Ig G2) to RANK ligand (RANKL). It blocks interaction of RANKL to RANK. This is given subcutaneously either every 3 months (6, 14 or 30 mg) or every 6 months (14, 60, 100 or 210 mg). Bone marrow density is increased after the use of Denosumab.

Side effects of Denosumab are arthralgia, back pain, hypertension and nasopharyngitis.

Denosumab is also being used for treatment of Rheumatoid arthritis. (discussed in chapter 35 under rheumatoid arthritis)

Teriparatide

This is latest drug to be used for treatment of osteoporosis. Teriparatide was approved by FDA on Nov. 26, 2002 to treat osteoporosis in postmenopausal women and in men with hypogonadal or idiopathic osteoporosis, who have high risk for fractures.

This is synthetic form of human PTH. This is the only anabolic agent available for treatment of osteoporosis, while others are catabolic agents. This is first drug to cause new bone formation.

Dose: FDA has approved 20 mcg/day by subcutaneous route to be given in thigh or abdomen. Treatment should be given for 18–24 months. Concurrent use of biphosphonate should be avoided.

Tereparatide comes in a preloaded pen with 28 doses. This should be kept in refrigerator. New needle should be used for each injection. Daily dose is required because body eliminates it very quickly.

Among patients with glucocorticoid induced osteoporosis who were at high risk of fracture, bone marrow density is increased more in patients receiving teriparatide than in those receiving alendronate. (Ref. New England Journal of medicine Nov. 2007)

Indications:

Teriparatide is indicated in following conditions:

1. Severe osteoporosis with compression fracture.
2. Repeated fractures despite prolonged use of biphosphonate.
3. T score < –3.5 on Bone marrow density.
4. Osteoporotic patients taking high dose of prednisolone for prolonged time.

Contraindication

Teriparatide is contra indicated in following conditions:

1. Children and adolescents.
2. Bone cancer.
3. Patient receiving radiation therapy.
4. Pagets disease.
5. Hypercalcemia and hyperparathyroidism.
6. Pregnant and lactating mother.
7. Gout.

Side Effects

- Dizziness
- Nausea
- Heart burn
- Diarrhoea
- Headache
- Leg cramps
- Weakness
- Depression
- Hypotension (while standing) can occur with initial few doses.

Cost of Teriparatide: $ 516 per month.

CHAPTER

26 Scurvy

- Scurvy
- Gout
- Fluorosis
- Hypoparathyroidism
- Pseudohypoparathyroidism
- Hypophosphatasia

SCURVY

This is a nutritional deficiency disorder caused by vitamin C deficiency. Scurvy is also known as **Scorbutus.** Tissue and cells which are mesodermal in origin are primarily affected in scurvy.

Aetiology

Infants of age group 5 months to 10 months which are artificially fed are more prone to develop scurvy. Exclusive breast feeding may also develop scurvy in infants if vitamin D is not supplemented. Combination of scurvy and rickets is known as **Barton's Disease.** Elderly people may also develop scurvy if their diet is devoid of vitamin C.

Pathology

Capillary haemorrhage

It commonly occurs beneath mucous membrane as the cohesive property of matrix of connective tissue and endothelium is impaired. Cunjuctiva, gum, skin, intestine, kidney and bladder are other sites where haemorrhage can occur.

Subperiosteal haemorrhage

It may cause ballooning out of periosteum thus giving false impression of bone tumor. This blood is usually converted into fibrous tissue.

Supplementation of vitamin C may ossify this blood later on.

Metaphyseal haemorrhage

It can interfere with growth of osteoblastic tissue.

Wimberger line

This is calcified cartilage which encircles the epiphysis. It is visile as dense line on X-ray.

Scurvy line

It is translucent zone in metaphysis adjacent to white line of frankle, seen in X-ray.

White line of Frankel

It is broad layer of calcified cartilage between epiphysis and metaphysis.

Pelkan spur

It is a bony spur usually arising from medial border of metaphysis at it's junction with epiphysis.

Osteogenesis is impaired while osteoclasis continues. Bone show **ground glass appearance** in X-ray as trabeculae are thinned and poorly visible.

In infants **pathological fractures** occur through metaphysis, while in adults it occurs through diaphysis.

Teeth become loose due to porosis of alveolar bone. Enamel is not affected. Haemorrhage occurs in pulp as well as in gums. So gums are swollen. Papillae between teeth are also swollen known as **Scurvy buds.**

Clinical Features

If the diet is deficient in vitamin C continuously for 2-3 months; following clinical manifestations start to appear:

1. Gum bleeding occurs usually from upper central incisor teeth. Teeth become loose and brittle. Enamel is not affected.
2. Petechiae or echymosis.
3. Haematemesis or haematuria may be seen.
4. Chronic disease presents with anorexia, weight loss, secondary anemia, fever and pneumonia. Sometimes it may be fatal if not treated properly.
5. Pseudoparalysis is a distinctive clinical feature. Infant presents with voluntary immobilization of extremities as the muscles are in spasm. If infant attempts to move the limbs, it causes excruciating pain in limb due to spasm. Infant is pale, febrile and restless. He may present with night cry.
6. Subperiosteal haemorrhage persists as fixed, palpable and painful swelling over the bone.
7. Epiphyseal fracture sepration is commonly seen at lower end femur, upper end of tibia and humerus.
8. Metaphyseal fracture is seen in infant while adult patient shows diaphyseal fracture.
9. Typical costchondral sepration is present. Sharp anterior ends form **scorbutic rosary** in contrast to rounded prominence in rachitic rosary.

Investigations

Blood level of vitamin C is less than 0.5 mg. (normal 1 mg/dl)

X-ray Findings

Scurvy has classical radiological features as follows:

1. **Wimberger line** is dense line encircling the epiphysis is caused by calcification of cartilage.
2. **Scurvy line** is translucent zone in metaphysis.
3. **White line of Frankel** is a broad layer of calcified cartilage in between epiphysis and metaphysis.
4. **Pelkan spur** is a bony spur usually arises from medial border of metaphysis at its junction with epiphysis.
5. Cortex is thin.
6. Subperiosteal haemorrhage and fractures are seen.
7. Ground glass appearance of bone due to thin trabeculation.
8. Epiphyseal fracture separation is also seen.
9. Angulation is seen at costochondral junction and vertebral ends of ribs.

Treatment

Supplementation of vitamin C in form of fruit juice can be given. Tablet of vitamin C is also given. Processed milk should be stopped. No attempt should be taken to reduce the fracture and it should be immobilized. Iron and folic acid can be given to correct anemia.

Differential Diagnosis

Rickets

In rickets; we do not find dense zone of calcification. Metaphyseal cupping is seen.

Acute poliomyelitis

It is pure motor neurone disease. Bony abnormality is not seen. Meningeal sign may be seen.

Acute osteomylitis

Patient is febrile and may also present with localized pain, raised temperature and raised leukocyte count.

Osteogenesis imperfecta

It presents with diaphyseal fracture while metaphyseal fractures are seen in scurvy.

Luetic osteochondritis

In this condition children of less than 3 months age are affected. Mother often has history of repeated abortions. Mother is sero positive.

GOUT

This is a hereditary metabolic disorder, which presents with hyperuricemia, tophi deposits, arthritis, nephritis, renal calculi and cardiovascular lesion. This is predominantly seen in male patients of 30–40 years of age and usually seen in family.

Pathogenesis

In acute gout; urate crystals are deposited in synovial fluid where they induce inflammatory reaction. Granulocytes migrate into joint and phagocytose urate crystal and release a glycoprotein that aggravates inflammation by releasing lysosomal enzyme and by increasing lactic acid production. Lysosomal enzyme destroys the joint. Increased production of lactic acid decreases the local ph leading to precipitation of more urate crystal in local area. Most common joint to be affected is first metatarsophalangeal joint of big toe. Gout may also cause fibrous ankylosis and granular fibrosis. If death occurs due to gout, it is either due to coronary or cerebral vascular disease or nephrosclerosis with uremia.

Predisposing Factors

1. Prolonged walk.
2. Liver extract drugs.
3. High fatty diet.
4. Operative procedures.
5. Prolonged exposure to cold.
6. Withdrawl of ACTH.

Clinical Features

Most common presentation is painful, swollen, red hot, tender first metatarsophalangeal joint of big toe. Pain frequently occurs during night and disturbs the sleep. Other joints to be involved are knee, ankle, wrist and elbow. Mild attack resolves within 2 days, while severe attack may lasts for 7 days. Patient may also present with small deposits of urate crystal in ear lobule known as tophi. Later patient may develop arthritic changes that can cripple the patient.

Diagnostic Features of Gout

GOUT can be diagnosed by following features:

1. Hyperuricemia
2. Frequent attack of pain with interval of freedom from pain.
3. Family history of gout
4. Urate calculus
5. Response to colchicin.

Investigations

1. Hyperuricemia >5 mg/dl. (normal plasma urate level is 1–4 mg/dl).
2. Decreased urinary ketosteroid is less than 3 mg/day is a constant feature.

3. **Murexide test.** Add nitric acid to tophi or synovial fluid of a patient of gout and then evaporate it. Now moisture it with ammonium hydroxide, a purple color is developed due to formation of murexide. This test is positive in gout.

X-ray Findings

Following three radiological features are commonly seen in GOUT:

1. Destruction of cartilage
2. Reduced joint space
3. Punched out appearance in bone as urate crystals replace the bony structure.

Treatment

Acute attack

Colchicine is drug of choice in acute attack. NSAID can be used as strong anti-inflammatory drug, while intraarticular soluble steroid can provide symptomatic relief. Colchicine (Colhidone/Goutnic) is given 1 mg orally followed by 0.25 mg 1–3 hourly till control of acute attack is achieved or diarrhea occurs. Patient gets so dramatic relief that it can be used as a diagnostic test. Maintenance dose (0.5–1 mg/day) is given for 1-2 months.

Colchicine inhibits the release of glycoprotein and subsequent events. It dose not affect the phagocytosis of urate crystal.

Chronic Gout

Patient of gout can be divided into under excretor and over producer. Probenecid or sufinpyrazone (uricosuric drug) are used in under excretor. Allopurinol is preferably used in over producer. Allopurinol can be used in both.

Probenecid and sufinpyrazone are equally effective. Both are neither analgesic nor anti-inflammatory. Probenecid is started 250 mg 1 B.D. for one week then 500mg 1 B.D. (maximum dose is 1 gm 1B.D.)

Sulfinpyrazone is started with 100–200 mg 1 B.D. Then it is increased gradually depending upon response. (maximum dose is 800 mg/day)

Allopurinol (short acting) is competitive inhibitor of xanthine oxidase. Its major active metabolite alloxanthine (oxypurine) is long acting non competitive inhibitor. It is started with 100 mg 1 OD; gradually increased to a maintenance dose of 300 mg/day. Its maximum dose is 600 mg/day.

Surgical procedure

This is indicated when conservative treatment has failed and joint shows destructive changes. Following procedures can be done:

1. Excision of gouty lesion.
2. Surgical stabilization of joint in functional position.
3. Immobilization of affected joint will lessen the chance of joint destruction.

Complications

1. Urate crystal may cause renal failure and haematuria.
2. Chronic glomerulonephritis and interstitial nephritis may lead to uremia and death.
3. Hypertension and arteriosclerosis.

Conditions of Secondary Hyperuricemia

There are a lot of conditions which can cause hyperuricemia:

1. Leukemia
2. Lymphoma
3. Polycythemia
4. Thiazide
5. Furosemide
6. Pyrazinamide
7. Ethambutol
8. Levadopa
9. Clofibrate

PSEUDOGOUT

This is arthropathy of larger joints (mainly knee joint) in which calcium pyrophosphate is deposited in joints. This condition is less severe than gout.

FLUOROSIS

Fluorosis is an endemic disease of Punjab, Andhra and Tamilnadu states. It occurs due to excessive ingestion of fluoride in drinking water (1 ppm). This leads to excess of deposition of calcium in bone and soft tissue.

Clinical Features

Patient presents with mottled enamel of teeth, usually in upper incisor teeth. Later teeth fall off. This condition is known as **dental fluorosis.**

Later patient presents with backache and stiffness in spine with tingling numbness in limb. Posterior spinal ligament is calcified, which may compress the cord leading to paraparesis. This condition is known as **skeletal fluorosis.**

X-ray Findings

Calcification of posterior spinal ligament or ischiopubic rami/sacroiliac ligament/interosseous membrane of forearm is seen.

Lab Findings

1. Raised serum fluoride level
2. Raised urine and drinking water level of fluoride
3. Raised level of fluoride is seen in bone biopsy.

Treatment

Best treatment is prevention. Defluorinated water should be used.

PRIMARY HYPERPARATHYROIDISM

In this condition excess of PTH is secreted (by a parathyroid adenoma) leading to increased number of osteoclasts and fibrous replacement of bone marrow. This condition leads to hypophosphatemia and hypercalcemia. Alkaline phosphatase level is increased. Conditons in which primary hyperparathyroidism occur are osteitis fibrosa cystica, parathyrotoxicosis and Von-reckling hausen disease.

Clinical Features

Patient presents with severe low bachache, generalized muscular weakness, hypotonia and limb deformity. Patient may also present with pathological fracture and delayed union, polyuria, polydypsia and renal calculi.

Brown tumor is not a true tumor; instead it is a localized accumulation of haemorrhage, blood pigment and reactive masses of osteoclasts in a spindle cell stroma.

Radiological Features

Following radiological features may be present:

1. Bony deformity and pathological fractures.
2. Cyst in skeleton and marrow fibrosis.
3. Pin head stippling in skull.
4. Collapse of vertebrae and ballooned disc.
5. **Subperiosteal resorption of phalanx** and lateral end of clavicle.

Lab Findings

Blood investigations show following findings:

1. Hypercalcemia
2. Hypercalciuria
3. Hyperphosphaturia
4. Hypophosphatemia
5. High alkaline phosphatase

Treatment

Parathyroidectomy is treatment of choice provided renal function and serum alkaline phosphatase level should be normal.

Differential Diagnosis

1. Osteomalacia (marrow fibrosis is absent)
2. Osteoporosis (marrow fibrosis is absent)
3. Sarcoidosis (hypercalcemia)
4. Vitamin D intoxication (hypercalcemia)

SECONDARY HYPERPARATHYROIDISM

To compensate prolonged hypocalcemia, parathyroid gland undergoes hyperplasia. So PTH secretion increases. This condition is known as secondary hyperparathyroidism and seen in CRF, malabsorption, osteomalacia and rickets.

TERTIARY HYPERPARATHYROIDISM

In these conditions continuos stimulation of parathyroid causes adenoma formation and autonomous PTH secretion. Serum calcium is raised while PTH is not suppressed. Plasma phosphate and alkaline phosphatase is high. Renal impairment is a associated feature.

HYPOPARATHYROIDISM

Hypoparathyroidism is clinically characterized by twitching, carpopaedal spasm, laryngeal spasm, convulsion, positive chvostek sign and trousseau sign. Accidental removal of parathyroid gland during thyroidectomy results into hypoparathyroidism. Patient suffers from hypocalcemia and hypophosphatemia.

Treatment

1. Parathyroid hormone should be given. Alternatively 2–4 ml dihydrotachysterol can be given orally. It's dose is regulated by Sulkowitch test.
2. Milk is contraindicated due to its high phosphorus content.
3. Calcium gluconate injection can be given to treat tetany.
4. Magnesium sulfate infusion can restore the calcium level to normal.

PSEUDOHYPOPARATHYROIDISM

Congenital deficiency of adenyl cyclase causes this rare disease. In this condition target organ like kidney and bone do not respond to hormone while PTH production is adequate. Patient has short stature and short metacarpal on ulnar side. If we give parathyroid extract to patient typical clinical and blood chemistry changes fail to develop.

Lab Findings

1. Urinary excretion of c-AMP is decreased or absent.
2. Urinary phosphorus is reduced.

Treatment

Dehydrotachysterol and vitamin D2 is given to treat this condition.

HYPOPHOSPHATASIA

In this condition patient presents with persistent low serum alkaline phosphatase level resembling with rickets. Severe cases are fatal.

Clinical Features

1. Failure to gain weight.
2. Walking and dentition are delayed.
3. Frequent vomiting.
4. Short bones.
5. Thickend epiphysis and beaded ribs.
6. Prone to develop fractures around metaphysis.
7. Unsteady gait.
8. Impaired vision due to craniostenosis.

9. Premature loss of deciduous teeth.
10. Skull is soft and becomes leather like.

Investigations

1. Low alkaline phosphatase level.
2. Urinary excretion of phosphoethanolamine is increased.
3. X-ray shows demineralization of bone.

Treatment

Correction of serum phosphate level is treatment of choice. It should not be taken lightly as severe cases are fatal.

CHAPTER

27 Congenital Diseases

- Congenital talipes equino varus
- Acquired talipes equino varus
- Congenital dislocation of hip
- Bilateral CDH
- Sprengel's deformity
- Torticollis
- Cleidocranial dysostosis
- Congenital coxa vara
- Congenital pseudoarthrosis of tibia
- Madelung's deformity
- Klippel-feil syndrome
- Congenital deformities of hand
- Congenital absence of radius
- Congenital absence of fibula
- Proximal femoral focal deficiency
- Congenital dislocation of knee
- Congenital absence of patella

CONGENITAL TALIPES EQUINO VARUS

CTEV (Club foot)

CTEV is a gross deformity of foot and presents since birth. Word talipes is derived from latin language which means ankle bone, whereas pes means foot. In this deformity adduction and inversion are combinedly present, known as varus.

In CTEV; foot is small and bean shaped with a smaller heel. Tendoachillis is contracted. Splaying is seen in forefoot.

B.N. Sinha index explains severity of forefoot adduction. Normally ratio of medial to lateral border of foot is 1.2. In CTEV this ratio is reversed i.e. lateral to medial border ratio becomes 1.2. This index was described by Prof. B.N. Sinha (KGMC). Skin creases are present posteriorly above the heel and medially at the forefoot and hindfoot junction. Callosities are present over dorsolateral aspect of foot. Bony prominence may also be seen at this place. Wasting of calf muscle is also seen. Ratio of muscle belly to tendon is reversed from 2:1 to 1:2.

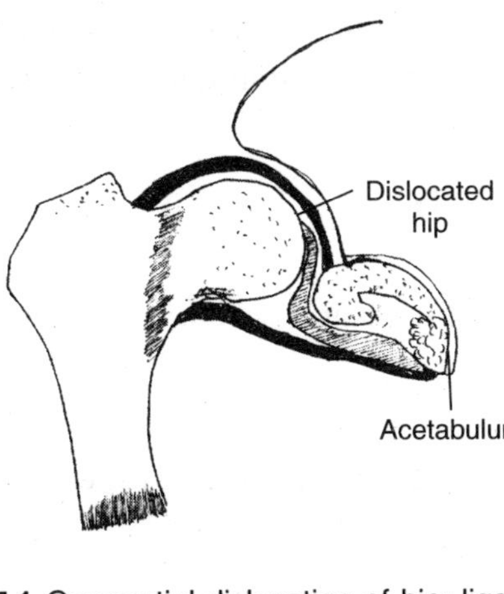

Fig. 27.1 Congential dislocation of hip: ligamentum teres and acetbular labrum is hypertrophied

Applied Anatomy of Foot

Following joints are significant due to their corresponding deformities:

Plantar flexion is seen at **ankle joint.**

Inversion is seen at **subtalar joint.**

Adduction is seen at **midtarsal joint.**

Head of talus faces inferomedially and its neck is angulated while calcaneum is small and concave medially.

Major Ligaments of Foot

Deltoid ligament

This is also known as medial collateral ligament of ankle. In surgery of CTEV, superficial part (tibionavicular, tibiocalcaneal and posterior tibiotalar ligament) of ligament is excised while deep part (anterior tibiotalar ligament) is left behind.

Talocalcaneal ligament

This is also known as interosseous ligament that connects talus and calcaneum. This ligament is also released in posteromedial soft tissue release operation of CTEV.

Spring ligament

This ligament connects anterior end of calcaneum to navicular.

Capsular ligament

Capsular ligament of naviculo-cuneiform, ligament between cuneiform and first metatarsal joint are also released.

Terminology

Equinus

Foot is fixed in plantar flexion and patient walks on toes.

Calcaneus

Foot is fixed in dorsiflexion and patient walks on heel.

Varus

Foot is fixed in inversion and adduction at midtarsal joint. Sole of foot faces medially (inward).

Valgus

Foot is abducted and everted at midtarsal joint. Sole faces outward.

Planus

Longitudinal arch of foot is flattened.

Splay

Transverse arch of foot is flattened.

Cavus

Exaggerated longitudinal arch of foot is known as cavus.

Mobile CTEV

Deformities of foot can be partially corrected.

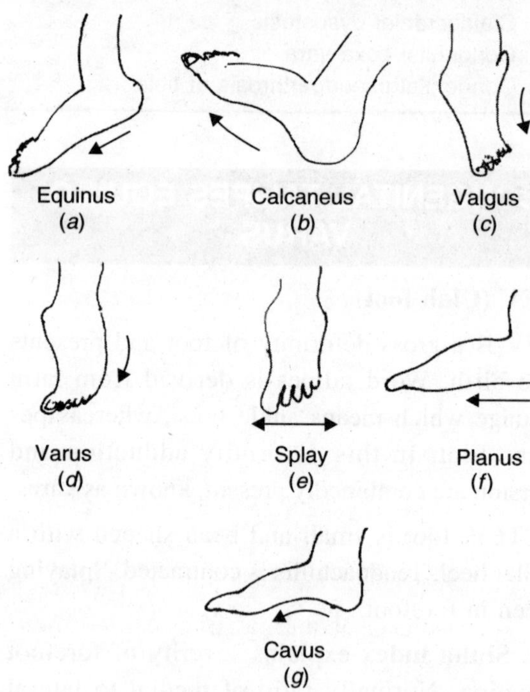

Fig. 27.2 Types of foot deformity

Rigid CTEV

Deformities can be hardly corrected or only one component of deformity can be corrected.

Resistant CTEV

If CTEV does not respond to treatment, it is known as resistant CTEV.

Relapse CTEV

If deformity recurs inspite of getting adequate treatment; it is called as relapse CTEV.

Neglected CTEV

If patient has not taken any treatment for a long time; it is known as neglected CTEV.

Etiology of CTEV

Idiopathic is commonest cause.

Neurogenic

1. Spina bifida occulta
2. Meningocoele
3. Meningomyelocoele
4. Diastematomyelia
5. Cerebral palsy

Myopathic

Arthrogryposis multiplex congenital

Osteopathic

Congenital absence of fibula is a common example.

Theories of Etiology

1. Intrauterine compression, forcing the foot against the uterine wall, thus creating deformity in foot.
2. Arrest in foetal development.
3. Dysplasia of muscles that causes muscle imbalance.
4. Abnormal tendon insertion particularly tibialis anterior.

ACQUIRED TALIPES EQUINO VARUS

This is characterized by following features:

1. Deformities take time to develop and appear late in life.
2. Muscle wasting is seen in various muscle groups.
3. Deformities can be corrected if treated prior to development of contracture.
4. History suggestive of polio is present (URI, high grade pyrexia and paralysis).

Etiology (Acquired Talipes Equino Varus)

1. Commonest cause is poliomyelitis.
2. Local contracture of foot due to burn or infection.
3. Lateral popliteal nerve palsy.
4. Freidrich's ataxia.
5. Peroneal muscle dystrophy.

Pathology

Bony changes

Neck of talus is angulated in such a way that the head of talus faces downward and medially. Calcaneum is small and concave medially.

Deformities	**Joints**
Equinus	Ankle joint
Inversion	Subtalar joint
Forefoot adduction	Midtarsal joint
Forefoot cavus	Midtarsal joint

Changes in muscles and tendon

Posteromedial muscle group is contracted.

Tendoachillis is at posterior aspect while tibialis posterior, Flexor digitorum longus and flexor hallucis are situated at medial aspect of leg.

CHAPTER 27

Changes in capsule and ligament

Posterior capsule of ankle, subtalar, talofibular and calcaneofibular joints are contracted.

Ligaments

Following 3 ligaments at **medial aspect** of leg are contracted:

1. Talonavicular ligament
2. Deltoid ligament
3. Spring ligament

Following 3 structures at plantar aspect are also contracted:

1. Plantar fascia
2. Plantar ligament
3. Interosseous ligament between talus and calcaneum

Skin changes

1. Deep medial crease
2. Dimple at lateral aspect of ankle and midfoot

Secondary changes

Development of callosities and bursae over bony prominence or at lateral aspect of foot are common.

Clinical Features

Child can present in OPD in following periods:

1. At birth (deformity is mild and also known as postural equinovarus).
2. Early infancy period.
3. Late infancy and early childhood.
4. Late childhood.

Examination Findings

To rule out CTEV, just dorsiflex the foot till dorsum touches anterior aspect of shin of tibia. If it is possible, CTEV can be ruled out.

Examination findings have been discussed under heading of club foot earlier.

General Examination

1. Spine must always be examined to look any evidence of open neural tube defect e.g. spina bifida, meningomyelocoele.
2. Look for tuft of hair or naevus or lipomatous mass at low back in case of spina bifida occulta.
3. Midline soft tissue mass is suggestive of meningocoele or meningomyelocoele.
4. Always look for other congenital anomalies e.g. cleft lip, supernumerary digits. So always look at limbs, face, chest and abdomen.
5. Congenital dislocation of hip should be looked for.

Indications of X-ray

1. Neglected CTEV (To look for bony changes e.g. superior articulating surface of talus is partially out of ankle mortis that may change the preoperative planning of surgeon)
2. Tripple arthrodesis.
3. To detect Kite angle. (Angle between long axis of talus and calcaneum is called as Kite angle. Normally it is >35 degree. In CTEV this angle is reduced)

Treatment

1. Start the treatment as soon as possible or from the day one of seeing patient.
2. First 3 weeks since birth are called golden period for treatment because in this period relaxin hormone remains in circulation that keeps the ligaments relaxed. So they are amenable to stretching.
3. In new born child skin is not mature enough for plaster so mother should be taught about repeated stretching and corrective manipulation of foot 5–6 times in a day or

while at every time of feeding till 2–4 weeks.

4. Treatment for the age group of 1 month to 3 years is repeated stretching and corrective manipulation followed by retention of correction in AKPOP cast till over correction is achieved. Knee is kept at 90 degree of flexion. To check over correction just tickle the sole. if dorsiflexion and adduction both are present it means over correction is achieved. BKPOP cast usually slips like a socks, so always apply AKPOP cast. It can also take care of internal tibial torsion deformity if present in child.
5. Sequence of correction starts from Adduction-Inversion-Equinus. If we do not follow this sequence, child will develop **Rocker bottom foot**. (convexity develops at sole of foot).
6. Aim of treatment is to provide painless, mobile and cosmetically normal appearing foot.
7. After achieving the correction Denis-Brown splint or Night shoes are prescribed to patient of less than walking age group. These shoes should be worn throughout day and night and can be removed 4–5 times in a day to clean and manipulate the foot. Both the shoes are connected by a connecting bar which is connected in such a way that dynamic correction of deformity occurs while child kicks his leg.
8. Orthopaedic boot with straight and stiff border, with outside crooked and elongated heel are prescribed to child of more than walking age group. Forefoot adduction is corrected by straight and stiff medial border. Correction of varus is maintained by outside crooked and elongated heel. Denis Brown splint can be prescribed to these children during night time. These orthopaedic shoes should be used till bony maturity has achieved. (till 10–12 years of age).

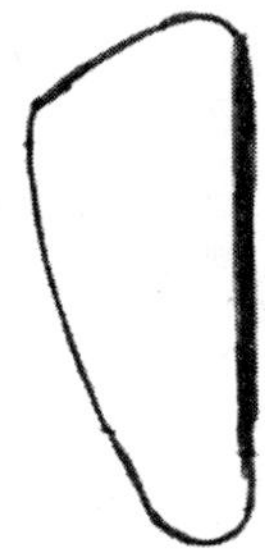

Fig. 27.3 (*a*) Left shoe with straight stiff inner border

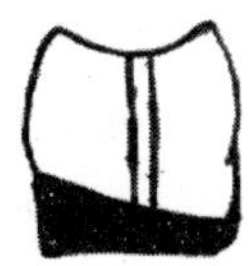

Fig. 27.3 (*b*) Lateral shoe raise (Left shoe)

Complications

Conservative treatment can have following complications:

1. Recurrence of CTEV
2. Plaster sore
3. Painful and stiff foot
4. Table top talus (Flat toped talus) can occur due to osteochondral compression fracture of talus.
5. Rocker bottom foot.
6. Neurovascular deficit of foot.

Surgical Treatment

Posteromedial Soft Tissue Release (PMSTR)

This operation can be done upto 3 years of age.

Following **posterior structures** are released:

1. Lenghtening of tendoachillis by Z-plasty.
2. Posterior capsulotomy of ankle and subtalar joint.

3. Release of posterior talofibular and calcaneofibular ligament.

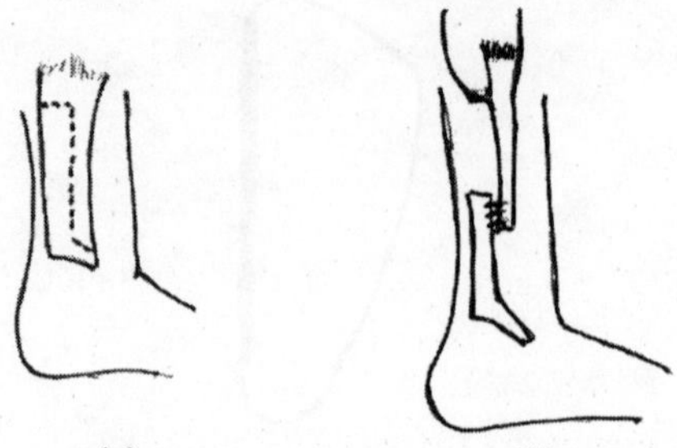

Fig. 27.4 Z-plasty of tendoachillis

Following **medial structures** are released:

1. Lengthening of tendons of
   A. Tibialis posterior
   B. Flexor digitorum longus
   C. Flexor hallucis longus
2. Three ligaments are released:
   A. Talonavicular ligament
   B. Deltoid ligament (superficial ligament)
   C. Spring ligament
3. Capsule of naviculocuneiform and cuneiform-first metatarsal joint are released. Interosseous talocalcaneal ligament are also released.

Steindler's Release

Plantar release

Extraperiosteal release of structure from medial calcaneal tuberosity is known as Steindler's release. Following structures are released:

1. Plantar apponeurosis
2. Flexor hallucis brevis
3. Abductor hallucis
4. Abductor digiti quinti minimi

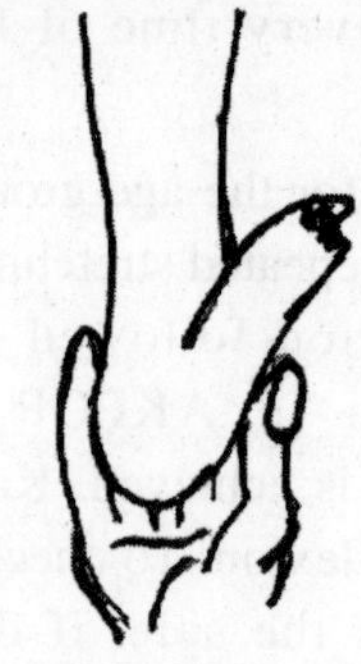

Fig. 27.5 Normally dorsum of foot can be made to touch, shin of leg

Limited soft tissue release

If only one component of deformity remains after conservative treatment, limited (selective) soft tissue release can be done e.g. posterior release for equinus, medial release for adduction and plantar release for cavus deformity.

Tendon Transfer

At the age of 5 years, tendon transfer can be done. Tibialis anterior can be transferred to outer side of foot.

Dwyer's Osteotomy

This osteotomy is done **at the age of 3 years** to correct the varus at heel. Before the age of 3 years it is not recommended as the calcaneum is cartilaginous. This is an open wedge osteotomy of calcaneum by which varus of heel can be corrected.

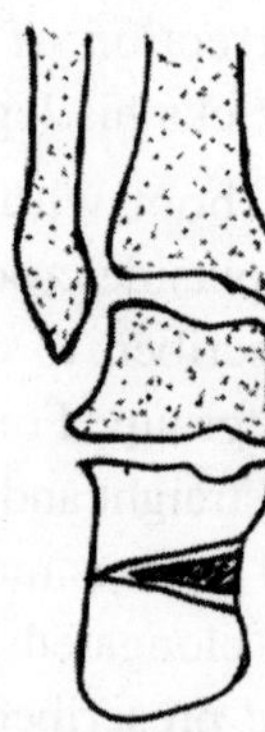

Fig. 27.6 Dwyer's osteotomy

Evan's Procedure

This surgery is performed at the age of **4–8 years.** This procedure is indicated in neglected or recurrent CTEV. In this procedure calcaneocuboid fusion is done along with posteromedial soft tissue release. Calcaneocuboid fusion restricts the growth on lateral side of foot, leading to gradual correction of deformity.

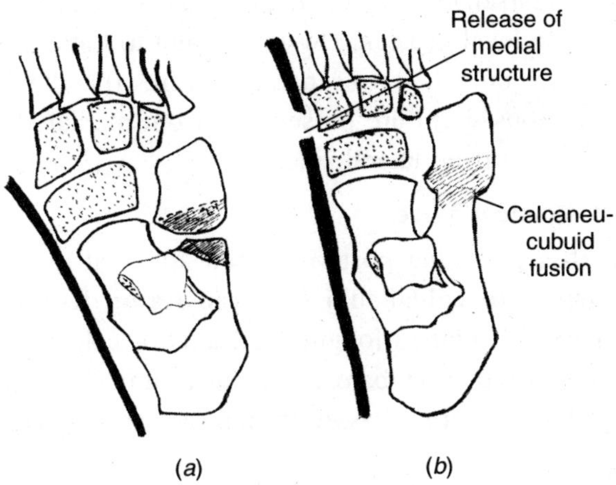

Fig. 27.7 Evan's procedure

Wedge Tarsectomy

This procedure is performed **at the age of 8–11 years.** Indication of this operation is neglected CTEV. In this operation triangular wedge of bone is removed from midtarsal area with its base facing toward dorsolateral side. After removing the wedge foot is brought in plantigrade position.

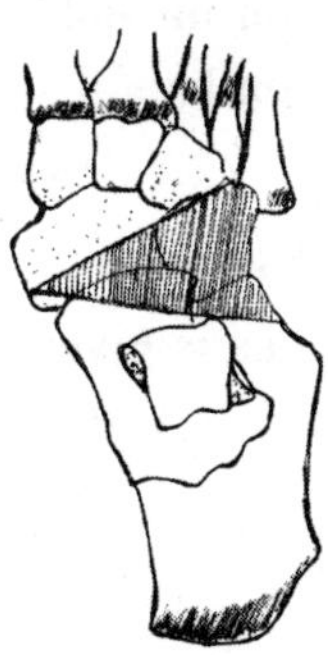

Fig. 27.8 Dorsolateral wedge tarsectomy

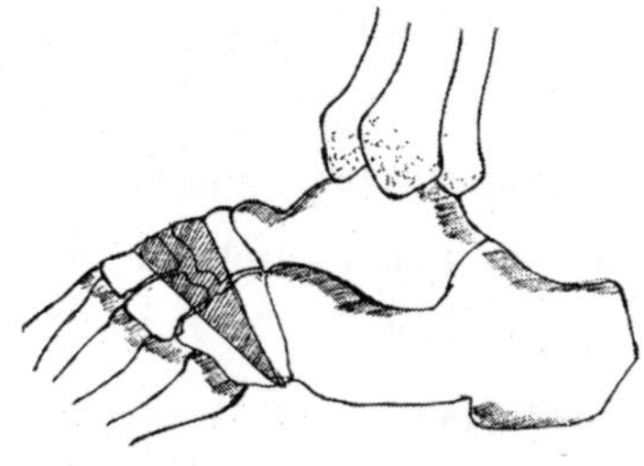

Fig. 27.9 Lateral view of wedge tarsectomy

Triple Arthrodesis

This is indicated in patients of more than 12 years of age. In this procedure 3 joints are fused; subtalar, calcaneocuboid and talonavicular.

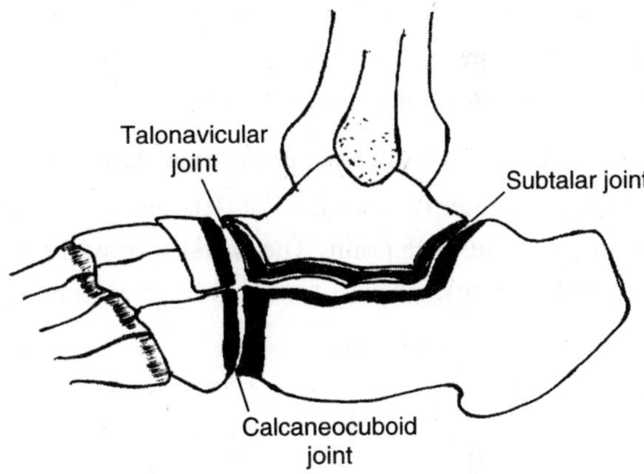

Fig. 27.10 Triple arthrodesis of ankle joint

Joshi's External Stabilization System (Jess)

JESS frame is designed by Dr. B.B. Joshi (Bombay). The principle of controlled differential distraction is applied to correct all the aspect of deformities by gradual, sequential stretching of soft tissue by Kirschner wires anchored in bone. Jess is applied in children of more than 6 years age usually. But this frame is successfully used in all presentation of CTEV in children between the age of 3 months to their adulthood.

Advantages of Jess

1. It causes lengthening of all contracted tissue, preventing histogenesis witout cutting and with minimal scaring of tissue.

2. No further shortening of foot in revision cases.
3. Magnitude of correction is controlled.
4. Results are much suppled as compared with surgical release.

Indications of Jess

1. All such cases of congenital and acquired talipes equino varus that can not be corrected by conservative treatment.
2. Relapse cases of CTEV.
3. Arthrogryposis multiplex congenita.
4. Late presentation of cases.
5. Adjunct to surgical treatment for realignment of skeleton and to minimize bone resection and shortening of foot.

Scoring for Pre-operative Clinical Assessment

This assessment comprises of 10 features. Each feature carries one point. The worst foot will have 10 points, while normal foot will have zero point.

These are the 10 features:

1. Calf atrophy
2. Medial or posterior crease
3. Cavus
4. Curved lateral border
5. Posterior displacement of fibula
6. Fixed equinus
7. Navicular fixed to medial malleolus
8. Os calcis fixed to tibia
9. No midtarsal mobility
10. Fixed forefoot supination

Assembly Planning

1. Length of outer border is measured to judge the size of distractor required.
2. Length and diameter of tibia is measured to select the size of tibiocalcaneal distractor and tibiometatarsal connecting rod.

Operative Procedure

Tibial Wires

Two parallel transfixing K-wires are passed in tibia perpendicular to its longitudinal axis from lateral to medial side. Occasionally a vertical tibial wire is passed anteroposteriorly.

Metatarsal Wires

One transfixing wire is passed from first metatarsal, engaging at least 5th and 1st metatarsal at the level of neck. Do not attempt to flatten the transvers arch. Two separate K wires (parallel to previous wire) are passed one from medial side and one from lateral side.

Calcaneal Wires

After palpating posterior tibial artery at medial aspect of calcaneum two transfixing K-wires perpendicular to longitudinal axis of calcaneum are passed into tuberosity of calcaneum. One axial calcaneal wire is passed from posterior to anterior aspect.

Assembly is connected by Z-rods.

Distraction Schedule

1. Medial tibiocalcaneal and medial calcaneometatarsal distractor nobs are rotated clockwise upto 90 degree 6 hourly thus 360 degree in 24 hours. Lateral counterparts are rotated in clockwise direction upto 90 degree 12 hourly, thus 180 degree in 24 hours.
2. Calcaneometatarsal distraction derotates calcaneum on medial side 0.2mm every 6 hourly and on lateral side 0.2mm every 12 hourly.

Static Phase of Assembly

Period of 3–6 weeks is given to this assembly as a static phase to allow soft tissue mobilization in elongated position.

Complications of Jess

Application of jess can develop following complications:

1. Contamination
2. Jamming of distractor
3. Temporary oedema
4. Superficial pin tract infection
5. Flexion contracture of toes
6. Linear skin necrosis
7. Loosening of linking joint
8. Under correction
9. Rocker bottom foot

CONGENITAL DISLOCATION OF HIP

CDH is common in western countries. In Asian countries it is uncommon due to existing culture of mother carrying her child on the side of their waist.

Etiology

Females are more commonly affected.

(Female to male ratio is 9:1)

1. **Maternal relaxin hormone** induced laxity plays a major role in etiology of CDH. Relaxin hormone crosses placenta and enters foetus. It acts on joints of foetus to produce laxity; thus predisposing CDH.
2. **Heredity** also plays a role in etiology of CDH. Hereditary conditions in which joints are lax become more prone for CDH.
3. **Breech presentation** has more chances of developing CDH. Ratio of development of CDH in breech and vertex presentation is 10:1.

Pathological Anatomy

Word dysplastic hip is also used for these congenital malformations of hip. Underlying pathology of CDH is either faulty development of acetabulum presenting with dislocation at birth or joint laxity presenting dislocation after birth. Pathological changes seen in CDH are as follows:

1. Shallow and small acetabular fossa.
2. Acetabular roof is oblique or even vertical.
3. Superior acetabular pole is grooved and irregular.
4. Femoral head is enlarged and dislocated upward and laterally.
5. Femoral neck is anteverted.
6. Ligamentum teres may be elongated/ hypertrophied/degenerated/attenuated or absent.
7. Adductor muscles are usually shortened.
8. Capsule of hip joint is also shortened.
9. Inverted limbus is also seen.

Clinical Features

(Neonate and infant)

1. Extra skin crease along the medial aspect of thigh is seen in unilateral cases, while widening of perineum is seen in bilateral cases.
2. Limited abduction in flexed hip.
3. Barlow test, Ortoloni test and telescopy test are positive.
4. Walking is delayed and limping is present.

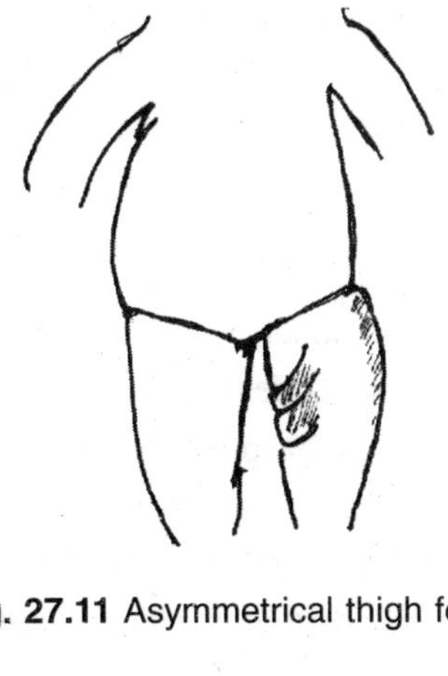

Fig. 27.11 Asymmetrical thigh folds

CHAPTER 27

Barlow Test

Examiner should stand facing toward perineum of patient. During examination; both the hip joints should be flexed at 90 degree with both the knees fully flexed. Both the hips should be completely adducted. Now exert a downward pressure along the axis of femur with little fingers placed over greater trochanter. If the hip is dislocatable femoral head will be heard to roll over posterior rim of acetabulum as a distict cluck sound. In second phase of test both the hips are gradually abducted. Little fingers placed over greater trochanter are pushed inward simultaneously. Sound of click can be felt at head of femur during its reduction into acetabulum.

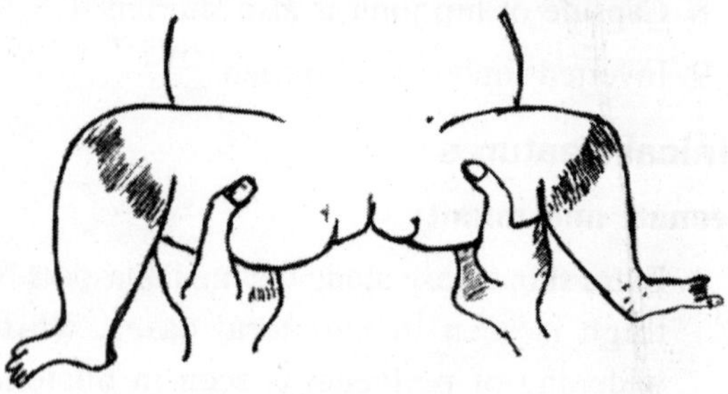

Fig. 27.12 Barlow's test

Ortoloni Test

In this test both hips and knees are flexed and thigh of affected side is gradually abducted. This test is, second phase of Barlow test in which a click of entrance will be felt as femoral head slips into acetabulum and a click of exit will be felt as it quits the acetabulum.

Telescopy Test

Patient lies supine on table. Now fix the pelvis with one hand that touches greater trochanter. Now flex the hip upto 90 degree and knee is grasped with other hand. Now push the thigh downward along the axis of femur. Previous hand notes whether greater trochanter is moving downward. This test is also positive in charcot joint.

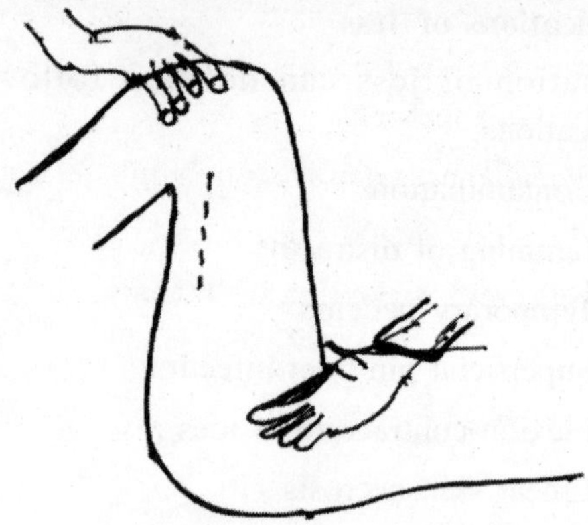

Fig. 27.13 Telescopy test

Galeazzi Sign

Hight of both knees are compared after flexing the hips upto 70 degree and knees upto 135 degree. On affected side, hight of knee is reduced.

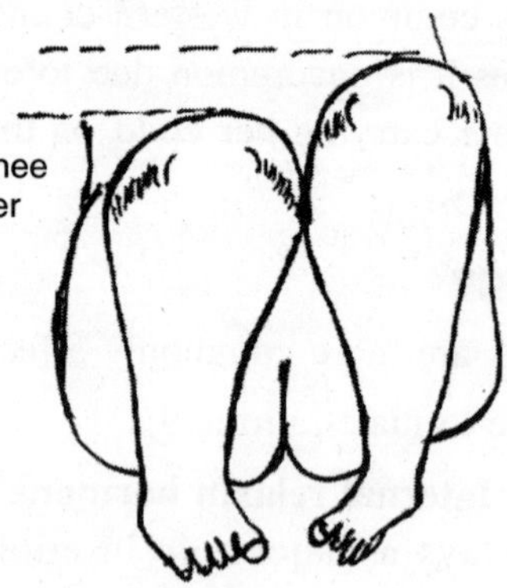

Fig. 27.14 Galeazzi sign

Clinical Features In Childhood

1. Increased lordosis, with undue protrusion of abdomen anteriorly and buttock posteriorly.
2. Space just below the perineum is widened.
3. In unilateral cases groove between labia and thigh (females) is asymmetrical.
4. Additional skin crease on medial side of thigh.
5. Movements at hip are painless.
6. Abduction and rotation movements at hip are restricted.

7. Vascular sign of narath is positive. (Femoral pulse can not be felt due to dislocation of head of femur)
8. Trendlenberg gait is seen in unilateral cases.
9. Waddling gait is present in bilateral cases.
10. Skin fold is present at gluteal region.

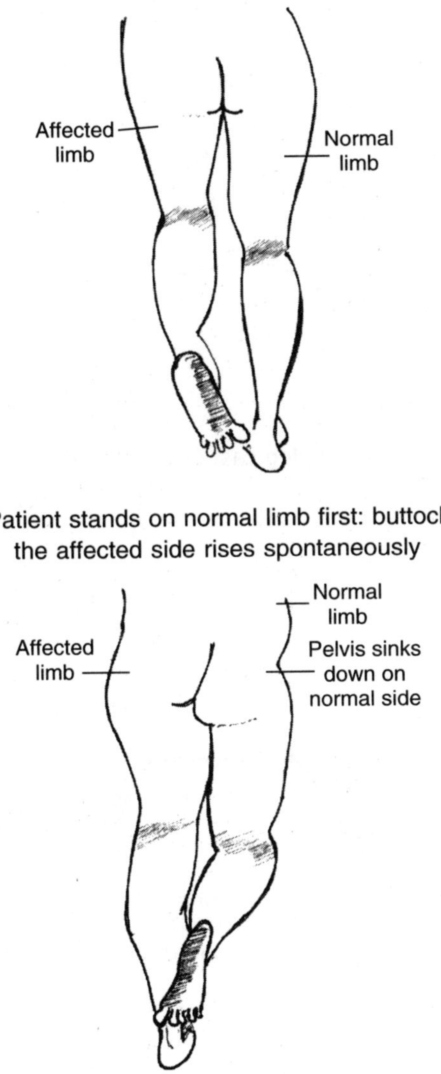

(*a*) Patient stands on normal limb first: buttock on the affected side rises spontaneously

(*b*) Patient stands on affected limb; pelvis on normal side sinks down

Fig. 27.15 Trendlenberg test

Investigations

Arthrography

Injection of 3 ml diodone into joint can determine the presence of limbus or hour glass contraction of capsule.

X-ray Findings

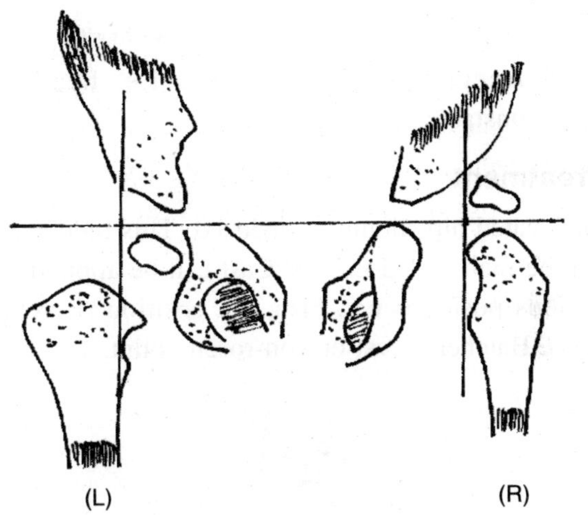

Fig. 27.16 Radiological appearance of CDH: upper femoral epiphysis on (R) side lies above the horizontal line and outside at vertical line.

1. Upper epiphysis of femur is usually smaller.
2. Neck is anteverted and clearly not seen due to superimposition.
3. Shenton line is distorted.
4. **Perkin's lines** are drawn to detect the pathology. A horizontal line is drawn through triradiate cartilage and a vertical line is drawn down from the outer edge of acetabulum on both sides. Normaly upper femoral epiphysis lies medial to vertical line and below horizontal line. But in CDH it becomes reverse.
5. **Von-rosen** lines can also detect the pathology. X-ray is taken with both hips in 45 degree abduction and internal rotation.

Now line along the axis of femoral shaft is extended upward. Normally it will touch the acetabular roof, while in CDH it will strike the pelvis above the top of acetabulum.

6. Acetabular angle is increased from 22 degree to 40 or 45 degree.
7. Head lies in upper and outer quadrant.
8. Acetabulofemoral space is increased.
9. Acetabular index is >30 i.e. head is unstable.

Treatment

Dislocated hip should be reduced. This reduction can be maintained in cast. Cast can be applied in various positions e.g. Frog leg position (Lorenz cast), Batchelor cast or von-rosen splint.

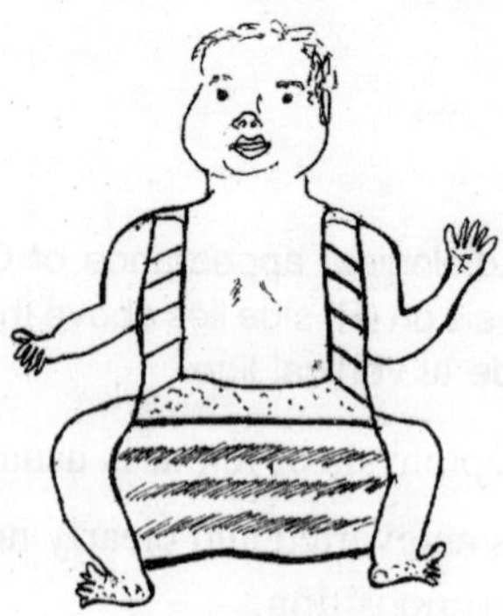

(*a*) Frazka pillow

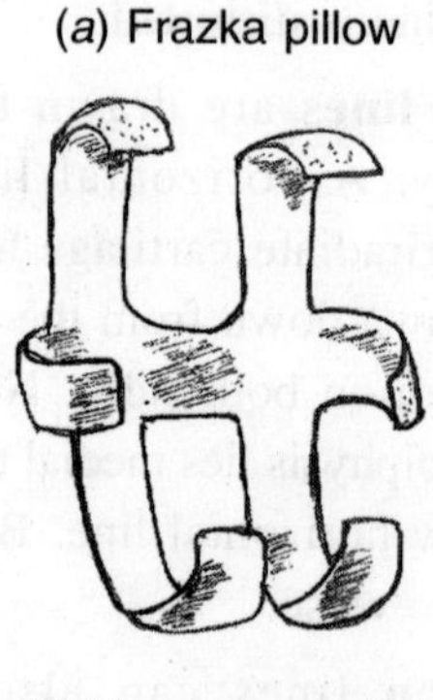

(*b*) Von rosen splint

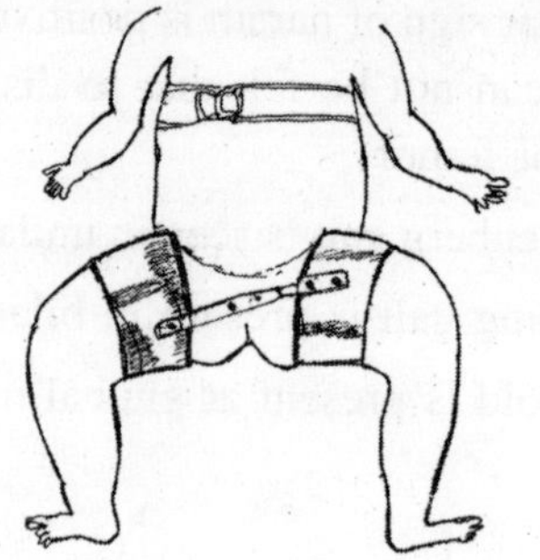

(*c*) Craig splint

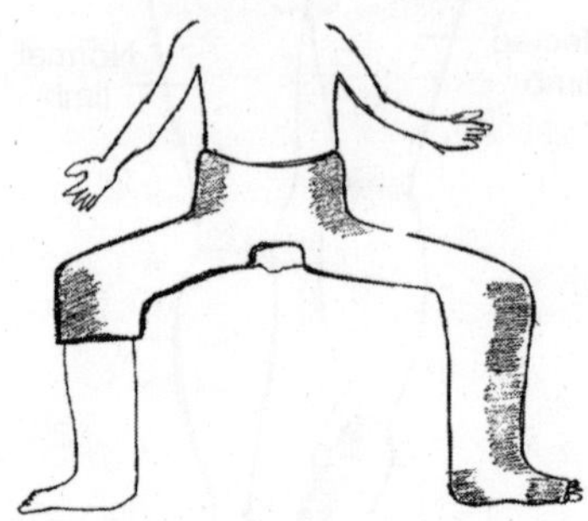

(*d*) Frog leg cast (Lorenz cast)

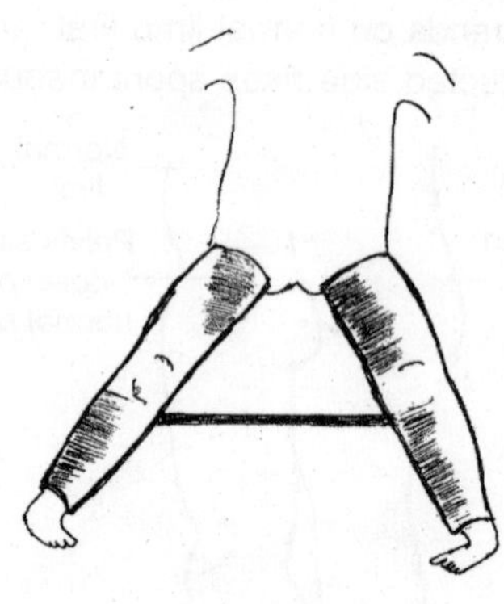

(*e*) Batchelor's cast

Fig. 27.17 Various type of treatment for CDH

Human position is the preferred position of immobilization. Hips are flexed at more than 90 degree with 30–60 degree abduction. This position decreases the chances of avascular necrosis.

Upto Age of 1 Year

Bilateral dislocation can be reduced at same time by closed manipulation. Maintenance of reduction can be achieved by frog leg/batchelor cast or von rosen splint. This immobilization can be done for 3 months to 1 year depending on progress of treatment.

1 Year to 3 Years

Closed reduction is preferred in this age group. After reduction femoral head should rest deeply and concentrically within its socket. An arthrogram will rule out the limbus into acetabular cavity. Limbus can be removed either by surgery or by application of traction (in abduction for several weeks).

If closed reduction fails open reduction must be done and redirection of acetabulum (by innominate osteotomy of salter or pericapsular osteotomy of pemberton) or reconstruction of acetabular roof (by chiari osteotomy) must be strongly considered if a tendency to subluxation is present.

Marked anteversion of femoral neck is corrected by rotation osteotomy.

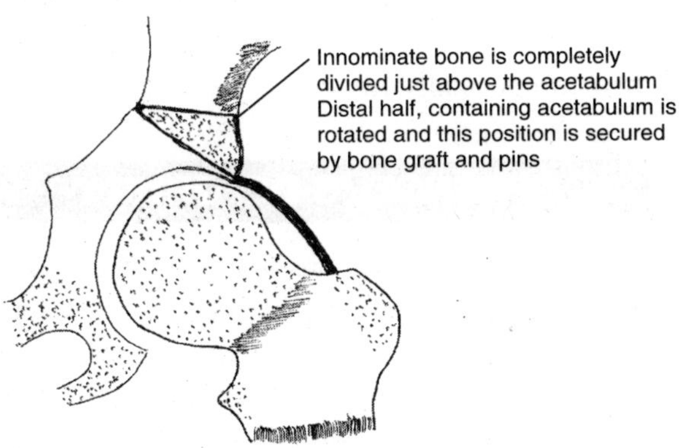

Fig. 27.18 Salter's osteotomy (performed between 1½ to 6 years of age)

After the Age of 3 Years

Surgical correction is treatment of choice. Preoperative Brayant traction is used in children while sliding skin traction with Thomas knee splint is used for older children. This traction is applied for several days to weeks to facilitate the reduction.

After the age of 4 years reconstruction of acetabular roof is mandatory by **chiari osteotomy.** This is a pelvic displacement osteotomy in which iliac bone is divided transversly immediately above acetabulum and fragment along with acetabulum is displaced medially.

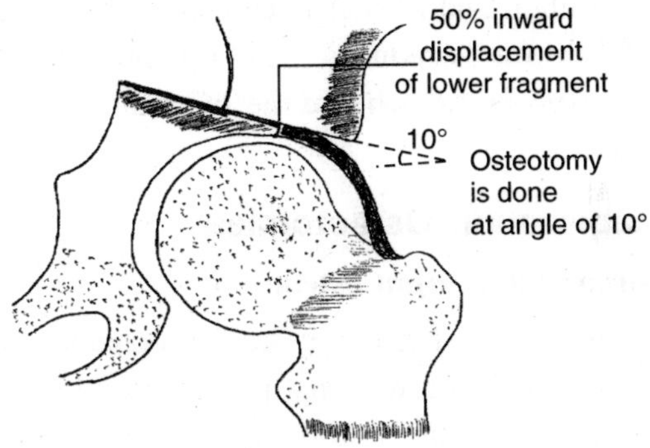

Fig. 27.19 Chiari's osteotomy: Performed after 4-5 years of age. Osteotomy is done just above the capsular attachment.

Pemberton Pericapsular Osteotomy

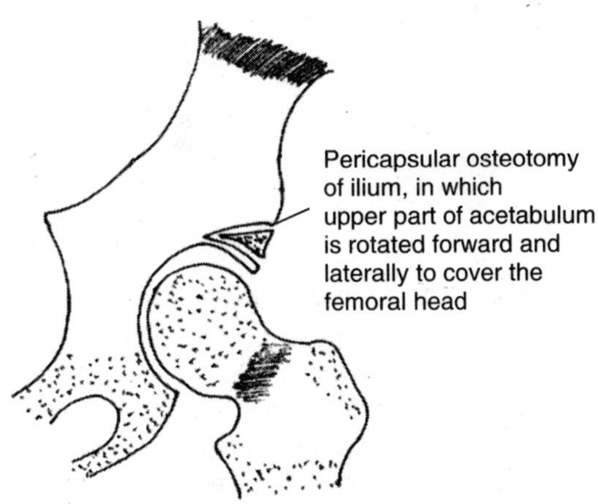

Fig. 27.20 Pemberton's osteotomy: It should be done preferably at 1 year of age and should be before 4 years of age

CHAPTER 27

This osteotomy is done after the age of 1 year but before 4 years of age. In this procedure roof of acetabulum is deflected downward over the femoral head with the fulcrum at the triradiate cartilage of pelvis.

Shelf operation

This operation is indicated when instability of hip becomes symptomatic. This is done between the age of 5–10 years. In this procedure femoral head is brought forward to a point just above the acetabulum and a shelf is constructed. Pelvic tilt and lordosis is reduced. This operation is likely to be successful when done over the age of 10 years.

Stabilization Osteotomies

Lorenz bifurcation osteotomy

A long oblique osteotomy in subtrochanteric area is done in such a way that proximal end of distal fragment rests at the level of acetabulum. Large raw surface of osteotomised bones are opposed to each other in such a way that union takes place in this angulated position quickly. A cast is applied for 3 months.

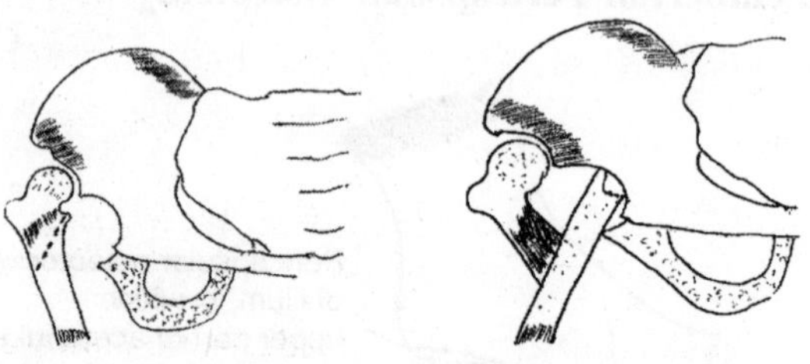

Fig. 27.21 Lorenz bifurcation osteotomy (*a*) This is a long oblique osteotomy in subtrochanteric area ; (*b*) Proximal end of distal fragment lies at the level of acetabulum, while, raw surface of osteotomized bones opposed to each other, so that union takes place in angular position.

Schanz osteotomy

This is done in older children. This is triple innomonate osteotomy usually done when pubic symphysis and triradiate cartilage are fused.

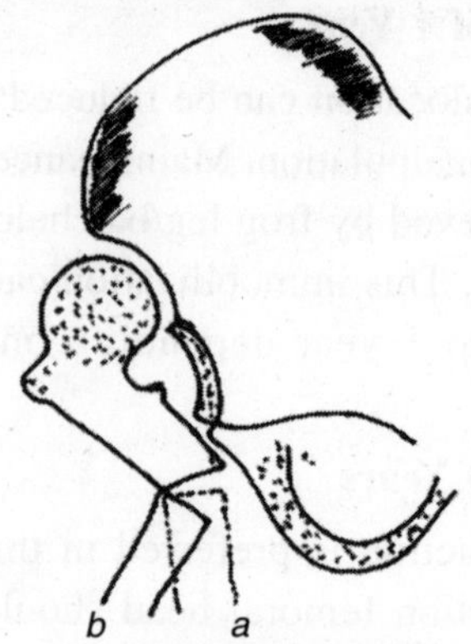

Fig. 27.22 Shanz osteotomy: Femur is sectioned transversely at the lower border of pelvis. Proximal angled inward, until it rest fragment is against the side wall of pelvis. Distal fragment can be kept in most acceptable position (*a*) or in hyperabduction, (*b*) indicated for shortening and instabilty.

Old Subluxation of Hip

In young patient cup arthroplasty or hip resurfacing procedure will provide stability and relief of pain. At later age total hip replacement is the procedure of choice.

BILATERAL CDH

In these cases treatment is not done due to less noticeable limp. Along with that these patients live their life normally till 40–50 years of age.

SPRENGEL'S DEFORMITY

This clinical condition was first described by Otto Sprengel. This is congenital anomaly of scapula in which scapula lies at a higher level and consists of permanent elevation of shoulder girdle. It is also known as **undescended scapula.**

Etiology

At the time of development, limb buds fail to descent at the level of thorax resulting in a permanently high shoulder girdle. Scapula becomes small in vertical diameter and appears broad.

Clinical Features

1. It is a painless condition.
2. Shoulder girdle and scapula appear at a higher level.
3. Neck may appear short if condition is bilateral.
4. Scapula is rotated counterclockwise and inferior angle is displaced toward spine.
5. Inferior angle of scapula does not rotate outward during the abduction of arm.
6. Sometimes patient may also have cervicothoracic scoliosis or torticollis with sprengel's deformity.

Treatment

1. Surgical treatment is indicated for cosmetic purpose only.
2. It should be done during childhood period.
3. It may cause traction on brachial plexus.
4. Surgical treatment includes Z-plastic osteotomy of clavicle. Completely denuded scapula is freed for displacement.

TORTICOLLIS

This is a rotational deformity of neck that produces turning and tilting deformity of head. This is also known as **wry neck.** Congenital toricollis is most common type of permanent torticollis.

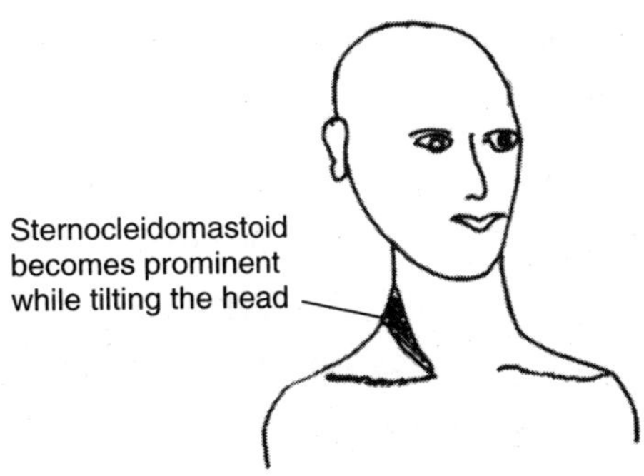

Fig. 27.23 Torticollis

Aetiology

1. Congenital
2. Traumatic
3. Infective (Tuberculosis of spine, tonsillitis, labyrynthitis and infection of atlantoaxial joint)
4. Cervical disc prolapse
5. Spasmodic torticollis
6. Paralytic torticollis
7. Myositis
8. Neuritis of 11th nerve
9. Rheumatoid arthritis.

Congenital Torticollis

This type of torticollis is present since birth and commonly seen in children with breech presentation. Sternomastoid tumor is common mode of presentation in infants. This tumor is nothing but fibrosis of sternomastoid muscle that occurs due to ischaemic necrosis of an end artery that supplies middle part of this muscle and is a branch of superior thyroid artery. This end artery is blocked by a birth trauma e.g. breech presentation or by forceps application. Ischaemic muscle is swollen and presents like a tumor.

Clinical Features

1. Child presents with swelling of sternomastoid muscle.
2. Head is tilted to one side while child looks to opposite site.
3. Sternomastoid becomes tight to the side where head tilts.
4. Facial changes can be seen.
5. Macular changes in retina may be seen.
6. Squint may be an associated finding.

X-ray Finding

No positive finding is seen in X-ray.

Treatment

1. Passive stretching of sternocleidomastoid is helpful. Sometime splintage can also be applied.
2. Chronic cases may require release of sternomastoid muscle at one or both sites.
3. Retention of corrected position is maintained on Callot's cast.
4. Bipolar release of muscle, Ferkel's modified bipolar release and Z-plasty are other surgical procedures that can be tried in older children.

CLEIDOCRANIAL DYSOSTOSIS

This is a congenital deformity in which clavicles are absent and membranous bones have faulty development. Patient lives his life normally and requires no treatment. Clavicular part of trapezius and anterior fibres of deltoid are absent.

Clinical Features

1. Clavicles are absent on both sides.
2. Shoulders are drooping and can be approximated voluntarily.
3. Anterior fontanelle are large and do not close.
4. Maxilla is hypoplastic and small.
5. Sometimes mild degree of hydrocephalus is also present.
6. Dentition may be delayed or deficient.
7. Pubic bones may have deficient ossification.
8. Spina bifida is commonly seen.

X-ray Findings

1. Aplasia of both clavicles.
2. Maxilla is hypoplastic.
3. Anterior fontanelles are open.
4. Ossification at the base of skull is normal.
5. Mandible is normal.
6. Sometimes deficient ossification of pubic bones can be seen.
7. Congenital coax vara is an associated finding.

Treatment

As patient has no disability so he does not require any treatment. These patients live their life normally.

CONGENITAL COXA VARA

Reduction of neck shaft angle of femur is known as coxa vara. Normal neck shaft angle ranges 120–140 degree in infants. In this condition acuteness of neck shaft angle progressively increases. Neck becomes short, epiphyseal plates are vertically placed. Greater trochanter is beak shaped and extends upward toward ileum. Head of femur is normal. Later acetabulum may show secondary degenerative changes.

Etiology

1. Congenital
2. Traumatic
3. Infective
4. Slipped upper femoral epiphysis

Clinical Features

1. Painless limp.
2. Progressive limitation of abduction and internal rotation of hip.
3. Shortening of lower limb.
4. Lumbar lordosis is increased.
5. Trendlenberg test is positive.
6. Telescopy test is negative.
7. Bilateral cases will show waddling gait.
8. Greater trochanter lies above Nelaton's line.

X-ray Findings

1. An oblique defect resembling as nonunion appears at vertically placed epiphyseal plate. Later it produces inverted V or Y defect.
2. X-ray shows large head, short neck and beak shaped greater trochanter.
3. Head appears to be slipped downward.

Treatment

1. Subtrochanteric osteotomy.
2. Y Shaped osteotomy of Pauwel.

CONGENITAL PSEUDOARTHROSIS OF TIBIA

This is an idiopathic congenital condition in which continuity of tibia is disrupted at the junction of middle and lower third of it's shaft. This produces abnormal mobility and gives the impression of a false joint. This is associated with neurofibromatosis and fibrous dysplasia in 40% cases.

X-ray Findings

Bone formation is absent at the junction of middle and distal third of shaft of tibia.

Treatment

Various modes of treatment are as follows:

1. Stabilization either by dual onlay graft or intramedullary nail or by external fixator.
2. Osteogenesis stimulation either by electrical stimulation or by bone transplant.
3. Above knee POP cast can be applied with the knee in 45 degree of flexion.

MADELUNG'S DEFORMITY

This is the deformity at wrist which develops during puberty between 10–15 years of age. Male to female ratio is 1:4. This deformity is bilateral in majority of cases.

It consists of dorsal subluxation of ulna and volar tilting of lower end of radius that brings carpal bones forward. Asymmetrical growth of epiphyseal plate of lower end of radius is responsible for this deformity.

Etiology

Etiology of this deformity is damage to epiphyseal plate of distal end of radius that may occur due to trauma, infection or rickets.

Clinical Features

1. Mild pain at wrist.
2. Distal end of ulna becomes prominent dorsally.
3. Volar subluxation of hand.
4. Volar and ulnar angulation of lower end of radius.
5. Dorsiflexion, abduction and supination may be limited.
6. A sound of click may be heard during rotation, flexion and extension of wrist. It is caused by slipping of extensor carpi ulnaris over ulnar styloid process.

Treatment

Surgery is avoided until bone growth is complete. This is indicated for severe deformity and persistent pain. Two types of surgeries can be done:

Darrach's procedure is performed in skeletally mature patients.

Milch Resection is done in skeletally immature patients. In this procedure wedge osteotomy is done at distal end of radius and lower end of ulna is excised subperiosteally. Ulnar styloid process and ulnar collateral ligament are left behind intact.

Tenodesis of distal radioulnar joint restores the stability of joint.

Surgery has few complications e.g. recurrence of deformity and unimproved range of motion.

KLIPPEL-FEIL SYNDROME

1. This is a congenital condition in which cervical vertebrae are fused since birth.
2. This is also known as **Brevicollis.**
3. Number of vertebrae may be reduced.
4. Child presents with short neck, restricted neck motion, low hair line and neurological features.
5. Scoliosis, kyphosis or torticollis may also be associated with deformity of cervical vertaebrae.
6. Sometimes patient may also develop prominent skin folds on either side of neck known as **Pterigeum colli.**
7. It is treated by traction and immobilization by cervical collar or cast.
8. Surgical treatment includes removal of cervical and first 3 thoracic ribs.
9. Pterigeum colli is corrected by Z-plasty.
10. Pott's spine and congenital torticollis are two diseases that should be kept in mind in differential diagnosis.

CONGENITAL DEFORMITIES OF HAND

Syndactylism

Syndactylism is most common deformity of hand in which patient presents with joined fingers. It is commonly seen between middle and ring fingers. In foot it is common between second and third toes.

In this condition two fingers are joined by skin known as web. If this web is present between all fingers it is called as **Mitten hand**. Webbing may involve partial or complete length of digits.

Treatment

Syndactylism is treated surgically by following operations:

1. Free full thickness graft.
2. Flap operation (Didol procedure).

Brachydactylism

This is a mandelian dominant, hereditary condition. In this condition patient presents with **short fingers** which may be either due to decreased length or decreased numbers of phalanx. Sometimes it may also be due to short metacarpal.

Brachydactylism is treated surgically by fusion of distal joint to improve function of pinch and grasp.

Polydactylism

Reduplication of fingers is known as polydactylism. It is commonly seen in distal phalanx of thumb known as bifid thumb. Three types of polydactylism are seen as follows:

1. Extrafleshy mass with absent bones, cartilage and tendon.
2. Duplicaton of digits.
3. Digit with its own metacarpal.

Treatment

1. Excision
2. Bilhout-cloquet operation.

Symphalangism

Fused metacarpophalangeal joints are known as symphalangism. Arthrodesis in partially flexed position is treatment of choice.

Lobster Claw Hand

This is characterized by following features:

1. This is also known as **cleft hand**.
2. V shaped cleft divides hand into two parts.
3. This cleft tapers proximally.
4. True thumb is absent.
5. Divided each part has webbed fingers.

6. Middle finger and metacarpal are missing.
7. This is an extremely rare condition.

Thumb Clutched Hand

This type of hand has congenital absence of extensor pollicis longus, pollex varus. Clasped thumb and flexion adduction deformity of hand are other findings.

Megalodactylism

1. This is also known as macrodactylism.
2. This is congenital hypertrophy of digits or hand.
3. This is common in second and third fingers.

CONGENITAL ABSENCE OF RADIUS

This is a congenital condition in which radius is absent and is associated with club hand. Other findings are as follows:

1. Ulna is short, broad and bowed with concavity toward radial side.
2. Carpal bones on lateral aspect of wrist may be absent or fused with each other.
3. Contracture of muscle (commonly brachioradialis) is seen.
4. This condition is treated by release of contracture, gradual stretching and splinting. Sometimes it may require osteotomy of ulna. Wrist can be arthrodesed in functional position.

CONGENITAL ABSENCE OF FIBULA

This is also known as proximal fibular hemimilia. This is treated by making the foot in plantigrade position. This is of 3 types as follows:

Type 1: Fibula is partially absent on one side.

Type 2: Entire fibula is absent. Tibia is bowed. Equinovalgus at foot is present

Type 3: Along with absence of fibula, other congenital deformities are also present. Fibula may be absent on both sides.

PROXIMAL FEMORAL FOCAL DEFICIENCY

1. This is a congenital deformity in which head, neck and trochanter are cartilaginous in origin and attached to diaphysis through a pseudoarthrosis.
2. Patient can not bear weight on affected side, leading to severe coxa vara deformity.
3. Femur is short. Hip is unstable and presents with flexion, abduction and external rotation contracture.
4. Limb length discrepancy can be treated by early symes amputation as soon as child starts walking and an end bearing prosthesis is applied.

CONGENITAL DISLOCATION OF KNEE

This condition is also known as congenital genu recurvatum. Knee is dislocated since birth and leg can be approximated to anterior aspect of thigh. Upper end of tibia comes to lie anterolateral to femur. Patella may be absent or smaller in size. Length of quadriceps tendon and iliotibial band are shortened. This is of two types as follows:

1.**Traumatic**

It is more common and occurs due to malpositioning of foetus in uterus or due to fibrofatty degeneration of quadriceps.

2.**Primary Embryogenic Type**

This has some associated defect e.g. club foot or hair lip.

Treatment

1. Repeated manipulation and cast application to provide gradual flexion at knee joint is the goal of conservative treatment.
2. Surgical treatment includes subcutaneous tenotomy of iliotibial band or lengthening/ sectioning of quadriceps tendon.

CONGENITAL ABSENCE OF PATELLA

In this condition patella is displaced laterally or anterolaterally to laterl femoral condyle. Tibia is externally rotated. Child may present with pain and instability. In old age it may cuase severe degenerative arthritis with reduction in joint space. This is treated either by cast or by **Conri's operation.**

CHAPTER

28 Developmental Diseases

- Marble bone disease
- Osteogenesis imperfecta
- Achondroplasia
- Mafucci disease
- Ollier disease
- Osteopoikilosis
- Engelmann's disease
- Pycnodysostosis
- Exostosis
- Melorrheostosis
- Observation hip

MARBLE BONE DISEASE

This is also known as Albers-shonberg disease or chalk bone disease. This is a rare developmental disorder of unknown etiology in which bony architecture converts into marble appearance. Bones are as brittle as chalk.

Pathological Features

1. New bone continues to deposit over unresorbed calcified cartilage or primary spongiosa.
2. Metaphysis are wide and bones are club shaped due to failure of remodelling unit.
3. Cranial foramina get bony encroachment leading to optic atrophy, deafness and facial nerve palsy. **Mandible is not affected.**
4. Medullary canal is obliterated.
5. Haversian canals are rare.
6. Osteoclasts are normal or may be absent while osteoblasts are normal or increased.
7. Shallow pituitary fosa.
8. Air sinuses are converted into dense bone or sinuses may be absent. Skull diploes are fused as one.
9. Insufficient development of bone marrow.

Clinical Features

Patient may present with following clinical features:

1. Bone is as hard as marble and as brittle as chalk.
2. Transverse fractures are seen which heal slowly.
3. Secondary anemia occurs due to insufficient development of bone marrow.
4. Optic atrophy, occular/facial palsy and deafness can occur due to encroachment of cranial foramina.
5. Hydrocephalus may be seen as a complication.

6. Progressive osteoporosis is a common feature which starts during gestation and continues till longitudinal growth stops.
7. Disease is fatal within 2 years if it appears at birth. Secondary anemia is a prognostic factor.

Radiological Features

X-ray will show following radiological features:

1. Club shaped metaphysis.
2. Small pituitary fossa. Posterior clinoid processes are thick.
3. Air sinuses are either absent or dense.
4. Maximum density of skull is seen at its base.
5. Maxilla is affected while mandible escapes.

OSTEOGENESIS IMPERFECTA

This is a hereditary developmental disorder with classical features of fragile bone, deafness, blue sclera, laxity of joint and tendency to improve with age. It is also known as periosteal dysplasia, Fragilitas ossium and idiopathic osteopsathyrosis. Prenatal cases are mandellian recessive while postnatal cases are inherited as dominant. Triad of osteogenesis imperfecta, otosclerosis and blue sclera is also known as Vander Hoeve Syndrome.

Pathological Features

1. Failure of osteoblast formation is a primary defect, leading to minimum osteoid formation.
2. Bone has thick periosteum while cambium layer is thin.
3. Skull fontanelles close late.
4. Epiphysis is bulbous. Bones are short and thin.
5. Transverse trabeculae are absent.
6. Fracture heals with abundant callus.
7. Skull is thin and globular.
8. Scoliosis is frequently seen.
9. Vertebrae are biconcave, shallow and translucent.

Classification

Prenatal (foetal) type

At birth multiple fractures are present in body. Skull has a feeling of membranous bag of bones. This type is severe and infant may be stillborn or may die at birth.

Infantile type

In this type multiple fractures are seen but as the child grows tendency of fracture reduces provided child survives. Appearance of skull resembles with hydrocephalus.

Adolescent type

This type is also known as osteogenesis-imperfecta tarda. No fracture is seen at birth. Child is normal but fracture can occur due to trivial trauma. As child grows, tendency to frcture is lost.

Clinical Features

This is a developmental disease. Child may presents with following features:

1. Child presents with multiple fractures that heal rapidly with abundant callus.
2. Deafness can occur due to coexistent otosclerosis usually present in third decade of life.
3. Blue sclera.
4. Laxity of joint with feeble musculature.
5. Poorly calcified decidous teeth.
6. Dwarfism.
7. Broad skull.

Investigations

1. Blood chemistry is normal.
2. Amniocentesis is helpful in making prenatal diagnosis of osteogenesis imperfecta by measurement of inorganic pyrophosphate as it's level is raised 3.4 to 3.7 times the normal level. Normal value of inorganic

pyrophosphate upto 14 weeks of gestation is 6 micro gm/dl; 15–24 weeks 18 micro gm/dl and 25 weeks onward 13 micro gm/dl.

X-ray Findings

1. Bones are osteoporotic.
2. Cortices are thin with bulbous end.
3. Vertebrae are biconcave, translucent and shallow.
4. Skull is thin.
5. Fracture healing is seen with abundant callus.
6. Transverse trabeculatios are absent.
7. Bony deformities are seen.

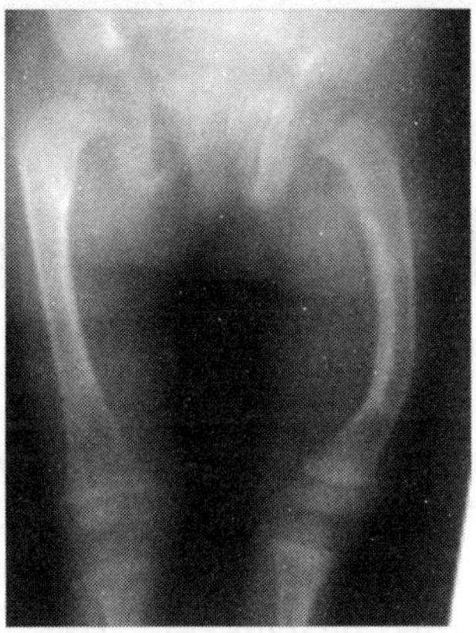

Fig. 28.1 Deformed femur in osteogenesis imperfecta

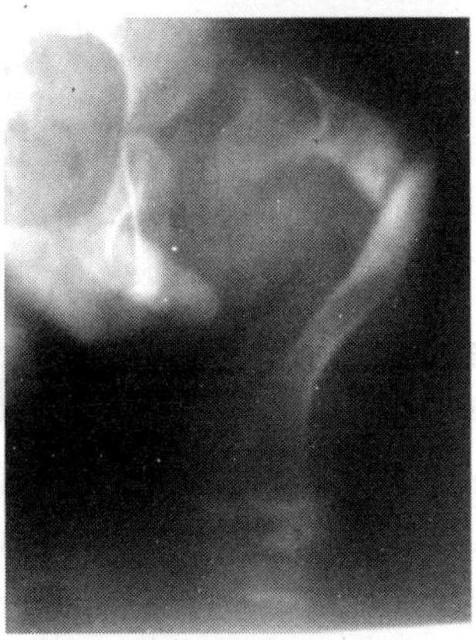

Fig. 28.2 Pathological fracture in osteogenesis imperfecta

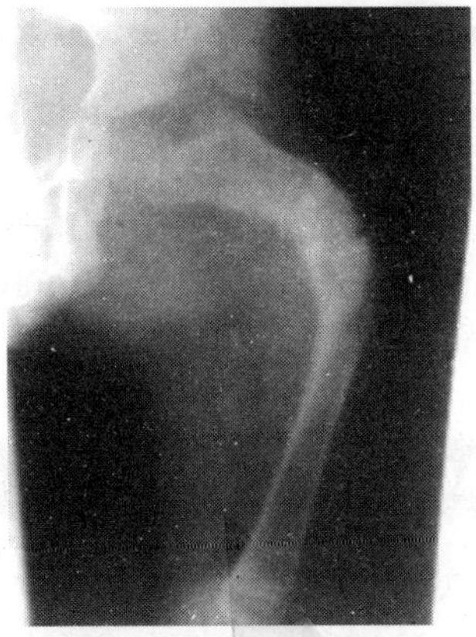

Fig. 28.3 Pathological fracture in osteogenesis imperfecta

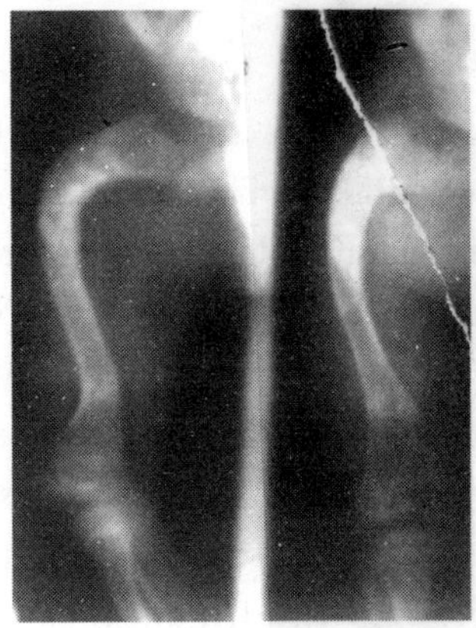

Fig. 28.4 Deformed femur (A.P. and lateral view) in osteogenesis imperfecta

Treatment

Child should be protected as he has tendency to get fractures easily due to trivial trauma. Excess of vitamin D administration can cause decalcification. Estrogen and androgen can also be given. Following surgical treatments are common:

Sofield osteotomy

Multiple osteotomies are done through the shaft and metaphysis. Then these fragments are threaded on an intramedullary nail. Results are excellent, union occurs rapidly.

William's method

In this method an extension is fixed to distal end of intramedullary nail; then it is inserted in retrograde manner thus driving the nail through the heel.

Baily and Duboy method

Belly used telescopic intramedullary nail that elongates as the growth occurs thus preventing the bony deformities.

ACHONDROPLASIA

This is a generalized bone disorder caused by disturbance of enchondral ossification at epiphyseal growth plate; chiefly affecting long bones e.g. humerus and femur.

Clinical Features

Patient is dwarf soon after birth. History of prematurity or still birth is frequent. This disorder affects the extremities. Upper limbs are so short that they hardly reach upto upper 1/3rd of thigh. Hands are short and broad and have typical triradiant appearance. Fingers are short and divergent. Fibula is not affected. These patients have superior muscle power in comparison to normal person. Intelligence and sexual development are normal. Buttocks are prominent, pelvis is tilted forward and lumbar lordosis is exaggerated. Patient walks with a rolling gait. Head is brachycephalic with prominent forehead. Chest is flat and small. Ribs are short. These patients have increased risk of cord and nerve root compression due to spinal stenosis.

X-ray Findings

1. Shortened long bones.
2. Ribs are short. Sternum is broad and thick.
3. Scapula and ileum is rectangular.
4. Skull is large.
5. Foramen magnum is small and tunnel shaped.

Treatment

Hight of patient can be increased by Illizarov's method.

Causes of Dwarfism

1. Achondroplasia
2. Diaphyseal achlasia
3. Dyschondroplasia
4. Cretinism
5. Multiple epiphyseal dysplasia
6. Malnutrition
7. Hurler, hunter syndrome and marquio disease.

MAFUCCI DISEASE

It comprises of dyschondroplasia with cavernous haemangioma and phlebolith in soft tissue.

OLLIER DISEASE

This disease is also known as multiple enchondromas or Dyschondroplasia. Patient presents with masses of unossified cartilages in metaphysis of long bones commonly at growing ends (e.g. knee, distal end of ulna, radius, upper end of humerus, phalanx and iliac crest). This disease involves one half of body. i.e. This disease is unilateral. Patient is normal at birth. Later patient presents with shortening of bones, valgus or varus deformity and multiple enchondromas of phalanx. Ulna is smaller than radius. Fractures are not so common but it may be seen in hand sometimes.

OSTEOPOIKILOSIS

Patient is usually asymptomatic but in X-ray multiple radiodense spots are seen in multiple bones that exist throught life. These spots are commonly seen in pelvis. Cancellous bone is predominantly affected, while shaft of bone is unaffected. These spots may also be seen in skull, ribs and spine. This disease is also known as **Osteopathia condensans disseminate.**

ENGELMANN'S DISEASE

Engelmann's disease is of unknown etiology that presents with symmetrical fusiform enlargement and sclerosis of shaft of long bones, usually seen in childhood before 7 years of age. Child has poor musculature, retarded dentition and walks with waddling gait. Puberty is late. Genitalia and secondary sex characters are poorly developed. X-ray shows fusiform enlargement of diaphysis, widened cortex. Encroachment of medullary canal can be seen. This disease should be differentiated from caffey disease as later is seen before 6 months of age. Mandible is affected. Increased bone density is unilateral. This is also known as Progressive diaphyseal dysplasia/hyperostosis.

PYCNODYSOSTOSIS

This disease is genetic and is inherited as autosomal recessive trait resembling with cliedocranial dysostosis, characterized by short stature, dysplasia of skull and outer end of clavicles, obtuse mandibular hypoplasia, partial or total aplasia of distal phalanges and increased density of skeleton.

Clinical Features

History of repeated fractures due to trivial trauma is common. Fracture of mandible can occur during tooth extraction. Anterior fontanelles and skull sutures remain open till adulthood. Patient also presents with proptosis. Spinal deformities like kyphosis and spondylolisthesis are common.

X-ray Findings

1. Wide distal end of femur. (Erlenmeyer flask deformity)
2. Distal phalanges are short.
3. Obtuse mandibular angle is approaching 180 degree.

EXOSTOSIS

Exostosis is an outpouching of cortex, clinically presenting as bony out growth which may or may not be tender and uncommonly may turn malignant. If it arises adjacent to nerve it may produce numbness, paresthesia and muscle weakness. Complicated exostosis can present as fracture, bursitis, shortening/bowing of bone, pressure on nerve/tendon and sarcomatous degeneration. Exostosis is a benign growth. Malignant changes are characterized by rapidly increasing swelling, sudden origin of pain and irregular cartilaginous cap on X-ray with osteoblastic foci. Exostosis may arise by failure of development or failed osteoblastic activity or due to deficiency of perichondrium.

Exostosis first occur near epiphyseal cartilage, later metaphysis is affected. Metaphysis is uniformly enlarged producing trumpet like appearance on X-ray. Common sites for development of exostosis are lower end femur and radius, upper end of radius and tibia. This does not arise from membranous bone. This should be removed when it cause deformity, compresses nerve or when it undergoes malignant changes.

MELORRHEOSTOSIS

Melorheostosis is a disease of unknown etiology occurring in childhood in which bone resembles the **flow of candle drippings.** This is also known as Leri type of osteopetrosis. Clinically patient presents with dull aching pain, limitation of motion or bony deformity and shortening of limbs.

Sympathetic ischaemic phenomenon may produce swelling, skin changes, coldness and increased perspiration. Lower extremity is affected more than the upper. It usually involves one limb. X-ray shows flow of radioopaque substance in bone. Sympathetectomy may be helpful in case of sympathetic ischaemia.

OBSERVATION HIP

This is transient synovitis of hip which is commonly seen between 5–10 years of age. Child presents with pain and stiffness at hip. Symptoms disappear within 2-3 weeks if patient takes adequate bed rest. X-ray and ESR are normal.

CHAPTER

29 Regional Diseases

- Genu varum
- Genu valgum
- Genu recurvatum
- Tibia vara
- Dislocation of patella
- Congenital dislocation of patella
- Recurrent dislocation of patella
- Larson-Johansson disease
- Osgood-Schlatter disease
- Chondromalacia patellae
- Slipped femoral capital epiphysis
- Leg-calve-perthes disease
- Pes cavus
- Flat foot
- Hammer toe
- Hallux valgus (bunion)
- Hallux rigidus
- Hallux varus
- Dorsal bunion
- Plantar fascitis and calcaneal spur
- Sever's disease
- Tarsal tunnel syndrome
- Frozen shoulder
- Tennis elbow
- Golfer's elbow
- Student's elbow
- Elbow tunnel syndrome
- Dequervain's disease
- Dupuytren's contracture
- Trigger finger
- Bursitis
- Ganglion
- Loose bodies
- Carpal tunnel syndrome
- Meralgia paraesthetica
- Impingement syndrome
- Bennet's lesion
- Popliteal cyst
- Cervical rib

GENU VARUM

Definition

This is defined as lateral angulation of knee joint with medial deviation of longitudinal axis of femur and tibia. Genu varum involves tibia or femur alone or tibia and fibula both.

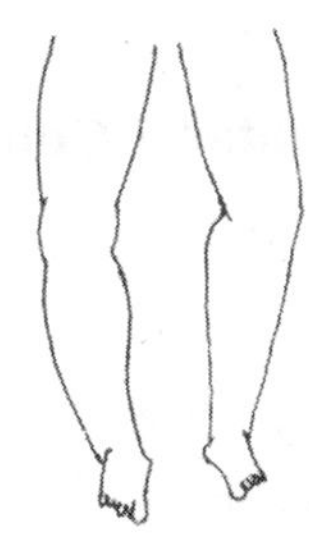

Fig. 29.1 Genu varum

Associated Findings

1. Internal torsion of lower end of tibia.
2. Intoeing of bilateral feet.
3. Patella faces outward.
4. Medial structures of knee are tight while lateral structures are lax.

Aetiology

1. Rickets is most common cause of genu varum.
2. Injury to medial part of upper tibial epiphyseal plate leads to unilateral deformity.
3. Certain posture is also a predisposing factor for development of genu varum e.g. infant lying in prone position.
4. Position with thighs abducted and toes turned inward, can also cause genu varum.

Causes of Bilateral Genu Varum

Physiological (upto 4 years of age)

Pathological

- Congenital
- Metabolic
- Developmental
- Endocrinal
- Osteoarthritis
- Occupational
- Bount's disease
- Paget's disease

Causes of Unilateral Genu Varum

- Growth disturbances of upper tibial epiphysis.
- Trauma to epiphysis.
- Tumor of lower end of femur and upper end of tibia.
- Infection e.g. osteomyelitis.

Clinical Features

1. Patient presents with lateral angulation of knee.
2. Associated deformities are also seen.
3. Plumb line test is performed. In this test a line is drawn from ASIS to centre of patella. If this line is extended downward it will strike at medial malleolus normally but in genu varum medial malleolus lies medial to this line.
4. Measurement of distance between two knees is more than 3 cm. In children it is measured in supine position with knees extended and patella facing toward ceiling. Both malleoli should touch each other. Now distance between two knees is measured. If it is more than 3 cm it hints toward genu varum. In adults this distance is measured in X-ray of both knees which is taken on large single plate in standing position.

Treatment

1. In less than 4 years of age conservative treatment is adviced. Knee-ankle-foot orthosis with medial bar and lateral strap is used for walking.
2. During growing period lateral epiphyseal stapling is adviced.
3. If patient has achieved skeletal maturity supracondylar medial open or lateral closed wedge osteotomy is done.

GENU VALGUM

Definition

Medial angulation of knee with outward deviation of longitudinal axis of both femur and tibia is known as genu valgum deformity. It can be unilateral or bilateral. Due to pull of biceps femoris and tensor fascia lata, lower end of femur and tibia are externally rotated. As a result lower end of tibia, develops compensatory internal tibial torsion deformity.

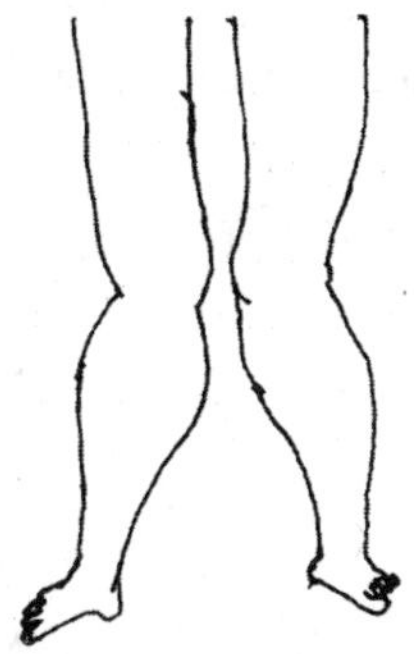

Fig. 29.2 Genu valgum
(Intermalleolar distance is increased)

Associated Findings

1. Internal torsion of distal end of tibia.
2. Pronated and flat foot.
3. Shortening of lateral structures (biceps femoris, iliotibial band and peroneal nerve) and lengthening of medial structure (medial collateral ligament) at knee.
4. Lateral subluxation/dislocation of patella.

Aetiology

Unilateral genu valgum is commonly seen in case of trauma, tumor and osteomyelitis. Bilateral genu valgum is seen in following conditions:

- Physiological genu valgum is seen in 60–70% of children upto 2 years of age and it disappears by the age of 4 years.
- Traumatic (fracture dislocation of epiphysis or fracture through outer portion of epiphyseal plate)
- Idiopathic
- Congenital
- Rickets (Metabolic)
- Developmental epiphyseal dysplasia
- Degenerative
- Inflammatory
- Endocrinal (Thyroid dysfunction)

Clinical Features

1. Deformity at knee is the only complaint.
2. Associated findings may be seen.
3. Intermalleolar distance is more than 10 cm. (normal 8–10 cm)
4. **Knee flexion test** is performed in which patient is asked to lie on a couch. Now his knee is flexed. If deformity disappears it means cause is in lower end of femur. If deformity does not disappear it means cause is in upper end of tibia.
5. Plumb line test is performed. Draw a line from ASIS to centre of patella. If this line is extended downward it will strike medial malleolus normally. But in this condition medial malleolus will remain outside of this line.

X-ray Findings

X-ray of both knee to be taken on single large plate in standing position with both knees in approximation. Angle between femoral and tibial shaft can be measured on X-ray plate. Normally it is 6 degree. Angle of more than 6 degree indicates genu valgum deformity.

Treatment

Conservative treatment is indicated for mild cases. Medial border of shoe is raised from 3/16th inch-1/4th inch. Knock knee brace with a lateral bar and inner strap to be worn round the clock.

Surgical treatment is indicated for severe cases. This is decided on the basis of X-ray findings of epiphyseal plate. If lateral part of epiphyseal plate is intact it will contribute to longitudinal growth at a slower rate. In this condition stapling is done at medial part of epiphyseal plate. This will arrest growth at medial side but allows at lateral side, thus helping in correction of deformity.

Osteotomy must be done after epiphysis have fused. Medial closed wedge osteotomy is done if limb is long. Lateral open wedge osteotomy is done if limb is short.

- No treatment is required for less than 4 years of age.
- 4–10 years: Medial heel is raised by 3/16th to 1/4th inch. Knock knee brace (with lateral iron bar and inner strap) to be worn round the clock.
- 10–14 years: Epiphysis is stapled at the medial portion of epiphyseal plate.
- 14–16 years: Wait and watch till skeletal maturity because it is too early for osteotomy and too late for stapling.
- >16 years: Osteotomy can be done as epiphysis has fused at this age. Medial close wedge osteotomy is done if limb is long. Lateral closed wedge osteotomy is done if limb is short.

GENU RECURVATUM

Backward bowing of knee is known as genu recurvatum. In this condition epiphyseal plate of lower end of femur and upper end of tibia show retarded activity.

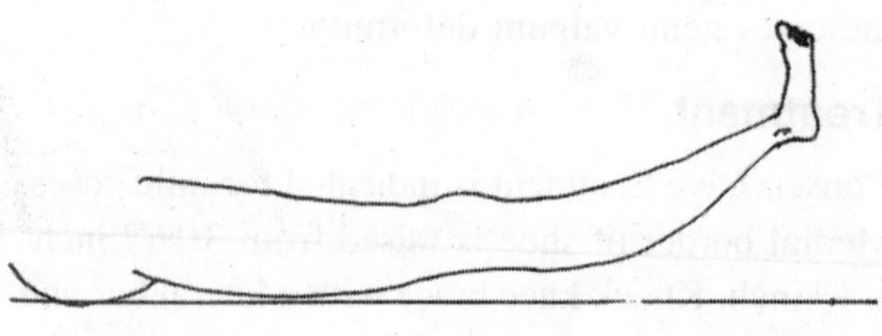

Fig. 29.3 Genu recurvatum

Aetiology

1. Quadriceps contracture is commonest cause.
2. Muscle imbalance e.g. polio and equinus deformity of foot.
3. Congenital disorders.
4. Malunited fracture of knee.

Clinical Features

1. It is commonly seen in females and identical twins. It is usually bilateral.
2. Patient usually presents with limited knee flexion.
3. Proximal part of patella shows dense contracted quadriceps that can be palpated.
4. Patella is slightly high riding in position.
5. It may be associated with dislocation of patella.

Treatment

Correction of this deformity requires surgery. Osteotomy is done in proximal part of tibia, just below the attachment of patellar tendon. Postoperatively AKPOP cylinder cast is applied for 3 months. Weight bearing is not allowed during this period. Quadriceps plasty and proximal release of rectus femoris are other methods of treatment.

TIBIA VARA

This is also known as Blount's disease or Erlacher's disease or osteochondrosis deformans tibiae. This is a developmental condition in which enchondral ossification at the proximal end of tibia, mainly at posteromedial aspect and at medial part of epiphyseal ossification centre is disturbed. This is most common in infant and children. In this condition diaphysis remains straight, while varus angulation develops at upper end of tibial metaphysis. 50% of infantile type cases are bilateral. Adolescent type is unilateral.

Associated Findings

- Internal torsion of tibia
- Stretched lateral collateral ligament
- Longitudinal growth is retarded in neglected case.

Aetiology

This is idiopathic in nature and commonly seen in West indies and West Africa.

Clinical Features

1. Tibia vara can be noticed when child starts standing and walking i.e. between 1–3 years of age. This is known as infantile type.
2. Three types of tibia vara can be found on examination: sharp medial angulation of tibia at metaphysis, internal tibial torsion and pes planovalgus.
3. Bony hard non tender prominence is palpable at medial part of epiphysiometaphyseal junction of tibia.

X-ray Findings

Poor development of ossification centre at posteromedial aspect of medial tibial condyle produces a dip deformity which is responsible for joint instability. It is visible on X-ray. This dip deformity is known as **Siffert-katz sign.**

Treatment

If the deformity is more than 30 degree, osteotomy is the treatment of choice. 3 types of osteotomy can be done as follows:

- **Curved osteotomy of tibia with oblique osteotomy of fibula.** This is indicated when deformity exceeds 10 degree.
- **Curved osteotomy of tibia and oblique osteotomy of fibula. Epiphysiodesis of lateral part of tibial growth plate and upper end of fibula.** It is done after 9 years of age.
- **Osteotomy and elevation of medial tibial condyle and epiphysiodesis of lateral part of tibial growth plate and upper end of fibula.** This is indicated in excessive ligamentous laxity.

DISLOCATION OF PATELLA

Patella dislocates due to contraction of quadriceps muscle which tends to displace it laterally. This dislocation is prevented by strong vastus medialis, medial capsule and retinacula.

Aetiology

Most common cause is trauma. Rarely it may dislocate spontaneously.

Pathology

- Capsule is torn.
- Upto a certain extent musle attachment at medial edge of patella is torn.
- Articular cartilage may be damaged. Old cases may show degenerative changes.

Treatment

Basic principle is to realign quadriceps mechanism. Dislocation should be reduced followed by AKPOP cast to be applied.

Complications

Osteoarthritic changes are likely to develop if not treated properly.

CONGENITAL DISLOCATION OF PATELLA

It is very difficult to diagnose it at birth. Child presents with external rotation of leg. Patella is displaced laterally over lateral condyle of femur where it can be palpated. Genu valgum may be associated. Valgus deformity should be corrected as a first phase of treatment. Later osteotomy at supracondylar area and internal rotation of tibia is required. X-ray does not show patella as ossification starts after 2 years.

RECURRENT DISLOCATION OF PATELLA

Recurrent dislocation of patella is commonly seen in children and adolescent. Displacement takes place laterally. It can cause degeneration of articular surface.

Predisposing Factors

1. Patella alta
2. Shallow lateral femoral condyle
3. Genu valgum
4. Hypoplastic patella
5. High riding patella due to elongated patellar tendon
6. External tibial torsion
7. Insufficient vastus medialis
8. Shallow patellar groove
9. Lax medial capsule
10. Tight lateral structures and lax medial patellar retinaculum
11. Genu recurvatum.

Clinical Features

1. Patient presents with bony prominence at lateral aspect of knee due to lateral displacement of patella.
2. Knee is held in mild flexion.
3. Tenderness is present at lateral aspect of patella.
4. Old cases may show atrophy of vastus medialis and contracture of iliotibial band.
5. Associated features e.g. genu valgum, genu recurvatum and external tibial torsion may be present.

X-ray Findings

X-ray should be taken in standing position and full extension. X-ray will show lateral dislocation of patella. Old cases may show degenerative changes at medial facet of patella and at patellofemoral joint. These degenerative changes have been divided into 5 types on the basis of X-ray findings as follows:

Type 1: It consists of fibrillation and heaping up of articular cartilage which is confined upto medial facet of patella.

Type 2: Small loose body may be present. Medial facet shows degenerative changes.

Type 3: Degenerative changes are present in patella and femur. X-ray shows bony spur at femur and patella.

Type 4: This shows frank patellofemoral osteoarthritis.

Type 5: This shows generalized osteoarthritis of knee joint.

Treatment

Patella is relocated by extending the knee and flexing hip. This relaxes quadriceps muscle thus helping in reduction of patella over lateral condyle. After this AKPOP cast is applied in full extension for 6 weeks to allow healing of capsule. Patient is adviced graduated quadriceps exercise.

Surgical Methods

Basic principle of surgery is to align quadriceps apparatus to more medial position. Following surgical methods are common:

1. **Hauser Method**

This is most effective method where tibial tubercle and patellar tendon are transplanted medially and distally.

2. **Elmslie-Trillat Method**

Lateral knee structures are released. Tuberosity is transferred medially. Medial structures are plicated.

3. **Galleaze Procedure**

Semitendinosus tendon is tenodesed to patella.

Other Methods

1. Campbell operation
2. Goldthwaite-Roulex operation
3. Albee's operation
4. West and Sotohall operation
5. Houghston procedure

LARSON-JOHANSSON DISEASE

1. Osteoarthritis of patella (usually lower pole) is known as Larson-Johansson disease.
2. This is commonly seen between the ages of 10–14 years.
3. Pain, swelling and inability to kneel and run are main complaints. Tenderness is present at lower pole of patella.
4. Extension of knee is painful.
5. This is associated with Osgood-Schlatter disease.
6. Early X-ray findings are normal. Later it may show blurring and irregularity of bone.
7. It heals spontaneously. However AKPOP cylinder cast is applied to get retinaculum symptoms.

OSGOOD-SCHLATTER DISEASE

Osteochondritis of tibial tubercle is known as Osgood-Schlatter disease. In this condition tibial tubercle may be avulsed.

Aetiology

1. Trauma is a common predisposing factor.
2. Repeated flexion of knee against tight quadriceps.
3. Rapid growth period of puberty particularly in boys.

Clinical Features

1. Pain, swelling and tenderness at tibial tubercle.
2. Active extension of knee (against resistance) is painful.
3. Difficulty in climbing upstairs and running.
4. Kneeling is painful.

X-ray Findings

1. Multiple fragmented areas of ossification are seen.
2. Soft tissue around patellar tendon may be seen.
3. Irregular areas of ossification or well circumscribed bone may be present in patellar tendon.

Treatment

Above knee POP cylinder cast in full extension is best conservative treatment. As far as surgical treatment is concern, drill holes are made into main bone through tibial tubercle. This procedure facilitates rapid vascularization. Bone graft is kept into these drill holes.

Complication

Failure of union of tubercle to tibia is most common complication.

Differential Diagnosis

Larson-Johansson disease is main differential diagnosis.

CHONDROMALACIA PATELLAE

Softening of articular cartilage of patella due to aetiology of diverse origin is known as chondromalacia patellae.

Types

- Adolescent type—primary and secondary.
- Adult type.

Primary Adolescent Type

This is idiopathic in nature and more common in females. (male:female 2:3). This is characterized by softening of articular cartilage of patella without known cause.

Pathology

Pathological changes are seen in 4 stages as follows:

Stage 1: Surface of cartilage is elevated. This is known as 'Blistering'.

Stage 2: Fissure reaches upto subchondral bone.

Stage 3: Extensive fibrillation and loss of cartilage gives a crabmeat appearance.

Stage 4: Subchondral bone is exposed due to thining and complete loss of cartilage.

Clinical Features

Diffuse type of pain at anterior or anteromedial aspect of knee which is aggravated during flexion of knee. Patient has difficulty in going up and down stairs due to pain.

Cinema sign

If patient sits for a long time with knee kept in flexion it causes pain, which is relieved by extension of knee.

Outerbridge's Grading

It has been divided into 4 grades as follows:

1. Soft and swollen patella
2. Fissuring of patella
3. Crabmeat appearance (Fibrillation is seen)
4. Subchondral bone is exposed and erosive changes are seen.

Treatment

- Spontaneous recovery is seen in majority of cases so it should be treated conservatively.
- Patient should be adviced quadriceps resistance exercises.
- AKPOP cast may give temporary relief to patient.
- If conservative treatment is fruitless, surgical treatment is recommended.

Following surgical treatment are helpful: medial plication of patellar tendon, shaving of articular cartilage and excision of lesion.

Secondary Adolescent Type

This is most commonly caused by trauma. Its pathology shows a lesion at the medial ridge that extends outward mediolaterally in a ellipsoid fashion.

Clinical Features

1. Patient complaints of severe pain while climbing upstairs.
2. He also has sensation of instability and buckling.
3. Feel of patella going out. (lateral displacement of patella)

X-ray Findings

X-ray may show associated findings e.g. patella alta or lateral subluxation of patella.

Treatment

Superficial shaving of cartilage can be done through arthroscope leaving behind basal layer of healing cartilage. Extensive damage to cartilage can be managed by enblock excision with drilling of exposed subchondral bone.

SLIPPED FEMORAL CAPITAL EPIPHYSIS

This is also known as adolescent coxa vara or epiphysiolisthesis. This was first described by Muller. In this condition capital epiphysis is displaced downward and backward resulting into external rotation deformity of hip. This slipping causes avascular necrosis of femoral head and chondrolysis leading to painful and stiff hip. Later on hip joint becomes incongruous, resulting into degenerative arthritis.

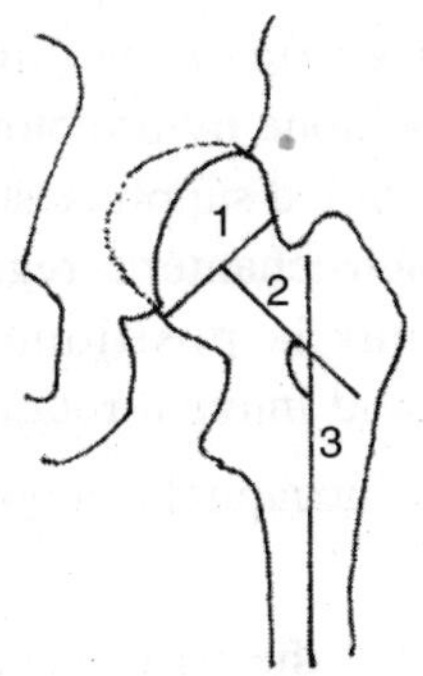

Grade I (Mild): Neck is displaced; less than 1/3rd diameter of femoral head **or** head shaft angle deviates from normal by 30° or less

Grade II (Moderate): Neck is displaced 1/3rd—1/2 of diameter of femoral head **or** head shaft angle deviates from normal 30–60°

Grade III (Severe): Neck is displaced > ½ of diameter of femoral head or head shaft angle deviates > 60°

Fig. 29.4 Slipped capital femoral epiphysis

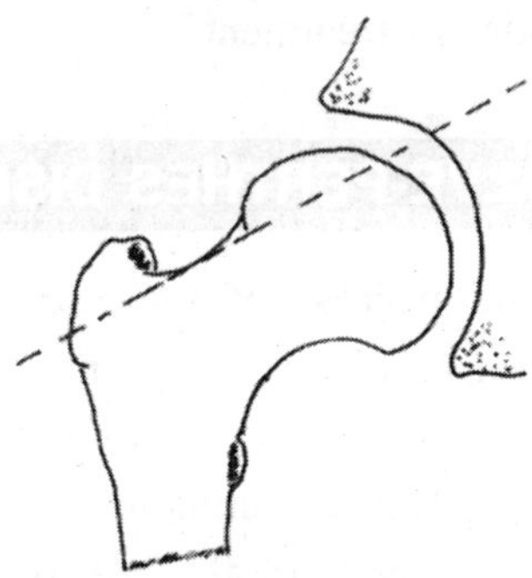

Fig. 29.5 Normal femoral epiphysis

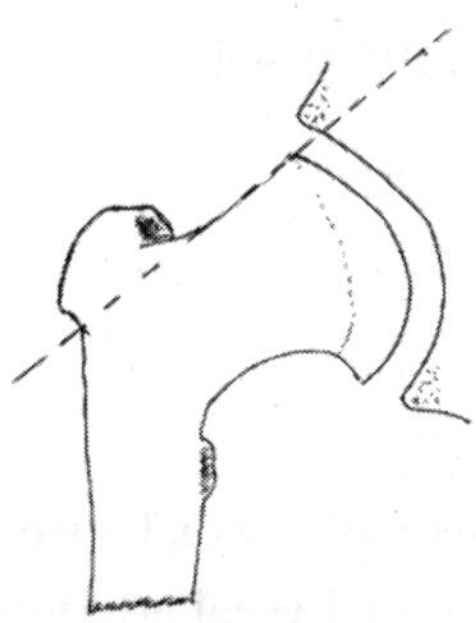

Fig. 29.6 Slipped capital epiphysis shows positive Trethowan's sign

Aetiology

1. Actual cause is not known.
2. Trauma may be a predisposing factor.
3. Growth hormone and estrogen also play some role in its aetiology.
4. Thinning of periosteum during adolescence, makes periosteal covering stretched and unable to withstand the shearing force.
5. Frolich type of obesity is also a predisposing factor.

Pathology

1. Epiphysis is displaced downward and backward leading to varus deformity. It also causes adduction and external rotation at hip joint.
2. Displacement takes place through hypertrophied mature cartilage.
3. Synovial membrane is grossly swollen, odematous, hyperemic and villous. Later this membrane becomes less vascular and more fibrotic and inelastic.
4. Later avascular necrosis develops in head of femur.
5. Degeneration and erosion of articular cartilage cause chondrolysis.
6. Gross displacement of epiphysis causes limitation of abduction and internal rotation of hip.

Clinical Features

This is commonly seen in adolescent age group between 10–17 years. Males are predominantly affected. Left hip is more commonly affected than right.

Patient presents in following three clinical stages:

Stage of Preslipping

In this stage patient develops mild discomfort at hip after doing some activity which subsides after rest. This stage does not have any objective findings.

Stage of Chronic Slipping

Patient has severe pain and antalgic gait. Tenderness is present at hip joint. Abduction and internal rotation at hip is limited leading to adduction and external rotation deformity at hip. Real shortening occurs due to upward displacement of femur.

Trendlenberg test is positive. Patient presents with waddling gait in bilateral severe slipping of epiphysis.

Stage of Fixed Deformity

Pain and muscle spasm is absent. Adduction and external rotation deformity is seen at hip. Limping is present. Limb is shortened.

X-ray Findings

X-ray are taken in AP. And lateral views. Lateral view should be taken in frog leg position. In this position hip should be flexed to 90 degree and abducted to 45 degree.

Following findings are seen:

1. Globular swelling of joint capsule.
2. Irregular widening of epiphyseal line.
3. Decalcification of epiphyseal border of metaphysis.
4. Shenton line is broken.
5. Trethowan's sign is positive i.e. if we draw a line along the superior border of neck, it will transect the femoral head above it.

Treatment

1. Abstinence from weight bearing is mandatory for the treatment. It means that patient has to take absolute bed rest.
2. Muscle spasm can be relieved by longitudinal traction, combined with medial rotation.
3. Surgery is treatment of choice. Principle of surgery is to restore positioning of femoral head, concentrically within acetabulum. This can be done by osteotomy away from epiphyseal blood supply. Osteotomy can be done at subtrochanteric region. After this distal femur is positioned in flexion, abduction and internal rotation.
4. Cuneiform subcapital osteotomy gives best result.
5. Osteotomy at the base of femoral neck is suitable only for extreme degree of slip. This osteotomy is maintained on 1½ hip spica for 2 months.
6. Trochanteric osteotomy can also be done which is of following three types:
   - Ball and socket type
   - High subtrochanteric type
   - Measured biplane intertrochanteric type

Epiphysiodesis and osteoplasty of femoral neck are other modes of treatment.

LEG-CALVE-PERTHES DISEASE

This is avascular necrosis of ossification centre of capital femoral epiphysis; also known as Coxa plana or osteochondritis juvenilis deformans or pseudocoxalgia. This is commonly seen between 3–12 years of age. Peak age is 6 years. Waldenstrom was the first person to describe this clinical entity. It is predominantly seen in male. Male to female ratio is 4:1.

Aetiology

Aetiology of coxa plana is described by two hypothesis:

Tureta's Hypothesis

According to this hypothesis between the ages of 4–8 years lateral epiphyseal artery (single arterial supply) is exposed to compression by strong lateral rotator muscles.

Caffey's Hypothesis

According to this Tureta's theory is not compatible as coxa plana is predominantly seen in male child, while arterial supply is similar in both sexes.

Pathological Changes

1. Stage of synovitis lasting for 1–3 weeks.
2. Stage of AVN lasting for 6 months to 1 year.
3. Stage of regeneration seen between 2-3 years.
4. Stage of healing shows cup shaped defect. X-ray shows gage sign i.e. superior part of neck becomes prominent on X-ray.
5. Hypertrophy of greater trochanter. Along with this greater trochanter is elevated thus impairing the power of abductor muscles. This makes trendlenberg test positive.

Clinical Features

1. Earliest symptom is limp.
2. Antalgic gait
3. Vague pain that may radiate to groin or knee. Pain is relieved by rest.
4. Abduction and internal rotation are predominantly restricted. Other movements are also restricted.
5. Atrophy of gluteal and thigh muscles.
6. Muscle spasm is also present.
7. Slight shortening may be seen.

X-ray Findings

1. Waldenstrom sign is seen. (head socket distance is increased)
2. Gage sign is also seen. (superior aspect of neck becomes prominent)
3. Tear drop phenomenon
4. Rarefaction
5. Thickened epiphyseal plate
6. Bulging of joint capsule
7. Osteoporosis of metaphysis.

Principles of Treatment

Following principles should be considered while treating such cases:

- Head and acetabular congruity should be maintained.
- Containment of head into acetabulum is must.
- Bed rest and traction should be considered.
- Weight bearing should be encouraged in abduction.
- Hip joint movements should be continued.

Modalities of Treatment

- Recumbent conservative treatment with bilateral traction.
- Ambulation abduction brace is very helpful.
- Subtrochanteric derotation and varus osteotomy.
- Innominae osteotomy.
- Penetration of growth plates by drill holes.

PES CAVUS

This is also known as Cavus foot, claw foot and congenital pes cavus. This is characterized by excessive high longitudinal plantar arch caused by equinus position of forefoot in relation to hind foot.

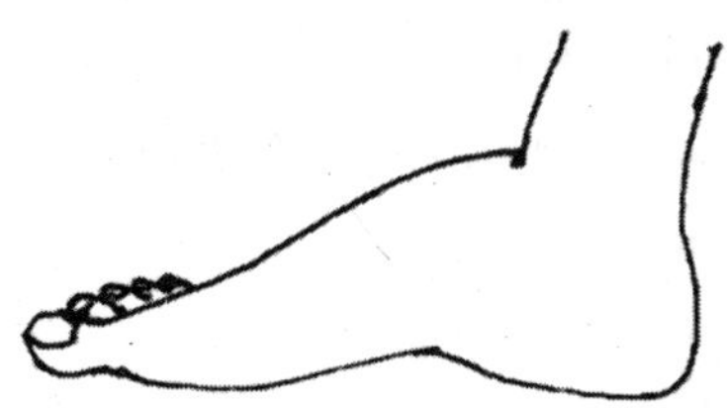

Fig. 29.7 Normal foot

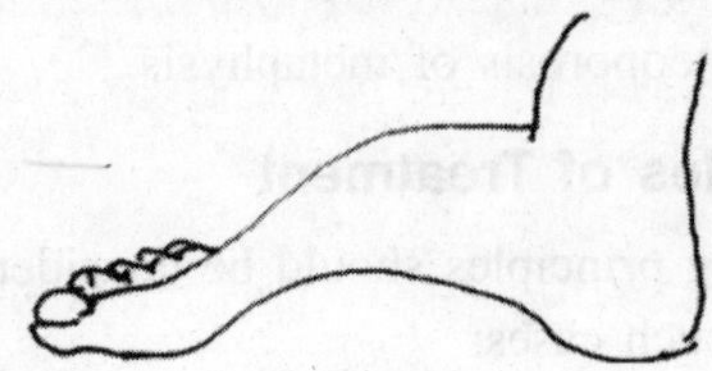

Fig. 29.8 Pes cavus

Aetiology

There are three aetiologies which can cause pes cavus:

1. Obscure cavus foot
2. Paralytic disease e.g. poliomyelitis
3. Neurological disease or developmental deformity of spine.

Classification

This is classified into two types as follows:

Primary

This is idiopathic in nature and seen after 3 years of age. This is most common type and often associated with spina bifida occulta.

Secondary

This is caused by following aetiologies:

- Spinocerebellar hereditary degeneration.
- Poliomyelitis
- Freidrich's ataxia
- Diastematomyelia
- Cauda equina tumor
- Cerebral palsy
- Spina bifida
- Charcot, Marrie-Tooth disease
- Trauma
- Muscular dystrophy
- CTEV
- Plantar fibromatosis

Components of Pes Cavus

Pes cavus has following four components:

1. Dropping of forefoot
2. Contracture of plantar fascia
3. Varus of heel
4. Clawing of toes

Types

1. Simple pes cavus
2. Pescavovarus
3. Calcaneocavus
4. Equinocavovarus

Clinical Features

1. Excessive high longitudinal arch.
2. Thick plantar fascia.
3. First metatarsal drop and pronation.
4. MP joint show cockup deformity of all toes.
5. Flexion deformity of all interphalangeal joints.
6. Heel is in varus.

X-ray Findings

Talocalcaneal angle is decreased.

Treatment

First Degree Cavus

It can be treated by daily manipulation, exercises, dorsiflexion, and anterior arch bar in shoe and night splint.

Second Degree Cavus

This can be treated by transfer of EHL to neck of first metatarsal. Equinus deformity can be treated by Jones tenosuspension procedure.

Third Degree Cavus

Extensor or shift procedure and posterior calcaneal osteotomy are popular methods to correct this type of pes cavus.

Fourth Degree Cavus

This can be treated by following methods:

- Japa's osteotomy of tarsals
- Anterior tarsal wedge osteotomy
- Fusion of first metatarsocuneiform navicular joint.

Fifth Degree Cavus

This can be treated by bone wedge resection or triple arthrodesis.

FLAT FOOT

This is also known as pes planus. It is caused by partial or complete loss of longitudinal arch. In this condition entire talus angulates forward, downward and medialy. Forefoot is in abduction and slight supination. Navicular and head of talus becomes prominent on medial aspect of foot. Calcaneum is everted (valgus). Deltoid, plantar and spring ligaments are stretched. Dorsal and lateral ligaments are contracted.

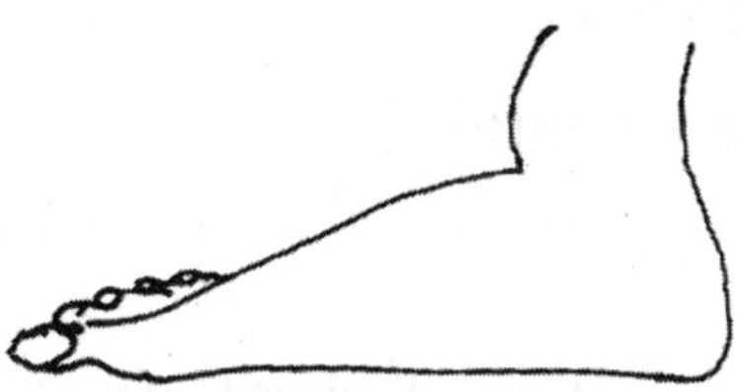

Fig. 29.9 Flat foot

Classification

Congenital

1. Hypermobile flatfoot
2. Rigid flatfoot with tarsal anomalies.

Acquired

1. Osseous
2. Ligamentous
3. Muscle imbalance
4. Postural/static
5. Arthritic

Clinical Features

1. Discomfort and burning sensation in feet are common complaints.
2. Patient becomes fatigue easily.
3. Pain becomes more severe while standing, than walking or running.
4. Tenderness is present below medial malleolus or at plantar ligament.
5. Patient avoids use of heel before the ball of foot to avoid strain on plantar ligament.

X-ray Findings

X-rays are taken in weight bearing position. Superior, inferior, lateral and oblique projection views are taken. X-ray shows the following findings:

1. Medial displacement and anterior projection of head of talus.
2. Divergence of long axis of talus from calcaneum.
3. Longitudinal arch is flattened.
4. Talus is pointed downward.

Treatment

Principle of treatment is to relieve ligamentous tension and transfer the body weight to lateral side of foot. Flat foot can be treated conservatively by following methods:

- Arch support (Whitman type) as a shoe insert.
- Shoes with Thomas heel or ¼ inch wedge on medial border of heel.
- Non weight bearing exercises can be performed in hot tub bath i.e. plantar flexion of toes. Heel to toe walking is also adviced.
- Surgical treatment is adviced in case of severe deformity and disability. Arthrodesis is treatment of choice and should be done around 15 years of age, but not before 10 years.

HAMMER TOE

Flexion deformity of proximal interphalangeal joint most commonly at second toe is called hammer toe. Tips of toes are pointed downward. MP joint is not hyperextended.

This is most commonly congenital and often bilateral. Metatarsal head is depressed and a callus is present at its plantar aspect.

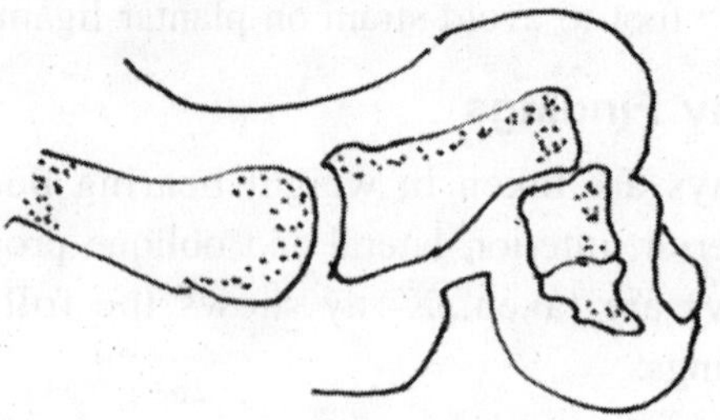

Fig. 29.10 Hammer toe

Treatment

Early deformities can be treated by adhesive strapping. Mother can manipulate the toes into extension frequently.

Surgical treatment is reserved for severe deformity. In this method dorsal callus is excised. Head of proximal phalanx and base of distal phalanx are excised. Toes are straightened by K wires. K wires are kept inserted into phalanx till fusion becomes complete.

HALLUX VALGUS (BUNION)

This is a deformity of great toe which is deflected laterally plus a bony prominence at medial aspect of first metatarsal head and neck.

Aetiology

1. Hereditary
2. Pressure caused by narrow shoes.
3. Wedging of medial cuneiform.

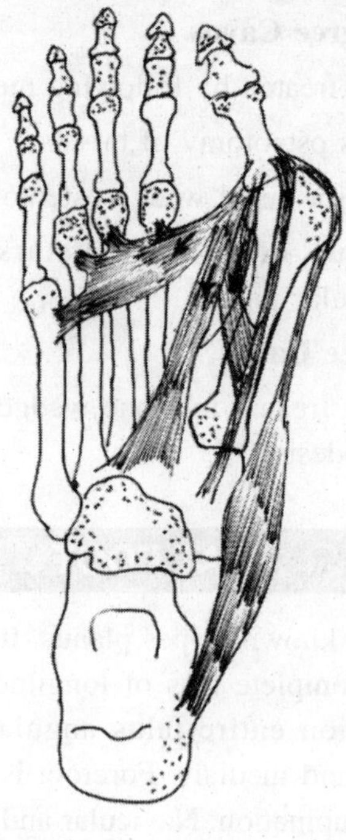

Fig. 29.11 Hallux valgus mechanism of muscle pull that maintains valgus deformity of great toe

4. Degenerative arthritis of first MP joint of foot.
5. Flat foot.

Clinical Features

1. Patient present with laterally deflected great toe.
2. Second toe is displaced dorsally, by great toe, thus it develops hammer toe deformity.
3. Foot becomes flat.
4. Heel is in valgus.

Treatment

A shoe with enlarged toe portion can be adviced. To relieve pressure around exostosis a thick felt ring can be applied.

If conservative treatment fails, surgical treatment is required. Following surgical treatments are available:

- Mc Bride's soft tissue surgery

- Bone excision procedure
- Arthroplasty or arthrodesis of MP joint.
- Sling procedure
- Osteotomy of first metatarsal or proximal phalanx.

HALLUX RIGIDUS

- This is painful restricted motion of great toe (mainly dorsiflexion of metatarsophalangeal joint) that leads to degenerative arthritis later in life.
- Patient walks with short stepped hopping gait.
- Plantar flexion is normal.
- Interphalangeal joint is hypermobile.
- Great toe is excessively long.
- Failure to conservative treatment requires surgical treatment.
- Hallux rigidus can be surgically corrected by Lambrinudi procedure, Keller's arthroplasty, Flexible implant arthroplasty and Arthrodesis of MP joint.

HALLUX VARUS

This is a congenital anomaly in which great toe is deflected medially.

DORSAL BUNION

This is a condition which is characterized by dorsiflexion of first metatarsal and plantarflexion of great toe. A painful dorsal prominence develops at metatarsal head while walking and weight bearing.

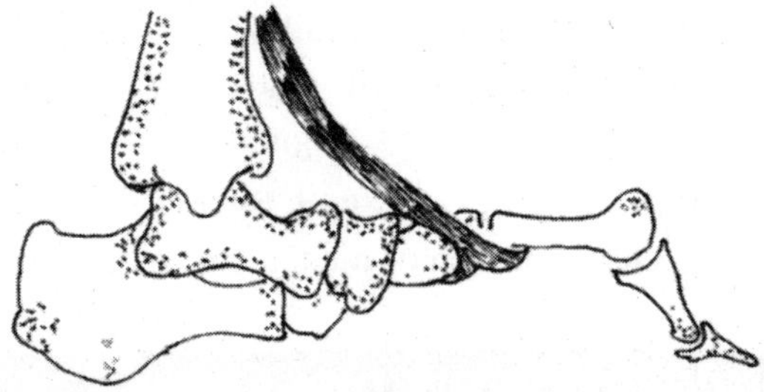

Fig. 29.12 Dorsal bunion

Treatment

Tibialis anterior can be transferred either to cuneiform or to tibialis posterior.

PLANTAR FASCITIS AND CALCANEAL SPUR

A bony prominence develops at plantar aspect of calcaneum, known as calcaneal spur. Bursa overlying it becomes inflamed known as plantar fascitis. It can also cause strain of fibres of plantar fascia.

Clinical Features

1. Patient complaints of pain at under surface of heel while standing and walking. This pain is relieved by rest.
2. Tenderness is present at the site of spur.
3. Sometimes patient may present with mild swelling at plantar aspect of foot.

X-ray Findings

A bony spur may be seen on X-ray.

Treatment

1. Bed rest
2. Contrast foot bath
3. Local injection of corticosteroid
4. Shoe with silicon heel provides tremendous relief from pain.

5. Surgical treatment includes excision of spur and resection of part of plantar apponeurosis at it's origin.
6. Pain can be relieved by resection of posterior branch of medial calcaneal nerve.

SEVER'S DISEASE

This is also known as calcaneal epiphysitis. This is an inflammation of epiphysis of posterior part of calcaneum.

Clinical Features

1. This is commonly seen between age of 11 and 14 years of age.
2. Males are predominantly affected than females.
3. Pain is experienced while standing on toes and while using low heel.
4. Patient walks with short steps.
5. Tenderness is present at mediolateral aspect of tendocalcaneal attachment.

Treatment

Treatment is conservative. AKPOP cast can be applied with knee in flexion and foot in equinus. Physiotherapy has no role.

TARSAL TUNNEL SYNDROME

This is a compression neuropathy of posterior tibial nerve.

Clinical Features

1. Nocturnal burning pain in foot that awakes the patient from sleep is classical feature. Hanging the legs over the edge of bed relieves the pain.
2. Tingling and numbness in toes and distal part of foot which is aggravated by prolonged standing and walking. This is relieved by taking rest.
3. Sensory loss is present in distribution area of medial and lateral plantar nerve.
4. Tinel sign may be positive.
5. Two points discrimination is diminished.

Treatment

Local injection of steroid provides temporary relief. Surgical decompression of nerve is effective.

FROZEN SHOULDER

This is a clinical condition in which shoulder becomes stiff and patient presents with painful restriction of both active and passive movement at shoulder joint. External rotation is most commonly affected. This is also known as periarthritis shoulder or adhesive capsulitis.

Aetiology

Local Causes

1. Rotator cuff tendinitis
2. Bicipital tendinitis
3. Fracture dislocation at shoulder
4. Prolonged immobilization of shoulder
5. Muscle imbalance.

Generalized Causes

1. Diabetes
2. Frozen hand shoulder syndrome
3. Reflex sympathetic dystrophy.

Pathology

Rotator cuff and long head of biceps become stretched due to repeated overhead activity of shoulder and to abduction movement.

This kind of repeated strain causes inflammation of capsule. Later capsule becomes fibrosed and thickened that leads to loss of movement at shoulder. Repeated movement at shoulder can break fibrosis which can bring back active movement at shoulder joint.

Clinical Features

1. This is more common between 50–60 years of age.
2. Females are more commonly affected.
3. Patient presents with pain and stiffness at shoulder joint.
4. Active and passive movements at shoulder are restricted.
5. Restriction of external rotation movement is characteristic.
6. Arm is held in internal rotation.

Treatment

1. Hot saline fomentation at shoulder gives tremendous relief.
2. Analgesics are given in the form of NSAID.
3. Intraarticular corticosteroid injections can be helpful.
4. Physiotherapy is most important aspect of treatment. Regular and disciplined exercises increase the range of motion at shoulder. Shoulder wheel and pendulum exercises are very helpful. Active and passive movements should be performed.
5. Short wave diathermy and ultrasonic therapy is helpful in severe cases.

Surgical Treatment

1. This is indicated when pain is severe and persistent.
2. Subacromial bursa is resected. Intraarticular biceps tendon is released. This is cut at its origin at glenoid rim.
3. Extraarticular tendon is elevated after cutting transverse humeral ligament.

TENNIS ELBOW

This is a clinical condition in which tendinous origin of common wrist extensor is affected that causes pain at the tip of lateral condyle of humerus. This is commonly seen in tennis players.

Aetiology

1. Tear in common extensor origin. (epicondylitis).
2. Inflammation of adventitious bursa between radiohumeral joint and common extensor origin.
3. Hypertrophy of synovial fringe between capitulum and radial head.
4. Calcification is common extensor origin.

Clinical Features

Patient complaints of pain at the tip of lateral condyle of elbow which aggravates while doing daily activity e.g. wringing a towel, while getting up from a chair, while lifting a jug from its mouth and while sweeping the floor. On examination tenderness is present at tip of lateral condyle of humerus. Following tests are positive in this condition:

Cozen Test

To perform this test, keep the elbow in full extension then extend the wrist against resistance. This will elicit pain at lateral condyle of humerus.

Mill's Manoeuver

In this test elbow is kept extended. Now passively flex the wrist and pronate forearm. This will cause pain at lateral condyle.

Wringing Test

Ask the patient to wring a towel. This will elicit pain at lateral condyle.

Jug Test

Ask the patient to lift a jug full of water from its mouth. This will also elicit pain at lateral condyle.

Chair Test

Ask the patient to get up from a chair with both hands firmly gripping and pressing the arm of chair. This will also elicit pain at lateral condyle.

Rolling Pin Test

Rolling the dough for preparing round bread will also elicit pain at same site.

Stirfry Test

Stirfrying causes pain at tip of lateral condyle of humerus.

Broom's Manoeuver

Holding a broom firmly to sweep floor also causes pain at tip of condyle of humerus.

Treatment

Conservative treatment consists of rest to joint by elbow strap, hot saline fomentation, ultrasonic therapy and local injections of anaesthetics/ steroids are helpful. Failed conservative treatment requires surgical treatment.

Following two surgical treatments are popular:

- Release of epicondylar muscle percutaneously.
- Excision of proximal portion of annular ligament and release of common extensor origin also gives relief from pain. This also involves excision of bursa and synovial fringes.

GOLFER'S ELBOW

This is a clinical condition that affects tendinous insertion of common flexors of hand. This is also known as epitrochleitis.

Clinical Features

Patient presents with pain at medial condyle of elbow and difficulty in activity of daily living.

Test for Golfer's Elbow

Keep the elbow in extension and forearm in supination. Now ask the patient to make a fist and then to flex it against resistance. This will elicit pain at medial epicondyle. Pain aggravates by a valgus stress to elbow in extension.

Treatment

This is treated conservatively by means of hot saline fomentation, analgesics and ultrasonic therapy. Surgically it can be treated by percutaneous release of medial epicondyle muscle.

STUDENT'S ELBOW

This is a clinical condition in olecranon bursa undergoes chronic inflammation. This is also known as olecranon bursitis. It is predisposed by repeated minor trauma or by deposition of microcrystal or by keeping the elbow repeatedly over table.

Clinical Features

Patient presents with pain and mild swelling at the tip of elbow.

Treatment

Aspiration should be done and should be sent for culture and sensitivity to rule possibility of infection. NSAID and local injections of steroid may provide symptomatic relief.

ELBOW TUNNEL SYNDROME

This is uncommon condition affecting ulnar nerve. This nerve is involved between two heads of flexor carpi ulnaris. This is seen in osteoarthritis of elbow in which ulnar nerve is injured by osteophytes.

DEQUERVAIN'S DISEASE

This is tenovaginitis of common sheath of abductor pollicis longus and extensor pollicis brevis tendons.

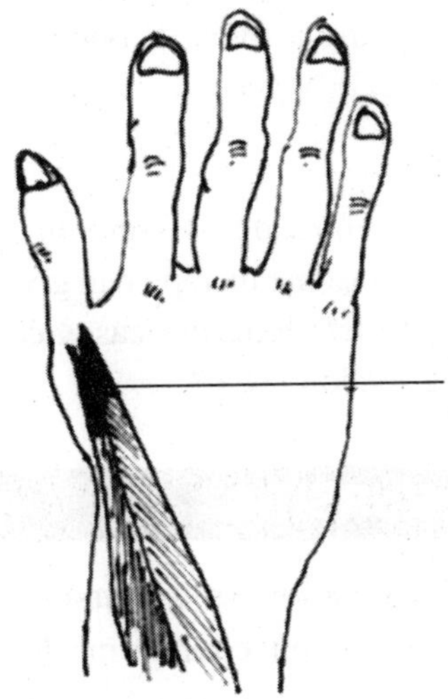

Fig. 29.13 Dequervain's disease

Clinical Features

Patient presents with pain and swelling at radial styloid process. Tenderness is present at radial styloid.

Abduction of thumb across the palm and forced ulnar deviation causes pain at radial styloid process.

Finkelstein Test

This test is perfomed in Dequervain's disease. Patient is asked to pronate his forearm with flexed elbow. Now ask him to make a fist. After this, deviate his fist toward ulnar side. This will result in pain at the site of insertion of APL and EPB.

Treatment

This can be treated conservatively by means of ultrasonic therapy, local injections of steroids and creppe bandage application.

Surgical treatment is indicated in extreme cases in which tenon sheath is excised.

DUPUYTREN'S CONTRACTURE

This is contracture of palmar aponeurosis which leads to flexion deformity of ring and little finger at M.P. and PIP joint. Palmaris aponeurosis is continuation of palmaris longus tendon.

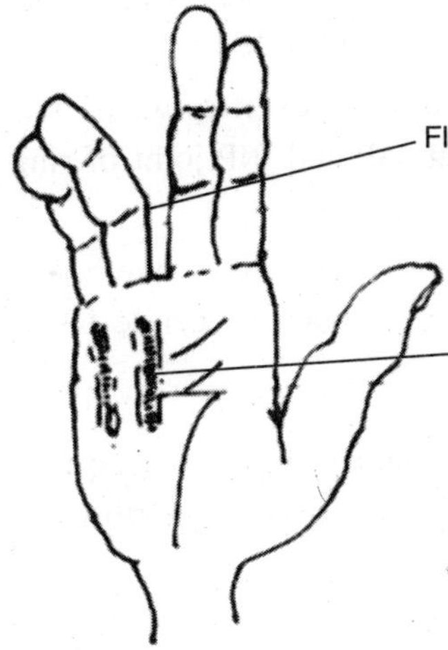

Fig. 29.14 Dupuytren's contracture

Aetiology

Dupuytren's contracture can develop in following conditions:

1. Hereditary
2. Cirrhosis
3. Epilepsy
4. Drug induced: Phenylhydantoin.
5. Chronic alcoholics.
6. Trauma.

Pathogenesis

Palmaris aponeurosis is continuation of palmaris longus tendon. This tendon divides into 4 slips one for each finger. These slips binds with fibrous flexor sheath and extends up to middle phalanx. In this condition aponeurosis is thickened due to fibroplasia. Subcutaneous fat is reduced. Later contracture develops in aponeurosis which brings MP and PIP joint into flexion deformity.

Clinical Features

1. This is usually seen before 40 years of age.

2. Males are more commonly affected than female.
3. Initially patient may present with thickening at base of ring and little finger.
4. Later patient presents with flexion deformity at MP and PIP joint of ring and little finger.
5. Uncommonly patient may have associated thickening of plantar and penile fascia.

Treatment

Mild deformity usually does not require any treatment. Radiotherapy may be helpful in early phase of disease.

Most common surgery is subtotal excision of palmar aponeurosis.

TRIGGER FINGER

This is a clinical condition in which digital fibrous sheath is constricted in such a way that flexion tendon can not glide freely. In this condition finger moves like trigger of a pistol. Finger become locked in flexed position and can only be extended by applying a force.

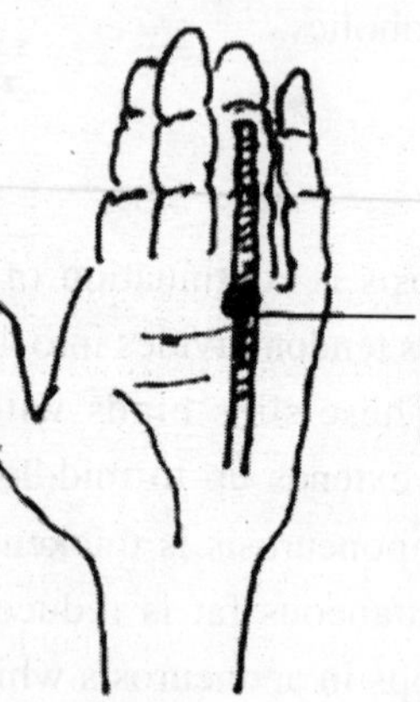

Fig. 29.15 Trigger finger

Clinical Features

Patient presents with pain during extension of finger. Finger becomes locked in flexed position and extends on applying a force. It opens like a trigger of pistol.

Treatment

Local injections of hydrocortisone provide tremendous relief. Ultrasonic therapy can give you only symptomatic relief. Extreme cases can be treated by spiltting tendon sheath.

BURSITIS

Inflammation of bursa is known as bursitis. It is caused by either bacterial infection or mechanical irritation. Examples of irritative bursitis are prepatellar bursitis (housemaid knee), ishial bursitis (weaver's bottom), olecranon bursitis (student elbow), infrapatellar bursitis (clergyman' knee), bursitis at lateral malleolus (taylor's ankle).

GANGLION

This is pseudomucinous degeneration of tendon sheath or joint capsule. Patient presents with localized swelling which may or may not be painful. Common sites of ganglion are wrist, forearm and foot. This is multiloculated and can be relieved by aspiration of cyst.

LOOSE BODIES

Loose bodies may arise from three following sites:

1. Synovial fluid
2. Synovial membrane
3. Bone

Synovial Fluid

These are fibrinous loose bodies which develop due to haemorrhagic or inflammatory effusion. This is commonly seen in tuberculosis of joints. These loose bodies are known as melon-seed bodies.

Synovial membrane

These loose bodies originate from within villous synovial processes. This is also known as osteochondromatosis.

Bone

This type results from fracture or detachment of osteophytes. This is commonly seen in osteoarthritis, osteomyelitis and osteochondritis dessicans.

CARPAL TUNNEL SYNDROME

This is compression neuropathy of median nerve while it passes beneath flexor retinaculum. This results due to narrowing of carpal tunnel. This is commonly seen in rheumatoid arthritis, pregnancy and as a complication of colles's fracture. Women of 40–60 years of age are commonly affected.

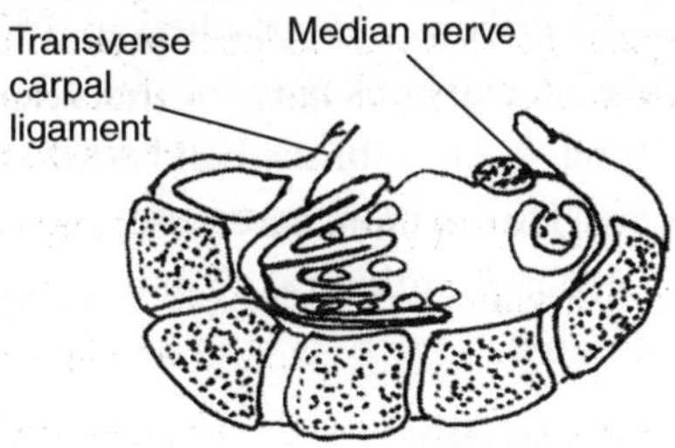

(*a*) Decompressed carpal tunnel

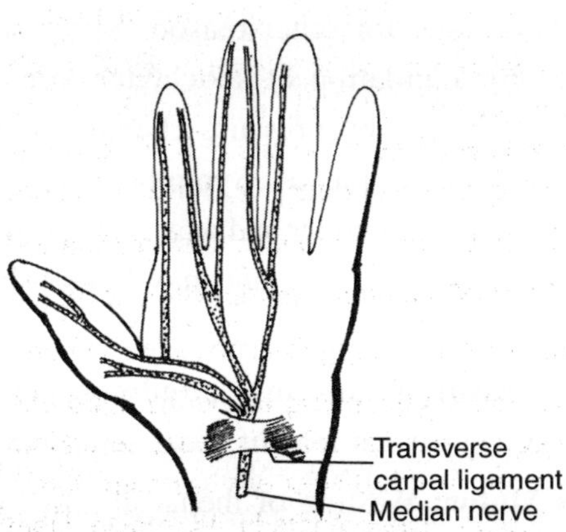

(*b*) Compression of median nerve in carpal tunnel syndrome

Fig. 29.16 Carpal tunnel syndrome

Aetiology

Idiopathic This is most common cause.

Inflammatory

- Rheumatoid arthritis
- Osteoarthritis of wrist

Endocrinal

- Myxoedema
- Acromegaly

Post-traumatic

- Colles's fracture

Clinical Features

Patient presents with progressive weakness and impairment of fine movements. Tingling, numbness or discomfort in thumb and medial two and half fingers are common features. This is most commonly seen while sleeping.

Phalen test

This test is also known as wrist flexion test. Patient is asked to flex the wrist. Patient will feel tingling numbness in distribution area of median nerve. These symptoms subside as soon as wrist is straightend.

Treatment

Symptoms can be relieved by dividing flexor retinaculum.

MERALGIA PARAESTHETICA

This is a clinical condition which is caused by compression of lateral cutaneous nerve of thigh just medial to anterior superior iliac spine. This can be treated conservatively by analgesics and injections of hydrocortisone.

IMPINGEMENT SYNDROME

This is a clinical syndrome in which rotator cuff muscles are impinged under coracoacromial arch.

Patient presents with pain, stiffness at shoulder and restricted movement (painful arc of 60–120 degree abduction). This is also known as painful arc syndrome.

This clinical syndrome has been divided into following 3 stages **(Neer's staging)**:

1. Stage of oedema and haemorrhage.
   (< 25 years of age)
2. Stage of fibrosis, tendinitis and partial tear.
   (25–40 years of age)
3. Stage of complete rotator cuff tears.
   (> 40 years of age)

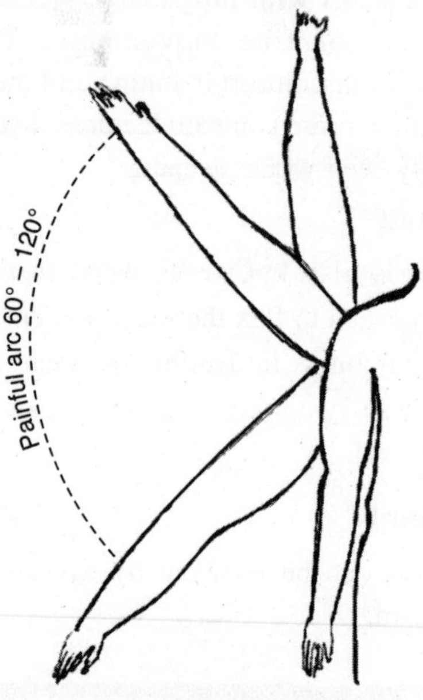

Fig. 29.17 Painful arc syndrome

Treatment

Stage 1 can be treated conservatively by analgesics, ultrasonic therapy and intra-articular injections of steroid. Stage 2 is treated by bursectomy and division of coracoacromial ligament. Stage 3 can be treated by anterior acromioplasty and rotator cuff repair. Stage 2 and 3 can be treated arthroscopically as well as by open surgery.

BENNET'S LESION

Sometimes triceps tendon is injured at its insertion due to a traction injury. This area later undergoes calcification. This condition is known as Bennet's lesion.

POPLITEAL CYST

This is herniation of synovial membrane at popliteal fossa. This can be seen in osteoarthritis (Baker cyst) and rheumatoid arthritis. Patient presents with painless localized swelling in midline of popliteal fossa. Due to high recurrence rate it is not recommended for excision.

CERVICAL RIB

This is an additional rib which takes origin from 7th cervical vertebra and attached to 1st rib near to insertion of scalenous anterior muscle. Anterior part of rib has a just fibrous band while posterior part is bony. This is most commonly seen on right side and usually unilateral. Young females are usually affected.

Clinical Features

Mostly it is asymptomatic and incidently detected on X-ray done for other reason. Symptoms are caused by angulation of subclavian artery over cervical rib and by pressure changes of lowest trunk of brachial plexus. Symptoms are relieved by elevation of shoulder and aggravated by pulling the arm downward. Patient may have following features:

- **Sensory:** Tingling, numbness and pain along medial side of hand and forearm.
- **Motor:** Wasting of thenar and hypothenar muscles leading to **claw hand.** Power of hand may be lost.

- **Vasomotor:** Circulatory impairment and sweating of hand are main features which sometime may lead to gangrene.
- **Adson test:** This test is positive. In this test patient is asked to sit on a stool and to take a deep breath. Turn his face to affected side. Now feel pulsation of radial artery on wrist. Pulse will be obliterated.

Treatment

Cervical rib excision is only required if symptoms are severe and not relieved by conservative treatment.

CHAPTER

30 Pott's Spine

- Pott's spine (tuberculosis of spine)
- Multi drug resistant tuberculosis (MDRTB) in orthopaedics
- Pott's paraplegia
- Seddon's classification of pott's paraplegia
- Signs and symptoms

POTT'S SPINE (TUBERCULOSIS OF SPINE)

Tuberculosis of spine is known as Pott's spine as it was detected by Sir Percivial Pott. Spine is most common part of skeletal system to be affected by tuberculosis. (50% of all cases)

Lower thoracic and lumbar vertebrae are more commonly affected due to following reasons:

- Abundant spongy tissue is present within vertebral body.
- Weight bearing capacity is more at this area.
- These vertebrae are more mobile.

Embryology of Vertebra

Lower half of one vertebra, intervertebral disc and upper half of next vertebra develop from each pair of sclerotome, which has common blood supply. So the infection that reaches to these arteries involves embryological section, as seen in paradiscal type of tuberculosis.

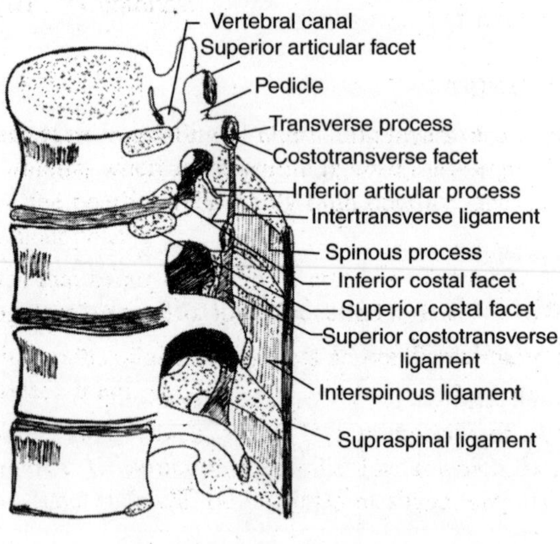

Fig. 30.1 Anatomy of vertebral column (Lateral view)

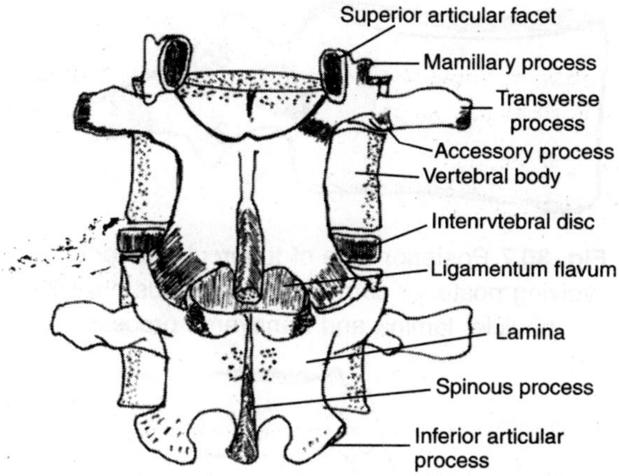

Fig. 30.2 Posterior view of L_3 and L_4 vertebrae

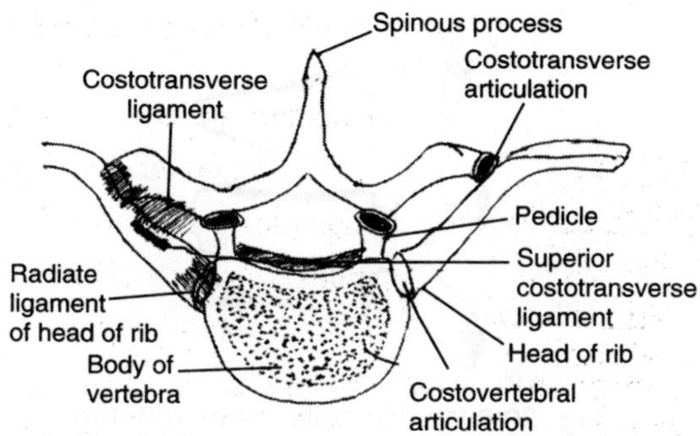

Fig. 30.3 Thoracic vertebra with rib attachment

Cord-Segment Level

Spinal cord terminates at lower end of L1 vertebra and from here it continues as dural sac containing a bunch of nerve roots known as cauda equina. Cauda equina ends at S2 vertebra.

Relationship between Spinal Segment and Cord Segment

Spinal segment	Cord segment
C1-C7	Add 1
T1-T6	Add 2
T7 8 9	Add 3
T10	All dorsal segment over
T12	All lumbar segment over
L1	All sacral segment over
Below L1	Cauda equina

Pathology

Tuberculosis of spine is always secondary and spreads by haematogenous route from lungs or lymph nodes. It reaches the vertebra via Batson plexus (paravertebral plexus of veins).

Tubercular infection causes endarteritis which later on causes marrow devitalisation. Hyperemia causes destruction of lamellae. Later osteoporosis develops at this place. As a result vertebrae are compressed. Anterior wedge compression is more common due to normal kyphotic curvature in thoracic spine. Exudative reaction is seen in vertebrae while caseative reaction is rare.

Cold Abscess

Non pyogenic infection leads to formation of cold abscess. It consists of caseous material, WBC, serum, tubercular bacilli and granulation tissue. Signs of inflammation are absent in cold abscess. This may travel beneath anterior longitudinal ligament (Prevertebral abscess). If it travels posteriorly, it may compress spinal cord more commonly in thoracic area because spinal canal is narrow in this area. Cold abscess may travel through areas of least resistance e.g. along the fascial plane, blood vessels and nerves. When it travels on the sides of vertebra it is known as paravertebral abscess.

Classification of Vertebral Tuberculosis

Vertebral tuberculosis has been classified into following five types:

1. Paradiscal
2. Central type
3. Anterior (periosteal) type
4. Posterior type
5. True tubercular arthritis

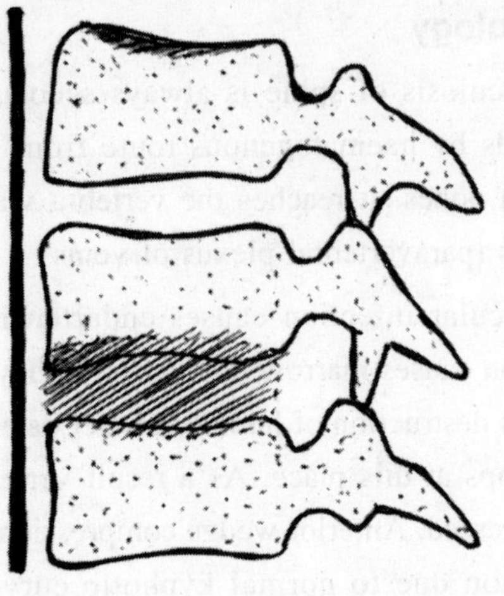

Fig. 30.4 Paradiscal type of tuberculosis

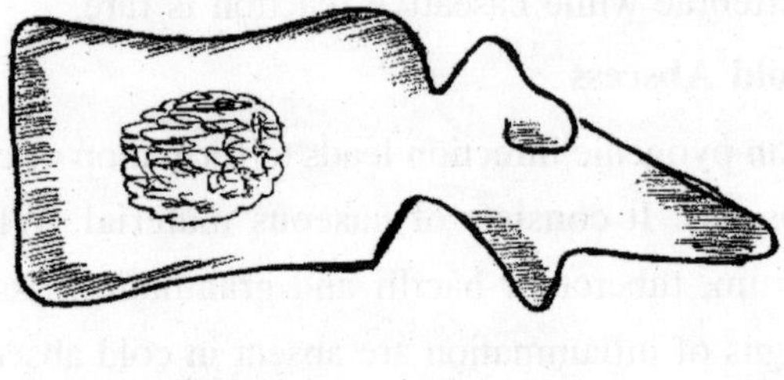

Fig. 30.5 Central type of tuberculosis vertebrae

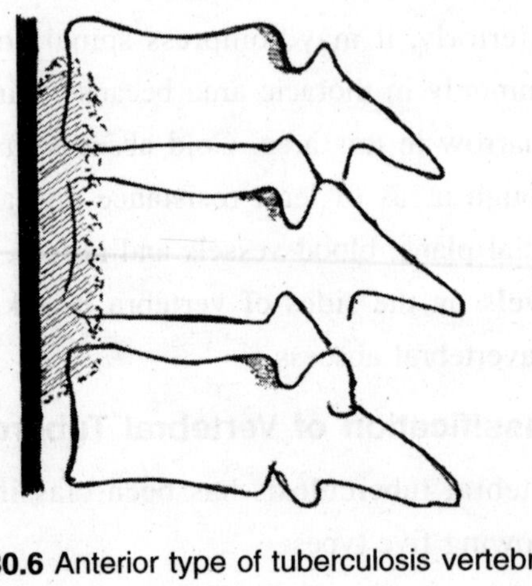

Fig. 30.6 Anterior type of tuberculosis vertebrae

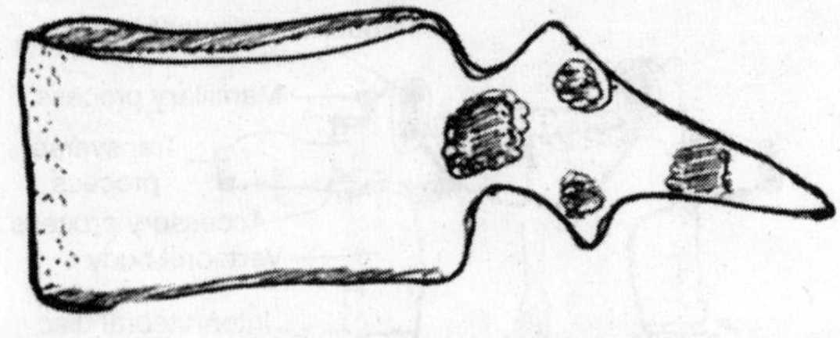

Fig. 30.7 Posterior type of tuberculosis vertebra involving posterior complex e.g. spinous process, pedicle, lamina and transverse process

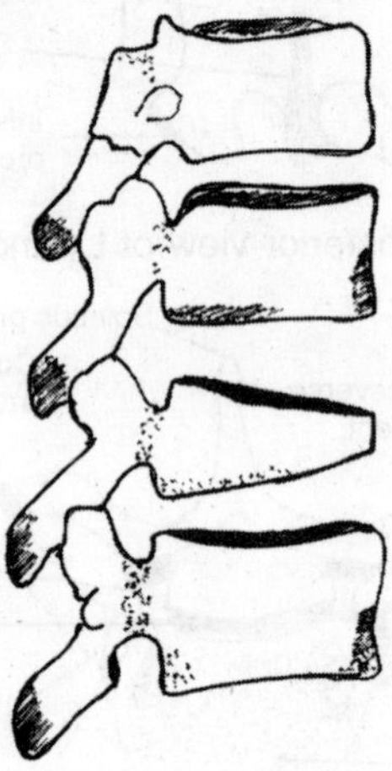

Fig. 30.8 Wedge collapse of vertebra

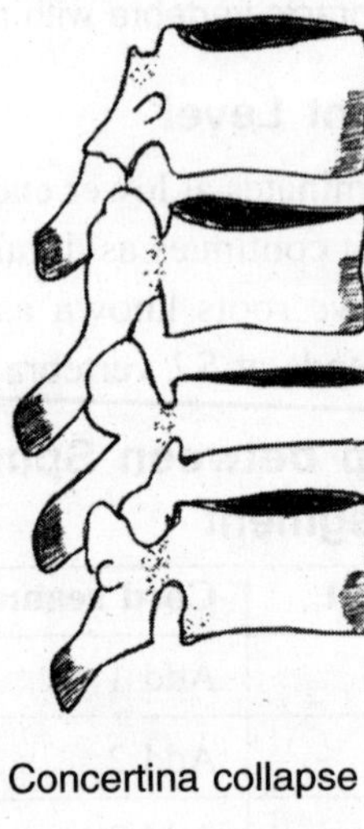

Fig. 30.9 Concertina collapse of vertebra

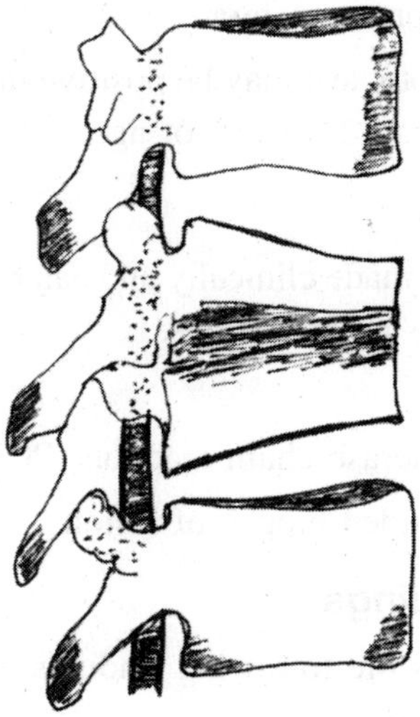

Fig. 30.10 Formation of internal Gibbus by collapse of two vertebrae

Paradiscal Type

In this type intervertebral disc along with contiguous areas of 2 adjacent vertebrae are involved. This is commonest type.

Central Type

Central part of vertebral body is involved that leads to collapse of vertebra (wedging/concertina). Intervertebral disc is normal.

Anterior Type

Anterior surface of vertebral body is involved. Infection spreads through anterior longitudinal ligament.

Posterior Type

In this type pedicle, lamina, transverse and spinous process are involved.

True Tubercular Arthritis

This type of lesion is usually seen in atlantoaxial and atlanto-oocipital joint.

Clinical Features

Patient presents with following clinical features:

Backache

Patient complaints of diffuse pain at lower back. This pain is mild to moderate and may radiate along the nerve root.

Stiff Spine

This is second commonest complaint of patient. Stiffness occurs due to spasm of paravertebral muscle. This is a protective phenomenon that protects movement at affected vertebra.

Cold Abscess

Cold abscess is a collection of WBC, serum, caseous material, granulation tissue and tubercular bacilli. This is called cold because it does not show any feature of inflammation. Cold abscess may travel the following track:

At cervical spine

- Retropharyngeal
- Parapharyngeal
- Posterior triangle of neck
- Sternocleidomastoid (posterior border)
- Axilla

At thoracic spine

- Mediastinal abscess
- Paravertebral abscess
- Anterior chest wall
- Mid axillary line
- Posterior chest wall

At lumbar spine

- Prevertebral abscess
- Paravertebral abscess
- Lumbar abscess
- Psoas abscess
- Femoral triangle
- Gluteal abscess
- Petit's angle

Deformities of Spine

Patient may present with three types of kyphosis:

Gibbus: It is formed by fusion of 2-3 spinous processes, which become prominent.

Knuckle: Only one spinous process becomes prominent.

Kyphosis: Vertebral column shows diffuse roundening. This is most common deformity. It constitutes 95% of all deformities.

Paraplegia

If adequate treatment is not given for pott's spine it may result in paraplegia.

Miscellaneous

Malaise, fever, weight loss, loss of appetite and letharginess are other features of pott's spine.

Examination Findings

Short Step Gait

During a routine walk, even a small jerk produces pain in tuberculous vertebra. So to avoid these jerks patient walks with short steps. If cervical spine is affected patient supports his head with both hands and rotates his body to look sideways.

Deformities

Following deformities can be observed in pott's spine; kyphosis 95%, scoliosis 5% and lordosis (uncommon).

Cold Abscess

This can present as paravertebral swelling. (site of cold abscess is discussed earlier). This is fluctuant cold swelling and aspiration shows pus collection.

Bony Tenderness

Bony tenderness can be elicited over the side of spinous processes.

Movements of Spine

Movements of spine may be restricted (flexion, lateral flexion, rotation and extension).

Neurological Findings

Patient will have sensory motor deficit depending upon the level of lesion in spine.

Lab Findings

- Anemia
- Lymphocytosis
- Raised ESR
- Hypoprotienaemia
- Mantoux test may be positive in children of less than 2-3 years of age.

Diagnosis

Diagnosis is made clinically and can be confirmed by following investigations:

1. Elisa
2. Polymerase chain reaction (PCR)
3. CT-guided biopsy of lesion

X-ray Findings

X-ray shows the following findings:

1. **Reduced disc space**

This is earliest and important sign seen in X-ray. Disc space is reduced because bacteria affect disc as well as contiguous areas of two adjacent vertebrae.

2. **Collapse of vertebrae**

Two types of collapse can be seen:

Wedging collapse

- Anterior part of vertebra is compressed that results into wedging.
- This happens because line of weight bearing passes anterior to dorsal vertebrae.

Concertina collapse

Vertebra is uniformly compressed (central body collapse)

3. **Paravertebral shadow**

- This shadow is suggestive of cold abscess. This may have fusiform or globular shape.
- Soft tissue shadow (thickness of more than 4 mm) in front of C3 vertebra is suggestive of retropharyngeal abscess.
- Prominent psoas shadow in X-ray of abdomen indicates toward psoas abscess.
- Mediastinum becomes wide due to abscess collection.

- Diffuse rarefaction of vertebra is seen in X-ray.
- Anterior part of vertebral body shows erosion similar to aneurysm of aorta. So this is also known as **Aneurysmal sign.**
- **Skipped lesion.** If more than one tuberculous lesion is present with one or more normal vertebra in between these two lesions, it is known as Skipped lesion. This is visible on X-ray.

CT-SCAN

Following findings can be detected in CT-scan:

- Paravertebral abscess
- Extent of destruction of vertebra
- Level of nerve compression
- Spinal tumor syndrome
- Fine calcification of soft tissue

MRI

MRI can detect the level of cord compression. Paravertebral abscess can also be detected.

USG

It can detect size and quantity of cold abscess.

Gallium Scan

This investigation is helpful in dessiminated tuberculosis.

Treatment

Bed rest

Patient is adviced bed rest during the active phase of disease. This is also necessary to prevent further collapse or dislocation of vertebra. Bed rest is recommended at least for 3-4 weeks.

Antitubercular Treatment

According to latest WHO schedule Rifampicin 600mg, INH (300 mg for <50 kg, 600 mg for >50 kg), Pyrazinamide (1500 mg for <50 kg and 2000 mg for >50 kg) and Ethambutol (1000 mg for <50 kg and1600 mg for >50 kg) are given for two months in a new case (**Intensive phase, total 24 doses** of each drug). These drugs are taken thrice in a week. After two months Pyrazinamide and Ethambutol are stopped while Rifampicin and INH are continued for next 4 months (**continuation phase, total 54 doses** of each drug). During this treatment patient should be watched for side effects of drugs. These possible side effects should be explained to the patient. Liver function test should be checked if required. Response of ATT starts within 3–4 weeks. Pain and other constitutional features subside gradually.

Injectable streptomycin can be given to hospitalized patient but less preferred in these days due to toxicity.

High Protein Diet

High protein diet is necessary for these patients. Albumin can be given by intravenous route.

Aspiration of cold abscess

Cold abscess is aspirated through an antigravity insertion method. Needle should be entered through a zig-zag tract. Abscess is drained and it's wall are currettaged and closed without a drain.

Gradual mobilization

If patient improves and does not show any feature of neurological complication, he can be mobilized with the help of suitable brace according to level of spinal tuberculosis. ASH brace is given for dorsolumbar spine while cervical collar is given for cervical spine tuberculosis. Brace is recommended for 18–24 months and then discarded.

Follow up X-ray and ESR

After 3 months a follow up X-ray of spine and ESR to be done to see the response of treatment.

Complications of Pott's Spine

- Paraplegia
- Cold abscess

- Multiple sinuses
- Amyloidosis
- Secondary infections.

Differential Diagnosis

1. Traumatic spine with or without neurological deficit

- Intervertebral disc space is normal in X-ray.
- Paravertebral shadow is absent.
- Wedging of vertebra is seen in X-ray.
- Patient will give history of trauma.

2. Prolapse intervertebral disc

- History of low backache with radiculopathy is present.
- Examination will show irregular LMN type of paralysis in lower limbs. Ankle jerks are absent on both sides. Hypoaesthesia is present in corresponding dermatome.
- SLR and Laseque test are positive.
- Bragard sign and contralateral SLRT are positive.

3. Ankylosing spondylitis

- Patient presents with painful stiff spine. Pain becomes severe in night or early in morning. Pain is relieved by walking.
- Gaenslen test, Fleche test and pump handle tests are positive.
- X-ray shows characteristic picture of bamboo spine with evidence of enthesopathy, squaring of vertebrae, syndesmophytes and loss of lordosis.
- HLA B-27 is positive.

4. Secondaries

- This usually involves pedicle.
- History suggestive of primary tumor elsewhere in the body will be present.
- Intervertebral disc space is normal in X-ray.

MULTI DRUG RESISTANT TUBERCULOSIS (MDRTB) IN ORTHOPAEDICS

Pathologically multiple drug resistant patients are those who show infecting organisms resistant to INH and Rifampicin with or without resistance to other antitubercular drug.

Clinically if the patient is not responding to ATT (multi drug therapy) within 4–6 months they are known as multi drug resistant.

These patient presents with deterioration of disease and development of sinus, cold abscess and ulcer. Followup X-ray and MRI may show deterioration of features upto 2–4 months of treatment. If deterioration continues beyond 5–6 months of treatment it means pathology is different or it may be refractory tuberculosis.

Once the diagnosis of MDR is sure, we can start second line drug under close observation. Second line drugs are PAS, thiacetazone, ethionamide, cycloserine, capreomycin, kanamycin, fluroquinolone, clofazimine, amikacin and minocycline.

Immunomodulator drug e.g. Levamisol 150 mg can be given for 3 consecutive days at weekly interval. Total 45 tablets are given. These tablets are given at night.

Injections of DPT and BCG can also be effective. 2–5% cases may show recurrence of tuberculosis within 20 years after healing of lesion. It may be due to prolonged use of steroid, malnutrition, diabetes, immunodeficiency or any surgical procedure/trauma. These patients are treated by newer chemotherapeutic drugs which may be given upto 1–1½ years.

POTT'S PARAPLEGIA

If pott's spine is not treated, it may result in pott's paraplegia. Dorsal spine is commonest area to be affected because spinal canal is narrowest in this area.

SEDDON'S CLASSIFICATION OF POTT'S PARAPLEGIA

Early (Slow) Onset Paraplegia

In this type paraplegia occurs within 2 years of onset of disease.

Late (Rapid) onset paraplegia

This type of paraplegia is seen after 2 years of onset of disease, once it had healed.

Pathology

Basic pathology is that the cord is compressed in vertebral canal by following mechanism:

(*a*) **Inflammatory oedema**

Vascular stasis and toxins released from tubercular infection produce inflammatory odema.

(*b*) **Tubercular osteitis and extradural pus**

This is most common mechanism in which tubercular osteitis of vertebral bodies and extradural pus cause compression of cord from anterior aspect.

(*c*) **Sequestra and Internal Gibbus**

Avascular part of diseased vertebra produces sequestra which compress the cord. Bony ridge formation on anterior wall of spinal canal occurs due to angulation of tuberculous spine. This is known as internal gibbus.

(*d*) **Peridural fibrosis**

Tubercular granulation tissue lies in a thick layer outside the dura and causes peridural fibrosis. This peridural fibrosis causes recurrence of paraplegia.

(*e*) **Infarction of Spinal cord**

The causes of infarction of spinal cord are endarteritis, periarteritis or thrombosis of anterior spinal artery. This infarction causes irreversible paralysis.

(*f*) **Extradural granuloma and Tuberculoma**

These patient presents as a case of spinal tumor syndrome. These lesions do not show any radiological evidence of tuberculosis of vertebra.

SIGNS AND SYMPTOMS

Slow Onset Paraplegia

Slow onset paraplegia shows following findings:

1. Spontaneous twitching of muscles in lower limb is a common feature.
2. Clumsiness while walking.
3. Plantar reflex is extensor.
4. Reflexes are exaggerated.
5. Sustained clonus of ankle and patella.
6. Motor functions are impaired earlier than sensory functions. Motor functions are more affected in comparison to sensory functions.

Rapid Onset Paraplegia

This paraplegia presents in following stages:

1. **Spastic motor paraparesis**

This tubercular paraplegia is usually spastic to start with.

2. **Spastic paraplegia in extension**

Normal corticospinal inhibition is lost which leads to increased tone of muscles, resulting into paraplegia in extension.

3. **Spastic paraplegia in flexion**

Absence of paraspinal tract and corticospinal tract functions leads to paraplegia in flexion.

4. **Areflexic paraplegia**

In extremely severe cases all spasticity disappears and paralysis becomes flaccid. This causes anaesthesia and loss of sphincter control.

5. **Complete flaccid paralysis**

Sudden and complete damage to cord stops all transmission across the cord and patient presents as he is in spinal shock.

Stages of Pott's Paraplegia

Stage 1

- Patient can walk.
- He is not aware of motor weakness.
- Ankle clonus is present.
- Plantar reflex is extensor.

Stage 2

- Patient presents, with clumsiness, incordination and spasticity while walking.
- He is aware of weakness but manages to walk with or without support.
- All signs of spastic paresis are present.

Stage 3

- Patient is bed ridden and can not walk.
- Examination shows paraplegia in extension.
- Sensory deficit is less than 50%.

Stage 4

- Patient can not walk.
- Paraplegia in flexion.
- Severe muscle spasm.
- Complete loss of sensation with sphincter disturbances.

Investigations

- X-ray findings are already discussed earlier.
- CT-scan shows types of vertebral destruction, paravertebral soft tissue, abscess and aetiology of paraplegia i.e. pus and sequestra etc.

Treatment

Conservative

- Absolute bed rest is adviced to patient.
- Anti tubercular treatment is started according to latest WHO schedule.
- Two hourly side to side turning.
- Car of bladder bowel and back is mandatory.
- Neurological examination is done at regular interval to see any improvement or deterioration in muscle power.
- If patient responds to ATT, treatment is continued.
- Once patient has gained sufficient power, brace is adviced for 6–12 months.

Surgical Treatment

Before jumping to surgical treatment you should be sure that you have ruled out all possibilities of multidrug resistant tuberculosis.

Indications

1. Pott's spine converting into pott's paraplegia.
2. Failure of conservative treatment.
3. Rapid onset paraplegia.
4. Recurrent paraplegia.
5. Painful paraplegia due to spasm or nerve root compression.
6. Paraplegia occurring in old age.

Rare Indications

1. Spinal tumor syndrome.
2. Posterior spinal disease leading to paraplegia.

Operative Procedures

Anterolateral decompression

Spine is opened through lateral approach then we reach to front and side of cord. This is most common surgical procedure to be performed. In this operation rib, transverse process, pedicle and part of vertebral body are removed. Lamina and facet joints are left intact.

Costo transversectomy

In this operation transverse process of vertebra along with 2 inch of rib are removed. This facilitates drainage of pus.

Hongkong operation (Pedicle debridement and Arthrodesis)

This operation is performed through transthoracic or transperitoneal approach. In this process dead and diseased vertebra is removed and raw area is filled by a rib graft. There are no chances of development of kyphosis after this operation. This operation provides quick healing of disease.

Laminectomy

Indications of this operation are spinal tumor syndrome and posterior spinal disease. In this procedure lamina is removed.

Good Prognostic Factors

- Children
- Motor paralysis
- Acute onset paraplegia

Bad Prognostic Factors

- Long standing paraplegia
- Bladder bowel incontinence
- Sudden progress of paraplegia

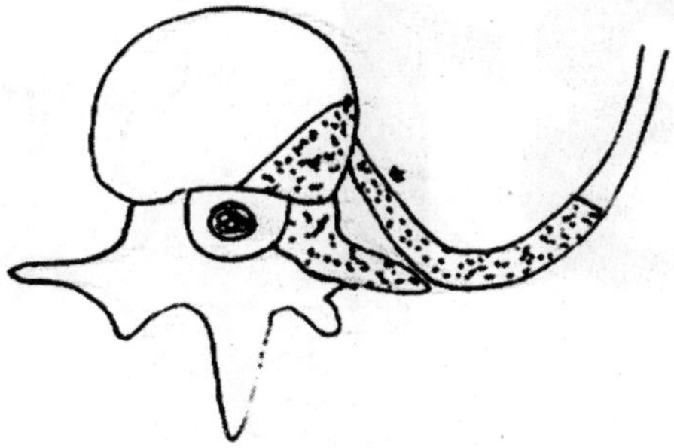

Fig. 30.11 Anterolateral decompression

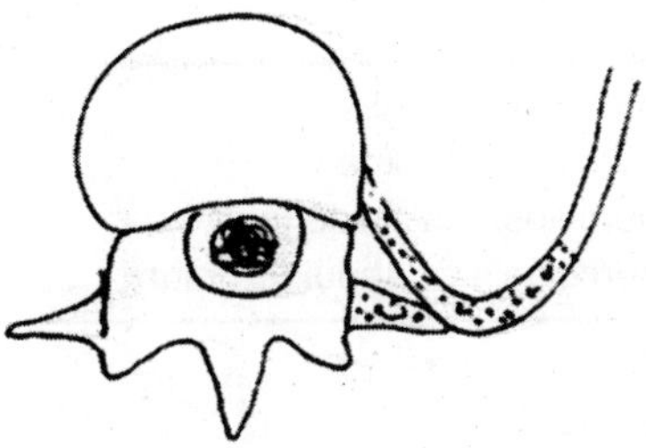

Fig. 30.12 Costo transversectomy

CHAPTER

31 Tuberculosis of Hip

- Tuberculosis of hip
- Tuberculosis of knee
- Tuberculosis of ankle joint
- Tuberculosis of shoulder joint
- Tuberculosis of elbow joint
- Tuberculosis of wrist joint
- Tubercular osteomyelitis without joint involvement

TUBERCULOSIS OF HIP

Tuberculosis of hip is very common in our country. 15% of all cases of skeletal tuberculosis constitute cases of tuberculous hip. This is commonly seen between 10–30 years of age.

Pathology

Initial focus of infection may begin in acetabular roof, epiphysis, Babock's triangle (metaphysis) or in greater trochanter. Uncommonly it may begin in synovial membrane. If disease starts in upper end of femur, joint will be involved early because upper end of femur is intracapsular. Joint involvement is late if disease starts in acetabular roof. Child presents with a few symptoms and attends OPD when extensive destruction of bone has occurred. Tubercle formation, giant cell and lymphocytes are seen under microscope. Tubercle coalesces and undergoes caseation thus forms a cold abscess.

Cold abscess may form at the following sites:

- Within the joint
- Femoral triangle
- Medial, lateral or posterior aspect of thigh
- Ischiorectal fossa
- Pelvis
- Inguinal region

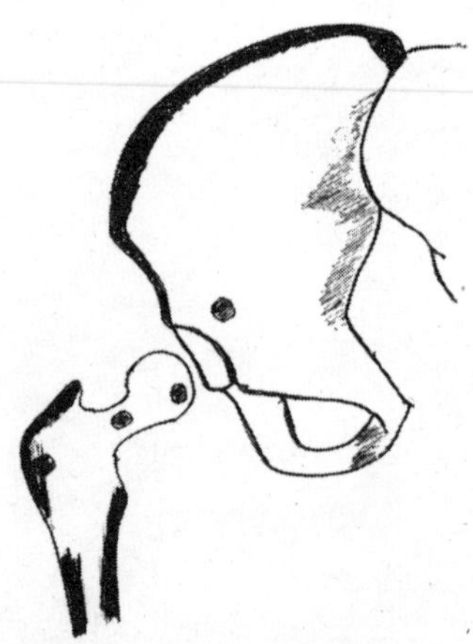

Fig. 31.1 Pathology of tuberculous hip shows initial foci of infection

Once tubercular infection starts in the joint synovial membrane undergoes hypertrophy which in turn causes Pannus formation. This pannus destroys articular cartilage and leads to fibrous ankylosis of hip. Rarely bony ankylosis takes place. Multiple cavitations are seen in femoral head and acetabulum.

Coxa magna

If the disease occurs in growing age, chronic hyperemia causes enlargement of femoral head epiphysis and metaphysis. This condition is known as Coxa magna.

Coxa brevia

Gross reduction in blood supply of femoral head and its physis may cause reduction in size of femoral head and neck. This condition is known as Coxa brevia.

Fibrous ankylosis

If healing starts in stage of advanced arthritis, condition will result into fibrous ankylosis. In fibrous ankylosis slight movements are present at joint which cause pain. Muscle spasm is also present. Deformity turns more severe with passage of time.

Bony ankylosis does not occur in tubercular hip.

Stages of Tuberculous Hip

Stage of Synovitis (FABER)

This is a **stage of apparent lengthening.** In this stage effusion occurs within the joint. This keeps the joint in position of maximum capacity i.e. flexion, abduction and external rotation. Flexion and abduction is mild while external rotation becomes obvious. Flexion is compensated by lumbar lordosis and by lifting the pelvis forward. Abduction is compensated by tilting of pelvis downward and by scoliosis of spine with convexity toward affected side. This stage causes apparent lengthening of limb. On examination both the limbs are equal in length. Patient does not come to OPD in this stage.

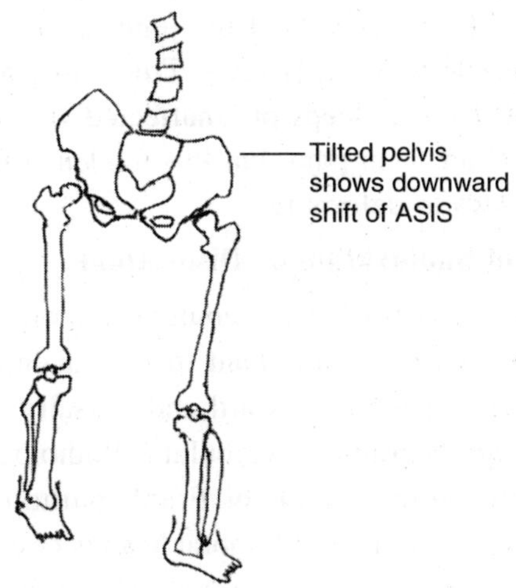

Fig. 31.2 Abduction deformity in T.B. hip

Stage of Arthritis (FADIR)

This is a **stage of apparent shortening.** In this stage, effusion subsides and articular cartilage becomes involved. This leads to spasm of adductor and flexor group of muscles. This condition becomes very painful so joint takes the attitude of slight flexion, adduction and internal rotation. This stage causes apparent shortening. On examination both the limbs are of equal length.

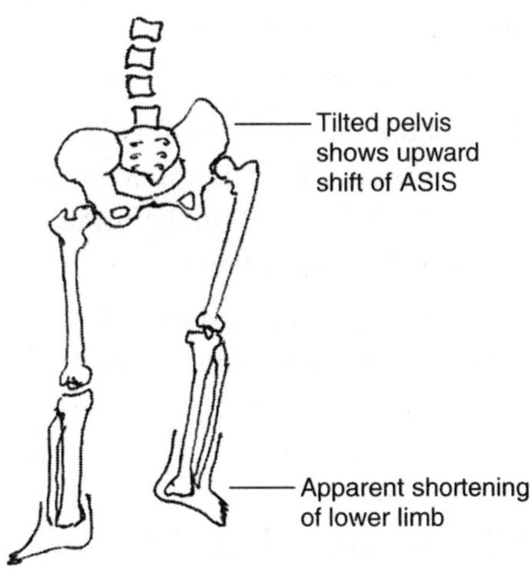

Fig. 31.3 Adduction deformity of hip in T.B. hip

Stage of Erosion (FADIR)

This is a **stage of true shortening.** In this stage articular cartilage of femoral head is grossly destroyed. Movements at the joint are restricted and muscle wasting is seen. True shortening is present. Patient sleeps on unaffected side of hip to get relief from pain, but this tendency further contributes to deformity.

Stage of Subluxation or Dislocation

Severe destruction of acetabulum, femoral head, capsule and ligaments lead to displacement of upper end of femur upward and dorsally within wandering/migrating acetabulum. Radiologically shenton's line is broken. Frank pathological posterior dislocation of femoral head is rare. Head of femur may protrude through acetabulum, the condition known as **Protrusion acetabuli.** Radiologically patient may present as mortar and pestle appearance. In this condition femoral head and neck are grossly damaged and collapsed. Head becomes smaller in size and is contained in enlarged acetabulum.

Clinical Features

Patient presents with the following clinical features:

1. Tuberculosis of hip is commonly seen in the age group of 10–30 years.
2. Stiffness at hip joint is the earliest symptom.
3. Patient presents with painful hip joint along with limping. Pain is referred to medial aspect of knee. Pain becomes severe towards the end of day.
4. Child has peculiar history of night cry. It happens due to rubbing of both diseased surfaces during the movement at joint which occurs due to muscle relaxation during sleep.
5. Antalgic gait is a painful gait in which patient walks with a short stance phase.
6. Marked muscle wasting is seen around thigh and hip joint.
7. Swelling/fullness is present around hip joint.
8. Discharging sinus may or may not be present in groin or near greater trochanter.
9. Muscle spasm can be observed in lower abdominal muscle and adductor compartment of thigh.
10. 8% patient present with palpable cold abscess with or without discharging sinus.
11. Tenderness is present at femoral triangle or elicited during bitrochanteric compression.

Flexion Deformity

Flexion is the position of maximum joint capacity so patient keeps hip joint in flexed position. Later on soft tissue contracture converts it into fixed flexion deformity. Lumbar lordosis is increased to bring the limb on ground. Fixed flexion deformity is concealed by this exaggerated lordosis. **Thomas test** is used to find out the degree of fixed flexion deformity. In this test patient lies supine on hard bed. Now pass your hand beneath lumbar spine of patient. You will find a gap between bed and lumbar spine of patient. Now flex the sound hip till lumbar lordosis disappears. Now a hand can not be insinuated beneath lumbar spine of patient in this position. Affected joint will come into position of fixed flexion deformity. Now measure the angle between the axis of thigh and bed. This will be angle of fixed flexion deformity. (See Fig. 41.4; chapter of Clinical Methods)

Adduction/Abduction deformity

These deformities can be concealed by compensatory tilt of pelvis. Ask the patient to lie supine on a hard bed. Now draw a line connecting both ASIS. If this line is horizontal it means pelvis is square and there is no adduction or abduction deformity. If affected pelvis is higher it means adduction deformity is present. Lower level of ASIS shows abduction deformity. (See Fig. 41.6; chapter of Clinical Methods)

To measure the angle of deformity you will have to make pelvis square by moving the affected limb in the direction of deformity. Now draw a vertical line from hip joint. Angle formed between this vertical line and axis of affected limb will indicate the degree of adduction or abduction deformity.

Shortening of Limb

To measure the shortening of lower limb, normal limb must be kept in identical position of affected limb. Now measure this limb from ASIS to tip of medial malleolus. Apparent length can be measured from xiphisternum or manubrium sterni to tip of medial malleolus.

External/Internal rotation deformity

Direction of patella will indicate rotational deformity. Normally patella remains in slight lateral rotation in supine position. If patella is pointing superior and medially it means limb is in internal rotation deformity and vice versa.

- Movements at hip joint (both active and passive) should be examined.
- Head of femur should be palpated to find out dislocated hip.

Investigations

- Anemia, raised ESR and lymphocytosis are haematological findings.
- Synovial fluid analysis can be done for protein, sugar and lymphocytes.
- Synovial biopsy
- Mantoux test
- Arthrography

X-ray Findings

- Hazziness around hip joint is earliest finding.
- Joint space is reduced due to destruction of cartilage.
- Joint is destroyed due to arthritic changes so head of femur comes to lie in ileum. This condition is known as **wandering acetabulum.**
- Head of femur threatens to protrude through acetabulum into pelvic cavity. This condition is known as **Protrusio acetabuli.**
- Femoral head and neck are badly damaged, collapsed and become smaller in size (pestle) and contained in wider acetabular cavity (mortar). This condition is known as **Mortar & pestle.**
- Subluxation is seen in X-ray. Complete posterior dislocation is uncommon.
- Perthes type of head femur occurs due to its collapse which appears dense on X-ray.
- Head of femur becomes small and atrophic.

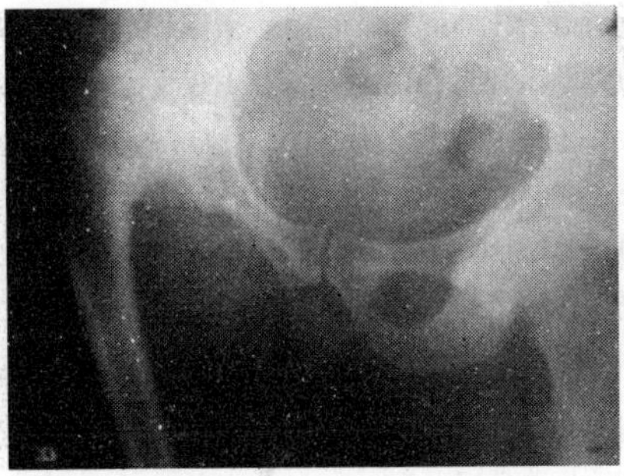

Fig. 31.4 Tuberculous hip. Femoral head is destroyed and protruding into acetabulum

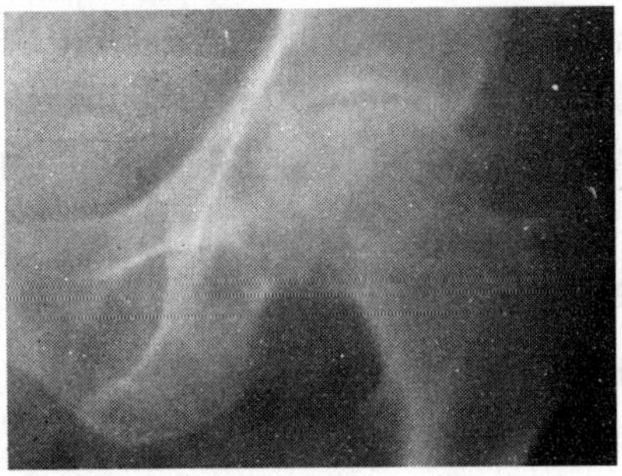

Fig. 31.5 Femoral head is deformed

Treatment

Stage of synovitis and arthritis

After confirmation of diagnosis of tuberculosis, start triple drug therapy of ATT. Bilateral traction is must otherwise traction applied on affected side will increase abduction deformity further. Patient can be made ambulatory after 4–6 months of conservative treatment. Weight bearing is not allowed in first 3 months of ambulation. After this period partial weight bearing is allowed for further 3 months. After 1 year of conservative treatment crutches/calipers can be discarded. After 1½ to 2 years of conservative treatment unprotected weight bearing can be allowed.

Failure of conservative treatment requires synovectomy or debridement of affected joint. After 3–6 months of operation protected ambulation is allowed.

Stage of advanced arthritis

Bilateral traction and triple drug therapy is continued. Gross fibrous ankylosis occurs in advanced arthritis. If ankylosis is in accepted position (5–10 degree of external rotation; 10 degree of flexion in children and 30 degree in adults) a hip spica can be applied in this position for 6–9 months.

Partial weight bearing is allowed first in single hip spica after 6 months of onset of treat of treatment. After this period of 6 months, crutches or calipers are adviced for about 2 years.

If ankylosis is not in accepted position, a corrective osteotomy and or an arthrodesis can be done. Partial weight bearing is allowed after 6 months of treatment. Crutch and caliper are adviced for 2 years.

Indications of Surgery

Osteotomy

This is indicated if sound ankylosis is in bad position. High femoral corrective osteotomy is done nearest to joint.

Arthrodesis

Arthrodesis is indicated in adult patient with painful (unsound) fibrous ankylosis with active or healed disease.

Two types of arthrodesis can be done; ischiofemoral and ileofemoral arthrodesis.

Excisional Arthroplasty

If skeletal maturity is achieved at hip joint Girdle stone excisional arthroplasty can be done in healed or active disease. Drawbacks of this procedure are shortening of limb (3.5–5 cm) and instability of joint.

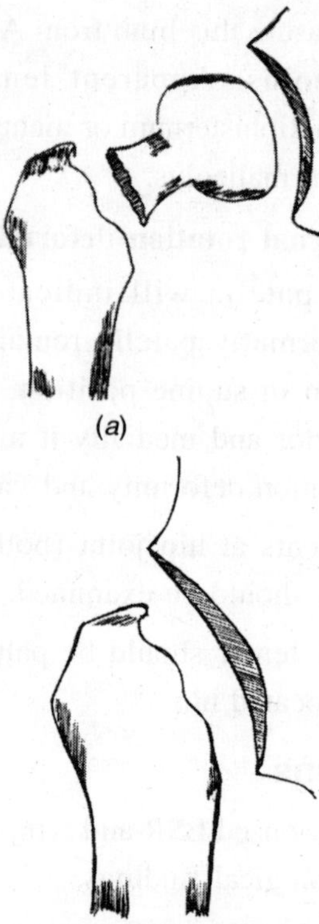

Fig. 31.6 Girdle stone arthroplasty of hip

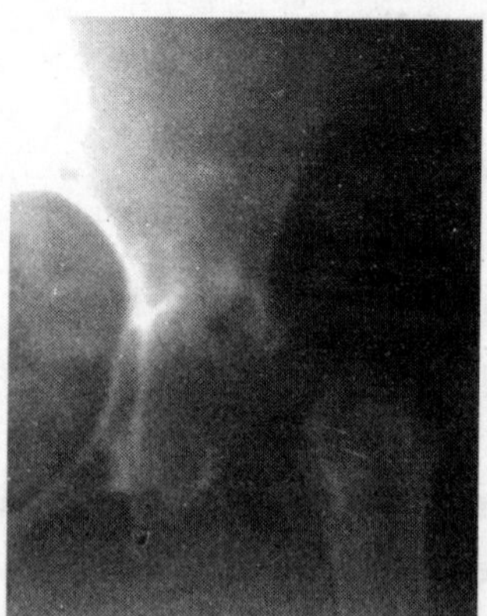

Fig. 31.7 Girdle stone arthroplasty of hip

Joint Replacement Arthroplasty

This operation is indicated at least 10 years after the last evidence of active infection or drainage.

Differential Diagnosis

Children

Congenital Dislocation of Hip

This is present since birth but detected when child starts walking. Child walks with painless limp. Telescopy test is positive. X-ray can confirm diagnosis.

Perthes Disease

Child walks with painless limp with minimum limitation of abduction and internal rotation. Children of 5–10 years of age are commonly affected.

Congenital Coxa Vara

Abduction and internal rotation are limited. Child walks with painless limp. Diagnosis can be confirmed by X-ray.

Adults

- Osteoarthritis
- Rheumatoid arthritis.

TUBERCULOSIS OF KNEE

Knee joint is third common site of skeleton to be affected by tuberculosis. It constitutes 10% of all cases of skeletal tuberculosis.

Clinical Features

Patient of tuberculous knee may present with following features:

1. Patient presents with painful knee.
2. Swelling around knee is common feature. This occurs first at medial parapatellar fossa. This swelling is warm.
3. Boggy feel of thickened synovium is usually detected on examination. It can be rolled between finger and underlying femur. It can be easily felt on medial aspect of knee.
4. Overlying skin is stretched and it may take white appearance known as **Tumor alba**.
5. Joint line tenderness is present.
6. Patellar tap and cross fluctuation are present.
7. Quadriceps muscle shows marked atrophy.
8. Lyphadenopathy is also detected.
9. Joint movements are restricted.
10. Limb lengthening may be observed.
11. Night cries.
12. Cold abscess or sinus may be present at the time of examination.

Triple deformities of knee:

1. Flexion of knee
2. Posterolateral subluxation
3. Lateral rotation and abduction of tibia.

Frame knee

Premature fusion of physis around knee may produce frame knee.

Pathology

Tuberculosis of knee is always secondary and spreads by haematogenous route. Initial focus of infection starts in synovium or subchondral bone or juxtaarticular osseous area. Synovium becomes oedematous, congested and studded with tubercles. Joint fluid is increased. Pannus is formed which destroys articular cartilage leading to fibrous ankylosis. In children initial focus of infection may begin at metaphysis. With the progress of pathological changes triple deformity results at knee joint.

Investigations

Routine investigations should be done as in case of tuberculosis of hip.

X-ray Findings

- Joint space is increased.

- Diffuse osteoporosis of femur and tibia is seen in X-ray.
- Erosion of articular surface may be seen.
- Features of triple deformity will be seen in X-ray.

Treatment

- Below knee skin traction is applied. In children bilateral skin traction is applied.
- Anti tubercular treatment is started.
- Joint can be aspirated to reduce effusion in knee.
- INH and streptomycin can be given intraarticularly once in a week.
- Intermittent active and passive knee mobilization exercise should be done.
- After 3 months of this conservative treatment ambulation is allowed with the help of crutch or walker.
- After 1 year of treatment crutch or walker can be avoided.
- After 1½-2 years of treatment weight bearing ambulation is allowed.

Surgical Treatment

It is mandatory to start ATT preoperatively in every case.

- Stage of synovitis requires synovectomy.
- Stage of early arthritis requires removal of loose body, debries, pannus, and loose articular cartilage. It also needs synovectomy. Juxtaarticular foci are currettaged. This procedure is known as Joint debridement.
- Stage of advanced arthritis requires **Charnley's compression arthrodesis.** Arthrodesis of knee joint is done in functional position i.e. 5–10 degree of flexion and neutral rotation. In this procedure Steinman pins are used.
- **Supracondylar osteotomy** is indicated when knee presents in unacceptable position with painless range of movement of atleast 20 degree.
- **Arthroplasty** is not much popular method of surgical treatment.

Differential Diagnosis

1. Rheumatic arthritis (children)
2. Rheumatoid arthritis
3. Chronic traumatic synovitis
4. Synovioma/hamartoma/lipoma
5. Haemarthrosis
6. Subacute pyogenic arthritis
7. Villonodular synovitis
8. Synovial chondromatosis.

TUBERCULOSIS OF ANKLE JOINT

This joint is uncommonly affected by tuberculosis. It may start from synovium (in children), lower end of tibia, malleoli, talus and calcaneum. It includes less than 5% of all osteoarticular tuberculosis.

Clinical Features

1. Painful swelling at ankle joint is a common feature.
2. Patient walks with a limp.
3. Ankle joint may be held in plantar flexion.
4. Anterior dislocation of ankle can occur in chronic case.

X-ray Findings

1. Joint space is destroyed.
2. Marked osteoporosis is seen around ankle joint.

Treatment

1. Primary aim of treatment is to keep the joint in neutral (plantigrade) position.
2. Anti tubercular treatment should be started.
3. Below knee POP cast is applied.
4. Crutches are adviced for 2-3 months.
5. A heel can be attached to BKPOP cast for next 2 years.
6. If conservative treatment fails, synovectomy with or without joint debridement can be done in stage of synovitis and early arthritis.
7. Ankle arthrodesis in plantigrade position with suitable wedge resection of is the last but not least surgical treatment.

TUBERCULOSIS OF SHOULDER JOINT

This constitutes 1–2% of all cases of osteoarticular tuberculosis. Adults are commonly affected. Concomitantly pulmonary tuberculosis is also seen. Lesion may start in head of humerus, glenoid an uncommonly in synovium.

Clinical Features

Patient may present with following clinical features:

1. Painful limitation of abduction and external rotation of shoulder joint is commonly seen.
2. Marked wasting of muscle is observed. (Deltoid and supraspinatus).
3. Fibrous ankylosis can be seen later.
4. Carries sicca is a dry type of tuberculosis in which joint does not have effusion.
5. Cold abscess and sinus are rare features.

X-ray Findings

1. Rarefaction of bone is seen around joint.
2. Erosion of articular margins is seen.
3. Destruction of upper end of humerus or glenoid is seen.

Treatment

1. Shoulder should be immobilized by plaster spica in saluting position which is functional position. (70–90 degree of abduction, 30 degree forward flexion, 30 degree internal rotation). Spica is applied for 3 months.
2. ATT shoulder be started.
3. After 3 months spica is replaced by abduction frame in same functional position.
4. Intraarticular and extraarticular arthrodesis is surgical treatment which can be tried if conservative treatment fails.

TUBERCULOSIS OF ELBOW JOINT

1. It starts from olecranon or lower end of humerus, upper end of radius or from synovium.
2. This constitutes 2–5% of all cases of osteoarticular tuberculosis.

Clinical Features

Patient may present with following clinical features:

1. Painful and warm swelling at elbow is a common feature.
2. Movements are limited.
3. Elbow is usually kept in flexion.
4. Marked wasting of arm and forearm muscles is seen.
5. Lymph nodes at axilla and supratrochlear region are enlarged.
6. Rarely patient may present with posterior dislocation of elbow.

X-ray Findings

1. Areas of bone destruction are seen.
2. Generalized demineralization of bone is seen.

3. Sometimes subperiosteal bone formation may be seen.
4. Rarely pathological posterior dislocation of elbow can be seen.

Treatment

1. ATT is started.
2. AEPOP slab is applied with elbow joint in 90 degree flexion with forearm in midprone position.
3. Overuse of elbow joint should be avoided.
4. Excisional arthroplasty is indicated in advanced arthritis and gross ankylosis. This can also be done when elbow presents in unacceptable position after the disease has healed.
5. Arthrodesis is rarely required.

TUBERCULOSIS OF WRIST JOINT

This is commonly seen in adults. Wrist joint is not so common to be affected by tuberculosis. It starts from capitulum and lower end of radius.

Clinical Features

1. Pain, swelling, tenderness at joint and limitation of movements are common features.
2. Patient presents with wrist in plantar flexion deformity.
3. Carpal instability may be seen in advanced cases.
4. Lymph nodes are enlarged in axilla and supratrochlear area.

Treatment

1. Antitubercular treatment should be started.
2. Splintage to wrist joint is given in 10–15 degree of dorsiflexion and forearm in midprone position. This is adviced for 1-1½ years.
3. If conservative treatment fails, synovectomy can be done.
4. Darrach's procedure can be helpful. In this procedure lower ¼ of ulna is excised to create a gap pseudoarthrodesis which provides painless ranges of pronation and supination movements even after fusion of joint.

TUBERCULAR OSTEOMYELITIS WITHOUT JOINT INVOLVEMENT

This is uncommonly seen in long tubular bones. Patient presents with pain, swelling over bones, abscess, sinus formation and lymphadenopathy.

X-ray may show bone destruction, irregular cavities and honeycoomb appearance. Bone may show subperiosteal new bone formation. **Spina ventosa** is tuberculosis of phalanx of hand. X-ray shows new bone formation and lytic lesion. Phalanx becomes grossly swollen like a balloon. This is treated by ATT and rest to affected part.

CHAPTER

32 Poliomyelitis

- Poliomyelitis
- Post polio residual paralysis (PPRP)
- Cerebral palsy

POLIOMYELITIS

Poliomyelitis is a viral disease caused by enterovirus (RNA virus) most commonly by type-1.

Pathogenesis

Polio virus multiplies in intestine and reaches to regional lymph nodes in absence of local immunity. In presence of adequate and fast immune response, virus is neutralized and illness is aborted. Polio virus produces viraemia following that antibodies are produced. These antibodies predominantly act at extraneural proliferation of virus.

Polio virus commonly affects the following areas:

- Anterior horn cell
- Vestibular and cranial nerve nuclei
- Vital centre in medulla. Vermis and nuclei in the root of cerebellum.

White matter of spinal cord, cerebellar hemisphere and non motor part of cerebral cortex are usually not affected by polio virus.

Clinical Features

Polio has incubation period of 7–14 days and patient presents with following clinical features:

- Fever, headache and sore throat
- Nauses, vomiting, loss of appetite and abdominal pain.

Non Paralytic Poliomyelitis

- Neck rigidity
- Pain and stiffness at back and legs.
- TRIPOD SIGN is positive. Child can not sit up without support. He uses his hands behind him for taking support. Child writhes from side to side.
- KISS the KNEE test is positive. Patient can not kiss his knees due to stiff spine.
- HEAD DROP SIGN is positive.

Paralytic Poliomyelitis

This type is less common and has following forms:

1. Spinal form
2. Bulbospinal form
3. Encephalitic form

Spinal Form

- This type presents with asymmetrical paralysis.
- Autonomic nervous system is spared.
- Diaphragm and intercostal muscle paralysis may cause difficulty in respiration.
- Tremor, hyperesthesia, muscular pain and changes in deep tendon reflexes are other features of spinal form.

Bulbospinal Form

- This is a life threatening condition.
- Weakness occurs in soft palate, pharynx and vocal cord due to vagus nerve palsy.
- Hoarseness of voice with nasal tone is commonly seen.
- Dyspnoea.
- Dysphagia: child refuses to feed. Aspiration can occur and may cause atelectasis and pneumonia.

Encephalitic Form

- Delirium
- Child is irritable
- Disorientation
- Tremor or convulsions may be seen.

Investigations

CSF Examination

- Sugar and chlorides are normal
- Protein is raised
- Moderate increase in cells; initially polymorphs, later lymphocytes predominate.

Diagnosis

Diagnosis is mainly clinical and investigations are supportive in making of diagnosis.

Prognosis

Paralytic type may take 6 months to 2 years to recover. If paralysis persists beyond this period it means that it will stay throughout the life.

Treatment

- BED REST and good nursing care have most important role in treatment. Child should be nursed in prone position. Foot end of bed should be raised because child has difficulty in swallowing. Raised foot end of bed will allow gravity drainage of pooled secretion in pharynx.
- Intermittent suction to be done to clear pharyngeal secretion. Tracheostomy may be required if suction fails.
- Hot moist packs are used over muscles to relieve pain and spasm.
- Positioning of limbs should be done in position of optimum comfort and function.
- Physiotherapy
- Mechanical ventilator may be required in case of respiratory failure.

POST POLIO RESIDUAL PARALYSIS (PPRP)

Post polio residual paralysis can present with following deformities:

Deformities of Lower Extremity

1. Flexion abduction contracture of hip.
2. Paralytic dislocation of hip.
3. Paralysis of gluteal medius and maximus muscles.
4. Iliotibial band contracture produces 9 classical deformities as follows:

   I. Lumbar lordosis

   II. Pelvic obliquity

   III. Flexion abduction deformity of hip

IV. External rotation of femur
V. External rotation of tibia
VI. Posterolateral subluxation of tibia.
VII. Flexion and valgus deformity of knee.
VIII. Equinus
IX. Limb shortening.

Deformities of Spine

- Kyphosis
- Scoliosis
- Kyphoscoliosis

Deformities of Knee

- Quadriceps paralysis
- Flexion contracture of knee
- Genu recurvatum of knee
- Flail knee

Deformities of Ankle and Foot

- Equinus and equinovalgus
- Equinovarus and calcaneovalgus
- Pes cavus
- Flail foot
- Clawing of toes and foot
- Dorsal bunion

Deformities of Upper Limbs

- Serratus anterior paralysis
- Rhomboid and trapezius paralysis
- Deltoid paralysis

Surgical Treatment

Following surgeries may be required to correct the deformities:

- Tendon transfer
- Arthrodesis
- Osteotomy

Principles of Tendon Transfer

- Transferred muscle must be equal in power to paralyzed muscle.
- Tendon must pass through its own sheath or through the sheath of paralyzed muscle.
- Nerve and blood supply must be preserved and protected.
- Muscle must remain under normal physiological tension.
- Tendon must pass in a direct line from its muscle to the point of insertion.
- Bony operation must precede tendon transfer if possible.
- Contracture should be released prior to tendon transfer. Joint should be mobilized.
- Transfers must be attached to tendon or actual point of insertion of paralyzed muscle.

Surgical Treatment of Quadriceps Paralysis

- Before transferring the tendon all the deformities are corrected e.g. Flexion contracture of hip, knee, genu valgum and equinus deformity of foot.
- Muscles used for tendon transfer are biceps femoris, semitendinosus, sartorius and tensor fascia lata.
- It is mandatory to have good hip flexor for hamstring transfer.
- Biceps femoris is transferred from head of fibula to lateral side of patella.
- Semitendinosus is transferred to medial aspect of patella.
- Postoperatively a spica cast is applied with hip in full extension to relax hamstrings.
- Exercises are started after 3 weeks.

Treatment of Flexor Contracture of Knee

- Iliotibial band and lateral intermuscular septum is resected proximal to knee.
- In severe contracture posterior capsulotomy, fractional hamstring tenotomies/lengthening

and supracondylar osteotomy may be required.

Treatment of Paralytic Dislocation of Hip

- Dislocation of hip occurs due to muscle imbalance among weak abductor, extensor and normal flexor and abductor.
- Dislocation is reduced by abduction or traction in abduction. In late cases tenotomy may be required.
- Iliopsoas muscle transfer is done to correct muscle imbalance.
- Valgus deformity is corrected by varus femoral osteotomy.
- Joint acetabuloplasty can be done to provide stability to hip joint.
- In painful degenerated hip, arthrodesis is better option of treatment.

Treatment of Flail Hip

If hip joint has no muscle power, it is called flail hip. Patient presents with lurching gait. Extremity remains unstable.

Arthrodesis is best treatment for flail hip because it will improve gait as well as provide stability. It may eliminate need of external support to hip.

Treatment for Paralysis of Dorsiflexor of Ankle

Two surgical procedures can be performed for treatment of loss of dorsiflexor of ankle:

- Triple arthrodesis
- Posterior bone block of Campbell.

Treatment for Pes Cavus

Wedge osteotomy of tarsals is done to correct cavus deformity of foot.

Treatment for Clawing of Great Toe

Jones operation can be done to correct clawing of great toe. In this operation tendon of EHL is transferred to neck of first metatarsal.

Orthosis for Poliomyelitis

1. HKAFO

   This is used for deformity of hip, knee, ankle and foot.
2. Knee brace

   This is indicated in quadriceps paralysis. It keeps knee in extension.
3. Below knee brace
4. Single below knee brace
5. Foot drop splint
6. Spinal brace
7. Abdominal support

CEREBRAL PALSY

Definition

This is a non progressive neuromuscular disorder resulting from injury or disease of upper motor neuron at the level of cerebral cortex.

Aetiology

Aetiology of cerebral palsy can be divided into 3 types; prenatal, natal and postnatal as follows:

1. Faulty development of brain (Prenatal)
2. Birth trauma to brain (Natal)
   - Poorly applied forceps
   - Excessive uterine contracture
   - Excessive traction on neck
   - Birth anorexia due to excessive use of analgesics and anaesthetics.
3. Postnatal causes
   - Meningitis and encephalitis
   - Head injury

Clinical Features

- Delayed mile stone
- Mask facies
- Grimacing and drooling of saliva

- Difficult speech
- Incordinated movements
- Shoulder is abducted and internally rotated.
- Elbow is flexed and forearm is pronated.
- Wrist flexion and ulnar deviation is seen.
- Thumb in palm deformity.
- Fingers are flexed.
- Flexion, adduction and internal rotation deformity is seen at hip joint.
- Knee is flexed while ankle is plantar flexed.
- Equinovarus
- While standing, heels do not touch the ground.
- Clonus is present.
- Deep reflexes are exaggerated.
- Athetosis
- Mental retardation becomes evident during 2nd and 3rd year of life.

Treatment

Rehabilitation can be done by education, teaching and institutional care.

Temple Fay Method

Aim of this treatment is development and organization of automatic spinal reflex.

Drugs can be given to control seizure. (eg. Phenytoin, primidone or phenobarbitone and diazepam)

Amphetamine is given for hyperkinesis and behavioural disorders.

Orthopaedic Treatment

Aim of this treatment is prevention and correction of deformity.

- Adduction deformity of hip is corrected by adductor release and anterior abductor neurectomy.
- Flexion deformity of knee is corrected by various methods. (egger method, green method and keats method)
- Patellar advancement is done for elongated patellar tendon and in high riding patella.

Neurectomy (Stoffel operation)

In this surgical procedure main nerve trunk is exposed, motor nerve tract is isolated by electric nerve stimulation and then it is resected. It is helpful in reducing spasticity of muscle.

CHAPTER

33 Osteomyelitis

- Osteomyelitis
- Acute osteomyelitis
- Subacute osteomyelitis
- Chronic osteomyelitis
- Salmonella osteomyelitis
- Garre's osteomyelitis
- Brodie's abscess
- Tom Smith arthritis
- Septic arthritis
- Gonococcal arthritis
- Charcot's joint
- Syphillis in orthopaedics
  - Early congenital syphillis
  - Late congenital syphillis
  - Adult syphillis

OSTEOMYELITIS

Definition

Osteomyelitis is an infection of bone and bone marrow. It is caused by various microorganism.

Classification

- Acute osteomyelitis
- Subacute osteomyelitis
- Chronic osteomyelitis
- Acute on chronic osteomyelitis

ACUTE OSTEOMYELITIS

Duration of acute osteomyelitis is usually less than 2 weeks. Patient comes to hospital within 24–48 hours. This is subdivided into following two types:

1. Primary Acute Osteomyelitis

It is commonly seen in children. It spreads through haematogenous route.

2. Secondary Acute Osteomyelitis

When osteomyelitis develops following a compound fracture or operation it is known as secondary acute osteomyelitis. It is less severe than primary type.

Causative Organisms

- Staphylococcus aureus is commonest organism to cause acute osteomyelitis.
- Other organisms are streptococcus pneumococcus and *E. coli*.
- Salmonella causes osteomyelitis commonly in patients of sickle cell anemia and in diaphyseal osteomyelitis. It causes very severe osteomyelitis. Several bones including spine may be involved.

- Pseudomonas is common in puncture wounds and commonly seen in heroin addicts.
- Haemophillus influenza is commonly seen between the ages of 6 months to 4 years.
- Other organisms are Clostridium welchii, Coliform, Brucella, Treponema pallidum, Mycobacterium tuberculosis.
- Fungal osteomyelitis can be caused by Actinomycosis, Blastomycosis, Cryptomycosis and Coccidiodomycosis.

Aetiology

Age: It is predominantly seen in infants and children.

Sex: Male to female ratio is 4:1.

Site: Metaphysis of long bones toward the growing ends. Upper end of tibia and lower end of femur are common sites to be affected.

Foci of Infection: Boils and tonsillitis.

Organism: Haemolytic Staphylococcus aureus is most common organism.

Pathogenesis

Acute osteomyelitis is most commonly spreads through haematogenous route from a pre existing foci of infection (boils or tonsillitis). Infective embolus get lodged into small end arteries and capillaries situated in metaphysis. This metaphyseal area is highly vascularized part of bone. Here vessels are arranged in hair pin pattern which accounts for blood stasis. This blood stasis and hair pin arrangement of vessels allows bacteria to settle.

Other factors that make the metaphyseal zone a favourite site for acute osteomyelitis are maximum osteogenic activity, relative lack of phagocytosis in this area. Along with this metaphyseal zone is more prone to get trauma.

In most of the joints metaphysis is extraarticular but when it is intraarticular it leads to pyogenic arthritis. (hip joint)

Epiphyseal plate acts as a barrier, so the infection does not spread to adjacent joint. Joint capsule also prevents spread of pus into joint.

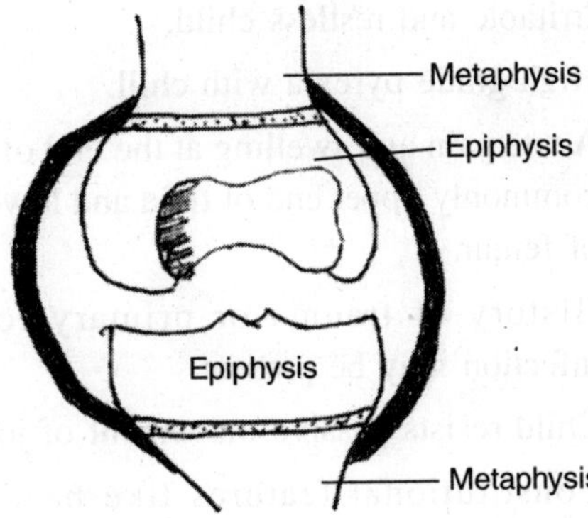

Fig. 33.1 Extraarticular metaphysis

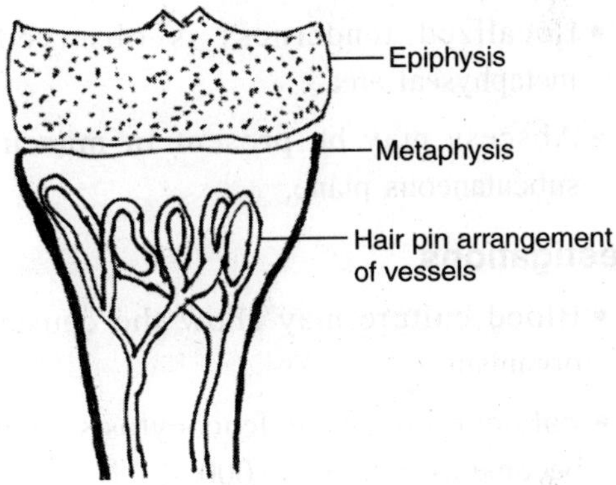

Fig. 33.2 Muscular anatomy of metaphyseal area of tibia

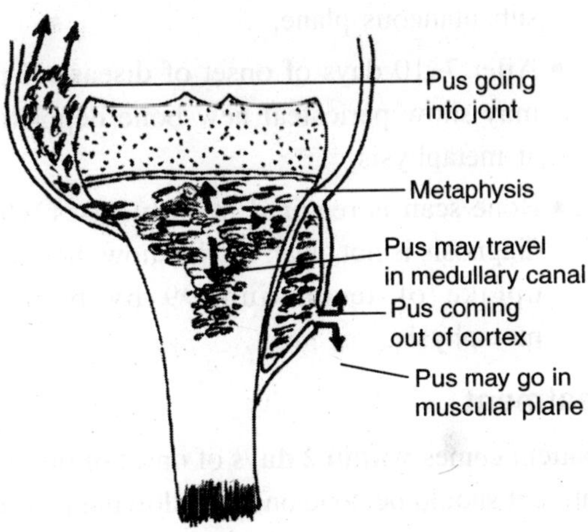

Fig. 33.3 Exudates spreading from metaphysis

Clinical Features

Patient of acute osteomyelitis may present with the following features:

- Irritable and restless child.
- High grade pyrexia with chill.
- Acute pain and swelling at the end of bone, commonly upper end of tibia and lower end of femur.
- History of trauma or primary foci of infection may be present.
- Child resists passive movement of joint.
- Constitutional features like headache, vomiting, convulsion and tachycardia may be present.
- Localized tenderness is observed at metaphyseal area.
- Abscess may be present in muscular/ subcutaneous plane.

Investigations

- Blood culture may show the causative organism.
- Polymorphonuclear leucocytosis. It may become as high as 30,000.
- ESR is raised.
- Aspiration may show pus in muscular or subcutaneous plane.
- After 7–10 days of onset of disease X-ray may show periosteal new bone deposition at metaphysis.
- Bone scan is required in early cases when diagnosis is not clear. It will show increased uptake of technetium-99 by bone at metaphysis.

Treatment

If patient comes **within 2 days** of onset of disease, treatment should be done on the following pattern:

- High dose systemic antibiotics
- Bed rest.
- Rest to affected part by slab or splint.
- Pencillin, cephalosporin and tetracycline are preferred until report of blood culture comes.
- Intravenous antibiotics are given for 15 days. Later we switch over to oral antibiotic which is given for 3 months.
- Intravenous fluid is given to correct dehydration.
- Temperature and pulse monitoring is done at regular interval.

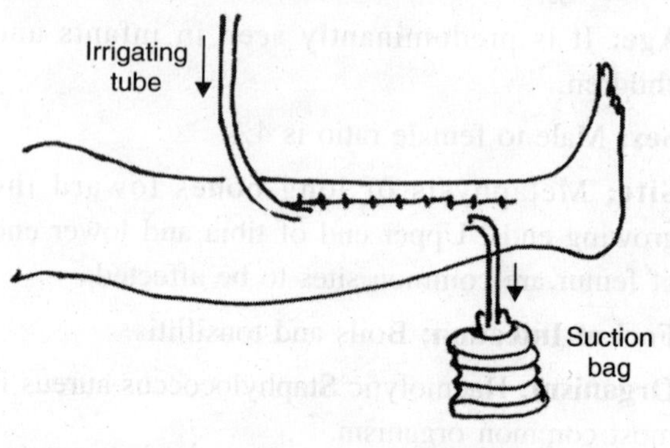

Fig. 33.4 Continuous suction irrigation

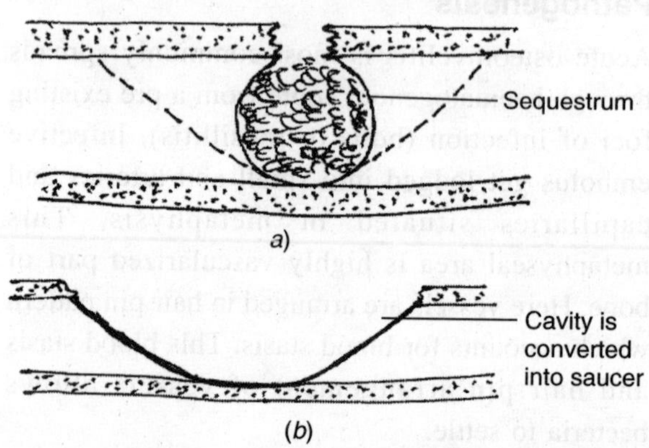

Fig. 33.5 Saucerization of bone

If patient comes **after 2 days** of onset of disease:

- In this stage patient usually does not get any treatment so pus collects in subperiosteal or muscular plane. This requires drainage of pus. Periosteum is incised longitudinally over the point of maximum tenderness.

Periosteum is stripped laterally for half an inch on both sides. Multiple drill holes are made until intraosseous exudate is localized. Currettage is avoided.

- Cavity is filled with plane gauge.
- To instill the antibiotics a catheter is placed into cavity.

Indications of Surgery

- A definite abscess is present.
- Failure of response to vigorous antibiotic treatment after 2-3 days.
- Patient comes after 2 days of onset of disease.

Differential Diagnosis

Acute Septic Arthritis

- Restricted and painful movements at joint.
- Swelling and tenderness is present at joint not over metaphysis.
- Muscle spasm is present.
- Aspiration will show purulent synovial fluid.

Scurvy

- Pain, tenderness and fever are absent.
- Subperiosteal haematoma may be seen as swelling.
- Child is malnourished.

Rheumatic Fever

- This involves multiple joints.
- Pain is fleeting type.
- It responds to salicylates and ACTH quickly.
- Antibiotic has no role.

Acute Poliomyelitis

- History of fever is present.
- Tenderness over muscle can be elicited.
- No tenderness is present at bone.

Ewing Tumor

- This tumor is confined to diaphysis of long bones.
- Fever, leukocytosis and subperiosteal bone deposition (onion peel appearance).
- It melts like snow while giving X-ray radiation.
- Diagnosis is confirmed by biopsy.

SUBACUTE OSTEOMYELITIS

This type of osteomyelitis is usually detected after 15 days of infection. Patient presents with pain with no other constitutional symptoms. It is caused by staphylococcus aureus. ESR and leukocyte count are raised. Blood culture is positive. Treatment is done by antibiotics.

CHRONIC OSTEOMYELITIS

If osteomyelitis persists for more than 3 weeks it is known as chronic osteomyelitis.

Causes

1. Following an acute osteomyelitis
2. Postoperative
3. Garre's osteomyelitis
4. Brodies abscess
5. Tuberculosis, syphyllis and fungal osteomyelitis.

Acute osteomyelitis may convert into chronic osteomyelitis due to following reasons:

1. Inadequate and late treatment of acute osteomyelitis results into pus collection into medullary cavity and beneath the periosteum. Later sequestrum is formed that provides a seat for persistent infection.
2. High virulence of organism.
3. Poor immunity status of host.

Sequestrum is a dead piece of bone surrounded by infected granulation tissue. Its inner surface is smooth while outer surface are rough. 3 types of sequestrum are known as follows:

1. **Ring Sequestrum**

This is seen around pintrack and amputation stump.

2. **Tubular Sequestrum**

This is a tube like hollow, dead bone. It is seen in haematogenous osteomyelitis and segmental fractures.

3. **Rice Grain Sequestrum**

This is seen in tuberculosis.

Involucrum is a new bone formation overlying the sequestrum.

Cloacae are openings in involucrum through which pus; exudates, bone debris and sequestrum find their way out to surface.

Clinical Features

Patient of chronic osteomyelitis will present with the following features:

- Chronic discharging sinus
- Mild to moderate pain
- History of bone pieces coming out of sinus tract.
- Examination findings include thickened irregular tender bone and stiffness at the adjacent joint.
- Fever is usually not seen in chronic stage.

Investigations

X-ray Findings

- Cortex is thick and irregular.
- Sclerosed cortex
- Rarefaction of bone
- Sequestrum
- Involucrum
- Cloacae
- Periosteal reaction.

Other Investigations

- Pus culture and sensitivity
- Sinogram is done to know the origin of sinus; from where it arises and also to localize the cavity that is not visible on X-ray.
- Hb, TLC, DLC, blood sugar and ESR.
- Bone scan can show the hot spot.

Treatment

Chronic osteomyelitis is managed by excision of sinus tract, sequestrectomy, curettage and saucerization. After this surgical procedure, limb is kept on continuous suction and irrigation system; in which an inlet tube goes into medullary cavity of bone carrying the irrigation fluid. This fluid comes out through an outlet tube.

When to perform sequestrectomy?

Follow up X-rays are done to see the involucrum synthesis. If sufficient involucrum is formed sequestrectomy can be done.

Why to do saucerization?

Bony cavity is converted into a saucer because pus collects inside the bony cavity and it does not come out of it. Pus is freely drained if saucerization is done.

How long saucerization should be done?

Currettage should be done until normal bone is seen and fresh bleeding starts from bone. Gentamicin impregnated beads can be used to fill the cavity.

Complications

Chronic osteomyelitis can have following complications:

- Damage to growth plate can lead to shortening.

- If vascularity of growth plate is increased, it can cause lengthening of limb.
- Deformity of limb can occur if growth plate is partially damaged.
- Flare up of infection
- Pathological fracture
- Joint stiffness
- Squamus cell carcinoma at sinus tract.
- Amyloidosis.

SALMONELLA OSTEOMYELITIS

This is usually seen after an episode of typhoid fever. Children with sickle cell anemia commoly suffer from salmonella osteomyelitis. 3 serotypes found in association with sickle cell anemia are Salmonella choleraesuis, Salmonella paraypħi B and Salmonella typhimurium. These are responsible for osteomyelitis associated with sickle cell anemia. Common features of salmonella osteomyelitis are as follows:

- Ulna, vertebrae and tibia are commonly affected bones.
- Sometimes it may become bilateral.
- Intestinal symptoms are absent.
- Characteristics of this osteomyelitis are that several bones may be affected at a time.
- Salmonella can be cultured from blood.
- Agglutination test is diagnostic.
- Chloremphenicol (3-4 gm/day in adult) is drug of choice.
- Ampicillin and penicillin can be used in high doses.
- X-ray shows diaphyseal sclerosis.

GARRE'S OSTEOMYELITIS

- This type of osteomyelitis does not have any discharging sinus. This is non suppurative sclerosing type of chronic osteomyelitis.
- This is common in children and young adults.
- Pain, fever and localized fusiform swelling are clinical features.
- Common bones affected are femur and tibia. Subperiosteal area is commonly affected.
- Osteosarcoma and Ewing tumor are differential diagnosis of this osteomyelitis.
- Blood culture is normal.
- This is treated conservatively by rest and broad spectrum antibiotics.
- This is also known as idiopathic cortical sclerosis.

BRODIE'S ABSCESS

This is a type of osteomyelitis in which a persistent, chronic abscess is formed which is surrounded by fibrous membrane and walled off by a ring of dense bone. Brodie's abscess has following features:

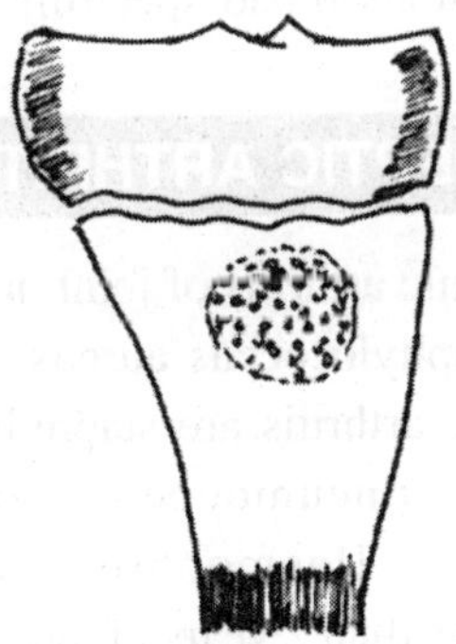

Fig. 33.6 Brodie's abscess

1. Upper end of tibia and lower end of femur are common sites. (at metaphysis)
2. This commonly affects 10–20 years of age group.

3. Patient presents with deep seated pain which becomes worse at night.
4. Joint may be swollen due to effusion. Tenderness is present at local area.
5. X-ray shows round area surrounded by zone of sclerosis.
6. It is treated by evacuation of pus followed by curettage. Cavity is filled with bone graft.

TOM SMITH ARTHRITIS

Septic arthritis of infants is known as Tom Smith arthritis. It is clinically similar to congenital dislocation of hip. Child presents with the following features:

1. Child presents with short legs, increased hip movement in all direction and positive telescopy test.
2. Septic arthritis completely destroys head of femur. Later abscess is formed that may burst out.
3. X-ray shows complete absence of head and neck of femur.
4. Treatment is conservative in the form of intravenous broad spectrum antibiotics.

SEPTIC ARTHRITIS

This is pyogenic arthritis of joint, most commonly caused by staphylococcus aureus. Other bacteria causing septic arthritis are staphylococcus albus, streptococci, pneumococci, gonococci and meningococci. Haemophillus influenzae is common in less than 2 years of age. Septic arthritis is most commonly seen in children. Most common joint to be involved are knee, hip (infants) and shoulder.

Modes of Infection

Septic arthritis has various modes of infections as follows:

- Haematogenous route is most common route of infection as primary foci of infection may lie elsewhere in body in the form of pyoderma, throat infection and septicemia.
- Secondary to adjacent osteomyelitis.
- Traumatic wounds.
- Intraarticular steroid injections.
- Umblical cord sepsis.

Pathology

Bacteria cause inflammatory reaction with migration of polymorphonuclear leukocytes and subsequent release of proteolytic enzymes in joint exudates.

Synovium becomes oedematous, congested and infilterated with polymorphonuclear leukocytes. Flakes of fibrin are deposited over linings of joint. Articular cartilage is destroyed by plasmin, cathepsin and prostglandins. Capsule and ligaments are destroyed by pus.

Pathology

Excruciating pain in swollen, red hot and tender joint with painful limp and high grade pyrexia are the classical features of septic arthritis. Child will not allow to touch his joint. If knee joint is involved, patella will become floating. If hip joint is involved, child will keep hip joint in flexion abduction and external rotation because this is the position of greatest relaxation of capsule.

Investigations

Septic arthritis needs following investigations to be done:

- Polymorphonuclear leukocytosis (50,000–100,000).
- Raised ESR >20 mm/hr
- C-reactive protein positive
- Blood culture

- Joint aspiration should be done and to be sent for culture sensitivity. Gram stain is positive.

X-ray Findings

- Soft tissue shadow is seen around the joint.
- In early stage joint space is increased but later joint space becomes narrow.
- Destruction of articular cartilage.
- Sometimes subluxation or dislocation of joint may be seen.

Treatment

- Merely joint aspiration is not useful in treatment as exudates rapidly reaccumulate. Repeated insertion of needle causes further infection to joint.

Arthrotomy and Drainage

Joint is opened on two sides to provide through and through gravity drainage. A drain can be kept inside for 24–48 hours to prevent premature closure. Do not suture the synovium. In case of gonococcal infection, surgical drainage is not required as it responds to penicillin.

Antibiotics

Parentral antibiotics are given for 6 weeks. Penicillin or cephalosporins are given by intravenous route. Cloxacillin can be given 0.25 gm–1 gm by intravenous route. Gentamicin 20 mg i/v b.i.d. can cover gram negative bacteria.

Immobilization of Joint

Joint is immobilized by applying skin traction. Traction immobilizes the joint and distracts the articular cartilage thus reducing the chances of pressure damage to joint.

- High protein diet should be given.
- Pathological dislocation of hip can be treated by subtrochanteric osteotomy or arthrodesis.
- Non functional ankylosis is treated by arthrodesis in functional position.

GONOCOCCAL ARTHRITIS

Gonococcal arthritis results after 3 weeks of acute gonorrheal urethritis. It is not as common as septic arthritis. This is polyarticular arthritis. Knee, wrist and ankle joints are commonly affected. Joint shows all signs of inflammation. Tenosynovitis in ankle and wrist is common. Patient suffers from high grade fever (104 degree F). Underlying pathology shows congested and oedematous synovium which is infilterated with polymorphonuclear leukocytes. Articular cartilage is digested by plasmin, cathepsin and PG's. Healing occurs by fibrosis of synovium leading to fibrous ankylosis. Bony ankylosis is uncommon.

Treatment

Treatment of choice is penicillin. Splintage provide immobilization and rest to joint. Splint is removed daily for passive joint motion. If joint have become ankylosed, arthroplasty can be done. When the joint shows degenerative arthritic changes or deformity, arthrodesis can be done in functional position.

CHARCOT'S JOINT

These are painless grossly swollen, flail joint with diffuse erythma around it. This is also known as neuropathic joints.

This condition is usually seen after 40 years of age and commonly involves knee, ankle hip, elbow, shoulder, wrist and intervertebral joints.

Syringomylia, tabes dorsalis and syphilis are common examples. Other examples are rheumatoid arthritis, intraarticular steroid injections, chronic liver disease, prolonged use of indomethamicin and traumatic division of sciatic nerve.

Underlying pathology shows thickened capsule, gross destruction of joint, loose bodies and osteophytes.

Charnley's compression arthrodesis is the treatment of choice.

SYPHILLIS IN ORTHOPAEDICS EARLY CONGENITAL SYPHILLIS

This clinical entity has been discussed here because it involves joints and bones. This is also known as **Parrot's pseudoparalysis.** Patient has following features:

1. Metaphyseal area is maximally involved due to richest capillary blood supply.
2. Child presents with grossly swollen tender joint soon after birth. Child is irritable and cries frequently.
3. Medulla is always affected.
4. Joints are so painful that child keeps the limbs immobile as though paralyzed. It is also known as Parrot's pseudoparalysis.
5. Keratitis, mucous patch, skin lesion and snuffel's are other associated features.
6. X-ray shows moath eaten appearance of metaphysis; saw toothed epiphysis and periosteal ossification of shaft of long bones.
7. If child survives, osseous involvement heals by itself.
8. Rickets and scurvy are differential diagnosis of early congenital syphillis.

Late Congenital Syphillis

This is also known as tertiary stage of congenital syphillis. Osteoblastic lesions are seen commonly at tibia and femur. Other features are as follows:

1. Periosteal bone formation typically over anterior aspect of tibia is known as **Saber shin.**
2. Bowing of shaft is usually not seen.
3. Outer table of skull may show nodular thickening.
4. Gummatous destruction of cortex is seen.
5. **Hutchinson triad** (interstitial keratitis, deformed incisor and 5th nerve deafness) is characteristic.
6. **Clutton joints** are usually seen between 8–18 years of age. These are painless effusion of both knees. If synovial fluid is aspirated it will rapidly refill.
7. X-ray shows no positive findings.

Adult Syphillis

50% Patient show bone and joint involvement. Patient presents with fixed non tender painless swelling of bone or skull. Other features are as follows:

1. Osteoblastic reaction is seen. Cortex becomes dense and thick.
2. Signs of acute inflammation are absent.
3. Gumma is infective material which may reach to subperiosteal space or medulla.
4. Infection is maximally seen at the ends of long bones.
5. Sequestrum is rarely seen.
6. Periosteitis of skull and long bones is commonly seen.
7. Outer table of skull is mainly involved. Later luetic meningitis may occur.
8. Gummatous arthritis may also occur later.
9. Early X-ray findings are negative but later it may show osteoblastic densities, thickened cortex, lace like subperiosteal new bone formation and moatheaten rarefaction of gumma.

CHAPTER

34 Infections of Hand

- Acute paronychium
- Whitlow (felon)
- Tenosynovitis
- Deep palmar abscess
- Other infections of hand

80% Hand infections are caused by Staph aureus and rest of them are caused by streptococcus. Such infections should be treated as an emergency as these are very painful and have chances of spreading proximally in body.

ACUTE PARONYCHIUM

This is most common infection of hand. This is an infection of nail fold (eponychium). It has other following features:

- Staph aureus is most common organism.
- This is caused by unsterile manicure instruments, hang nail or reckless pairing.
- Patient presents with painful swelling around the nail fold. Tenderness is present around nail fold.
- Acute paronychium is treated conservatively until suppuration has occurred. Pus is drained through vertical and lateral incision on one or both sides.
- If paronychium is not treated properly it can extend to pulp space.

WHITLOW (FELON)

This is infection of terminal pulp space. It is second most common infection of hand. This is transmitted through a pin prick. Digital artery enters into terminal pulp space and gives a branch to epiphysis of base of terminal phalanx. It has other following features:

- Patient presents with painful tender swollen terminal pulp space of index finger or thumb.
- This is treated conservatively. Suppuration is managed by incision and drainage at the centre of abscess. It can also be drained by lateral incision.
- If it is not treated well, it can produce osteomyelitis of distal phalanx or pyogenic arthritis of DIP joint. Uncommonly suppurative tenosynovitis can occur.

TENOSYNOVITIS

Tenosynovitis is an infection of fibrous sheath and synovial covering of flexor tendons of hand. If it is not treated it may cause permanent stiffness of fingers. Sometimes infection can spread upto a bursa.

Applied Anatomy

Hand has radial and ulnar bursa. Radial bursa covers synovial sheath of thumb, while ulnar bursa covers synovial sheath of rest of 4 fingers. Synovial sheath of index, middle and ring fingers extend upto transverse palmar crease. Synovial sheath of thumb and little finger extend 2-3 cm above the wrist.

Aetiology

Staph aureus or streptococcus pyogenes are common organisms that cause infection in tenosynovitis. Infection travels to tendon sheath through a penetrating injury. Rarely infection may travel from terminal pulp space.

Clinical Features

Tenosynovitis has following clinical features:

1. Pain and swelling in fingers is a common presentation.
2. Fingers are semiflexed and any movement at fingers causes pain.
3. **Kanavel sign** is positive i.e. area of maximum tenderness is present between transverse palmar creases. This sign becomes positive if ulnar bursa becomes infected.

Treatment

Infection is controlled with antibiotics. Abscess can be drained by transverse incision at distal palmar crease.

DEEP PALMAR ABSCESS

This clinical entity is rare. It constitutes only 1% of all infections of hand.

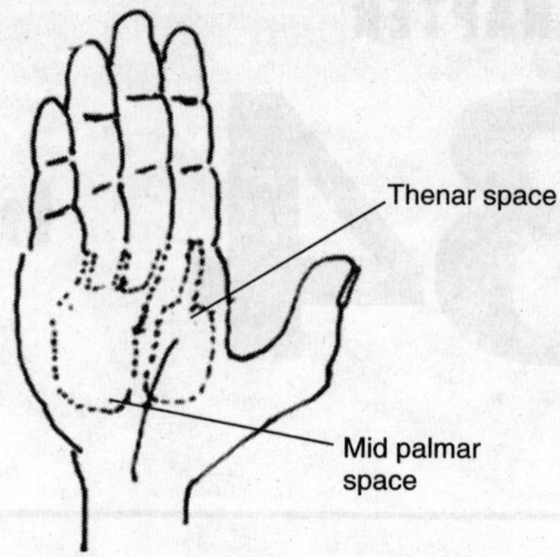

Fig. 34.1 Deep palmar abscess can occur in mid palmar or thenar space

Applied Anatomy

Deep palmar space has two halves; mid palmar space and thenar space. A fascia lies in its posterior relation which covers interossei. Laterally it has adductor pollicis muscle and medially metacarpal bones.

Clinical Features

Patient may present with following clinical features:

1. Intense throbbing pain in palm is usual presentation.
2. Mild swelling at volar aspect and gross swelling is seen at dorsal aspect. Grossly swollen hand resembles with **Frog hand**. Fingers are flexed.
3. Extension is painful at MP joint.
4. Extension at IP joint is painless.
5. Regional lymph nodes are enlarged.
6. Chronic infection may present as discharging sinus and stiff hand.

Treatment

Sometimes it can be controlled by antibiotics. Abscess is drained by central transverse incision at disatal palmar crease.

OTHER INFECTIONS OF HAND

- Apical subungual infection.
- Middle and proximal volar space infection.
- Web space infection.
- Infection at space of parona.
- Cellulitis
- Lymphangitis
- Superficial and deep aponeurotic infections.

CHAPTER 35 Osteoarthritis

- Osteoarthritis of knee
- Osteoarthritis of hip
- Rheumatoid arthritis
- Cervical spondylosis
- Approach to a case of arthritis (excluding O.A.)
- Juvenile rheumatoid arthritis

OSTEOARTHRITIS OF KNEE

Osteoarthritis of knee is a degenerative, non inflammatory joint disease, characterized clinically by early morning stiffness, difficulty in squatting, walking, climbing upstairs; pathologically by synovitis, effusion of joint, subchondral bone sclerosis, osteophytes formation, local degeneration of articular cartilage and deformed joint. It usually starts after 40 years of age with equal sex ratio.

Osteoarthritis commonly involves knee and hip joints. It also ***involves distal interphalangeal joint and carpometacarpal joint of thumb.*** *Metacarpophalangeal joints are spared.*

Pathology

Underlying pathology shows subchondral bone sclerosis, osteophytes formation, local degeneration of articular cartilage and deformed joint. In the matrix collagen fibres take vertebral position between deepening clefts thus producing fibrillary and fissured appearance. This is the hallmark of osteoarthritic cartilage.

Clinical Features

This is a very common condition in India and patient can present in OPD with following clinical features:

1. Early morning stiffness
2. Difficulty in squatting, climbing upstairs and walking. Patient has a lot of difficulty in getting up from a sitting posture.
3. Patient also has difficulty in using Indian toilet.
4. Mild swelling may be seen due to effusion.
5. Coarse crepitus may be felt.
6. Joint line tenderness may be present.

X-ray Findings

X-ray of knee can show the following findings:

1. Destruction of articular cartilage may cause reduced joint space.
2. Thickened subchondral bone (sclerosis)
3. Subchondral cyst.
4. Marginal osteochondral outgrowth forms osteophytes.

5. Loose bodies may also be seen.
6. Deformed and malaligned joint.

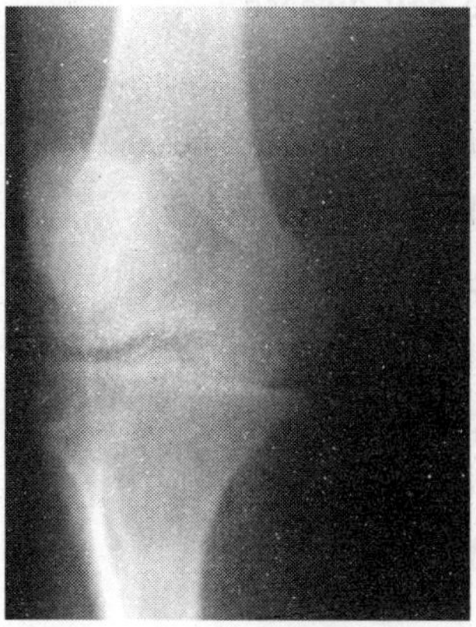

Fig. 35.1 Osteoarthritis of knee

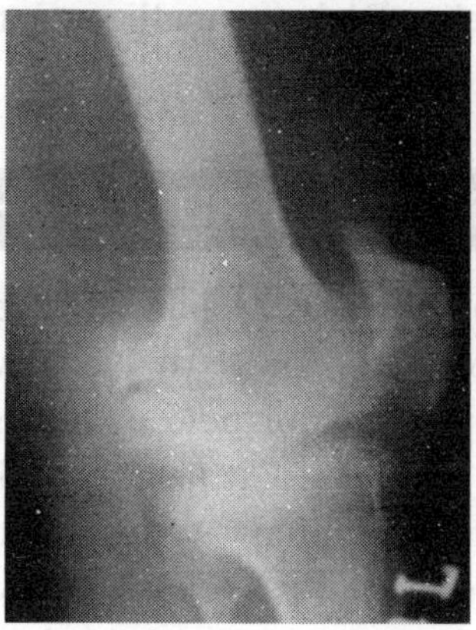

Fig. 35.2 Osteoarthritic changes in patella and knee joint

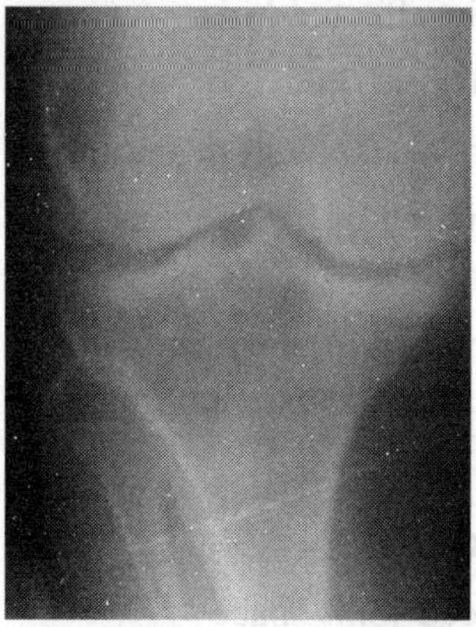

Fig. 35.3 Gross arthritic changes and reduced joint space

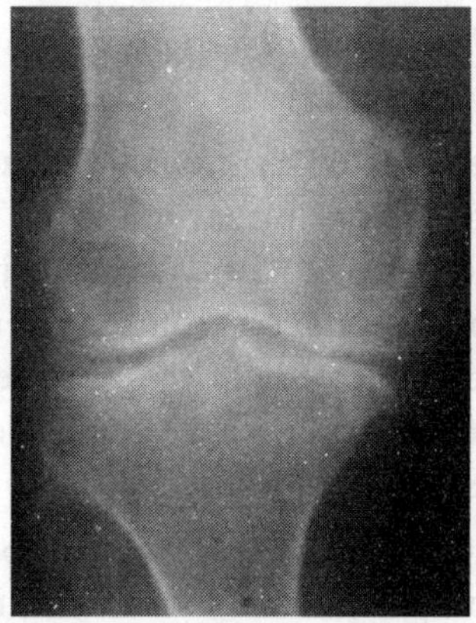

Fig. 35.4 Destruction of cartilage is seen

Treatment

Following conservative treatment can be tried in early cases of arthritis:

- Hot saline fomentation.
- Isometric quadriceps exercises.
- Reduction of body weight.
- Avoid squatting, climbing upstairs.
- Heat therapy to joint.
- Analgesics and muscle relaxant.
- Intraarticular injections of steroids can be tried.
- Arthroscopic lavage and removal of loose bodies gives pain relief for 4–6 months.
- **Chondrointin** and **glucosamine sulfate** also play important role in early cases of arthritis. They are supposed to help in biosynthesis of cartilage.
- ***Diacerein,*** *an anthraquinone derivative acts as analgesic, antipyretic, anti-inflammatory and slowly acting symptom modifying antiosteoarthritic drug. It inhibits production of IL-1 beta by monocytes. This in turn decreases collagenolytic activity in articular cartilage. (IL-1 triggers the articular injury). This also reduces ratio of chondroitin 6 sulphate to chondroitin 4 sulphate and increases lymphocyte*

membrane fluidity. This is given 50 mg twice in a day.

- Derivatives of hyluronan (Hylan G-F 20) can be given intraarticularly. This is an elastoviscous fluid containing hylan polymer produced from chicken coombs. This is indicated for the treatment of pain in osteoarthritis where analgesics become ineffective.
- Proximal tibial osteotomy can be done for unicompartmental osteoarthritis of knee with genu varum of less than 15 degree.
- If genu varum is more than 15 degree, distal tibial osteotomy will be helpful.

Total Knee Replacement (TKR)

Total knee replacement is indicated when all the conservative methods of treatment have failed and patient has persistent pain in knee. It is also indicated when both compartments of joint are destroyed and patient has genu varum >15 degree. Details of TKR have been discussed in chapter of joint replacement.

Computer Assisted TKR

Total knee replacement can also be done with the help of computer but it is not common in India.

Aetiology of Secondary Osteoarthritis

Developmental

- Slipped capital femoral epiphysis
- Perthes disease
- CDH

Traumatic

- Intraarticular fracture
- Meniscectomy
- Ehler denlos syndrome

Inflammatory

- Gout
- Septic arthritis
- Rheumatoid arthritis
- Haemophillia

Aseptic Necrosis

- Corticosteroid
- Sickle cell disease
- SLE
- Decompression sickness

Metabolic Disease

- Wilson disease
- Haemochromatosis
- Alkaptonuria
- Chondrocalcinosis
- Gaucher disease

Others

Paget's disease, Acromegaly, Tabes dorsalis, Syringomyelia, Diabetes mellitus, intraarticular acetabular labrum.

OSTEOARTHRITIS OF HIP

This is also known as Malum coxa senilis. This is next joint to knee to be involved in osteoarthritis. Superior pole of hip is typically affected in such cases. It has been divided into primary and secondary types. Aetiology of secondary osteoarthritis has been discussed earlier. Aetiology of primary osteoarthritis is not known.

Clinical Features

1. Pain in affected hip.
2. Stiffness of joint.
3. Patient walks with a limp.
4. Restriction of hip movements is a common feature.
5. Later patient may present with flexion adduction and external rotation deformity at hip joint.

X-ray Findings

1. Reduced joint space
2. Osteophytes, subchondral sclerosis and cyst are seen.

Treatment

Rest is given to joint. Heat therapy may be effective in such cases. NSAIDS and muscle relaxants are also helpful. Traction can be given in a stiff joint. Intraarticular steroid injections can provide significant relief from pain.

Surgical Treatment

- Coxa valga is treated by Pauwell's varus osteotomy.
- Adduction deformity of hip is corrected by valgus osteotomy.
- In advanced cases where osteophytes are formed MacMurray's displacement osteotomy is a better option. Osteotomy brings normal bony surface into line of weight transmission. It also changes line of weight.
- Late cases can be treated by cup arthroplasty, arthrodesis, hemireplacement arthroplasty and total hip replacement depending on condition of acetabulum and femoral head.

RHEUMATOID ARTHRITIS

It is chronic inflammatory disease of joints, characterized by symmetrical destructive and deforming polyarthritis with extraarticular manifestation.

Aetiology

Immnue complex composed of IgM activates complements and releases chemotactic factors for neutrophils. These inflammatory cells release lysosomal enzymes which damage synovium, cartilage and erode bone, while prostaglandins produced in process cause pain and vasodilatation. Inflammed synovium forms a **Pannus** (granulomatous mass that destroys cartilage, tendon and ligament). Autoantibodies are produced in synovial tissue in response to IgG. These antibodies are called as Rheumatoid factor. Those patients who have raised titre of Rh factor show poor prognosis.

Pathology

Rheumatoid arthritis principally affects small joints of hands, feet, ankle, wrist, knee, shoulder and elbow. **Distal interphalangeal joints are spared.** It principally involves PIP and MP joints. Rheumatoid arthritis shows a non specific inflammatory synovitis.

Following changes are seen in this synovitis:

- Marked hypertrophy of synovium with finger like projections.
- Proliferation of cells at synovial lining.
- Lymphocytic and plasma cell infiltration.
- Fibrinoid necrosis.

Synovium becomes highly inflammatory and vascularized and covers articular surface knows as Pannus (Mantle). Pannus fills joint space. Subsequent fibrosis and calcification may cause bony ankylosis. Periarticular soft tissue oedema, clinically presents as fusiform swelling of proximal interphalangeal joints.

Other pathological changes are also seen:

1. Nodular polymyositis
2. Subcutaneous nodules, usually over extensor surface of forearm. These are firm nontender rounded or oval masses upto 2 cm. Sometimes these nodules can also be seen over tendoachillis, back of skull, ischial tuberosity and tibia.
3. Acute necrotizing vasculitis of small and large arteries.
4. Fibrinous pleuritis or pericarditis.
5. Uveitis and keratoconjunctivitis.

Clinical Features

Patient may presents with following clinical features:

1. This is predominantly seen in females of 20–40 years of age.
2. Early morning stiffness of joint is characteristic.
3. Swelling in at least one joint continuously for not less than 6 weeks.
4. Symmetrical joint swelling.
5. Swelling of at least one other joint.
6. Subcutaneous nodule.
7. PIP joint shows typical fusiform swelling and stiffness.
8. MP joint shows flexed fingers which are deviated ulnarward.
9. **Swan neck deformity** shows hyperextension at PIP joint and flexion at DIP joint. It occurs because volar plate of PIP joint is ruptured.
10. **Boutonniere's deformity** shows flexion at PIP joint which is caused by rupture of central extensor expansion.
11. **Trigger finger/thumb**
12. Ankylosis can occur in late cases.
13. Muscular atrophy can occur around joint.
14. Cold and clammy extremities.
15. Skin is atrophic and glossy.
16. Thenar and hypothenar eminence show redness.
17. Sometimes psoriasis may be present.
18. Spleenomegaly and lymphadenopathy may be present.
19. Hip is flexed and adducted while knee is flexed.
20. Foot may show equinus, cavus/varus and clawing of toes.

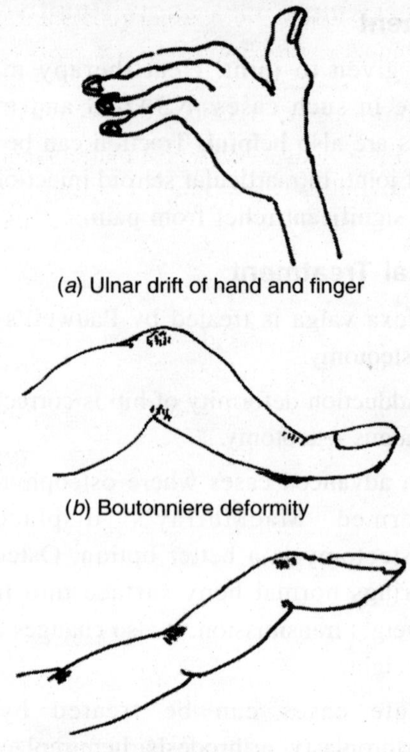

(*a*) Ulnar drift of hand and finger

(*b*) Boutonniere deformity

(*c*) Swan neck deformity

Fig. 35.5 Deformities in rheumatoid arthritis

Investigations

- Agglutination reaction (latex fixation test) is positive.
- Poor mucin clot.
- ESR is markedly raised.
- Rh factor is positive.
- Normocytic and normochromic anemia is seen.
- Anti CCP. This is microparticle enzyme immuno assay (MEIA) for semiquantitative determination of IgG class of autoantibodies specific to cyclic citrullin peptide (CCP) in human plasma and serum. This test provides additional diagnostic tool for diagnosis of rheumatoid arthritis. Normal value is 0–5 u/ml.

Diseases which may show Positive Rh Factor

Autoimmune diseases	Chronic infectious diseases
Rh. arthritis	Infectious mononucleosis
SLE	T.B.
Sjogren's syndrome	Leprosy
Systemic sclerosis	Kala-azar
Waldenstorm's macroglobulinaemia	Filariasis
Dermatomyositis	Bacterial endocarditis
Polymyositis	Infectious hepatitis
Cirrhosis of liver	Syphillis

X-ray Findings

Early stage shows osteoporosis, periarticular swelling and joint effusion. Later joint space is reduced. Bony destruction/deformities and ankylosis are also seen in X-ray.

Treatment

Principle of treatment is to keep inflammatory process at minimum, preservation of joint movements and prevention of secondary joint stiffness and deformity.

- Bed rest and high protein diet.
- Hot packs can be applied over joints.
- Joints can be immobilized by plaster splint, which must be intermittently removed daily to provide full range of movements to joint.
- Anemia can be corrected by haematinics and transfusion.
- Removal of infective foci.

Drugs to be used in Rheumatoid Arthritis

1. NSAIDS
2. DMARD (Disease modifying anti rheumatoid drugs)
3. Corticosteroids.

NSAIDS

Aspirin is drug of choice. It can be given 3–5 gm/day. Aspirin provides relief from pain, swelling and morning stiffness. Aspirin inhibits cyclooxygenase irreversibility by acetyling one of it's serine residue. Side effects of aspirin should always be kept in mind.

If aspirin fails to control the disease, Indomethacin should be given (25–50 mg BD-QID). Those patients who can not tolerate oral dose, a suppository can be given. Indomethacin is a highly potent inhibitor of PG synthesis and it suppresses neutrophil activity.

DMARD

Gold, d-pencillamine, chloroquine or hydroxychloroquine, sulfasalazine, leflunoamide, methotraxate, azathioprine and cyclosporine are disease modifying anti rheumatoid drugs.

Leflunomide

It inhibits proliferation of activated lymphocytes in active rheumatoid arthritis. It suppresses the arthritic symptoms and retards radiological progression of disease. In body leflunomide is converted into active metabolite, which inhibits dihydro-orotate dehydrogenase and pyramidine synthesis in actively dividing cells. Loading dose of 100 mg is given for 3 days followed by 20 mg 1OD. Drug shows its effect in 4 weeks. It is as effective as Mtx or sulfasalazine.

Methotraxate

Mtx is drug of choice among all DMARD. Mtx is dihydrofolate reductase inhibitor and acts as immunosuppressant and anti-inflammatory drug. Mtx inhibits cytokine production chemotaxis and cell mediated immune reaction. Mtx is preferred for initial treatment of rheumatoid arthritis and it provides rapid pain relief. If we forget its side effect it becomes much better drug than Leflunomide. This can be started with 2.5 mg tablet, 4 times in a week.

Sulfasalazine

It is primarily used for ulcerative colitis but it is also used for rheumatoid arthritis. It seems to suppress generation of superoxide radicles and cytokines elaboration by inflammatory cells. This drug is equally effective as hydroxychloroquine and better tolerated than gold or pencillamine.This is a good alternative of Mtx due to its less side effects and can be used in early and mild cases. It can be given 1–3 gm/day BD-TDS.

Corticosteroids

This can be used at any stage along with first line drug. They provide potent anti-inflammatory and immunosuppressant action. Intraarticular injections can be given.

Latest Treatment of Rheumatoid Arthritis

(Ref: Stanley B. Cohan, MD University of Texas south western medical school of Dallas)

Following group of drugs are being used for the treatment of Rheumatoid arthritis:

(A) *B cell-depleting therapies*

In this therapy following drugs are being used:

1. Rituximab
2. Ocrelizumab
3. Atacicept
4. TRU-015 (single chain polypeptide)
5. Humax (human monoclonal antibody to CD-20)
6. BR3-Fc

(B) *Cytokine inhibitors*

Following inhibitors are being used:

1. Infliximab
2. Golimumab
3. tgAAC 94
4. AME-527
5. Tocilizumab

(C) *Rank ligand inhibitors*

DENOSUMAB

(Ref: De siree vander Heijde M.D. coinvestigator and Professor in Rheumatology, Leiden University Medical Centre, Leiden Netherland, presented this study on 14th June 2007 of Annual European Congress of Rheumatology (EULAR)).

Denosumab is a fully human monoclonal antibody to RANK ligand (RANKL). In development of bone erosion, RANK is produced by activated T-cell and also synovial fibroblasts, thus leading to differentiation and activation of osteoclasts, which then invade the bone, and erosion is consequence, "Dr. van der Heijde said".

Mode of action of Denosumab in Rheumatoid arthritis is to block this osteoclasts activation pathway by binding to and sequestering RANKL. Further benefits of Denosumab includes high affinity for RANKL and no detectable binding to TNF-alpha, TNF-beta, TNF related apoptosis-including ligand (TRAIL) and CD 40 L.

Surgical Treatment of Rh Knee

- Early Rheumatoid arthritis is managed by synovectomy. It prevents progression of disease and prevents motion.
- Severe flexion contracture of knee is managed by supracondylar osteotomy.
- Varus or valgus deformity is corrected by corrective osteotomy.
- In bilateral advanced rheumatoid arthritis arthroplasty becomes treatment of choice. Medial collateral and posterior cruciate ligaments should be intact to perform arthroplasty.
- Arthrodesis is done when both knees are severely destroyed. In this case one knee

should be arthrodesed while other knee should undergo arthroplasty.

Surgical Treatment of Rh Hip

Total hip replacement is ideal procedure for middle aged patients. In this procedure hip is replaced by a complete prosthesis using both actabular and femoral component.

CERVICAL SPONDYLOSIS

This is a degenerative disease of cervical spine which shows osteoarthritic changes.

Clinical Features

Patient may presents with following clinical features:

1. Pain in cervical region which aggravates with activity and in standing position. It is relieved by lying down.
2. Stiffness in neck.
3. Radiculation in upper limbs with tingling numbness in arm, forearm and hand. Paresthesia occurs according to nerve root involvement.
4. Vertigo can occur due to vertibrobasilar syndrome.
5. Restriction of cervical motion in all direction except rotation.
6. Occipital headache.

Pathological Changes

Intervertebral disc undergoes degeneration leading to reduction in disc space and peripheral osteophyte formation. Later involvement of posterior intervertebral joint causes pain in neck. Osteophyte formation may cause nerve root compression and radicular pain in upper limbs. C5-6 is commonest joint to be involved in cervical spondylitis.

X-ray Findings

X-ray of cervical spine may show following findings:

1. Intervertebral disc space is reduced and commonly seen at C5-6 level.
2. Loss of cervical lordosis.
3. Osteophytes formation is also a common feature.
4. Oblique view may show narrowing of intervertebral foramen.

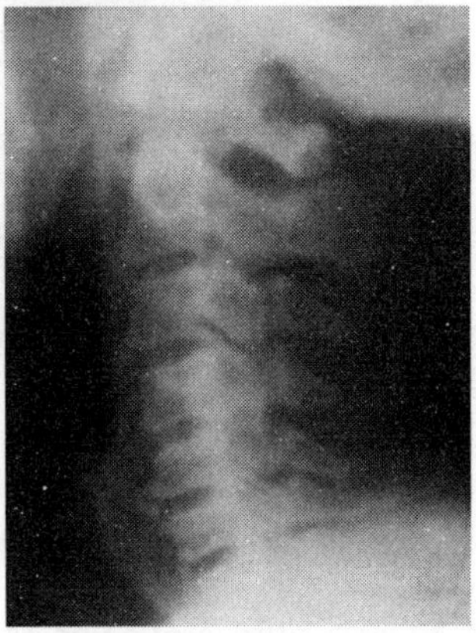

Fig. 35.6 Loss of cervical lordosis and arthritic changes in cervical spine

Treatment

- To lie on hard bed.
- Hot saline fomentation can be done at cervical area.
- A thin pillow should be adviced.
- Soft cervical collar should be adviced in case of loss of cervical lordosis.
- Cervical traction can be applied to provide relief from stiffness.
- Antiemetics are given in case of vertigo.
- Analgesics and muscle relaxant are also given.
- Short wave diathermy can also be given.

Differential Diagnosis

Following clinical conditions should be considered while treating a case of cervical spondylitis:

1. Cervical rib
2. Pancoast tumor
3. Cervical disc prolapse
4. Spinal cord tumor
5. Carpal tunnel syndrome

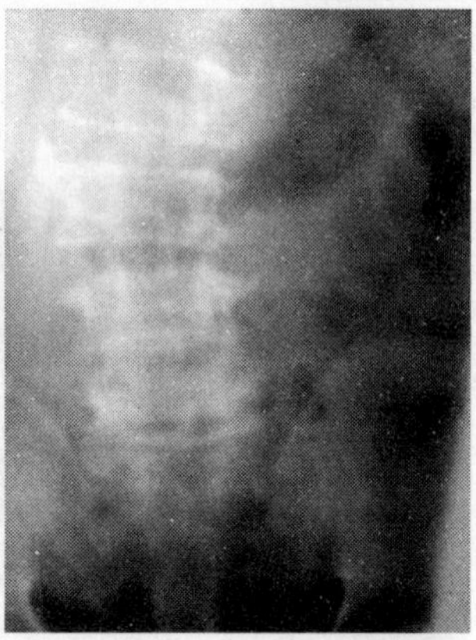

Fig. 35.7 Osteoarthritis of spine (A.P. view)

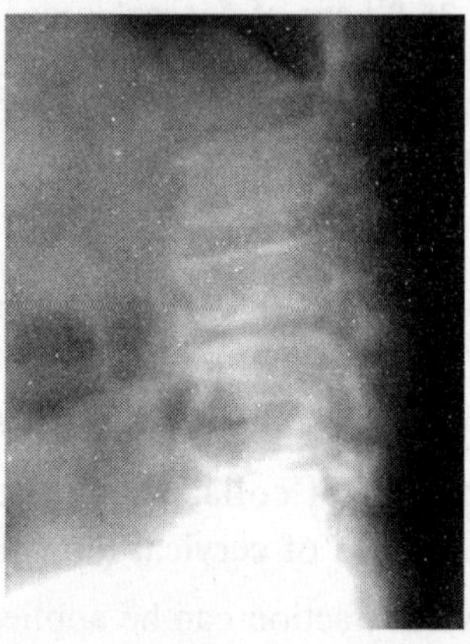

Fig. 35.8 Osteoarthritis of spine (lateral view)

APPROACH TO A CASE OF ARTHRITIS (EXCLUDING O.A.)

Arthritis with Fever	**Arthritis without Fever**
Monoarticular- Septic arthritis	**Monoarticular-*Acute*-** Traumatic/Haemophillia ***Chronic***-JRA
Polyarticular- ***Acute and Migratory-*** Rheumatic fever/Lyme's disease ***Acute and non migratory-*** JRA/SLE/Kawasaki's disease/sickle cell disease ***Chronic-*** JRA/SLE/Ankylosing spondylitis	**Polyarticular-** JRA/Ankylosing spondylitis/Sarcoidosis

Arthritis with rash	**Arthritis with aseptic meningitis**	**Arthritis with peripheral neuropathies**
JRA/SLE/ Kawasaki disease/Lyme's disease/PAN/ Acute rheumatic fever	SLE/JRA/ Lyme's disease	Lyme's disease/PAN

JUVENILE RHEUMATOID ARTHRITIS

This is inflammatory pathology of one or more joints which starts before the age of 6 years and persists at least for one and half months excluding other specific causes of arthritis.

Clinical Features

Patient usually presents with following three patterns:

1. 4 or < 4 joints involvement (pauciarticular)
2. 5 or > 5 joints involvement (polyarticular), within first six months of onset.
3. Systemic involvement.

Pauciarticular Type

- This is more common in females. Rh factor is negative. Antinuclear antibody is positive.
- Boys are affected after 8 years of age. Hip joint is commonly involved. Boys may have history of ankylosing spondylitis/psoriasis/ Reiter's disease. Rh factor and antinuclear antibody are negative.
- Knee, ankle and elbow joints are commonly affected.
- Small joints usually escape.

Polyarticular Type

- This is also more common in female.
- Rh factor may or may not be positive.
- Uveitis or low grade fever may be seen.
- Joints may develop flexion deformity.
- PIP joints are involved.

Systemic Type

- Systemic type is more common in boys.
- Patient may present with intermittent fever, evanescent maculopapular rash (with central clearing).
- Spleenomegaly and lymphadenopathy is seen.
- Interstitial lung disease and pericarditis may be present.
- ESR is raised.
- Rh factor is negative.
- Antinuclear antibody may be present.

Treatment

- NSAIDS (Naproxen/Ibruprofen/Piroxicam/ Indomethacin/Diclofenac) can be tried.
- Intraarticular corticosteroid (Triamcinolone/ Methylprednisolone) can be tried.

Complications

Patient may develop joint contracture, growth disturbances, anemia and chronic anterior uveitis.

CHAPTER

36 Bone Tumors

- Giant cell tumor (Osteoclastoma)
- Osteosarcoma
- Secondary osteosarcoma
- Paget sarcoma
- Parosteal osteosarcoma
- Ewing sarcoma
- Chondrosarcoma
- Aneurysmal bone cyst
- Unicameral bone cyst
- Osteoid osteoma
- Osteochondroma (Exostosis)
- Osteoma
- Textiloma
- Chondroma
- Chondroblastoma
- Chondromyxoid fibroma
- Osteoblastoma
- Reticulum cell sarcoma
- Haemangioma of bone
- Maffuci syndrome
- Fibrosarcoma
- Synovial sarcoma
- Multiple myeloma
- Chordoma
- Metastasis in bone

GIANT CELL TUMOR (OSTEOCLASTOMA)

Osteoclastoma is a benign but locally malignant tumor. It is an osteolytic tumor which originates from epiphysis. Osteoclastoma usually affects the people of 20–40 years of age. Male to female ratio is 1.5:1. Tumor gaint cells are seen under microscopy which is pathological hallmark of osteoclastoma.

Bones Commonly Involved in Osteoclastoma

1. Lower end of femur
2. Upper end of tibia and fibula
3. Lower end of radius
4. Lower end of ulna.

Clinical Features

Patient may present with following clinical features:

1. This is usually seen in 20–40 years of age.
2. Patient gives history of swelling in one half of bone for a longer duration. (Usually in months)
3. Pain is not a peculiar feature.
4. Joint movements are normal.
5. Skin overlying swelling is not shiny.
6. Swelling does not show any dilated veins over it.
7. Swelling is smooth.

8. Mild tenderness may be present over swelling.
9. Egg shell crackling may be felt on palpitation.
10. Effusion is not seen in the joint.
11. In advanced case a pathological fracture may be seen.
12. 1/3rd are benign, 1/3rd are locally malignant and 1/3rd are malignant.

Pathology

Gross

Tumor is reddish brown, friable, ragged. Tissues are filled with blood clots. Distortion of epiphyseal end is seen. Periosteal reaction is absent. Joint cavity is not involved in osteoclastoma.

Microscopy

Tumor giant cells are hallmark of GCT. These are present in large number. Size of these cells are large aid. These cells contain multiple number of nuclei usually more than 150. This tumor is covered by a fibrous capsule. Spindle cells are suggestive of malignant transformation.

Campanacci's Radiological Grading

Grade-1: Cystic lesion

Grade-2: Cortex is thin but there is no perforation of cortex.

Grade-3: Cortex is perforated and tumor is extended into soft tissue.

Investigations

- Complete haemogram
- X-ray of local area
- FNAC
- Biopsy

X-ray Findings

- Eccentrically situated lytic lesion at upper end of tibia/lower end of femur/lower end of radius.
- Cortex is thin and expanded.
- Joint is not involved and joint lines are intact.
- No periosteal reaction is seen.
- Soap bubble appearance.
- Calcification is not seen within the tumor.

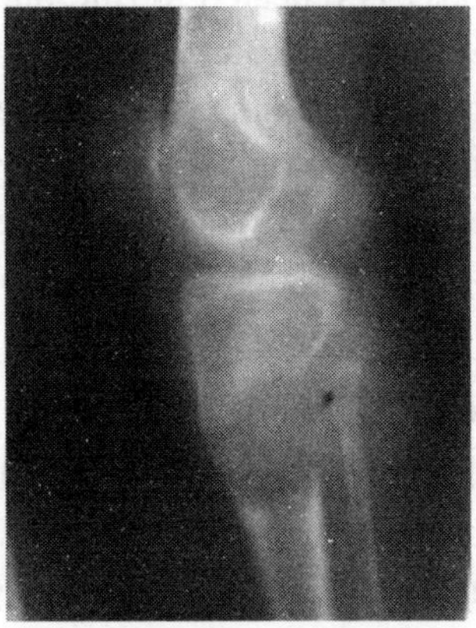

Fig. 36.1 Giant cell tumor of upper end of tibia

Biopsy

Biopsy is done to confirm the diagnosis. Findings are discussed under pathology of GCT.

Treatment

This tumor has a tendency of recurrence and along with that it is more invasive and aggrasive in nature. Surgery is the treatment of choice.

Surgical Treatment

Currettage and cryosurgery with bone cementation

This is the surgery of choice as this decreases the chance of malignancy from 15–18%. In this procedure repetitive freezing and thawing is done by liquid nitrogen. This destroys the tumor. Later bone cement can be filled up in vacant space left behind after excision of tumor.

After thorough curettage, liquid nitrogen is poured into cavity of tumor. Here temperature decreases up to –60 degree C at a time or up to –21 degree

C three times to ensure adequate cryonecrosis. Gelfoam sponge is used to seal the medullary canal. When liquid nitrogen is poured through a tunnel, gelfoam freezes and seals the medullary canal. Cavity can be filled with autogenous/homogenous, cancellous bone graft/fibular strut graft or methylmethacrylate. After 3–6 months of surgery biopsy is repeated to rule out recurrence. If biopsy is positive, cryosurgery should be repeated again. If malignant changes are observed ablation surgery can be sought. Complications of this surgery are skin necrosis, neuropraxia, prolonged healing, infection and pathological fracture.

Currettage and bone cementation

Whole of the tumor is currettaged and later cavity is filled with bone cement. Residual stromal cells and giant cells are destroyed by heat of polymerization. This procedure reduces the chances of recurrence.

Currettage and bone grafting

This procedure has high recurrence rate of 30%. In this procedure after doing the curettage, cavity is filled with bone graft.

Enblock excision

This is basically done in cases of recurrence. In this procedure, normal tissue of about 2 cm is also excised and cavity is filled with cancellous bone graft or freeze dried allograft or prosthesis.

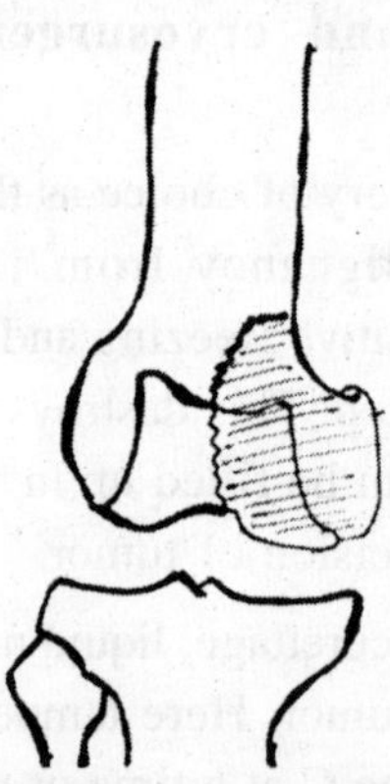

Fig. 36.2 Diagrammatic representation of giant cell tumor

Excision of Tumor and reconstruction

Following surgeries can be done under this method of treatment:

- Turnoplasty
- Arthrodesis
- Arthroplasty

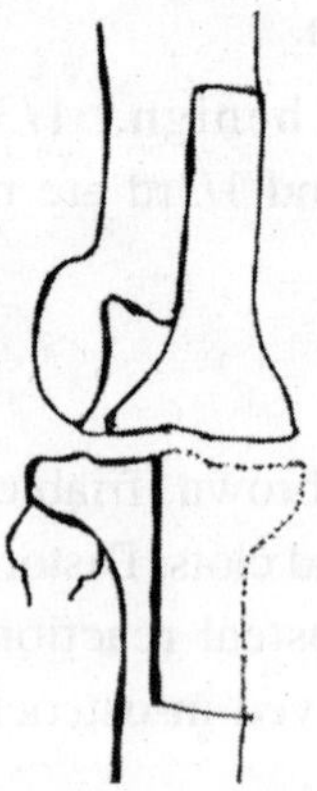

(*a*) Turnoplasty

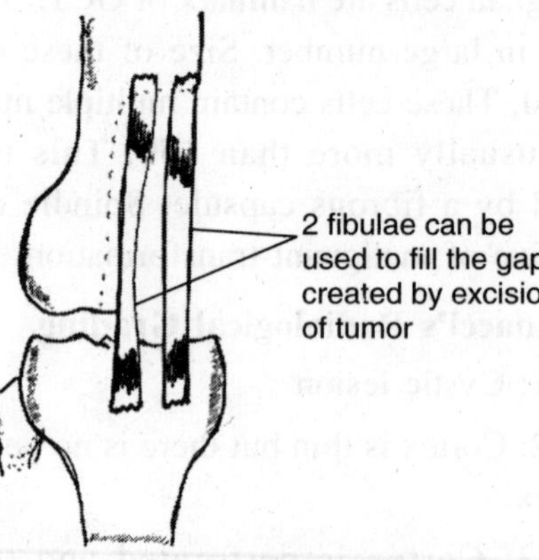

(*b*) Arthrodesis

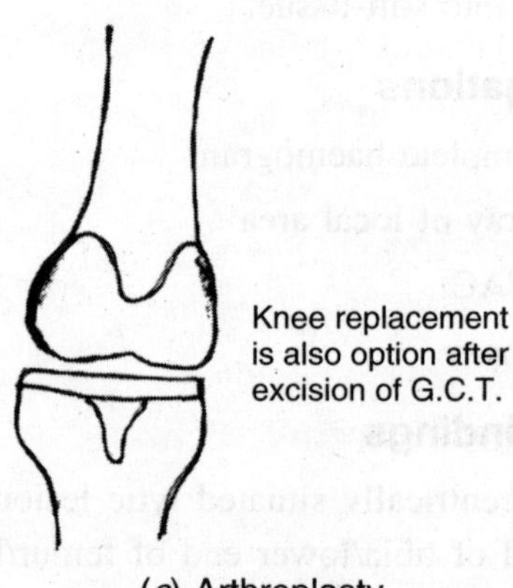

(*c*) Arthroplasty

Fig. 36.3

Turnoplasty

This procedure is indicated in GCT of lower end of femur and upper end of tibia. In case of femur, after excision of GCT, required length of tibia is taken and split in two halves. One half is turned upside down and fixed with left stump of femur. Femur bone can be used for osteoclastoma of tibia.

Arthrodesis

Fibula of both sides are taken and used to bridge the excised gap.

Arthroplasty

This is a reconstruction surgery which is done after excision of tumor. Reconstruction can be done by autograft, allograft or by a prosthesis.

GCT of lower end of radius

In this case lower end of radius is resected and reconstruction of wrist joint is done by using ipsilateral fibula.

Radiotherapy

This mode of treatment is given when tumor is present at vertebrae, spine, sacrum or pelvis. 1500–5000 rads can be given for 5–6 weeks. If radiotherapy is given to benign GCT it may produce malignant changes.

Differential Diagnosis

Following conditions should be considered while dealing with a case of osteoclastoma:

1. Chondroblastoma (benign)
2. Osteitis fibrosa
3. Aneurysmal bone cyst
4. Unicameral bone cyst
5. Nonossifying fibroma
6. Hyperparathyroidism
7. Chondromyxoid fibroma

OSTEOSARCOMA

Osteosarcoma is a highly malignant tumor of second decade, characterized by neoplastic osteoid formation and tumor tissue formation. This tumor arises from a common multipotential mesenchymal tissue and gives rise to fibroblastic, chondroblastic, osteolytic and osteoblastic type.

Aetiology

Age

It is commonly seen in 15–25 years of age group (primary type). Secondary osteosarcoma occurs beyond 45 years of age.

Sex

This tumor predominantly affects male population.

Predisposing factors

Oncogenic Virus

RNA virus which can produce bone tumor includes Harvey & Meloney mouse (murine) sarcoma virus.

DNA viruses are polyoma virus and SV-40 virus.

Radiation

Radiation of more than 2000 rads may produce osteosarcoma. Tumor appears after 3-4 years of exposure.

Chemicals

Following chemicals may produce osteosarcoma:

- 20-methylcholanthrene
- Cupric chelated N-hydroxy2-acetylamino-fluorene.
- Beryllium compound.

Sites of tumor origin

This tumor arises from metaphysis of long bone.

Table 36.1: Differential features of bone tumors

Features	Osteosarcoma	Ewing tumor	Osteoclastoma	Chondrosarcoma	Chondromyxoid fibroma	Multiple myeloma	Synovial sarcoma
Age	10–20 years	10–20 years	20–40 years	20–60 years	10–30 years	40–60 years	Any age usually 20–30 years
Origin	Metaphysis	Diaphysis	Originates from metaphysis quickly destroys epiphysis	Diaphysis or metaphysis of long bones	Metaphysis of large tubular bones of lower limb	Plasma cells	Synovial membrane of a joint tendon sheath or bursa
Bones	Lower end of femur, upper end of tibia, upper end of humerus	Femur, tibia fibula, humerus	Lower end of femur, upper end of tibia	Proximal end of femur and humerus illium, ribs and scapula	Femur and tibia	Skull and trunk bones	Knee, ankle or wrist joint
X-ray findings	Codman's triangle sun-ray appearance	Onion peel appearance	Soap-bubble appearance	Pop-corn or bread crumb appearance osteolytic lesion	Osteolytic lesiom	Punched out lesion in skull and pelvis produce silver beaten appearance, biconcave-vertebral bodies	Soft tissue shadow with hecks of calcification
Treatment	Primary lesion is treated by amputation followed by high dose megavoltage therapy	Radiation is treatement of choice	Excision	Low grade tumor wide excision high grade tumor radical margin excision	Tumor is locally excised and defect is filled with autogenous bone graft	Palliative	Local excision of tumor

Locations of Osteosarcoma

1. Lower end of femur (52%)
2. Upper end of tibia (20%)
3. Upper end of humerus (9%)

Pathology

Gross

Osteosarcoma takes origin from metaphysis of long bones. Destruction of inner cortex is seen that extends up to subperiosteal space. Area of destruction produces leg of mutton appearance. Tumor consistency varies from stony hard to soft gritty. Fibrous tumor is white, osseous tumor is yellowish white and tumor of cartilaginous origin is bluish white. Large vascular channels and areas of haemorrhage are seen. Neoplastic new bone formation occurs along the vessels and perpendicular to cortex thus creating **Sunburst appearance.** Reactive new bone formation occurs at subperiosteal space in a triangular area; known as **Codman's triangle.** Articular cartilage acts as a bar for extension of tumor into the joint. Haematogenous metastasis firstly occurs in lung.

Microscopic

Malignant characteristics are seen in stromal cells e.g. anisocytosis, poikilocytosis, nuclear pyknosis, pleomorphism and polyhedral contour. Peripheral zone of tumor shows best evidence of malignancy. Neoplastic osteoblastic areas are always seen. Calcification may be seen in malignant tumor cartilage. Small spindle cells are seen with hyperchromatic nuclei. Giant cells are also seen.

Classification

Clinical Classification

1. Primary osteosarcoma
2. Secondary osteosarcoma

Pathological Classification

1. Osteoblastic (sclerosing)
2. Osteolytic (telengiectatic)
3. Chondroblastic
4. Fibroblastic

Primary Osteosarcoma

- Premalignant conditions are not associated with it.
- This tumor occurs in the age group of 10-20 years.
- Primary osteosarcoma is less malignant than secondary type.

Secondary Osteosarcoma

- This osteosarcoma occurs when skeletal system is affected by benign tumors or if patient has generalized skeletal disorder.
- It is seen in Paget's disease, fibrous dysplasia, radiation exposure, multiple osteochondroma and multiple enchondromatosis.
- Secondary osteosarcoma is usually seen after 45 years of age.

Osteobalstic Osteosarcoma

- This is also known as Sclerosing osteosarcoma.
- It is associated with abundant tumor bone formation.
- Tumor spreads by early haematogenous metastasis.
- This is greyish white in colour.
- Consistency is in between fibrous tissues to bone.

Osteolytic Osteosarcoma

- It is known as telengiectatic osteosarcoma or malignant bone aneurysm.
- It shows little tumor bone formation.
- Pathological fractures are commonly seen which do not heal.
- Tumor exists subperiosteally.
- Inner cortex is motheaten.
- Slow growing tumor shows foreign body type giant cells while rapidly growing tumor shows multinucleated tumor giant cells.
- Transverse fractures are seen in metaphysis.

Clinical Features of Osteosarcoma

Osteosarcoma may present with the following features:

1. It is commonly seen between 10–20 years of age. This is also known as tumor of second decade.
2. Secondary osteosarcoma occurs beyond the age of 45 years.
3. Osteosarcoma arises from metaphysis of long bones.
4. Bones which are commonly affected in decreasing order of frequency are lower end of femur, upper end of tibia and upper end of humerus.
5. This tumor has gradual onset. Pain is the first symptom followed by swelling.
6. Pain becomes worst at night and gradually becomes more severe with the growth of tumor.

7. Patient may give history of trauma but it does not have any relation to aetiology of tumor.
8. On examination it is warm, tender palpable mass. It's consistency varies from firm to hard. Overlying skin is shiny and stretched. Premature veins are seen over skin.
9. Sometimes tumor becomes pulsatile which is known as telengeictatic osteosarcoma.
10. Skin overlying tumor never ulcerates.
11. When the tumor invades soft tissue and epiphysis, movements at the joint become limited.
12. Pathological fractures may be seen in osteosarcoma.
13. Weight loss and anemia are associated findings.

Prognosis

- This tumor is highly fatal. Patient dies within 2 years if he does not get any treatment.
- Pulmonary metastasis becomes evident usually 5-6 months after the onset of disease in 80% cases.
- Even after amputation 50% patients show pulmonary metastasis within 5 months.
- After detection of metastasis, death occurs within 6 months.
- 5–25% Patients show 5 years survival rate with or without metastasis.

Investigations

- Haemoglobin level is reduced. WBC, ESR is raised. Serum alkaline phosphatase is markedely increased but it is not diagnostic. It's level falls after removal of tumor but it rises again if metastasis spreads in the body.

X-ray Findings

- Tumor arising from metaphysis shows irregular destruction of bone.
- Erosion of cortex is seen.
- Periosteal neoplastic new bone formation is seen.
- Subperiosteal new bone formation occurs at the end of tumor in a triangular area which is known as **Codman's triangle.**
- New bone formation occurs along the Haversian canal which gives **Sun-ray appearance.**
- **Periosteal reaction** seen in osteosarcoma is different than seen in osteomyelitis because it is irregular in osteosarcoma and smooth in osteomyelitis.
- Pathological fractures may be seen in advanced cases.
- X-ray of chest shows pulmonary metastasis. CT-scan of chest is a better investigation to detect pulmonary metastasis.

Bone Scan

Bone scan can be done to rule out skip lesion or intramedullary spread of tumor.

MRI

MRI can detect soft tissue spread of tumor.

FNAC and Biopsy

FNAC and biopsy show the histopathological changes as described above.

Treatment Regimen

Following treatment regimen are applied for this tumor:

- Primary lesion is treated by amputation followed by high dose megavoltage therapy or vice versa.
- 1700 rads irradiation is given to lungs in 10 fractions in 15 days.
- Chemotherapy is started with Methotraxte, Adriamycin, Vincristine, Cyclophosphamide and Actinomycin-D.

Principles of Surgical Treatment

First of all diagnosis should be confirmed by biopsy. Now level of amputation should be determined. Mid thigh amputation is done if tumor involves lower end of femur, and upper end tibia. Disarticulation of hip or hind quarter amputation is done in tumor of upper end of femur. Fore quarter amputation is done in tumor of upper end of humerus. Time of surgery should be decided.

Treatment of Pulmonary Metastasis

- Microemboli are treated by chemotherapy.
- Tumor mass of lung is treated either by lobectomy or wedge resection.
- After every 3 months CT-scan of lung is done.

SECONDARY OSTEOSARCOMA

- It is highly malignant than primary tumor.
- This tumor is seen in people who are having benign tumor or generalized skeletal disease.
- Secondary osteosarcoma is seen in Paget's disease, fibrous dysplasia, radiation exposure and enchondroma.

PAGET SARCOMA

This is malignant transformation of Paget's disease. It is highly fatal and patient dies within 3 years. It has other following features:

- Common bones which are affected are femur, humerus, pelvis, skull and tibia in this frequency.
- Patient presents with severe pain radiating along the nerve root.
- Tumor mass is palpable and shows dilated veins over it.
- X-ray shows destructive changes in the cortex. Mixed areas of increased density and absorption are seen. X-ray chest shows metastatic lesion.
- Histopathological examination shows extremely hypercelluar stroma with hyperchromatic nuclei and marked pleomorphism. This tumor is predominantly osteoblastic or fibroblastic.
- Treatment consists of ablation or amputation as a palliative measure.

PAROSTEAL OSTEOSARCOMA

This is a low grade malignant tumor which takes origin within periosteum. It remains in intimate relationship to outer surface of periosteum. It has other following features:

- It is commonly seen between third and fourth decade.
- It takes origin from metaphyseal region of long tubular bone, commonly from lower end of femur and upper end of humerus.
- Patholgy shows hard lobulated encapsulated mass, firmly attached to underlying cotex by narrow or broad base. Microscopy shows all characteristics of malignancy.
- Clinically patient presents with painless localized bony hard swelling which is fixed to underlying bone. Skin overlying swelling is normal.
- X-ray shows longitudinally disposed radiolucent line usually 2-3 mm in width representing interposed periosteum. Tumor is bulky lobulated, oval/spherical with dense shadow at metaphyseal region of long bone density of tumor is more at it's base.
- Treatment is done by enblock excision. If shaft is also invaded segmental resection is done. High grade tumor is treated by

amputation or disarticulation. **Radiotherapy has no role in treatment.**

Prognosis

Near about 80% Tumor recur after simple excision and 50% Tumor recur after enblock excision.

EWING SARCOMA

Ewing sarcoma is a primary malignant bony tumor which arises from diaphysis of long bones. It is extremely radiosensitive. Stem cell for Ewing tumor is reticulum cell. Radiologically it is characterized by onion peel appearance.

Clinical Features

Patient of Ewing tumor may present with the following features:

1. It is commonly seen between **10–20 years of age.**
2. It is more common in males.
3. This tumor takes origin from **diaphysis of long bones.**
4. Common long bones affected are femur, tibia, fibula and humerus in decreasing order of frequency.
5. Patient presents with localized painful swelling at diaphysis of long bone. It is firm to hard in consistency.
6. Pain is intermittent and becomes worst at night. History of fever is also present which may give false impression of osteomyelitis.
7. This is firm to hard palpable tumor fixed to underlying bone. Swelling is red oedematous and shows dilated veins.
8. Constitutional reaction like fever, anemia and leukocytosis are also present.
9. Metastasis occurs through lymphatics and blood stream. Metastasis specially occurs in skull, vertebrae and ribs. **It metastasizes late to lungs.**

Pathology

This is a firm greyish white tumor encapsulated by fibrous tissue that sends septae into tumor and dividing it into lobules. Multiple layer of bones lie parallel to shaft. New bone formation occurs around vessels that extend radially from periosteum to shaft. This tumor is quite vascular and contains haemorrhagic foci. Cortex is also destroyed. Subperiosteal new bone formation occurs in layers producing onion peel appearance radiologically. This tumor surrounds a central clear area with no central fibril thus creating **pseudorosette pattern.**

Investigations

- Anemia and leucocytosis are frequently seen.
- Urine examination is done for vanillylmandelic acid (VMA).
- Glycogen stain can be done.

X-ray Findings

- It shows lytic lesion at diaphysis of long bones.
- Periosteal new bone formation occurs in layer producing **onion peel appearance** in X-ray.
- Cortical destruction may show moth eaten or cracked egg appearance.

Biopsy

Biopsy is essential to confirm the diagnosis.

Treatment

Ewing sarcoma can be treated by following methods:

- This tumor is extremely radiosensitive. Tumor melts like snow. Radiation is treatment of choice. Recurrence is common.
- Combined local radiotherapy and systemic chemotherapy is given to decrease the chances of recurrence.

- 6000 rads exposure is given to local tumor and to control metastasis.
- Vincristine, cyclophosfamide or ifosfamide and adriamycin are given at every 3-4 weeks. Such 12–18 cycles are given.
- New chemotherapy is used in the form of Ifosfamide, Cysplatinum and Epipodophyllin toxin.
- Surgical treatment can be done in the form of debulking of tumor or limb preservation surgery.

Prognosis

- Radiotherapy followed by amputation has 2 years survival rate.
- Chemotherapy, radiotherapy and amputation combinedly increase survival rate up to 3–5 years in 50–75% cases.

Differential Diagnosis

- Osteomyelitis
- Osteosarcoma
- Malignant lymphoma

All of these 3 conditions show onion peel appearance radiologically.

CHONDROSARCOMA

Chondrosarcoma is a slow growing cartilaginous malignant tumor which is predisposed by some antecedent lesion like enchondroma, olier disease, osteochondroma, hereditary multiple exostosis etc. It does not have osteoid formation unlike osteosarcoma.

Clinical Features

Chondrosarcoma may present with the following features:

1. This tumor can be seen between 10–80 years of age.
2. It is usually seen between 20–60 years or in 6th decade.
3. It is more common in male.
4. Proximal end of femur, proximal humeral shaft, innominate bone, ribs and scapula are commonly affected. It can also be seen in calcaneum.
5. Pain is not a prominent feature.
6. Central tumors are situated within metaphysis or diaphysis of long tubular bone. Central tumors are asymptomatic until pathological fracture occurs.
7. Chondrosarcoma is a palpable firm mass which is fixed to bone.
8. History of radiation may be present.
9. Metastasis occurs through blood vessels to lungs.
10. Diagnosis is confirmed by biopsy.

Investigations

- In contrast to osteosarcoma serum alkaline phosphatase is not raised.
- Chest X-ray may show metastasis in lungs.

X-ray Findings

- Tumor is seen within diaphysis or metaphysis of long tubular bones.
- Specks of calcification and ossification are surrounded by a zone of radiolucency.
- Erosion of cortex is seen.
- Slow growing tumors show greater degree of calcification while rapidly growing tumors show little or no calcification.
- X-ray shows fluffy cotton wool for making **popcorn or bread crumb appearance** due to calcification.

FNAC should be done to see cytological features.

Biopsy

Biopsy is main investigation to confirm the diagnosis. It may show the following findings:

- Lobulated, translucent bluish white cartilage is seen within spongiosa and medullary cavity.
- Specks of calcification are frequently seen in slow growing tumor.
- Cytological features of malignancy are seen. (hypercellularity, plumpness of nuclei or double nuclei, pleomorphism of cells and nuclei and hyperchromaism)
- High grade tumors show mitotic figures.

Treatment

- Low grade tumors are treated by wide excision. (hind quarter amputation for pelvic girdle, forequarter amputation for shoulder girdle tumor)
- Radical margin excision is done in high grade tumor.
- Role of chemotherapy and radiotherapy is controversial.

Prognosis

10 Years survival rate without recurrence or overt metastasis is mandatory. After 10 years of onset of tumor death is very unlikely.

ANEURYSMAL BONE CYST

This is a benign bone tumor also known as subperiosteal giant cell tumor or subperiosteal ossifying haematoma. Mass of vascular spaces are contained within a shell of periosteal new bone growing outward from bone.

Clinical Features

1. It is commonly seen in 10–30 years of age.
2. Males are predominantly affected.
3. It takes origin from metaphysis of long bones.
4. Upper end of humerus is commonly affected. Flat bones and vertebrae are less affected.
5. Pathological fracture is commonly seen.
6. Gradually progressive bony hard fixed swelling with mild pain is usual presentation of this tumor.
7. Joint movements may be limited.
8. Signs of nerve root compression may be seen if vertebrae are involved.

Pathology

This is a highly vascular tumor that bleeds profusely. Tumor shows reddish brown liver like friable mass. Blood filled spaces are enclosed within thin shell of bone. This tumor has its broad base attached to shaft of long bones. Soft tissues are displaced outward.

Microscopy

Microscopy shows following features:

- Multinucleate giant cells
- New bone formation
- Calcium deposits
- Periosteal new bone formation.

X-ray Findings

- X-ray shows expanded cystic ballooned out lesion in metaphyseal region of long bones. This tumor is eccentrically situated.
- Destruction of cortex is seen.
- Periosteal new bone formation can be seen.
- Tumor shows trabeculation within its substance.

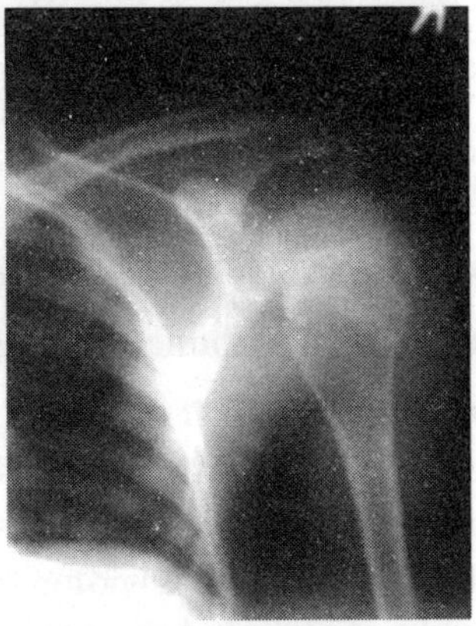

Fig. 36.4 Aneurysmal bone cyst

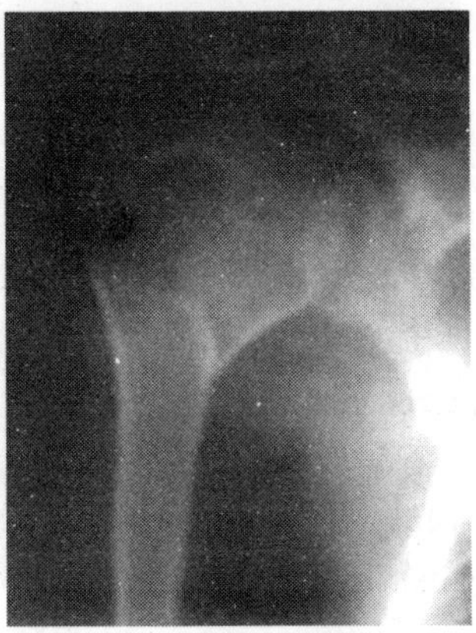

Fig. 36.5 Pathological fracture seen in aneurysmal bone cyst

Treatment

Currettage and bone grafting is mainstay of treatment.

UNICAMERAL BONE CYST

Unicameral bone cyst was first described by Jaffey and Lichtenstein. Unicameral word is made of latin word (unus:one; camera:vault). This is a tumor of first two decade of life. It takes origin at metaphyseal region of long tubular bones. Later it may migrate away from growth plate. Longitudinal growth may be disturbed if unicameral bone cyst involves epiphyseal growth plate.

Clinical Features

Patient can present with the following features:

1. This is commonly seen in between 5–15 years of age. It is rare after 20 years.
2. Male to female ratio is 2:1.
3. In children proximal end of humerus is involved while in adolescence proximal end of femur is involved.
4. It originates from metaphyseal region of long tubular bone. Later it migrates away from growth plate.
5. If femur is involved, calcar is usually preserved.
6. Illium, lower end of humerus and femur, tibia, talus, calcaneum, radius, ulna and ribs are uncommon sites to be involved.
7. This tumor is generally asymptomatic until **pathological fracture** occurs. This fracture **heals rapidly within a few weeks.**
8. On examination we find cystic swelling fixed to bone. Bony tenderness will be present if fracture occurs. Coxa vara may be present if femur is involved. If epiphyseal growth plate is involved growth disturbances will be seen.

Pathology

This tumor presents as fusiform expansile swelling which is filled with yellowish fluid. Periosteum is lifted away. Underlying bone is egg shell thin, semitransluscent and bluish in colour. It is easily penetrated.

Microscopy

Microscopy shows multilayered fibroblast containing multinucleated giant cells, foam cell containing lipid, haemosiderin and cholesterol crystal. Periosteal new bone formation may be evident.

Jaffey has classified this cyst into two categories; active and latent cyst. **Active cysts** are lying close to growth plate and continue to enlarge. **Latent cyst** exists away from growth plate.

X-ray Findings

X-ray shows radioluscent expansile cystic lesion in juxtaepiphyseal area of metaphysis which is sharply delimited from diaphysis. If femur is involved cyst will be present in subcapital area of neck that extends up to lesser trochanter. **Calcar is not involved.**

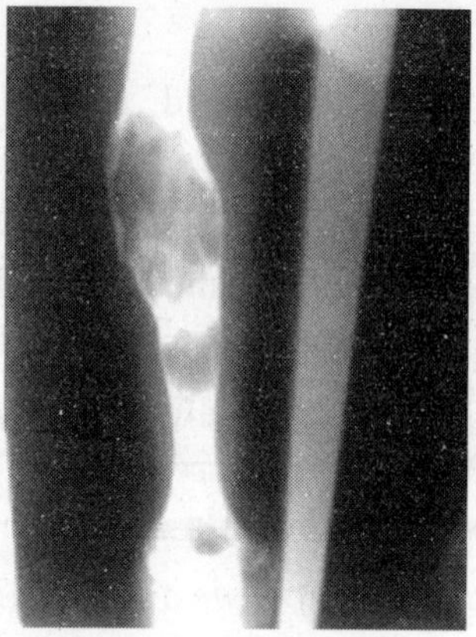

Fig. 36.6 Unicameral bone cyst (A.P. view)

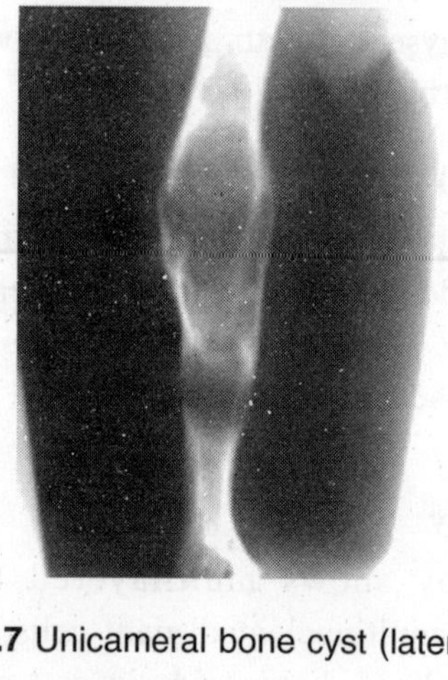

Fig. 36.7 Unicameral bone cyst (lateral view)

Treatment

Surgical excision of cyst is mainstay of treatment. This cyst can be managed with the following modes of surgeries:

Currettage and bone grafting

A small window is made into cortex and through that membranous lining is removed. This cavity is filled with autogenous bone graft. This mode of treatment has high recurrence rate.

Subtotal resection and bone grafting

In this procedure transverse section of bone is removed from 1 cm proximal and 1 cm distal to cyst. A portion of cyst wall is preserved to maintain length and alignment. Raw area is filled with autogenous cancellous bone graft. Periosteum is closed over the growth.

Total resection (Diaphysectomy) and bone grafting

Area of bone having cyst is excised followed by partial closure of periosteum. This creates a type of partial periosteal tube which is filled with cancellous bone graft.

Role of corticosteroids

If corticosteroids are injected into cyst, tremendous obliteration of cyst may occur. 40–80 mg of prednisolone is injected into small cyst while 200 mg prednisolone is injected into a large cyst. After 3-4 months X-ray is repeated to follow the case. If area of scanty osteogenesis is seen, intracystic injection of prednisolone can be repeated 5-6 times. It may take up to 3 years in obliteration of lesion.

Differential Diagnosis of Unicameral Bone Cyst

This cyst has following differential diagnosis:

Aneurysmal bone cyst

- It produces eccentric radiolucent defect on X-ray.
- Cortex is distended as well as eroded.
- Diagnosis is confirmed by biopsy.

Giant cell tumor

- It is an eccentric lytic lesion which does not involve the joint.

- Soap bubble appearance is seen on X-ray.
- Cortex is thinned out.
- Biopsy shows highly multinucleated giant cells.

Eosinophillic granuloma

- It commonly involve mid shaft of bone.
- It is very painful condition.
- Periosteal new bone formation is seen.
- Numerous eosinophils and histiocytes are seen in biopsy.

Enchondroma

- Common bones to be involved in this condition are metacarpal and metatarsal.
- It shows calcification within solid cartilaginous tumor.

Fibrous dysplasia

- This is an uncommon condition in which bony structure is replaced by avascular fibrous tissue. This can affect one (monostotic) or more than one bones (polyostotic). This lesion is situated within diaphysis. Epiphysis is not involved in this disease. Disease starts early in childhood and affects both sexes equally. This is usually asymptomatic and detected accidently in X-ray. Child may present with limp, pain or fracture. Females can present with vaginal bleed and sexual precocity. Bones are irregular and often bent. Bones may be fractured. **Shepherd crook deformity** of femur is characteristic and cause shortening of lower extremity. Hyperostosis develops at the base of skull which is responsible for asymmetry of head and face. Skin show large brown irregular patches in polyostotic fibrous dysplasia. Albright syndrome consists of unilateral polyostotic fibrous dysplasia, pigmentation and sexual precocity.
- It is also eccentrically situated radiolucent defect.
- X-ray shows ground glass appearance. Shepherd crook deformity is seen in femur. Harrison groove is seen in chest X-ray due rib fractures. Hyperostosis is seen at the base of skull. Pitutary fossa is normal.
- Serum calcium, phosphorus and alkaline phosphatase level are within normal limit. Alkaline phosphatase can be raised in severe cases.
- Biopsy is diagnostic.
- Most of the fractures heal spontaneously.

OSTEOID OSTEOMA

This is also known as **aspirin tumor,** because it quickly responds to conservative treatment by tablet of aspirin. This is therapeutic test for osteoid osteoma. This is a benign tumor of osseous origin. This tumor contains a nidus of less than 1 cm surrounded by reactive bone formation.

Clinical Features

Patient may present with the following clinical features:

1. This is commonly seen in between 10–25 years of age.
2. It is predominantly seen in male. (male:female = 2:1)
3. Tibia and femur are commonly affected.
4. Patient presents with pain which aggravates at night. This pain quickly responds to aspirin.
5. Shiny warm and tender swelling is present at tibia or femur.
6. Overlying skin is not stretched.
7. Uncommonly tumor may be present in spine.

Pathology

This tumor never contains cartilage. Irregular branching network of osteoid is seen. Vascular stroma shows fibroblast and osteoblast.

Investigations

Blood counts are negative.

X-ray findings

X-ray shows solitary rarefied small lesion <2 cm in diameter in cortex/subcortical area/subperiosteal area. This lesion is surrounded by thick and sclerotic bone.

CT-Scan

CT-scan can define the area of sclerotic bone and its entire nidus.

Treatment

Complete excision of nidus relieves the symptom.

Differential Diagnosis

1. Non suppurative osteomyelitis of Garre's.
2. Brodie's abscess.
3. Benign bone cyst
4. Chronic osteomyelitis with sequestrum.
5. Syphyllitic ossifying periosteitis.
6. Eosinophillic granuloma.

OSTEOCHONDROMA (EXOSTOSIS)

This is a commonest benign tumor of cartilaginous origin, composed of spongy bone covered by a cartilaginous cap. This is a **commonest benign bone tumor.**

Clinical Features

Patient of osteochondroma may present with the following clinical features:

1. Osteochondroma is seen in growing age and uncommon thereafter.
2. It is predominantly seen in males.
3. Favourite site of this tumor is at tendinous attachment of a strong muscle e.g. adductor magnus muscle. It is seen within metaphysis of long tubular bones especially around the knee. Other sites are ankle, hip, shoulder and elbow.
4. This tumor is usually asymptomatic. Symptoms develop due to overlying bursitis.
5. Patient presents with firm fixed nontender swelling which is fixed to bone. Overlying tissue is mobile.
6. Joint movement may be limited if the tumor is large and impinges on adjacent structures.

Pathology

Osteochondroma is a firm lobulated mass which is covered by fibrous tissue. It contains cancellous bone and fatty marrow. It also contains embryonic like cells. Matrix among the chondrocytes may show calcification.

Theory of Histogenesis

This tumor may be the result of perverted activity of periosteum which reverts to its role as perichondrium. It is to be noted that cambium layer of periosteum retains its ability to form cartilage and bone throughout the life.

X-ray Findings

- Outpouching of trabeculated bone at metaphysis is seen.
- Tumor may be sessile or pedunculated.
- Cartilage and capsule are only visible when they calcify.
- This tumor has cortical and medullary portion which are continuous with main bone.

Treatment

Complete excision of tumor is treatment of choice. Tendon above its point of attachment should be resected to prevent recurrence.

Surgical excision is done in following conditions:

- Joint interference
- Repeated painful bursitis
- Fracture of femur
- Malignant changes
- Pressure effect on neighbouring vessels.

OSTEOMA

This is slowly growing benign tumor which has following features:

- This is commonly seen in membranous bones of skull and face. Frontal bone is usually involved.
- Children are usually affected.
- Osteomas are usually external but may be intracranial, intranasal, intraorbital or within the sinus.
- This tumor does not produce any symptom. Only internal osteoma produces symptoms according to part where it is situated.
- Osteomas are nontender, hard, fixed swelling which may be sessile or pedunculated. Skin overlying swelling is freely mobile.
- Pathology shows dense compact bone covered by fibrous tissue.
- Multinucleated giant cells are seen.
- It does not undergo malignant changes.
- If it is found in skull it can be replaced by tantalum plate.

TEXTILOMA

This is a pseudotumor which is formed inside the soft tissue if a gauzepiece is left per-operatively.

CHONDROMA

This is a benign tumor of cartilaginous origin. This is also known as enchondroma or chondromyxoma. Chondroma is commonly seen in phalanges and humerus. This tumor is of more concern because it has chances of malignant transformation if situated in long bones. It causes destruction of cancellous bone.

Clinical Features

This tumor is seen between 10–50 years of age. This has other following features:

1. It involves metaphysis. Little finger is commonly involved.
2. Innominate and large long bones are uncommon to be involved.
3. It is usually asymptomatic except mild pain and swelling in phalanx. This bony swelling grows very slowly.
4. This is usually single lesion and rarely multiple.
5. Recurrence is seen in chondroma of long bones.

X-ray Findings

- X-ray shows translucent loculated or nonloculated area well demarcated from adjacent bone.
- Cortex is thin and expanded.
- In large long bones, cortex is not involved.
- Stippling of calcification along with striation of fibrous septae may be seen.
- This tumor does not show any new bone formation.

Pathology

This tumor is surrounded by a fibrous capsule. It is divided into lobules. Neoplastic tissue shows bluish white translucent cartilage and may also contain white areas of calcification. Most matured cartilage is found at the centre of femur.

Diagnosis

Circumscribed, rarefied and expanded lesion in phalanx is likely to be a case of enchondroma. If calcific stippling is seen it means diagnosis is confirmed.

Treatment

- Small tumors should be currettaged.
- Large tumors should be excised along with capsule to prevent recurrence.
- Chondroma of long bones and pelvis needs pelvic resection.

CHONDROBLASTOMA

Chondroblastoma is a benign cartilaginous tumor, found about the epiphyseal line, mainly in metaphysis. This tumor is cellular vascular and destroys the cancellous bone. Multiple calcium deposits are seen within the tumor.

Clinical Features

Patient of chondroblastoma has following clinical features:

1. It is commonly seen between 10–20 years of age.
2. Males are predominantly affected.
3. Pain, swelling, effusion and sometimes limping are clinical features.
4. It occurs toward the ends of long bone, around knee and upper end of humerus.
5. Its course is rapid from 1 month to 2 years.

Pathology

This is a dark red haemorrhagic friable tissue which shows yellow zones of calcification. Basic cell of chondroblastoma is reticulocytic cell with a tendency to differentiate into chondroblastic tissue and then into cartilage.

X-ray Findings

1. Rarefaction of epiphysis is seen.
2. Tumor is eccentrically situated either in metaphysis or epiphysis.
3. Cortex is thinned out but not perforated.

Treatment

Currettage and bone grafting is treatment of choice. Large tumors can be treated by excision but it is associated with recurrence rate of 25%. According to Copeland and Geschickter 50% tumor may become malignant.

CHONDROMYXOID FIBROMA

This is also known as fibromyxoid chondroma. It is least common benign cartilaginous tumor that takes origin from metaphyseal region of large tubular bone of lower limb. This tumor is composed of myxomatous substance and tissue.

Clinical Features

1. This is seen between 20–30 years of age.
2. Males and females are equally affected.
3. Metaphyseal region of large tubular bones of lower limb is affected. Uncommonly fibula, phalanx and calcaneum may be involved.
4. If this tumor appears before 10 years of age, symptoms will be more severe.
5. Metastasis and sarcomatous changes are not seen.

Pathology

This is a solid tumor mass of greyish or bluish colour. It's consistency is firm. Calcified areas are unusual. It is composed of lobulated or pseudolobulated areas of stellate cells. Nuclei are single oval and moderate in size.

X-ray Findings

1. X-ray shows eccentrically situated lytic lesion at metaphysis.
2. Cortex is expanded.
3. Triangular periosteal bone formation is seen at the base of tumor.
4. Medullary margins are sclerosed and scalloped.

Treatment

Tumor is locally excised and defect is filled with autogenous bone graft. Large tumors are treated by enblock excision.

OSTEOBLASTOMA

This tumor is commonly seen in spine and jaw. It does not occur in epiphysis. It takes origin either from diaphysis or metaphysis of long bones. Other features of this tumor are as follows:

- It is made up of vascular osteoid and new bone.
- It is commonly seen between 10–20 years of age.
- Patient presents with pain and localized swelling.
- X-ray shows radiolucent expansile lesion.
- It is treated by curettage.

RETICULUM CELL SARCOMA

- This is highly radiosensitive tumor which arises from marrow reticulum cells.
- Clinical and pathological features resemble with Ewing sarcoma.
- It is commonly seen in long bones but sometimes it can be seen in flat bones.
- Male population of 20–50 years of age is commonly affected.
- Patient may present with pathological fracture.

X-ray Findings

X-ray shows moth eaten appearance in bone.

Treatment

Radiotherapy is mainstay of treatment.

HAEMANGIOMA OF BONE

This is slowly growing benign tumor composed of masses of fully developed adult blood vessels. Vertebrae and skull are commonly affected.

Clinical Features

1. This is a tumor of young adult.
2. These are silent lesion.
3. Haemangioma usually develop in vertebrae between T4-L4.
4. In skull, haemangioma originates in meninges and scalp.
5. Patient may present with pain and neurological manifestation.

Pathology

Haemangioma is madeup of masses of blood vessels in a fibrous stroma. Periosteum is not perforated. Microscopy shows two types of haemangioma, Cavernous (more common) and capillary haemangioma.

X-ray Findings

Horizontal striations of vertebrae are lost. Vertical striation of vertebrae becomes more prominent.

Treatment

Radiotherapy is mainstay of treatment.

Differential Diagnosis

- Pott's spine
- Metastasis in bone.

MAFFUCI SYNDROME

This syndrome consists of dyschondroplasia (multiple enchondroma) and cavernous haemangioma. It is a hereditary condition.

FIBROSARCOMA

This is a malignant neoplasm which may originate in medullary cavity or in periosteum (periosteal fibrosarcoma). Basic cell of this tumor is fibroblast. It's histology is similar to fibrosarcoma arising from soft tissue structure. It produces blood born pulmonary metastasis.

Clinical Features

This tumor presents with the following features:

1. Fibrosarcoma occurs between 30–50 years of age.
2. Gradual onset of constant pain, which becomes severe at night with smooth firm, fixed swelling and sometimes pathological fracture are clinical features.
3. Long bones are commonly affected (femur). It can be seen in ribs, skull, vertebrae and mandible.
4. It takes origin from subperiosteal areas of diaphysis or metaphysis.
5. Metastasis spreads to lungs.

X-ray Findings

X-ray shows osteolytic lesion surrounded by reactive subperiosteal new bone. This reactive new bone formation may create Codman's triangle in slowly growing tumor.

Pathology

Fibrosarcoma is a firm, fibrous, glistening mass which is well encapsulated and lies beneath the elevated periosteum. Microscopy shows small oat cells resembling mesenchymal cells with scanty cytoplasm and small rounded nuclei with mitosis. Spindle cells are predominantly seen.

Treatment

Amputation is the only mode of cure. However fibrosarcomas are less malignant than osteogenic sarcoma.

SYNOVIAL SARCOMA

This is highly malignant tumor that takes origin from synovial membrane of a joint, tendon sheath, or a bursa. It is commonly seen in males of 20–30 years age. But it can occur at any age. It almost invariably lies outside the joint.

This is also known as synovial sarcomesothelioma or cancerous synovial tumor.

Clinical Features

Patient of synovial sarcoma may present with following features:

1. Male population of 20–30 years age group is generally affected but it can occur at any age.
2. It commonly occurs around knee in the soft tissue. (outside of joint)
3. Patient presents with painful swelling around knee joint.
4. Sometimes joint movements may be limited.
5. It grows very slowly and metastasizes to lungs.

Pathology

This is sharply circumscribed, rounded and lobulated tumor. Cut section shows blood stained or yellowish brown areas of necrosis.

Microscopy shows 3 patterns:

- Formation of tissue space
- Formation of cell tufts
- Epithelial like cells on a supporting stroma of compact bone.

X-ray Findings

X-ray shows a soft tissue shadow with flecks of calcification. Joint lines are intact. X-ray chest shows pulmonary metastasis.

Biopsy

Biopsy is diagnostic aid for synovial sarcoma.

Treatment

Local excision of tumor is done. If tumor has widespread involvement radical amputation is preferred.

MULTIPLE MYELOMA

This tumor arises from plasma cells of bone marrow also known as Plasmocytoma. In this condition plasma cells replace bone. This is commonly seen between 40–60 years of age. This tumor is also known as monoclonal gammopathy, solitary myeloma, myelomatosis or multiple myelomatosis.

Clinical Features

Multiple myeloma has following clinical features:

1. This tumor has multiple site involvement. Symptoms vary according to site.
2. Commonly patient presents with vague pain in lumbar and thoracic spine, chest and in ribs.
3. Generalized weakness and weight loss.
4. Pain may become severe.
5. Pathological fracture may be seen in vertebrae and ribs.
6. If tumor presses the spinal cord or nerve in the spinal canal, neurological symptoms may appear.
7. Signs of pathological fractures will be present.
8. Lumbar spine may become flattened due to collapse.
9. Increased roundening of dorsal spine.
10. Diffuse tender palpable swelling over sterum or ribs may be seen.
11. Movements at spine are painful.
12. Signs of neurological deficit will be present.

Prognosis

Multiple myeloma is a fatal disease due to extensive marrow replacement, severe anemia, thrombocytopenia and haemorrhage. Majority of cases die within 3 years and almost all in 5 years. Renal failure occurs due to tubular blockage by protein cast. (Myeloma kidney)

Lab Findings

Patient of multiple myeloma can show following laboratory findings:

- 30% Patients show Bence Jones protein.
- Serum globulin is raised.
- Serum calcium is also raised.
- ESR is increased.
- Serum alkaline phosphatase is low.
- Paper electrophoresis of serum and urine protein is mandatory. A single spike is found in alpha-2, beta and in gama region.
- Normocytic normochromic anemia.
- Bone marrow biopsy is diagnostic. It shows refractory anemia to iron, B12 and to folic acid.

- Increased total protein. A/G ratio is reversed.

Complications

- Pathological fracture.
- Spinal cord or nerve root compression.
- Progressive severe anemia and leucopenia in late stage.
- Renal failure.
- Immunological deficiency leading to severe bacterial infection.

Pathology

This is a red soft gelatinous mass which bleeds freely. This tumor lies within medulla of bone. Tumor breaks the cortex and extends beyond it.

Microscopy shows round typical cells with eccentrically placed nucleus with a nucleolus. Chromatin is arranged in spokes of wheel pattern. Cytoplasm is eosinophillic. Perinuclear halo typical of plasma cell is absent.

Plugs of protein are seen within the tubules of kidney. Metastatic calcium deposits are seen in kidney. Amyloidosis is seen in parenchymatous organs. Nodules are seen in lungs.

X-ray Findings

- Punched out lesions in skull and pelvis produce silver beaten appearance.
- Biconcave vertebral bodies.
- Collapse of vertebrae is seen.
- Extensive rarefaction of vertebrae may produce disappearing vertebrae. When pedicle is involved it is called as Pedicle sign.
- No reactive bone is seen.
- Osteolytic defect develops within interior of bone.

Treatment

- Treatment of this tumor is palliative.
- This is radiosensitive and pain is relieved.
- Chemotherapy is given in the form of steroid, melphalan, urethrane and cyclophosphamide. Cycles are repeated every 3-4 weeks for 6–12 weeks.
- If spinal nerve compression is present it is treated by laminectomy, removal of myelomatous tissue and postoperative radiation.
- Intramedullary fixation of fracture is not useful as diseased bone is soft and weak. It cannot hold implant.
- Solitary focus is surgically excised. Later radiotherapy is given.
- Solitary focus of vertebrae is treated by radiation alone.

CHORDOMA

This is a rare neoplasm of sacral spine and cranium. It is locally malignant. Metastasis spreads to regional lymph nodes very late. This tumor is derived from embryonic remnant of notochord. Sacrococcygeal region and sphenooccipital region are common sites for this tumor. Vertebral chordoma arises first within body and later extends to arch. Ultimately vertebra is collapsed.

Clinical Features

1. It is commonly seen after 40 years of age but can occur at any age.
2. Chordoma of sacrococcygeal region presents with pain in rectal area.
3. Obstinate constipation.
4. Urinary incontinence.
5. Sensory motor deficit may be seen in lower limbs.
6. Muscle weakness.
7. Chordoma presents as soft smooth mass at anterior or posterior aspect of sacrum.

Pathology

This is soft smooth gelatinous mass. It destroys the vertebrae and replaces it by tumor. Cortex is thinned and expanded.

X-ray Findings

X-ray shows osteolytic expansile lesion in sacrococcygeal region. Destruction of vertebral body and arch can be seen in X-ray.

Treatment

Chordoma in children is more radiosensitive than adults. Complete surgical excision is best choice.

Differential Diagnosis

- Chondrosarcoma
- Sacrococcygeal teratoma
- Tuberculosis of spine
- Carcinoma rectum

METASTASIS IN BONE

Metastasis is most common bone tumor in body. Carcinoma of breast (female) and carcinoma of lung are commonest tumor to metastasize in bone. Carcinoma prostate and thyroid also cause metastasis in bone.

Clinical Features

Patient may present with the following clinical features:

- Patient usually presents with bony pain most commonly at spine, ribs and extremities.
- Pathological fracture is also a known presentation.
- Patient may or may not be a case of primary malignancy.

Investigations

Bone scan is best investigation to trace metastasis in bones. Plain X-rays usually miss many secondaries.

ESR and serum calcium are raised. Carcinoma prostate shows raised serum acid phosphatase.

Treatment

Secondaries are treated symptomatically. Chemotherapy and radiotherapy can be given according to type of tumor.

CHAPTER

37 Diseases of Back

- Ankylosing spondylitis
- Prolapsed intervertebral disc
- Lumbar canal stenosis
- Scheuermann's disease
- Vertebra plana
- Spondylolisthesis
- Lumbar spondylosis
- Scoliosis
- Spina bifida
- Diastematomyelia
- Piriformis syndrome

ANKYLOSING SPONDYLITIS

This is an inflammatory disease of spine, sacroiliac joint and large joints of body like hip, knee and shoulder which leads to fibrous or bony ankylosis and deformities. This is commonly seen in 15–30 years of age. It is also known as Marie-Strumpell arthritis or Bechterew disease.

Aetiology

This is predominantly seen in male (male: female = 7:1). It is inherited in 70% cases. 90% Patients have association with HLA-B27 antigen.

Pathology

Along with fibrous and bony bridging destruction of articular cortices are also seen. Frequent ossification and calcification of particular tissues are seen. Anterior longitudinal ligament becomes calcified and show ossification. Bony bridges are formed in between vertebrae which creates **Bamboo spine** appearance in X-ray. Ankylosis of hip joint and apophyseal joint of spine are seen. Aorta and inferior vena cava may be ruptured due to forceful extension of spine.

Clinical Features

Patient may present with following clinical features:

1. Morning backache and stiffness in both sacroilac joint is a common feature which is relieved by activity and walking.
2. Stiffness and pain is progressive in nature. Pathology spreads through whole of spine within 6 months to 1 year.
3. Unilateral or bilateral radiculopathy in course of sciatic nerve can be seen.
4. Forward flexion of spine creates **Stooped-over position.** It occurs due to severe paraspinal muscle spasm in flexor group of muscles.
5. Entire back is rounded due to single kyphotic roundening of entire back.

6. Patient may present with several deformities e.g. flexion adduction deformity of hip, flexion deformity of knee and adduction and internal rotation deformity at shoulder.

Extra-articular features

7. Restricted chest expansion (<5 cm) is due to involvement of costovertebral joint.
8. Vital capacity is reduced and respiration is diaphragmatic.
9. Aortitis and iritis may be seen. Patient may also develop aortic incompetence.
10. Nongranulomatous anterior uveitis may develop prior to onset of or during the course of disease. This condition usually subsides within 2–6 weeks. Some cases may present with recurrent attack. Later patient may develop macular odema, cataract and glaucoma.
11. Pleural thicking and effusion may also be present sometimes.
12. Pleuropulmonary disease shows fibrobullous lesion in apical lobe due to aspergillosis.
13. Chin-on chest deformity is seen due to complete C1-C2 dislocation.

Fracture of cervical spine in ankylosing spondylitis

These fractures are chalk stick type separation in lower cervical spine. This is caused by trivial trauma. These fractures are seen in X-ray with difficulty. These fractures are highly unstable so it must be carefully managed. Traction is applied with utmost care and the line of traction must be in flexion due to existing deformity in spine. You should apply very light weight in traction. Acute fractures must be fixed either with external halo immobilization, internal fixation or both.

Clinical Signs of Sacroiliac joint involvement

1. Active SLR test produces pain at sacroiliac joint.
2. Tenderness is present at PSIS or deep in gluteal region.
3. Side to side compression of pelvis causes pain at sacroiliac joint.

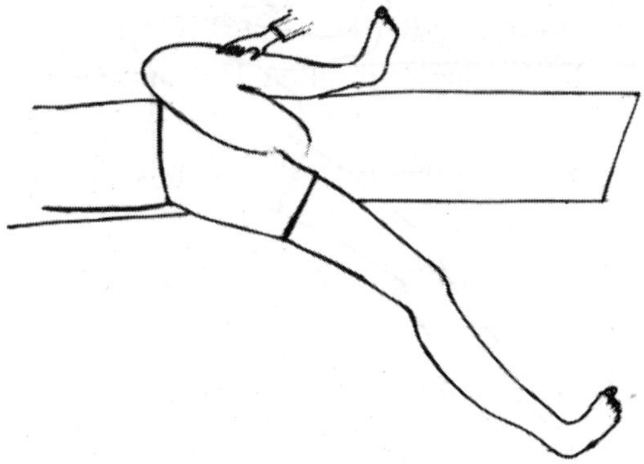

Fig. 37.1 Genslen test

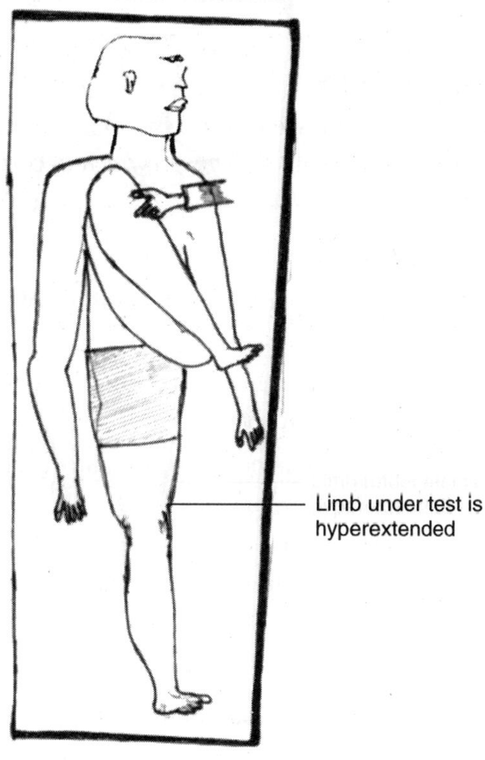

Fig. 37.2 Pump handle test

4. **Genslen test** is positive. In this test patient is asked to lie down on the table in such a way that his affected leg hangs down at the

edge of table thus hyperextending hip joint. Pre-requisite of this test is that pelvis should be fixed by flexing opposite hip and knee joints. This will create rotational strain at sacroiliac joint which is painful.

5. **Pump handle test** is positive. This test is done in supine position. Hip and knee joints are flexed in such a way that they come closer to opposite shoulder joint. It will produce pain on affected side.

Clinical signs of cervical spine involvement

Fleche test is positive. Patient stands with his back and heel against the wall. Ask him to touch the wall with back of his head without raising chin. If he is unable to touch the wall it means test is positive.

X-ray Findings

X-ray findings are seen after 3–6 months of onset of disease. *Following findings are seen according to site of involvement:*

Sacroiliac joint

- Patchy osteoporosis of distal third of both joint.
- Ill defined margins of sacroiliac joint with increased joint space.
- Multiple subchondral erosion may produce rosary effect.
- Calcification of sacroiliac and sacrotuberous ligaments can also be seen.
- **Enthesopathy** can also be seen. This is calcification at the attachment of muscle, tendon and ligament.

Lumbar spine

- Earliest sign is sharp squaring of anterior portion of vertebral bodies. Anterior concavity is lost.
- Loss of normal lumbar lordosis.
- Paravertbral ossification may be seen.
- Anterior longitudinal ligament is ossified. Bony bridges develop between vertebral bodies creating Bamboo spine appearance.

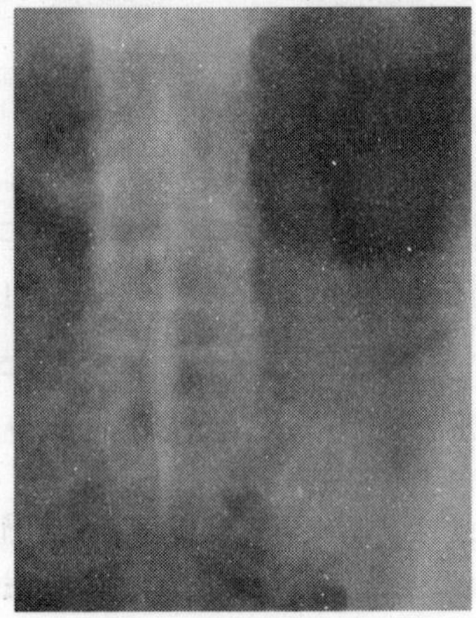

Fig. 37.3 Bamboo spine appearance in ankylosing spondylitis

Cervical spine

- Loss of cervical lordosis.
- Fusion of apophyseal joint.
- Occasionaly subluxation of atlantoaxial joint can be seen in forward flexion view of X-ray. Subluxation occurs due to destruction of transverse ligament.

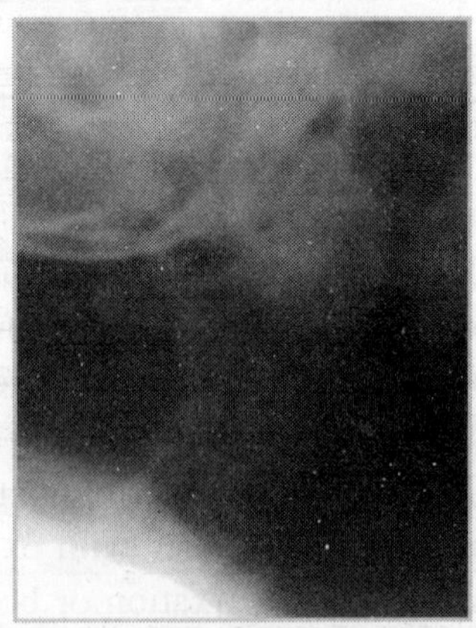

Fig. 37.4 Calcification of ligaments in cervical spine in ankylosing spondylitis

Hip joint

- Osteoporosis in both joints.
- Reduced joint space.
- Bony ankylosis may be seen at pubic symphysis.

MRI

MRI is a sensitive and specific tool to detect sacroilitis. It shows active inflammation in spine and SI joints.

Main use of MRI is to make early diagnosis and to distinguish active inflammatory axial disease from noninflammatory cause.

MRI can show inflammation, marrow oedema and pre-radiographic erosion of SI joints.

Investigations

Following investigations can be done in this pathology:

1. HLA-B27 antigen is positive in almost all cases.
2. Raised ESR and urinary 17 ketosteroid level.
3. Relative rise in mononuclear leukocytes.
4. Secondary anemia.

Treatment

- Patient should be adviced to lie on hard flat bed. Hyperextended position helps in straightening of spine.
- Deep breathing exercises should be adviced.
- Cervical traction provides relief from pain and spasm. Deformities in hip and knee should be corrected by traction.
- Hot moist packs provide relief from muscle spasm.
- Spinal jacket of plaster applied on Risser table helps patient in ambulation.
- Indomethacin is given 100–200 mg/day.
- Cortisone provides dramatic relief from inflammation and pain.
- Phenylbutazone can be given in acute cases for 1-2 weeks only. This is given 100–200 mg/day. It provides relief from pain.
- X-ray therapy also provides relief from pain. It's effect remains for 6 months.

Latest Treatment of Ankylosing Spondylitis

Infliximab

Infliximab is TNF-alpha blocking agent. It has strong and potent effect on almost all features of ankylosing spondylitis.

Infliximab is given 3–5 mg/kg body weight by infusion. Infusion takes 2-3 hours.

3 Induction doses of Infliximab are given at 0, 2 and 6 week. Thereafter 6 additional doses of maintenance (8 weekly infusion) in the first year of treatment are given.

This is very expansive drug. One vial of 100 mg costs around $-451.

Other TNF-alpha blocking agents are Etanercept and Adalimumab.

Refrence: Dr. Ghosh et al. (Calcutta)

Pamidronate

This is a biphosphonate and given intravenously 60 mg once in a month for 3 months.

Surgical Treatment

Total hip replacement provides good results in 90% cases. Hip contracture should be corrected first prior to replacement surgery.

Spinal osteotomy is done at the level of L2-3 or L3-4. A wedge of bone is removed from posterior element of spinal column. After this spine is forcibly hyperextended. Angle of wedge is equal to amount of correction.

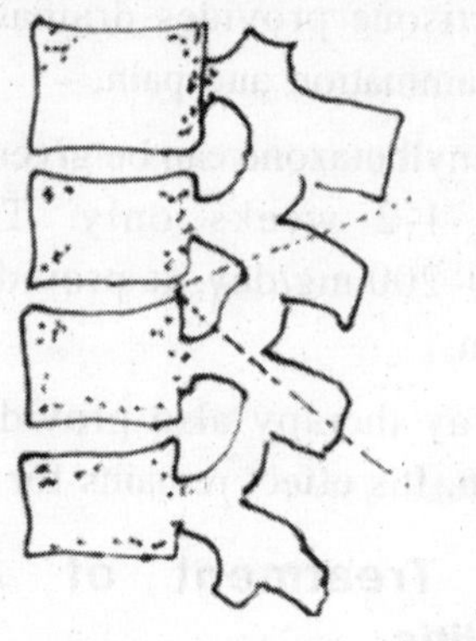

(*a*) Mechanism of spinal osteotomy

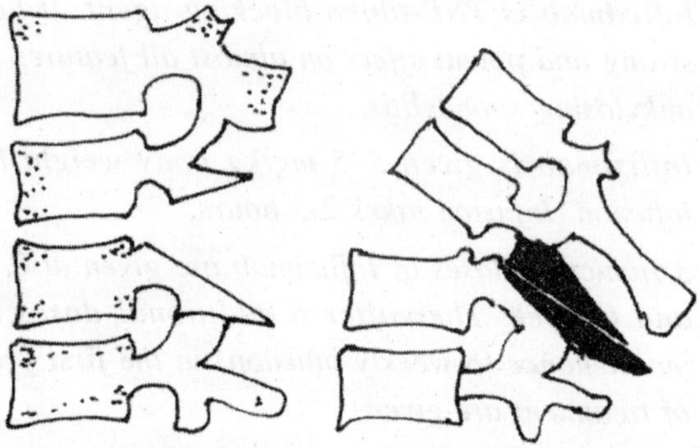

(*b*) (*c*)

Fig. 37.5 Osteotomy of spine wedge is excised with its apex at the anterior border of foramen

PROLAPSED INTERVERTEBRAL DISC

PIVD is a degenerative pathology that affects people of 20–40 years of age. Intervertebral disc protrudes through a rent in annulus fibrosus and later undergoes in brown degeneration. Brown pigment of unknown origin is deposited in annulus. This degenerative process is known as brown degeneration. Commonest level of disc prolapse is L4-5 in lumbar spine and C5-6 in cervical spine.

Intervertebral Disc

Human body has 23 discs in spine. Atlantoaxial articulation does not have disc. Discs of thoracic origin are thinnest, while discs at lumbar region are thickest. Disc lies in between two vertebrae. Each vertebra has superior and inferior cartilaginous end plate which show bony thickening at their peripheri known as **Randleiste of Schmorl.** It is absent posteriorly. Central portion of disc is semiliquid in nature, known as nucleus pulposus. It is surrounded by a thick ring of fibrous tissue known as annulus fibrosus (lamellous).

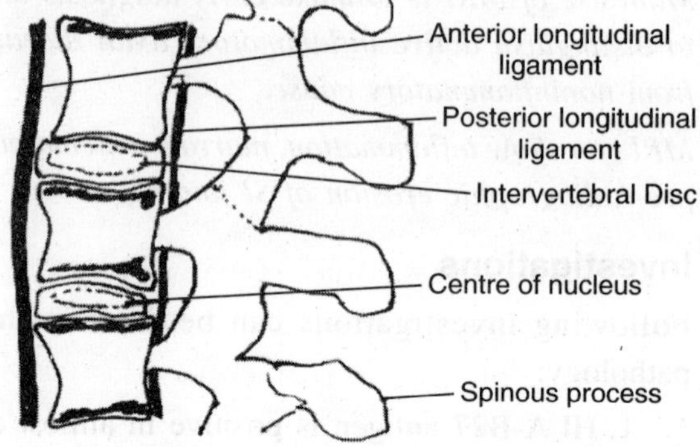

(*a*) Applied anatomy of disc

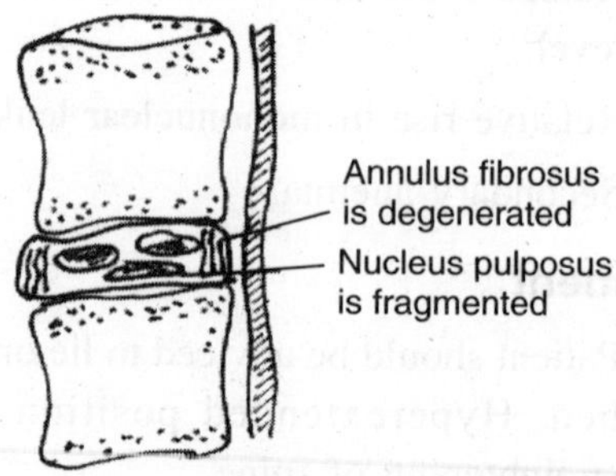

(*b*) Degeneration of disc

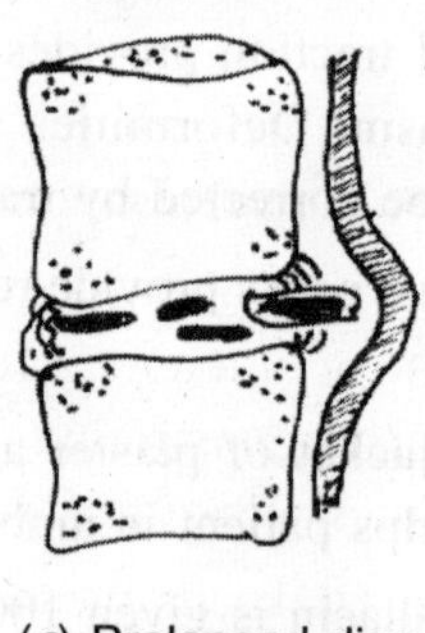

(*c*) Prolapsed disc

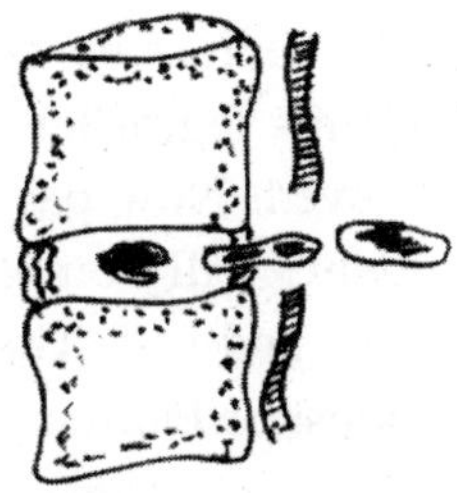

(*d*) Sequestrated disc

Fig. 37.6

Annulus fibrosus is strongest and thickest at anterolateral margin. As the age increases nucleus pulposus becomes granular and friable due to decreased water content in nucleus and due to increase in fibrous tissue, cartilage cells and amorphous material. Nucleus pulposus arises from endoderm, while annulus fibrosus arises from mesoderm.

Function of disc is to provide articulation (amphiarthrosis) which provides mobility to spine. It also acts as shock absorber. Superior and inferior end plate play the role of barrier between nucleus pulposus and vertebrae.

With advancing age cartilaginous end plate undergoes degenerative process and nucleus starts to bulge into bony end plate producing characteristic biconcave vertebrae. Sometimes bony end plates are broken and nuclear material enters into cancellous bone of vertebral body. It is later surrounded by reactive bone formation known as Schmorl node.

Pathology

After process of disc prolapse, nucleus pulposus undergo stages of degeneration, displacement and fibrosis.

Degeneration of nucleus pulposus causes its softening and fragmentation. Posterior part of annulus becomes weak. Later it disintegrates.

Annulus fibrosus keeps the nucleus inside disc where it faces positive pressure all the time. If annulus disintegrates it will give way to nucleus to come out. At this stage posterior ligament can not prevent protrusion of nucleus. This stage is known as displacement of nucleus pulposus.

After extrusion of nucleus it is fibrosed and calcified. Later osteophytes formation occurs at the site of stripping of posterior longitudinal ligament from vertebral body.

Types of Prolapse

Following types of prolapse are known:

1. Diffuse prolapse
2. Pedunculated prolapse
3. Sequestrated prolapse
4. Dissecting protrusion
5. Massive protrusion

Pathological changes in intervertebral joint

Due to prolapse of nucleus hight of disc is reduced. This hampers articulation in between posterior facet joints. These joints become incongruent and later cause degenerative arthritis.

Pathological changes in spinal canal

One or more nerve root is compressed in extrathecal course. Nerve root that leaves spinal canal below next vertebra is affected e.g., in L4-5 disc prolapse L5 nerve root is affected. Uncommonly cauda equina syndrome can occur due to massive disc protrusion in spinal canal.

Clinical Features

Disc prolapse usually occurs in the age of 20–40 years. History of weight lifting or sudden forward bending is usually present.

Low backache

Patient presents with severe low backache which is aggravated by forward bending, movement at spine, sitting and standing in same posture for prolonged period. Pain is relieved by rest.

Sciatica

Low backache is radiated into thigh, hip and leg along the distribtion of sciatic nerve root. L4-5 lesion causes pain at anterolateral aspect of leg and ankle. L2-3 compression causes pain at anterior aspect of thigh while compression at S1 nerve root causes pain in posterolateral aspect of calf and heel. Patient presents with neurological claudication phenomenon in which radiculopathy starts on walking. It is relieved by taking rest.

Paresthesia or numbness

Patient presents with paresthesia along the course of respective dermatome. At L4-5 level sensory deficit occurs over dorsum of foot and lateral aspect of leg. In L3-4 lesion sensory loss occurs over medial side of leg and at great toe. At L5-S1 level sensory loss occurs at lateral aspect of foot. Muscle weakness is also present. This motor weakness depends on nerve root affected. In L5 root weakness of EHL and dorsiflexor of foot is seen. L4 lesion presents with weakness of extensors of knee. S1 root lesion causes weakness of plantar flexor of foot.

Cauda equina syndrome

This is uncommonly seen when massive protrusion of disc in spinal canal produces pressure effect on intrathecal roots. In this syndrome bilateral ankle jerks are absent. Bowel and urinary incontinence is present. Sensations are reduced along the course of L4-5 dermatome. This is an irregular type of LMN paralysis.

Clinical Findings

1. Sciatic tilt (scoliosis). Patient stands in such a way that his body is tilted to one side while trunk shifts forward on pelvis.
2. Forward bending is restricted.
3. Diffuse tenderness is present at lumbosacral region.
4. **Straight leg raising** test is positive. In this test patient lies supine on a couch. His affected leg is raised with extended knee. If patient complaints of pain at the angle of 40 degree or less, this will be suggestive of nerve root compression i.e. positive test. Now bring this leg at lesser angle where pain is relieved. Now passively dorsiflex ankle. Patients will complaint of pain at back of thigh and calf. This test is known as Bragard test or Fazersztajn test.
5. **Well leg raising test.** If you lift the normal leg of patient, he will complaints of pain on affected side. This is suggestive of significant nerve root compression. It is also known as positive contralateral SLRT.
6. **Lasegue test** is also positive. Patient lies supine on a couch. His hip is flexed up to 90 degree with flexed knees. Now gradually extend knee, patient will complaints of pain over back of thigh or leg.

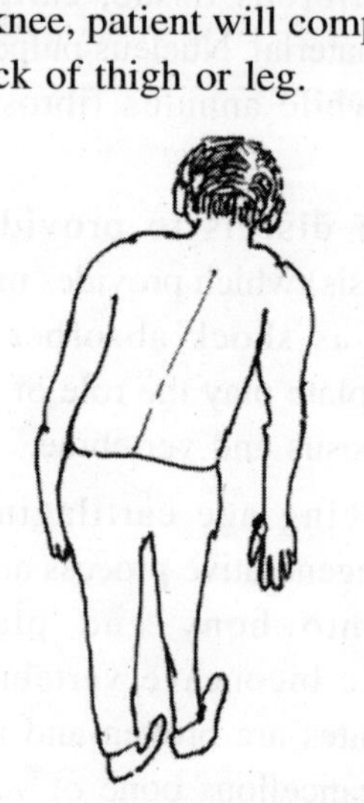

(a) Stooped posture

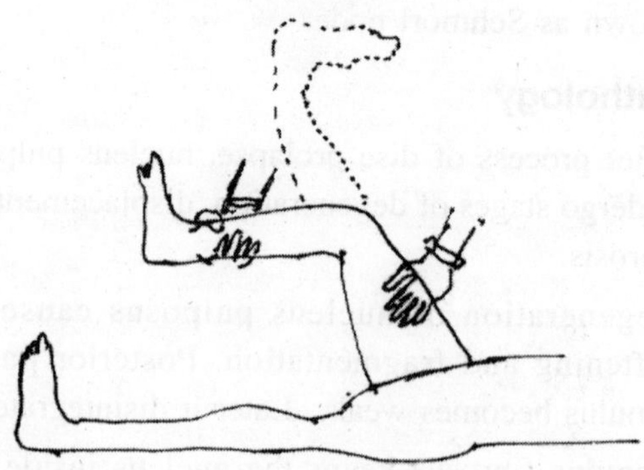

(b) Lasegue test

Fig. 37.7

Investigations

X-ray is nonspecific as no positive findings will be detected in X-ray. Late cases may show reduced disc space.

MRI

This is most effective and accurate investigation to detect level and type of prolapse. It is superior to CT-scan.

CT-SCAN

This is a noninvasive technique for accurate diagnosis of prolapsed intervertebral disc. It may also reveal similar condition like facet syndrome, spinal stenosis, extradural tumor and vertebral body destruction. In CT-scan normal concave contour of posterior border of disc appears flat or convex. Prethecal shadow between posterior border of disc and theca is not seen in prolapsed disc. Herniated disc material will be visible at the site of prolapse.

Myelography and EMG have become outdated investigations for diagnosis of prolapsed disc.

Treatment

Conservative

Prolapsed disc is a common clinical entity it can be treated by following conservative methods:

- Absolute bed rest on hard bed for 6 weeks is mandatory.
- Analgesics and muscle relaxants to provide relief from pain and muscle spasm.
- Hot saline fomentation and gentle arching excercises are helpful.
- Lumbar traction can also be applied.
- Transcutaneous electrical nerve stimulation may provide some relief from pain.
- **Chemonucleolysis** is a technique under X-ray control in which an enzyme chymopapin is injected into disc leading to dissolution and fibrosis of disc thus providing relief from symptoms. This is indicated where surgical treatment has failed. Chymopapin is a proteolytic enzyme that rapidly depolymerizes non collagenous protein which binds long chain mucopolysaccharides.

Surgical Treatment

Indications

1. Failed conservative treatment.
2. Cauda equina syndrome.
3. Severe sciatic tilt.

Types of Surgical procedures

Discectomy is treatment of choice either by open or endoscopic approach depending on surgeon's skill. However various surgical procedures for PIVD are as follows:

1. Fenestration operation

In this operation ligamentum flavum is excised that bridges two adjacent laminae.

2. Laminotomy

In this surgery fenestration procedure is done and along with that a hole is made in lamina.

3. Laminectomy

Bilateral laminae along with their spinous process are removed.

4. Hemilaminectomy

In this procedure unilateral lamina is removed.

5. Percutaneous discectomy

This method involves latest endoscopic removal of disc. In this method endoscopic removal of disc is done through a small percutaneous stab incision.

6. Laser discectomy

This is indicated in grade 1 and 2 disc prolapse. It was first done by Choy and asstt in 1986.

7. Endoscopic microdiscectomy

8. Posterior/Anterior lumbar interbody fusion (PLIF/ALIF)

9. Disc arthroplasty with artificial disc

LUMBAR CANAL STENOSIS

This is a clinical entity in which compression of cauda equina occurs due to narrow (lateral or antero-posterior) diameter of spinal canal with or without change in cross-sectional area. It is commonly seen in lumbar vertebrae. Constriction in spinal canal may compress one or more nerve root.

Clinical Features

Patient may present with following clinical features:

1. Low backache
2. Pain decreases by forward bending as length of canal increases by 2.2 mm.
3. Cauda equina claudication is usual presentation in lumbar canal stenosis. Patient presents with pain in buttocks and in lower limbs, usually elicited after walking. This pain is relieved by taking rest and by forward bending. Hypoasthesia or paraesthesia may also be seen. In contrast to ischaemic claudication there is no trophic changes and neurological deficit in cauda equina claudication. Pulses are normally felt.

Classification of Lumbar Canal Stenosis

Anatomical

- Lumbar (most common)
- Cervical
- Thoraic

Segmental

- Central
- Foraminal
- Lateral recess

Congenital

- Achondroplasia

Acquired

- Spondylitis
- Degenerative

Iatrogenic

- Inadequate treatment of stenosis
- Bone graft (used in surgery) may become hypertrophied.

Miscellaneous

- Kyphosis
- Scoliosis
- Flurosis
- Paget's disease
- Diffuse idiopathic skeletal hyperostosis (DISH)
- Spinal fracture

Investigations

Following investigations can be done in lumbar canal stenosis:

- Myelography may show waist like narrowing of dural sac at the level of facet joint.
- CT-scan and MRI should be done to rule out pathology.
- X-ray may show reduced interpedicle distance and reduced anteroposterior or mid sagittal diameter of vertebra. Facet joint may show it's hypertrophy and sclerosis. Interlaminar distance is reduced. Sometimes osteophytes and olesthesis may be seen.

Treatment

- Aim of treatment is to decompress narrow and constricted lumbar canal. So laminectomy is mainstay of treatment.
- Lateral canal stenosis can be treated by laminotomy, discectomy, foraminotomy and partial medial facetectomy.

- Sometimes osteotomy of inferior articular process may be required to remove hypertrophic elements.

SCHEUERMANN'S DISEASE

This is also known as adolescent kyphosis, epiphysitis of spine, juvenile round back, dorsum rotundum and osteochondritis deformans juvenilis dorsi.

This is osteochondritis of lower thoracic spine which leads to kyphotic deformity in adolescent period.

Pathology

Schmorl's nodes are formed by protrusion of disc material into soft yielding spongiosa thus leading to reduced intervertebral disc space. Deficiency of disc material causes increased flexion of thoracic spine with raised pressure on anterior part of vertebral body. Vertebrae become wedge shaped with narrow anterior end.

Aseptic necrosis and endocrinal factor (Frolich syndrome) also play an important role in etiology of this disease.

Clinical Features

Patient gives history of unusual strenuous physical activity followed by vague pain in lower thoracic spine which radiates laterally toward loins. It subsides with recumbence. Later patient develops kyphosis over lower thoracic spine.

Sometimes patient may also develop spastic paraplegia due to development of spinal extradural cyst. It produces slight sensory changes. Sphincter functions are normal.

X-ray Findings

Lateral view of lower thoracic spine shows irregularity and mottling at vertebrae. Deficient ossification of apophyseal ring (mainly anteriorly) can also be seen. Persistent transverse vascular groove beyond the normal time of obliteration at 6 years is peculiar feature in X-ray.

Compensatory increase in cervical and lumbar lordosis can be seen in X-ray. Kyphosis of lower thoracic spine is seen. Sometimes scoliosis may be present.

Treatment

Absolute bed rest in hyperextended position is best treatment. Spinal extension exercises should be done daily. A body cast may be applied in hyperextension to make patient ambulatory. Combined parentral therapy of androgen and estrogen is more effective. Milwaukee brace is better option of body cast because former can be removed at regular interval.

Surgical Treatment

Surgery is done only when patient suffers from severe progressive round back deformity, severe and disabling thoracic pain and in presence of signs of cord compression.

Prior to operation spine is mobilized by Cotrel head halter traction with a pelvic sling or halotemporal distraction.

Posterior spinal fusion supplemented with Harrington instrumentation is done when kyphosis is less than 70 degree and vertebral wedging is less than 10 degree. Anterior spinal fusion is done when kyphosis is more than 75 degree and apical vertebra is wedged more than 15 degree. Tight anterior longitudinal ligament is excised and several discs are removed.

VERTEBRA PLANA

(Calve's Disease of Spine)

This is a disease of children affecting single vertebra, characterized by rapid collapse and flattening of single vertebral body due to osteochondritis. Eosinophillic granuloma may be an etiological factor of this disease.

Clinical Features

Clinically it resembles pott's spine as child presents with pain, fatigue, night cry and muscle spasm. Tenderness is present at local area. Gradually kyphosis or scoliosis can develop. Symptoms disappear in about 2 months but deformity remains.

X-ray Findings

Flattened dense wafer like segment with deformity of spine is usual finding.

Treatment

Assuming eosinophillic granuloma an etiological factor, radiation is best treatment.

SPONDYLOLISTHESIS

(Spondylos=spine, olisthesis=to slip)

This is a slow anterior displacement of a vertebra at the lower lumbar spine. Interruption in continuity of pars interarticularis is essential lesion. It is commonly seen between L5-S1 and L4-5.

Spondylolysis

(Spondylos=spine, lysis=disintegrate)

If defect in pars interarticularis exists without forward slipping of vertebra it will be called as spondylolysis.

Spondylosis

(Spondylitis)

Spondylitis is a degenerative disease of spine which shows osteoarthritic changes.

Classification of Spondylolisthesis

Displastic

This is also known as congenital spondylolisthesis or lumbosacral subluxation or spondyloptysis. This type has structural deficiency of one articular process which occurs due to congenital deficiency of cephalad portion of sacrum or neural arch of L5. Usually there is absence or incomplete development of sacral articular process.

Isthmic

Essential lesion lies in pars interarticularis. It has 3 subtypes as follows:

(*a*) **Lytic type.** This is also known as true spondylolisthesis or spondylolytic spondylolisthesis. It is most common type and seen under 50 years of age. It has strong hereditary tendency. Gradual dissolution of pars interarticularis resulting into fatigue fracture of pars interarticularis is the main lesion.

(*b*) **Elongated pars without defect.** It shows fatigue micro fracture which contribute to elongated pars but without defect. Hereditary tendency is absent.

(*c*) **Acute pars fracture.** It is also known as spondylolysis as it is more often not associated with slip. No hereditary tendency is seen.

Degenerative

It is commonly seen at L4-5 level and degree of slip is not more than 30%. It has unstable paired zygoapophyseal joints. Intervertebral foramina are patent.

Traumatic

This type usually heals by immobilization. Vertebrae slip over due to trauma.

Pathologic

(*a*) **General:** Paget's disease, Alber's schonberg disease, Osteogenesis imperfecta.

(*b*) **Local:** Fatigue fracture occurs due to stress.

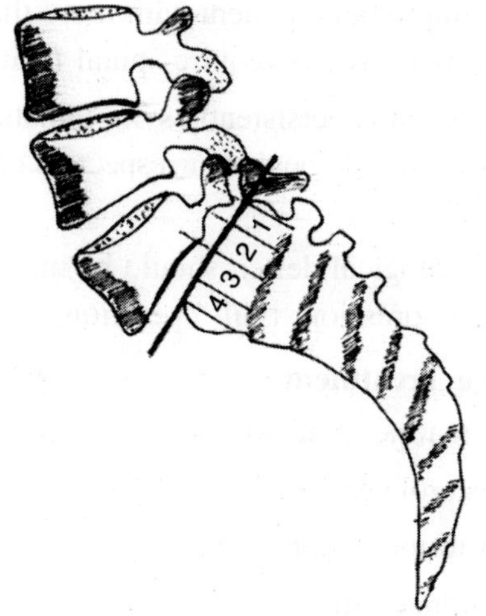

(*a*) Spondylolisthesis meyerding grading of spondylolisthesis

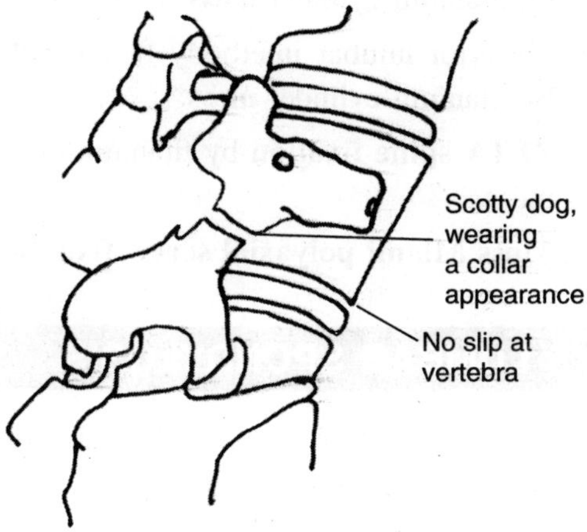

(*b*) Spondylolysis

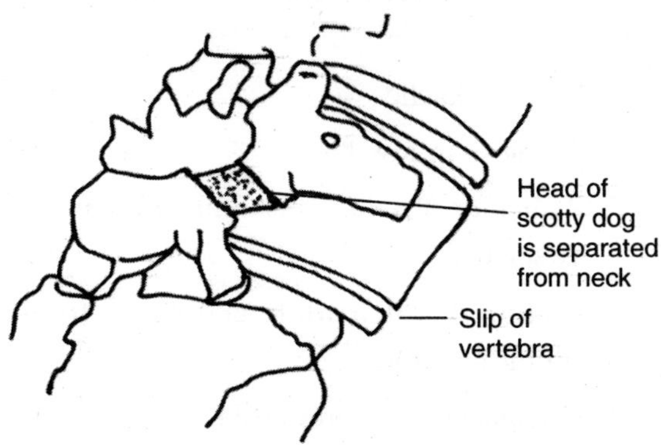

(*c*) Spondylolisthesis

Fig. 37.8

Causes of Spondylolisthesis

1. Separate ossification centre of each lateral mass.
2. Stress fracture, post natal fracture or birth fracture.
3. Impingement of articular process on pars interarticularis.
4. Stress and hereditary dysplasia.

Clinical Features

Patient may presents with following clinical features:

1. Low backache is a common feature which may be associated with radiculopathy in lower limbs. Pain is relieved by rest and aggravated by standing or walking.
2. Stiffness at low back.
3. Restricted forward bending.
4. Buttocks seem to be flattened.
5. Sacrum is more vertical.
6. Spinous process of L5 is palpable.
7. Patient walks with pelvic waddling gait.
8. SLR is restricted.
9. Laseque sign is positive.
10. Sign of nerve root compression are seen according to nerve root involvement.
11. In a female patient, labour is prolonged and may require caesarean section.

X-ray Findings

- X-ray shows forward displacement of lowermost vertebra, which carries forward spine above.
- Oblique view of spine shows **Scottish dog sign**. Neck of dog represents defect in isthmus (pars interarticularis) of vertebra.
- **Ullaman sign** is positive. If we draw a line from anterior surface of sacrum toward L5 vertebra it will project at or in front of

antero inferior angle of L5 vertebra normally. If this line intersects L5 vertebra, Ullaman's sign is said to be positive i.e. forward displacement of vertebra is present.

- **Lumbar index** is helpful in finding out severity or grading of spondylolisthesis. Lumbar index is inversely proportional to severity. Lowest index is seen in high grade olisthesis. Index of less than 100 means that posterior border of vertebra is less than anterior border.
- **Lumbar index=**Hight of posterior border of body/Hight of anterior border of body × 100.
- **Myelogram** will show partial or complete block at neural arch of L5 vertebra.
- **Meyerding grading system** is a radiological which classifies degree of slip of L5 vertebra into 4 grades from 1–4. 25% Displacement of L5 vertebra is seen in grade-1. 100% Displacement is seen in grade-4. Slip of vertebra does not occur after 20 years of age. If this occurs it will be due to operative intervention. Most rapid slip of vertebra is seen between the ages of 10–15 years.

Treatment

- If child is around 10 years of age, a lateral standing view of X-ray is taken at every 6 month till child becomes 15 years old. This is done because chances of progression of slip are more in first few years. If slip reaches up to 50%, spinal fusion becomes mandatory.
- Asymptomatic patient with 25% slip do not require any treatment.
- Asymptomatic patient with 50% slip requires avoidance of sport activity and weight lifting. If patient is not relieved spinal fusion should be done.
- Asymptomatic patient with more than 50% slip will always require spinal fusion.
- If patient is persistently symptomatic spinal fusion should be done irrespective of degree of slip.
- Neurological deficit should be managed by decompression. (Gill operation)

Operative Treatment

Surgical treatment includes following procedures:

1. Posterolateral fusion
2. Posterior fusion
3. Laminectomy
4. Laminectomy and intertransverse fusion
5. Anterior lumbar interbody fusion **(ALIF)** by titanium cylinder mess.
6. Posterior lumbar interbody fusion **(PLIF)** by titanium cylinder mess.
7. **ZETA spine fixation** by titanium cylinder mess.
8. **Moss Miami polyaxial screw fixation.**

LUMBAR SPONDYLOSIS

This is a degenerative disease of lumbar spine which shows osteoarthritic changes.

Clinical Features

Patient may present with following clinical features:

1. Low backache
2. Stiffness in low back
3. Radiculopathy in lower limbs may present as sciatica.
4. Feeling of catch while getting up from a sitting position.
5. Numbness and paresthesia.
6. Restricted SLR.

X-ray Findings

- Intervertebral disc space may be reduced.
- Osteophytes formation is commonly seen.
- Erosion of articular margin of vertebrae may also be seen.
- Lipping of vertebrae is also seen.
- Sometimes slipping of vertebra can be seen.

Treatment

Patient can be advised following instructions:

- To lie on hard bed.
- Hot saline fomentation at back.
- Spinal exercises.
- Lumbar corset should be worn.

SCOLIOSIS

Lateral or sideways deviation of spine is known as Scoliosis. Scoliosis causes disfigurement of body. Severe deformity may displace or compress viscera and may impair it's function. Scoliosis reduces life expectancy.

Aetiology

Most common cause of scoliosis is idiopathic (70%).

Types

1. Structural
2. Transient structural
3. Non structural.

1. Structural Scoliosis

(A) Idiopathic

- (*a*) Infantile
- (*b*) Juvenile
- (*c*) Adolescent

(B) Congenital

- (*a*) Vertebral (open and closed).
- (*b*) Extravertebral

(C) Neuromuscular

- (*a*) Neuropathic
- (*b*) Myopathic

(D) Neurofibromatosis

(E) Trauma

(F) Mesenchymal Disorder

2. Transient Structural Scoliosis

This is classified into following three types:

Sciatic Scoliosis

It is caused by pressure at nerve roots from a herniated disc. It is not true scoliosis.

Hysterical Scoliosis

This is a rare type.

Inflammatory Scoliosis

This is seen with perinephric abscess or similar infection.

3. Non Structural Scoliosis

This is classified into following two types:

Postural Scoliosis

It is commonly seen in adolescent girl in late years of first decade. Deformity disappears while lying down.

Compensatory Scoliosis

It is caused by leg length discrepancy. Pelvis dips down on short side.

Curves in Scoliosis

Primary curve

Lateral curvature of part of spine which develops first is known as Primary curve.

Secondary curve

Compensatory curvature of spine in opposite direction above and below primary curve is known as Secondary curve. It is a balancing response to primary curve.

Simple curve

If single deviation develops in spine it will be known as simple curve.

Compound curve

When displacement occurs in left and right direction, curve is known as compound.

Anatomical Types of Scoliosis

- Dorsal scoliosis
- Dorsolumbar scoliosis
- Lumbar scoliosis

Clinical Features

Scoliosis may present with following clinical features:

1. Patient presents with bony deformity over spine.
2. Backache and fatigue.
3. Patient may also show cardiopulmonary symptoms.
4. Neurological deficit may be present depending on compression of nerve root.

X-ray Findings

Measurement of curves can be done by Cobb's method and Risser Ferguson method.

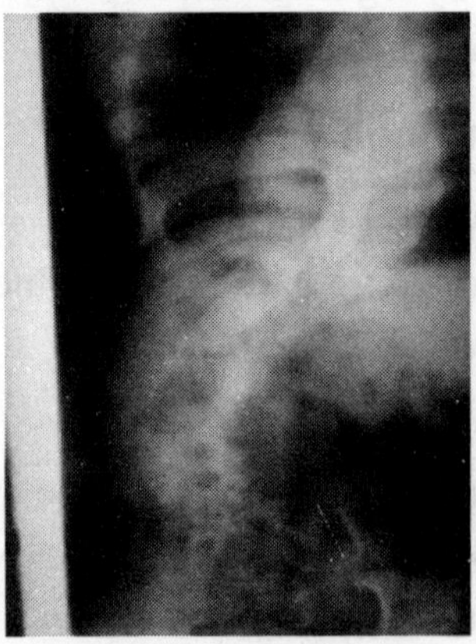

Fig. 37.9 Scoliosis

Cobb's angle

Cobb's angle can be measured in A.P. view of spine. A horizontal line is drawn at superior border of superior end vertebra. Second line is drawn at inferior border of inferior end vertebra. Now draw a perpendicular line from these two horizontal lines. Angle formed by these two intersecting lines is known as Cobb's angle.

Classification of curves by scoliosis research society

Group	Degree of angle
1	0–20
2	21–30
3	31–50
4	51–75
5	76–100
6	100–125
7	≥ 126

Risser Fergusson method

Mark a dot at the centre of upper end vertebra and lower end vertebra. One additional dot is marked at the centre of apical vertebra. Apical vertebra is situated at most wedging and deformity at the apex of curve. Now draw a straight line from dots in each end vertebra. Angle formed by these two intersecting lines is measured.

Risser's Sign

Fusion of iliac apophysis with iliac bone indicates completion of growth, so no chance of curve worsening. It is known as Risser's sign.

Rotation of Vertebra

Normally spinous process of vertebra lies at its centre in A.P. view of X-ray spine. If vertebra is rotated spinous process will be shifted to one side. Along with this both pedicles of vertebra will be asymmetrical.

Congenital Scoliosis

Following findings can be seen in congenital scoliosis:

- Wedging of vertebra
- Hemivertebra
- Unsegmented bar in between two vertebrae.
- Fused ribs.

Principle of Treatment

Aim of treatment is to correct and prevent deformity and to halt progression and impairment of cardiopulmonary function. Surgical treatment is postponed as long as possible provided that curve is not progressing and could be controlled by a suitable apparatus.

Following signs of growth stoppage should be looked for:

- Growth of iliac apophysis
- Wrist bone age
- Growth of vertebral apophyseal ring
- Menarche
- Body growth.

Milwaukee brace

This brace was designed by Blount and Schmidt. This is used for ambulatory and non-operative treatment of spinal curvature.

Indications of Milwaukee Brace

1. This is indicated as an ambulatory and non operative treatment of scoliosis.
2. During growing age.
3. It is also indicated in prevention of progression of deformity.
4. Curve not exceeding to 40 degree.
5. Until the end of growth spurt.

Indications of Surgical Treatment

1. Progressive curve
2. Trunk deformity

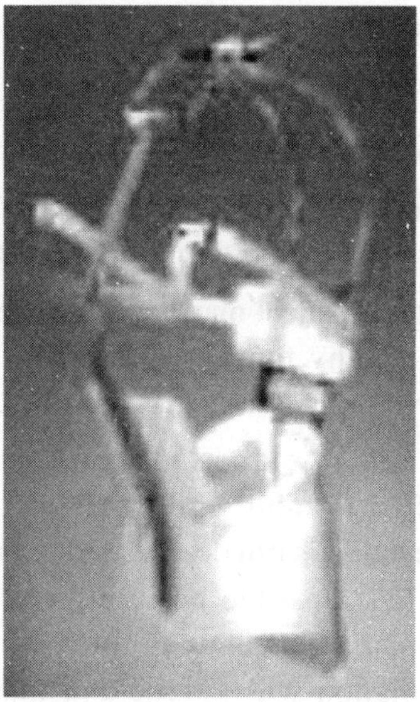

Fig. 37.10 Milwaukee brace

3. Painful deformity in older patient.
4. Impaired cardiopulmonary function.
5. Hereditary history of severe scoliosis.

Preoperative Treatment

Mobilization Exercises

- Gymnastic exercise
- Stretching exercise

Stretching

Longitudinal traction can be given by following measures:

- Head halter traction
- Pelvic halo cast
- Halofemoral distraction

Stretching can also be done by lateral traction and by over head suspension of arm and leg on convex side.

Milwaukee Brace

It is recommended for correction and maintenance of moderate flexible curve.

Forcible Corrective Stage

- Risser's turn buckle hinge

- Localizer's cast
- Corrective plaster jacket.

Surgical Treatment

First spinal fusion was performed by Dr. Russell Hibbs at New York orthopaedic hospital in 1911.

After surgery, patient may have little disability and can live healthy functional life with no fear of adult curve progression and disability.

Primary aim of scoliosis surgery is to achieve spinal fusion and stabilization of curve. Instrumentation is usually inserted in order to hold spine in best possible position, while fusion is accomplished. Without proper spinal fusion, instrumentation will fatigue and many times it fails completely.

In posterior approach paraspinal muscles are stripped from laminae of vertebra which are to be fused.

Most adolescent patients remain in hospital for 7-8 days while adults stay only slightly longer. Postoperative cast or brace is not necessary with new instrumentation technique. 2-3 weeks after surgery, patient can return to their work.

Strenuous exercise like bicycle riding is not recommended for first few months. Spinal fusion matures in one year. In second year it becomes hard lamellar bone.

Surgical procedures

Various surgical procedures can be adopted as follows:

- Spinal fusion by posterior or anterior approach followed by implantation of Harrington's rod.
- Dwyer's compression method.
- Luque-Hartshill system.

Indications of anterior instrumentation and interbody spine fusion

1. Severe paralytic scoliosis
2. Congenital or acquired absence of posterior elements.
3. Thoracic lordosis
4. Severe and rigid congenital scoliosis
5. Congenital kyphosis
6. Kyphoscoliosis

Different casts to be used in scoliosis

- Risser's localizer body cast
- Surcingle (Von lackum) cast
- Cotrel cast
- Transection jacket

SPINA BIFIDA

Definition

Spina bifida is a congenital anamoly that occurs due to failure of fusion of posterior part of spine resulting in a defect through which herniation of membrane and spinal cord may occur. In this condition only one vertebra is affected and mostly in lumbosacral region.

Embryology

Faulty mesenchymal formation leads to failure of tissue to fuse dorsally over the neural axis resulting in a bifid condition. Failure of mesenchyme to act normally impairs ability of ectoderm to invaginate properly and resulting in myelomeningocoele or encephalocoele.

Classification

1. Spina bifida occulta
2. Spina bifida aperta
   - Meningocoele
   - Meningomyelocoele
   - Syringomyelocoele
   - Myelocoele

Spina bifida occulta

- In this condition neural arches fail to unite posteriorly.
- Membrane or cord protrusion is not seen.
- This condition almost always occurs at lumbosacral region (S1 commonly).
- On examination we can find cicatrical thickening/dimple/tuft of hair/dilated vessels/fibrofatty tumor or naevolipoma at spine where bone is deficient.
- Skin is connected to spina theca by a fibrous band or membrane reunions. With growth of child, this membrane reunions pulls down the theca leading to symptoms e.g. backache, enuresis, foot drop, weakness of lower limb or sometimes paralysis of lower limb.
- Uncommonly child may be asymptomatic and he may be diagnosed while taking X-ray for another reason.

Treatment of spina bifida occulta

- Asymptomatic patient requires no treatment.
- Backache may be treated by analgesics and physiotherapy.
- Paralysis is managed by prevention and correction of deformity by tendon transfer/arthrodesis or by brace.
- Surgical treatment consists of laminectomy, opening of dura and exploration of spinal cord. A tight filum terminale is sectioned.
- Surgery is indicated in abnormal gait, deformity of foot, severe degree of spina bifida and low lying conus medullaris seen in myelography.

Spina Bifida Aperta

In this anomaly along with vertebral arches skin, meninges and cord are also involved. Sometimes nerve tube may be exposed in severe case. It is most commonly seen at dorsolumbar region.

Meningocoele

If meninges protrude out through the defect in spine the condition is known as meningocoele. It only contains CSF.

Meningomyelocoele

Meningomyelocoele has following features:

1. Meninges are protruded in this condition.
2. Normally developed spinal cord and cauda equina lie within sac and may be adherent to posterior part of sac.
3. Meningomyelocoele is commonly seen in living children.
4. This can be differentiated from meningocoele by transillumination test.
5. Transillumination test shows dark shadows of cord or nerve on transillumination.
6. Hydocephalus is often associated.

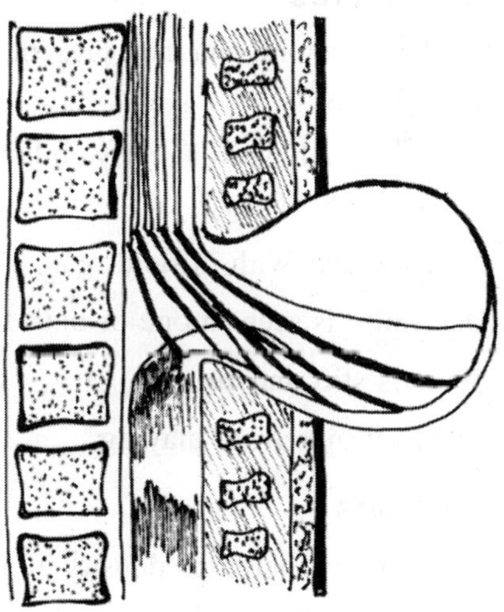

Fig. 37.11 Meningomyelocoele

Syringomyelocoele

In this clinical condition central canal of spinal cord is dilated. Cord lies within the sac and becomes adherent to posterior part of sac.

Myelocoele

This is commonest variety of spina bifida. This is a fatal condition. Child presents with paralytic deformity of foot and incontinence of urine and faeces. In this condition central canal of spinal cord opens out on surface and discharges CSF continuously. As far as treatment is concern basic defect (spina bifida) is treated. Prevention and correction of deformities is a better option. Urological treatment is required for incontinence of bladder.

DIASTEMATOMYELIA

This is longitudinal division of spinal cord or cauda equina into 2 portions each self contained within it's dural sheath by a bony cartilaginous or fibrous septum arising from posterior surface of vertebrae. This is a congenital malformation most commonly seen in lower thoracic and upper lumbar spine.

Clinical Features

Patient of diastematomyelia may present with the following features:

1. It is commonly seen in early childhood and growing age.
2. Patient walks with difficult gait.
3. Deformity is seen in one or both feet.
4. Spine is stiff and straight.
5. Child refrains from playing.

Investigations

- X-ray shows increased density in middle of widened spinal canal.
- CT-scan is more accurate in diagnosing the pathology.

Treatment

Laminectomy and freeing of nerve structure is main treatment.

PIRIFORMIS SYNDROME

This is entrapment of sciatic nerve by piriformis muscle as it passes through sciatic notch.

Causes:

1. Hypertrophy of piriformis muscle.
2. Vigorous exercise.
3. Trauma to hip.
4. Inflammation of piriformis.
5. Pseudoaneurysm of inferior gluteal artery.
6. Traumatic myositis ossificans.

Clinical Features

1. Pain at hip with radiation to thigh and leg.
2. Difficulty in walking.
3. Tenderness at sciatic notch.
4. Hypertrophied piriformis can be felt over hip and also laterally during per rectal examination.
5. SLR test is positive.
6. Lasegue test is also positive.

Management

MRI should be done to confirm hypertrophy of piriformis. This can be treated by physiotherapy, analgesics, ultrasonic therapy. If conservative methods fail, surgical release of piriformis can also be done.

CHAPTER

38 Muscular Dystrophies

- Duchenne's muscular dystrophy
- Werdnig Hoffman disease
- Landouzy-Dejerine dystrophy

DUCHENNE'S MUSCULAR DYSTROPHY

This is also known as pseudohypertrophic muscular dystrophy. This condition is seen in paediatric age group and x-linked recessive. Abnormal deletion gene is present at x-chromosome in cytogenetic band xp-21. This gene codes for dystrophic protein. This protein is present at peripheri of skeletal and smooth muscle fibre and in brain.

Clinical Features

Patient may present with following clinical features:

1. Normal perinatal history
2. Early development is normal.
3. Delayed walking
4. Child falls frequently while walking or running.
5. Waddling gait.
6. Lumbar lordosis is increased.
7. Difficulty in climbing upstairs. Child always use support of railing while climbing.
8. At the age of 4-5 years calf muscle may show hypertrophy.
9. Onset of disease in Backer's dystrophy is between 5–25 years of age.
10. **Gower sign** is positive i.e. child stands up as if climbing upon his body by supporting it with his hand. Positive sign indicates weakness of pelvic girdle muscle.
11. Atrophy of supraspinatus and sternal head of pectoralis major muscles are seen.
12. Glutei, calf muscle, deltoid, brachioradialis and tounge muscle may show pseudohypertrophy.
13. Occular, pharyngeal and masticating muscles are never involved.
14. Ambulation stops at the age of 12–14 years of age.
15. Patient dies in second decade of life. Cause of death is intercurrent infection or cardiac failure. (commonly seen in Duchenne type)

Investigations

- LDH5, CPK, SGOT, SGPT and aldolase are raised.
- EMG shows decreased amplitude and duration of motor unit potential.
- Muscle biopsy shows degenerative changes and varied size of central nuclei of muscle fibre.

Treatment

This condition does not have definitive treatment. Physiotherapy, exercise and use of tricycle help in ambulation. Tight fitting braces can prevent scoliosis. Cardiorespiratory complications are managed by conventional approach. Subcutaneous tenotomy can be done for severe contracture.

WERDNIG HOFFMAN DISEASE

This is autosomal recessive musculoskeletal disorder.

- Child presents with severe hypotonia, sluggish foetal movements and fasciculation of tounge.
- Child is alert.
- Poor cry. Feeding behaviour is also poor.
- Deep tendon reflexes are absent.
- Muscle biopsy is diagnostic which shows neurogenic type of atrophy.

LANDOUZY-DEJERINE DYSTROPHY

This is also known as facioscapulohumeral dystrophy. This is inherited as an autosomal dominant disease. This has following features:

- Disease affects children of puberty.
- It shows slowly progressive weakness of face, scapula and muscles around shoulder.
- Patient is unable to close eye forcefully, to whistle or hold air in oral cavity.
- Winging and elevation of scapula and foot drop are seen.
- This disease does not show hypertrophy of muscle.
- Sensorineural hearing loss is also seen.

CHAPTER

39 Arthroscopy

- Arthroscope
- Basic instruments
- Irrigation system
- Triangulation technique of arthroscopy
- Arthroscopic reconstruction of ACL
- Arthroscopy of knee
- Arthroscopy of hip
- Arthroscopy of ankle
- Arthroscopy of shoulder
- Arthroscopy of elbow

ARTHROSCOPE

Arthroscope is an optical instrument mend to see the structures inside a joint through a minimal portal entry.

This device can have following 3 types of basic optical lens system:

1. Rod-lens system (designed by Hopkins)
2. Classic thin lens system
3. Graded index (GRIN) lens system

Rod-lens system was designed by Prof. Hopkins of Redding, England. This is most commonly used optical system in modern arthroscope. In this system lens are thick compared to their diameter and air space between successive lenses is relatively small.

Fiberoptic arthroscope is made up of this rod-lens system which is surrounded by multiple light-conducting glass fibrils.

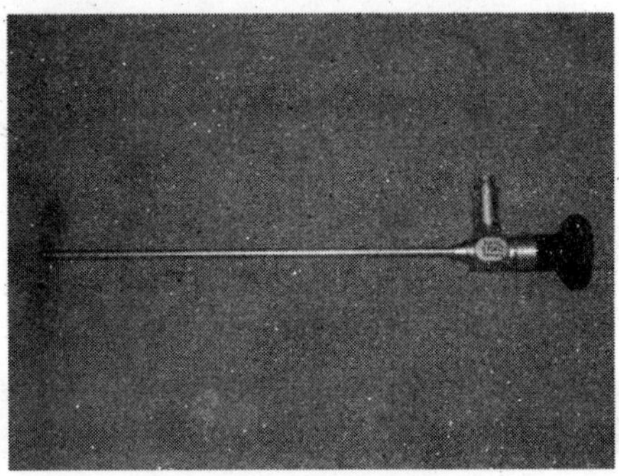

Fig. 39.1 Arthroscope

Features of arthroscope

Arthroscope has many features but following 3 features are most important because they determine the optical characteristics of arthroscope:

1. Angle of inclination
2. Field of view
3. Lens diameter

Angle between axis of arthroscope and a line perpendicular to surface of lens is known as angle of inclination. This angle has a range of 0–120 degree. Most commonly used angle is 25 and 30 degree. 70 and 90 degree are used to see structures around corner of a joint e.g., posterior compartment of knee.

Field of view is a viewing angle encompassed by lens. Wider is the view angle, easier is the orientation by observer. This angle varies according to type of arthroscope.

Diameter of lens varies from 1.7 to 7 mm. Most common size is 4 mm. 1.9 mm is used for wrist arthroscope. 2.7 mm is used for ankle arthroscope.

BASIC INSTRUMENTS

Basic instruments kit should have following:

1. Arthroscope (30 and 70 degree)
2. Probe and scissors
3. Basket (punch biopsy) forceps
4. Grasping forceps
5. Meniscus cutter and shaver
6. Arthroscopic knives.

IRRIGATION SYSTEM

Arthroscopy always needs irrigation and distension of joint by fluid. We can use ringer lactate or normal saline.

Ringer lactae is most commonly used fluid as it causes minimal synovial and articular surface changes. Other important aspect of ringer lactate is that it is physiological to human body.

If surgeon wants to use intra-articular electrocautry system he should evacuate the knee of either saline or ringer lactate and should irrigate and distend the knee with glycine (non electrolytic solution)

TRIANGULATION TECHNIQUE OF ARTHROSCOPY

This is basic arthroscopic technique in which 2 or more instruments are inserted into joint through separate portals and brought into optical field of arthroscope. Apex of triangle is made by tip of instrument and arthroscope.

ARTHROSCOPIC RECONSTRUCTION OF ACL

Arthroscopic reconstruction of anterior cruciate ligament can be done by taking following graft:

1. Patellar tendon
2. Semitendinosus
3. Gracillis

Graft can be autograft, allograft or an artificial graft. In this procedure an arthroscope is inserted into knee joint through a stab incision slightly away from lateral border of ligamentum patellae. On the opposite side, suction and drainage system is inserted into knee joint through a stab incision. First we thoroughly watch for ACL injury e.g. level of tear.

A graft can be taken from semitendinosus or Gracillis or both. This graft is prepared by suturing (ethibond) its end in such a way that it does not stick into the prepared tunnel in lateral condyle of femur. Length of this graft should be 8 cm. A tunnel is made in lateral condyle of femur. Prepared graft is taken into this tunnel. Proximal end of suture of graft is pulled out through shaft of femur on lateral side. Now proximal end of graft is fixed with screw into tunnel made into medial surface of lateral condyle. Fixation of graft can be checked by puling it's distal end. Distal end is fixed at upper end of tibia either by a screw or a metallic staple. Stability of knee is checked by anterior drawer test and Lachman test.

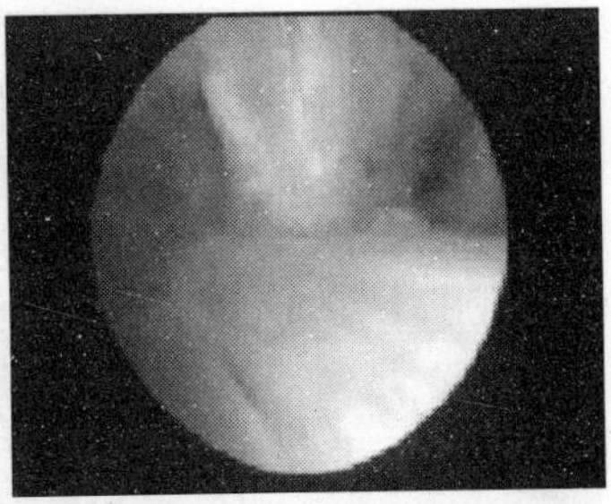

Fig. 39.2 Arthroscopic view of ACL and PCL

Advantages of Arthroscopy

Arthroscopic surgery has following advantages over arthrotomy:

1. Small incision
2. Patient can return to sedentary work immediately
3. Vigorous activities can be started within 1-2 weeks of arthroscopy
4. Less post-op pain
5. Faster rehabilitation
6. Improved accuracy of diagnosis
7. Hospital stay is reduced
8. Complications are less
9. Follow-up evaluation of patient is easy.

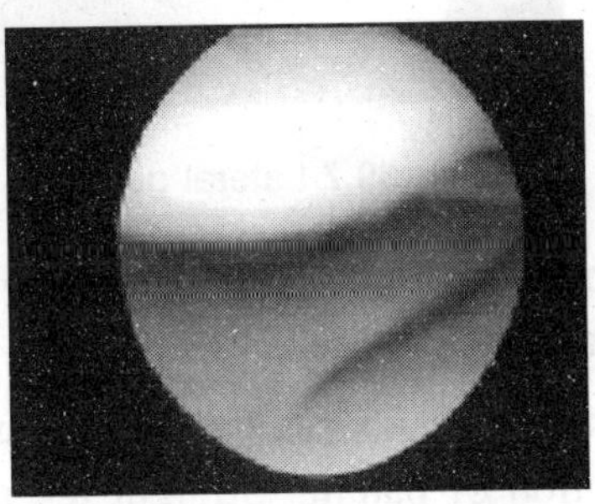

Fig. 39.3 Arthroscopic view of medial meniscus

Complications of Arthroscopy

Arthroscopic surgery can develop following complications:

1. Haemarthrosis (most common)
2. Infection
3. Thromboembolism
4. Anaesthetic complications
5. Failure of instruments
6. Reflex sympathetic dystrophy
7. Injury to ligament or nerve is less common.

ARTHROSCOPY OF KNEE

Indications

Arthroscopy of knee is indicated in following conditions:

Diagnostic

Arthroscopy of knee can be done to diagnose following conditions:

1. Injury to meniscus
2. ACL injury
3. PCL injury

Therapeutic

Therapeutic arthroscopy can be done in following conditions:

1. Menisectomy (partial/subtotal/total)
2. ACL reconstruction
3. PCL reconstruction
4. Repair of torn meniscus
5. Removal of loose bodies from knee
6. Arthroscopic management of osteochondritis dissecans of femoral condyle
7. Treatment of chondromalacia patella
8. Arthroscopic synovectomy in rheumatoid arthritis.
9. Arthroscopic evaluation of knee in fracture of anterior intercondylar eminence of tibia.
10. Arthroscopic examination of knee prior to tibial osteotomy.

Among the above therapeutic indications 1–4 indications are most common.

CHAPTER 39

Position of Patient

Patient is placed supine with his limb angled off the outer aspect of O.T. table. A lateral post should be applied so that surgeon can stand inside of abducted leg thus placing patient's ankle and foot on surgeon's hip and iliac crest.

Examination of lateral compartment of knee requires the assistant to keep leg in figure of four position.

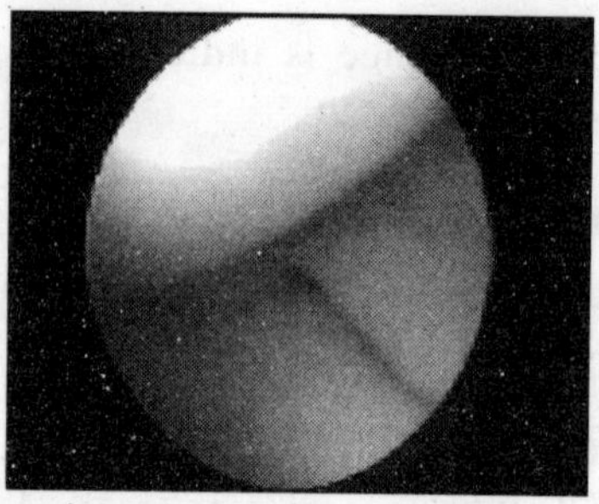

Fig. 39.4 Arthroscopic view of lateral meniscus

Portals for Arthroscopy

Arthroscope can be inserted into knee joint through following areas:

1. Anterolateral
2. Anteromedial
3. Posteromedial
4. Superolateral

Anterolateral portal is most commonly used for diagnostic arthroscopy.

Areas of Examination

Knee requires examination of following compartments:

1. Suprapatellar pouch and patellofemoral joint.
2. Medial gutter and medial compartment.
3. Lateral gutter and lateral compartment.
4. Intercondylar notch.
5. Posteromedial and posterolateral compartment.

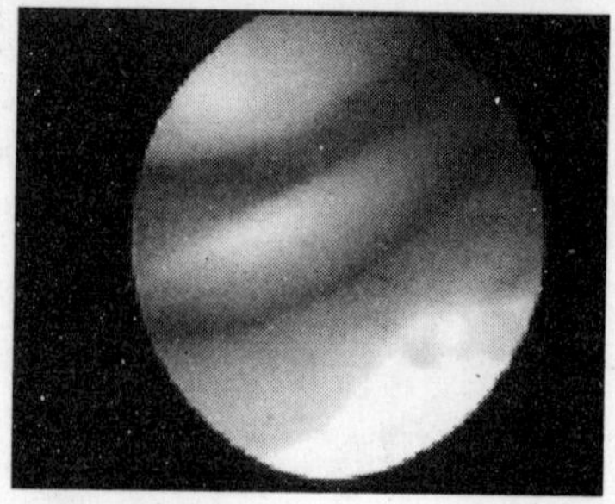

Fig. 39.5 Medial meniscus has turned up

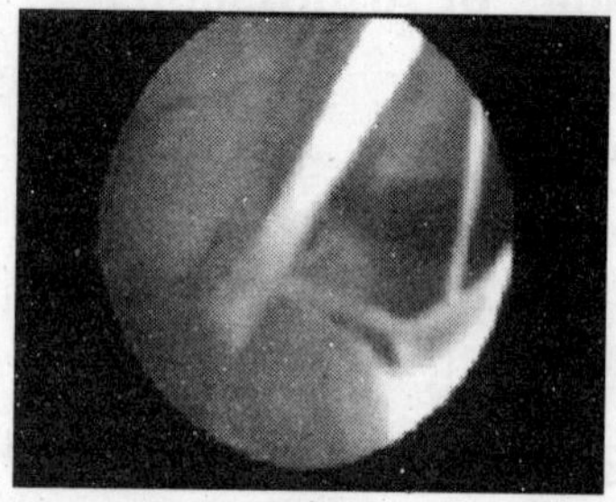

Fig. 39.6 Arthroscopic view of lateral compartment

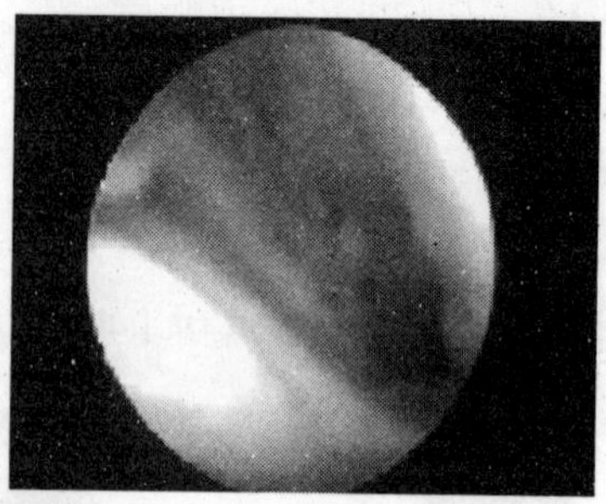

Fig. 39.7 Lateral gutter

Post-op Rehabilitation of ACL Reconstruction

Patient should be adviced for superior and inferior mobilization of patella. Straight leg rasing and quadriceps sets should be explained to patient. Active and passive knee flexion is adviced. Full range of passive extension is also done at knee joint. Patient is also adviced to sleep with knee brace in extension. Patient can return to sports activity after 6 months.

ARTHROSCOPY OF HIP

Indications

Arthroscopy of hip is not commonly done. This is indicated in following conditions:

1. Removal of loose bodies (most common)
2. Synovial biopsy
3. Synovectomy

ARTHROSCOPY OF ANKLE

Indications

This is also not commonly done. Arthroscopy of ankle is indicated in following conditions:

1. Treatment of osteochondritis dissecans of talus.
2. Transchondral fracture of talus.
3. Removal of loose bodies.
4. Synovectomy.

ARTHROSCOPY OF SHOULDER

Shoulder arthroscopy has become common in India.

Indications

Arthroscopy of shoulder is indicated in following conditions:

Diagnostic

Diagnostic arthroscopy of shoulder can be done in following conditions:

1. Identification of loose bodies.
2. Evaluation of primary rotator cuff impingement.
3. To detect any tear in rotator cuff.
4. To detect cause of recurrent dislocation of shoulder.

Therapeutic

Therapeutic arthroscopy of shoulder is indicated in following conditions:

1. Bankart's repair.
2. Acromioclavicular decompression in impingement syndrome.
3. Arthroscopic debridement and acrmioplasty can be done in case of rotator cuff tears.
4. Tear of glenoid labrum.
5. Biopsy.
6. Synovectomy.
7. Treatment of osteochondral lesion.

Position of Patient

Patient can be placed in following two positions:

1. Lateral decubitus position is commonly used position.
2. Beach-chair position.

Portals for Shoulder Arthroscopy

Arthroscope can be inserted into shoulder joint through following areas:

1. Anterior portal just anterior to superior acromioclavicular ligament.
2. Posterior portal just posterior to superior acrmioclavicular ligament.
3. Superior portal.
4. Lateral portal.
5. Posterolateral portal.
6. Anterolateral portal.

Among the above indications first 2 are commonly used portals.

ARTHROSCOPY OF ELBOW

Indications

Arthroscopy of elbow is indicated in following conditions:

1. Removal of loose bodies.
2. Radial head excision.
3. Idiopathic osteochondrosis of capitulum.
4. Osteochondritis dissecans.
5. Synovectomy.
6. Function of ulnar collateral ligament can also be evaluated by arthroscopy.

CHAPTER

40 Orthosis

- Amputation
- Prosthesis
- Orthosis

AMPUTATION

Removal of a part of limb through one or more bones is known as amputation.

Indications

This may be indicated in following conditions:

- Severe road traffic accident.
- Gas gangrene.
- Peripheral vascular disease.
- Diabetic foot.
- Bone tumors.
- Congenital anomalies.
- Nerve injuries.

Contraindication

- Ischaemic limb

Types

This is usually of two types as follows:

Closed Type

This is more commonly done procedure in which skin is closed primarily.

Open Type

This is also known as Guillotine type. In this type skin is not closed over stump. Later it is managed by secondary closure/plastic repair or revision of stump.

Procedure

Torniquet must be applied prior to surgery. Before inflation of tourniquet limb is elevated and esmarch bandage is wrapped tightly. Joint must be saved as much as possible. Skin over the stump must be mobile. Muscles should be cut distal to level of bone. Nerves should be brought distally into wound and resected with a sharp knife so that their ends retract well proximal to level of bone resection. All the major blood vessels should be doubly ligated. Edges of resected bone should be smooth. Excessive bone stripping should be avoided due to risk of ring sequestrum formation. A corrugated rubber drain is essential and to be kept for 48–72 hours.

Complications

- Phantom limb i.e. patient complaints of severe pain at part of limb which has been removed.

- Haematoma formation.
- Infection.
- Necrosis of skin folds.
- Neuroma formation.
- Deformity of joint.

PROSTHESIS

Prosthesis is an artificial device used to replace a part or whole of extremity. It can be used for cosmetic and functional purposes. Purpose of prosthesis is to transfer body weight to its socket and to provide normal locomotion. Patient is taught about pre-prosthetic preparation e.g., stump hygiene, excercises, strapping etc. Prosthesis is made up of 4 parts as follows:

1. **Socket**-to be fitted with stump.
2. **Suspension**-used to hold the socket to stump.
3. **Extension**-includes substitute joints.
4. **Terminal device.**

Common Prosthesis

Commonly used prosthesis are as follows:

- Patellar tendon bearing prosthesis
- Quadriceps socket prosthesis
- Shoe fillers
- Canadian Symes's prosthesis
- SACH foot—Solid ankle cushion heel.
- SAFE foot—Stationary attachment flexible endoskeleton.

Sach Foot

This foot is made up by a keel embedded in layers of rubber. This foot also has a break. Movements like inversion, eversion, dorsiflexion and plantar flexion are possible at this foot.

Safe Foot

This foot is madeup of semirigid polyurethrane elastomer keel. Other fetures of this foot are resilient heel wedge and rigid polyurethrane bolt block. Movements possible at this foot are plantar flexion, minimum dorsiflexion, inversion and eversion. Toes can be hyperextended.

ORTHOSIS

This is an artificial device which supports weak part of body. It is madeup of metal, wood steel, aluminium and plastic. Sometimes leather or carbon fibres are also used. Primary aim of orthosis is to prevent and correct deformity. It also reduces axial load and improves function of limb. It also provides relief from pain. Following types of orthosis are in use:

- HKAFO (Hip-knee-ankle-foot orthosis)
- KAFO (Knee-ankle-foot orthosis)
- AFO (Ankle-foot orthosis)
- KO (Knee-orthosis)
- FO (Foot-orthosis)
- CO (Cervical orthosis)
- WHO (Wrist-hand orthosis) for ulnar nerve lesion
- CTLSO (cervico-thoraco-lumbar sacral orthosis)
- Functional hand splint
- Mouth stick for holding objects like pen or brush

Lower limb orthotics can also be divided in two types:

1. Ambulatory

- Weight bearing
- Weight relieving e.g. Toranto brace (perthes disease), PTB orthosis (nonunion of tibia).

2. **Non ambulatory**

Parts of HKAFO

HKAFO has following parts:

- Pelvic band
- Hip joint unit
- Tuber band
- Thigh band
- Knee joint unit
- Calf band
- Ankle joint unit
- Stirrup split
- Stirrup plate

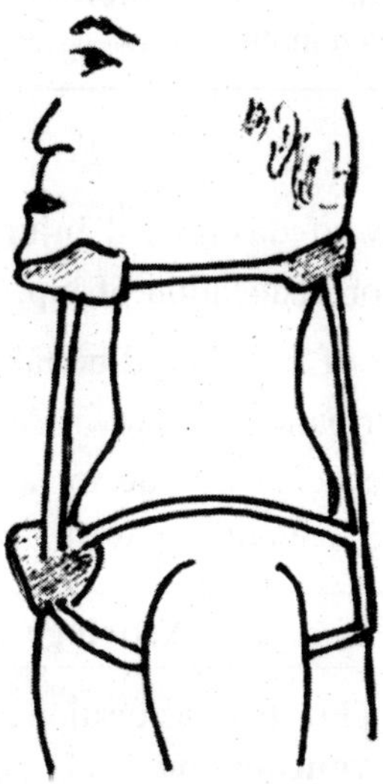

Fig. 40.1 Four post collar orthosis

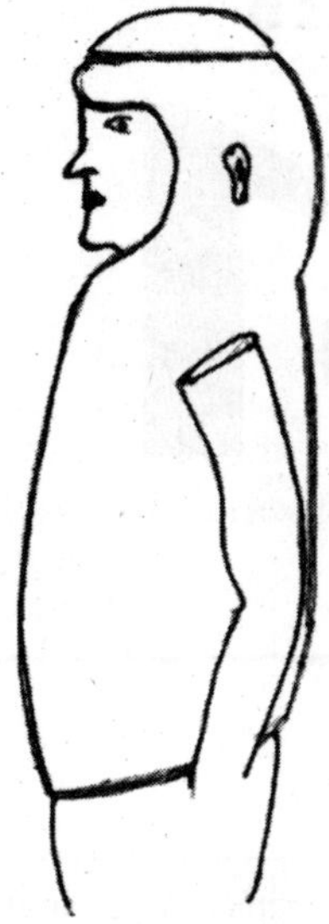

Fig. 40.2 Minerva jacket

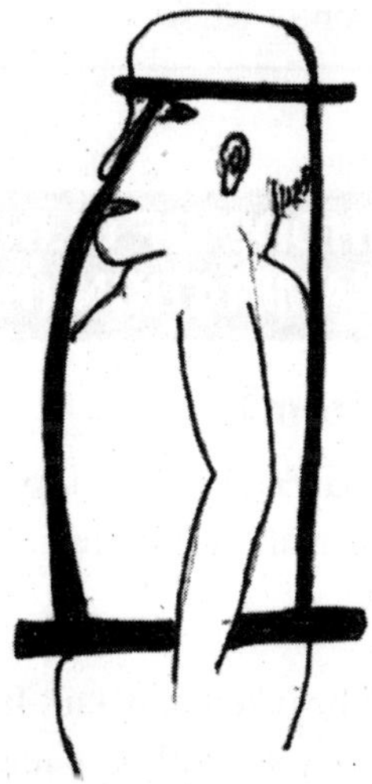

Fig. 40.3 Halo-Pelvic traction

CHAPTER

41 Clinical Methods

- Methods of clinical examination (Hip)
- Examination of knee
- Examination of shoulder
- Examination of elbow
- Examination of wrist
- Examination of spine
- Examination of bony swelling
- Local examination of swelling

METHODS OF CLINICAL EXAMINATION (HIP)

Applied Anatomy

Hip joint is a ball and socket type of joint which provides movements in multiaxial direction.

History

History should be taken in detail. It should include history of trauma as well as pathology affecting the joint.

Trauma

History of trauma should include following points:

1. Patient may give history of pain at groin/ trochanter. Pain may radiate to knee due to common nerve supply of hip and knee joint.
2. Swelling at scarpa's triangle occurs due to haematoma which is caused by fracture neck femur. Swelling at trochanter may be due to fracture at trochanter. Protruded swelling at hip may be due to dislocation of head of femur.
3. History of dashboard injury is found in posterior dislocation of hip.
4. History of fall should be taken clearly i.e., whether patient fell down due to fracture or fracture occurred due to fall. In impacted fracture, patient can walk.

Age	Aetiology
< 5 Years	Fracture/dislocation around hip are **uncommon.**
5–20 Years	Fracture neck femur can occur.
20–50 Years	Fracture neck femur, fracture pelvis and dislocation of hip are seen.
50–60 Years	Fracture neck femur is more common than intertrochanteric fracture.
> 60 Years	Intertrochanteric fracture is more common.

History of cold pathology

History of limp is very common in case of hip pathology which may be associated with pain. History of night cry may be found. This happens due to rubbing of joint cartilage. (If cartilage is damaged it will abolish protective muscle spasm which will cause striking of joint cartilage to each other.)

Age	Pathology
< 5 Years	CDH, Tom smith arthritis
5–10 Years	Perthes disease
10–15 Years	Slipped epiphysis
20–40 Years	Secondary osteoarthritis (T.B. hip, Ankylosing spondylitis)
> 40 Years	Primary osteoarthritis, Rheumatoid arthritis.

Pre-requisites for Examination

1. Patient should lie supine on a flat and hard couch.
2. Hips, lower limbs and abdomen should be fully exposed. In case of female patient genitalia should be covered with a narrow strip.

Inspection

Patient should be inspected on the basis of following points:

- Whether the patient can stand up or not.
- Can patient walk?
- Examine gait of patient e.g., antalgic or trendlenberg gait.
- Watch for lumbar lordosis or scoliotic spine.
- Watch for fixed flexion/abduction/adduction deformity and fixed external rotation deformity.
- Inspect for gluteal fold to rule out congenital dislocation of hip.
- Whether the patient can squat or sit cross leg.
- Watch for limp. Whether it is painful or painless?

Painful limp	Painless limp
Trauma	Post polio residual palsy of lower limb
Tuberculous hip	Congenital dislocation of hip
O.A. hip	Arthrodesed hip/knee/ankle joint

Gait

Normal walking comprises of two phases: stance phase and swing phase. Both of these phases are further divided into 3 phases as follows:

Stance phase

1. Heel stroke (heel strikes the ground)
2. Mid stance (foot is kept flat on ground)
3. Push off (foot is off the ground)

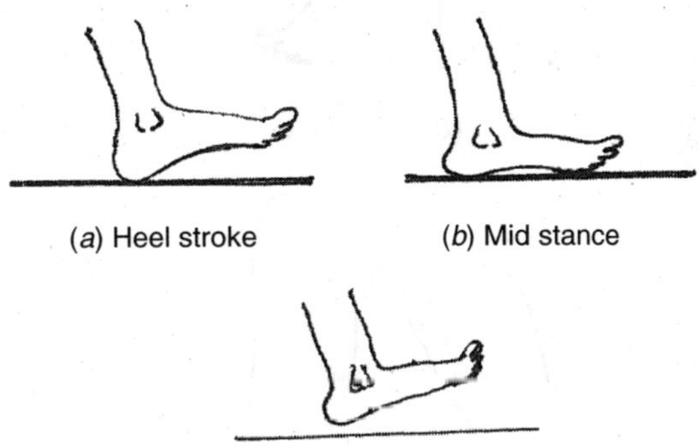

(*a*) Heel stroke (*b*) Mid stance (*c*) Push off

Fig. 41.1 Stance phase of walking

Swing phase

1. Acceleration phase (leg comes infront of body)
2. Swing through (leg is swinging forward)
3. Deceleration phase (swinging becomes slow and heel becomes ready to strike the ground)

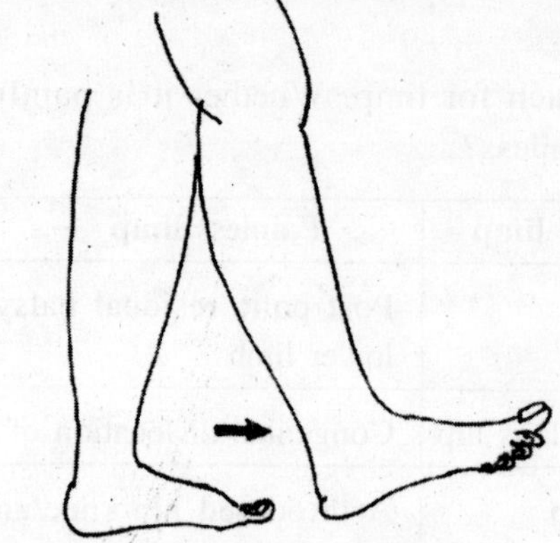

(*a*) Heel stroke

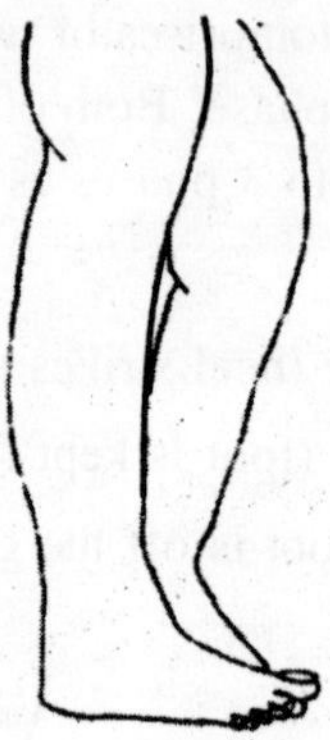

(*b*) Mid stance

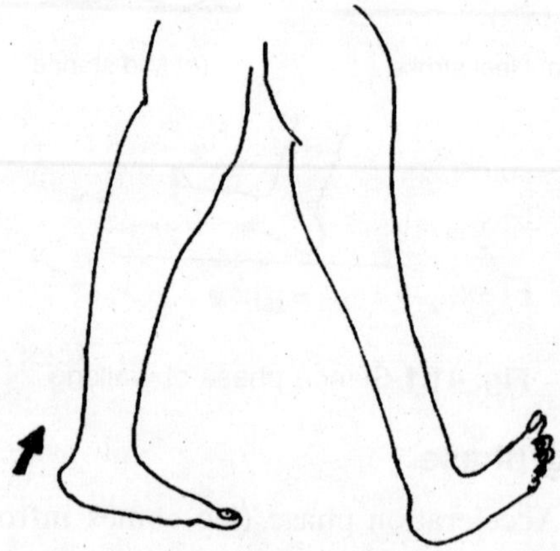

(*c*) Push off

Fig. 41.2 Stance phase

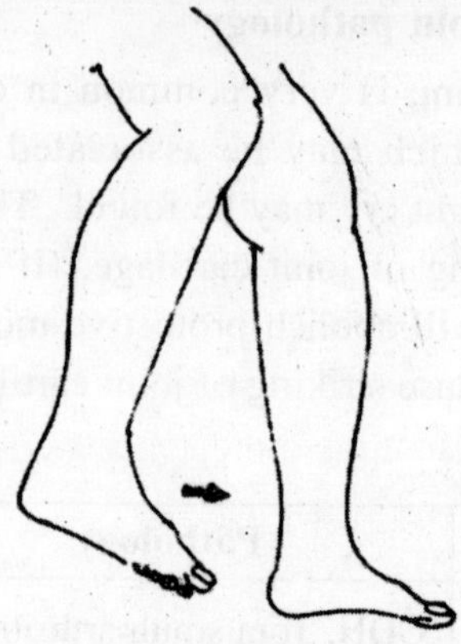

(*a*) Acceleration phase

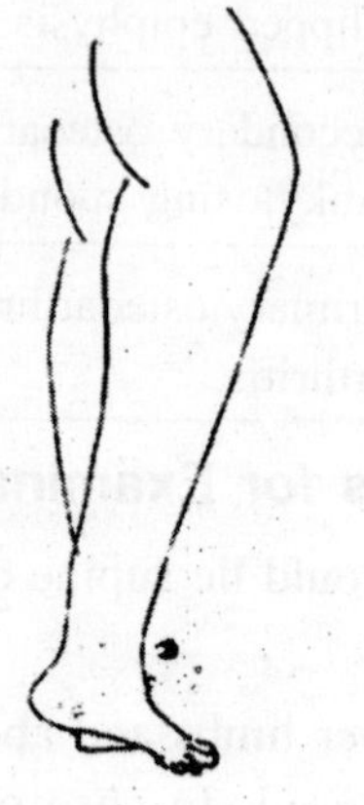

(*b*) Swing through

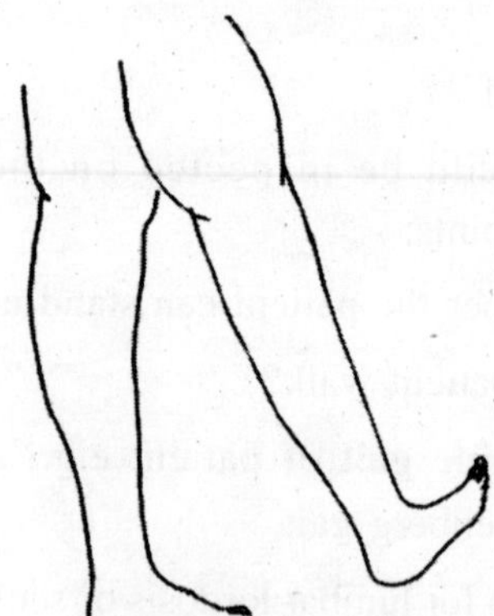

(*c*) Deceleration phase

Fig. 41.3 Swing phase

Attitude

An elder patient lying on a couch with lower limb in external rotation indicates fracture neck femur. If external rotation of lower limb is so much that lateral border of foot touches to bed it will be fracture intertrochanteric femur.

Young patient lying with hip in flexion adduction and internal rotation indicates posterior dislocation of hip while flexion abduction and external rotation of hip indicates anterior dislocation of hip.

In case of synovitis of hip patient presents in mild flexion, abduction and external rotation at hip. Along with this patient has apparent lengthening of limb.

All bony landmarks should be looked for e.g., ASIS, pubic symphysis, pubic tubercle, trochanter, iliac crest and posterior superior iliac spine.

We should also look for muscle wasting, swelling, sinus, ulcer and any visible pulsation.

Limb should be inspected for shortening and lengthening.

Palpation

Bony landmark can be marked by a marker or skin pencil.

Superficial Palpation

We should look for raised local temperature of skin, tenderness, anesthesia/hyperesthesia and venous prominence on sharp bony points.

Deep Palpation

Pulsation of femoral artery should be felt against bony surface (head of femur). In dislocation of hip (congenital or traumatic) this bony support is missing so pulsation of femoral artery cannot be felt. This is known as **vascular sign of narath.**

Hip should be palpated in all directions i.e., anterior, posterior, medial and lateral aspect. On anterior aspect tenderness should be elicited in scarpa's triangle. Head of femur should be palpated. In posterior dislocation of hip it will be at dorsum illi. It will be felt in groin in pubic type while in perineum in obturator type of dislocation.

Tenderness should be checked at lateral aspect of hip over trochanter. Touch tenderness hints toward inflammatory condition. Transmitted tenderness indicates trochanteric fracture, fracture neck femur, tuberculosis of hip and fracture acetabulum.

You should also look for cold abscess at scarpa's triangle, iliac fossa, gluteal area, subtrochanteric area and anteromedial aspect of mid thigh.

Lymph nodes should be palpated at inguinal and external illiac area.

Fixed Deformities

Three types of deformities are commonly seen at hip joint.

- Fixed flexion deformity
- Fixed abduction/adduction deformity
- Fixed external rotation deformity.

There are certain causes of fixed deformity:

- Muscle spasm
- Fibrotic contractures in periarticular soft tissue
- Destructive changes in joint.

If patient has fixed deformity he will adopt compensatory posture to conceal the deformity and to stabilize unstable hip and to hide limb length discrepancy.

Fixed Flexion Deformity

This deformity was detected by Sir Hugh Owen Thomas test. Patient is asked to lie supine on a couch with hard and flat surface. Now ask patient to extend his legs. He will do it by increasing lumbar lordosis. This lordosis can be checked by passing a hand beneath lumbar spine. In this test normal thigh is flexed (with bent knee) till lumbar lordosis completely disappears. This can be checked by passing a hand between lumbar spine

CHAPTER 41

and bed. Now angle between back of thigh and bed will be angle of fixed flexion deformity.

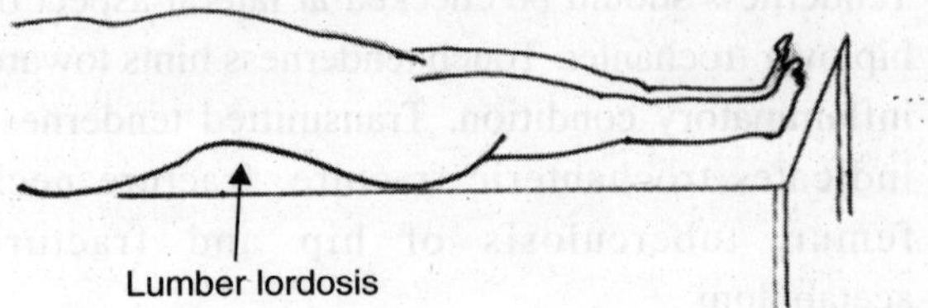

(*a*)

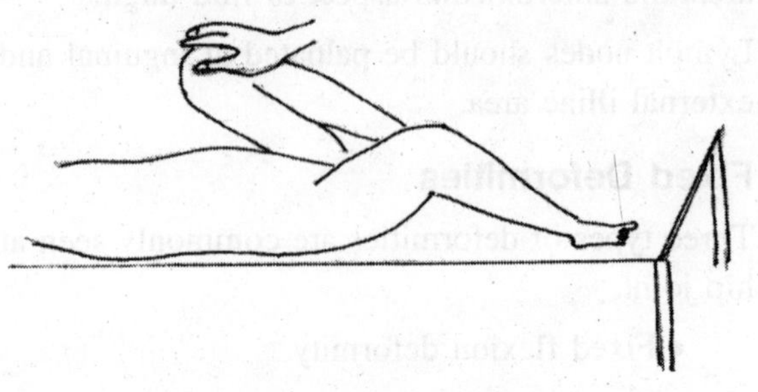

(*b*) Eliciting Thomas test for fixed flexion deformity at hip

Fig. 41.4 Measurement of fixed flexion deformity

Limitation of Thomas test

This test has following limitations:

1. This test cannot be done in bilateral fixed flexion deformity.
2. If we continue to flex normal thigh even after lordosis has disappeared, it will give fallacious result.
3. This test cannot be performed if knee is ankylosed.

Bilateral Fixed Flexion Deformity

To detect bilateral fixed flexion deformity patient is asked to lie in prone position on a couch in such a manner that his trunk remains on couch while his hips should be at the edge of couch. Now support both knees with hands from anterior aspect to avoid injury to patient. Now both hips should be passively extended till a resistance is felt. During this test no force should be applied. Angle between long axis of trunk and thigh will be angle of fixed flexion deformity.

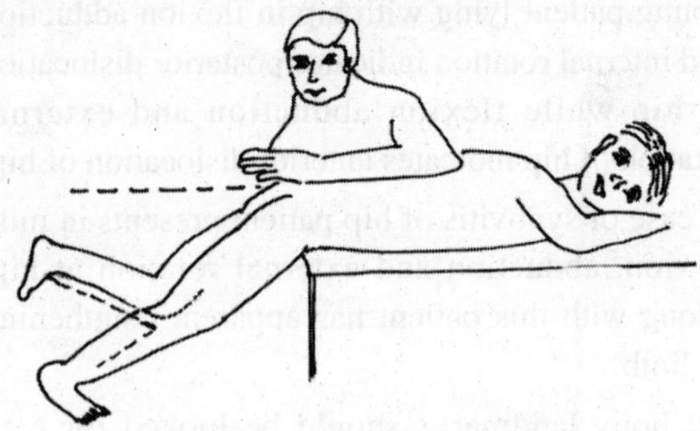

Fig. 41.5 Measurement of bilateral fixed flexion deformity

Fixed Abduction Deformity

In this deformity affected ASIS remains at lower level in comparison to normal side. To detect this deformity affected limb is further abducted till ipsilateral ASIS comes at the level of normal ASIS. Thus pelvis is squared up. Now a vertical line is drawn from ASIS. Angle formed between this vertical line and long axis of thigh will define angle of fixed abduction deformity.

Fixed Adduction Deformity

In this deformity affected ASIS remains at higher level in comparison to normal side. To detect this deformity affected limb is further adducted till ipsilateral ASIS comes to the level of normal ASIS. Thus pelvis is squared up. Now a vertical line is drawn from ASIS. Angle formed between this vertical line and long axis of thigh will define angle of deformity.

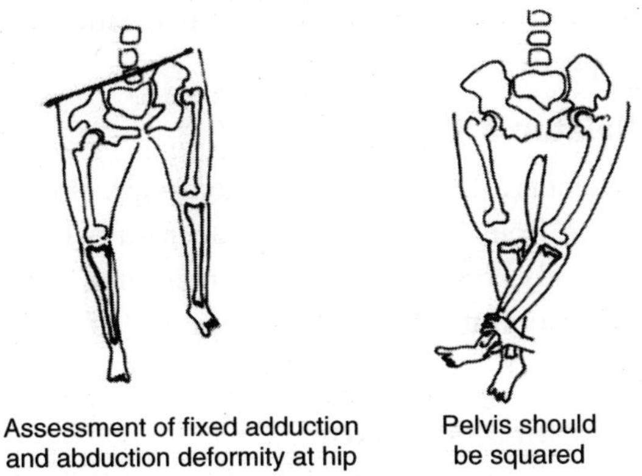

Fig. 41.6 Measurement of fixed adduction deformity

Movements at Hip

HIP-		
	Flexion (with knee extended)	0–90
	Flexion (with knee flexed)	0–120
	Extension	0–20
	Abduction-	0–45
	Adduction	0–30
	External rotation	0–45
	Internal rotation	0–30

Flexion

Flexion at hip is performed by illiacus and psoas muscle. To check this movement patient is asked to flex his thigh with knee fully flexed till thigh touches abdomen. Normal range of flexion with flexed thigh is 0–120 degree. During this maneuver other lower limb should be extended. Normal range of flexion with extended knee is 0–90 degree.

Extension

Extension of hip is performed by gluteal maximus and hamstring muscles. Range of extension at hip joint is 0–20 degree. This movement can be checked in prone as well as in lateral position. Pelvis should be fixed before checking movements. To check this movement patient is asked to take his lower limb backward with extended knee.

Adduction

Adduction at hip is performed by adductor (longus, brevis and magnus) muscles. Normal range of adduction at hip is 30 degree. To check this movement pelvis is held with hand in such a way that thumb rests at ASIS. Now patient is asked to move his lower limb inward till it crosses contralateral limb and thumb just appreciates movement at ASIS.

Abduction

Abduction is performed by gluteus medius and minimus muscles. Rang of abduction is 0–45 degree. Pre-requisite to check this movement is same as in adduction. In this test patient is asked to move out his extended lower limb till thumb feels movement at ASIS.

Measurements

Actual measurement should be done first in normal limb.

True Measurement

True measurement can be done in standing as well as in lying position. Pelvis should be squared up and both lower limbs should be in identical position. Limb is measured from ASIS to tip of medial malleolus.

Standing Position

Patient compensates **limb shortening** by abducting limb thus tilting pelvis downward on that side. Patient is asked to bring the abducted limb to a neutral position. He will bring it by lifting his heel. This will lift his pelvis upward. Now insert a wooden block beneath the foot at a level where pelvis becomes horizontal. Now measure the hight of wooden block which will indicate limb length discrepancy.

Pelvis remains at higher level in case of **limb lengthening**. In such case insert a measured wooden block beneath the opposite foot to bring pelvis at horizontal level. Height of wooden block will indicate limb length discrepancy.

Lying Position

Patient should be fully exposed and all bony land marks should be marked with a marker or skin pencil. Pelvis should be squared up by exaggerating the adduction or abduction deformity. Now normal limb is brought in identical position of affected limb. Metal end of measuring tape should be used to localize bony point. Metalic end of measuring tape should be slided over inguinal ligament toward ASIS. First bony resistance catching the metal tip should be marked. Now length is measured from ASIS to tip of medial malleolus.

Apparent Measurement

This should be done in lying position with affected limb in the line of trunk. Both lower limbs should be parrallel to each other. Measurement is done from xiphisternum/suprasternal notch to tip of malleolus. This measurement can signify any concealed fixed deformity of hip or limb length discrepancy.

Brayant's Triangle

Patient is asked to lie in supine position. Now draw a vertical line downward from ASIS. Another line is drawn from tip of ASIS to greater trochanter. Now a horizontal line is drawn from tip of greater trochanter which connects preivious line. Reduction in length of horizontal line indicates upward shift of greater trochanter which occur in fracture neck femur or separation of upper femoral epiphysis, dislocation of hip. Diminution or increase in length of second line hints of anterior or posterior dislocation of hip respectively.

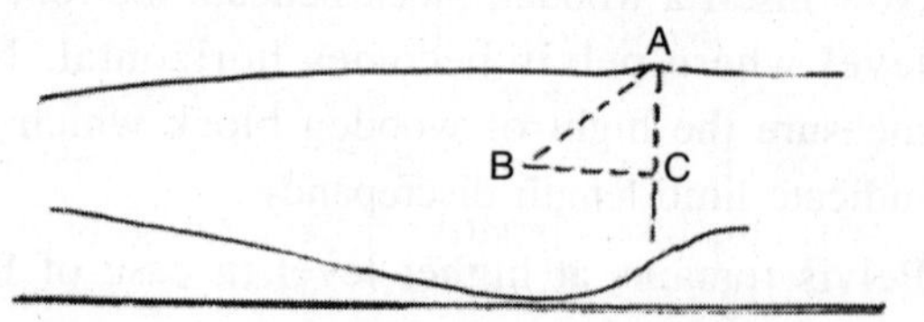

Fig. 41.7 Assessment of Brayant's triangle
A : ASIS; B : greater trochanter; C : Junction of 2 perpendicular lines

Nelaton's Line

Patient is asked to lie on his sound side. Now draw a line from ASIS to ischial tuberosity. This line normally crosses over greater trochanter. This line can demonstrate displacement of greater trochanter.

Schoemaker's Line

Patient lies in supine position. A line joining up of trochanter and anterior superior iliac spine is extended toward abdomen. Normally it will cross at or above umbilicus. If trochanter shifts upward line will cross below umbilicus. If patient has bilateral CDH or coxa vara, both lines will meet in centre and below umbilicus.

Chiene's Test

Lines joining tips of both trochanters and ASIS should be parrallel to each other normally. If trochanter shifts upward line will converge on that side.

Morris Bitrochanteric Test

If we draw lines from both trochanters to pubic symphysis, the distance of each line will be equal to each other normally.

Straight leg raising test

This is done in supine position. Patient is asked to raise his extended leg. Normally he can raise up to 90 degree.

SLR	Inference
30 degree	Dural stretch from disc herniation
45 degree	Sciatic irritation due to sacroilitis
70 degree	Lumbosacral involvement

Telescopy test

This test is done in supine position. To examine right hip use your left hand to hold hip while right hand is used to flex the knee and hip up to 90 degree. Right hand pushes down the thigh along its axis. Other hand feels whether greater trochanter is moving downward. This test is positive in congenital dislocation of hip, charcoat's joint and pathological dislocation of hip.

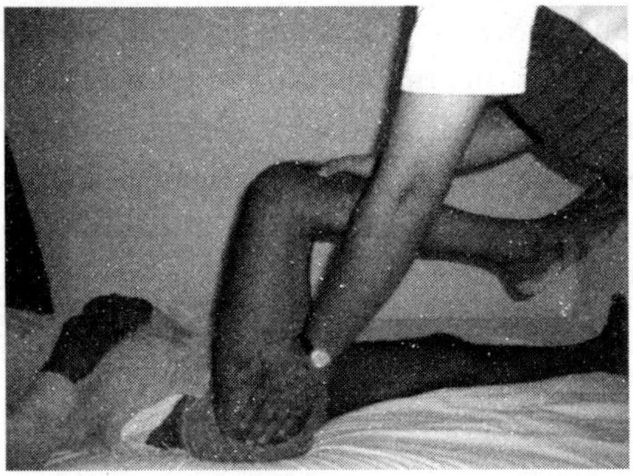

Fig. 41.8 Telescopy test

Ortolani's test

This test is done in supine position. Both hips and knees are fully flexed and gradually abducted. A click of entrance and will be felt as femoral head slips into acetabulum and a click of exit when it quits the acetabulum while pressure is released.

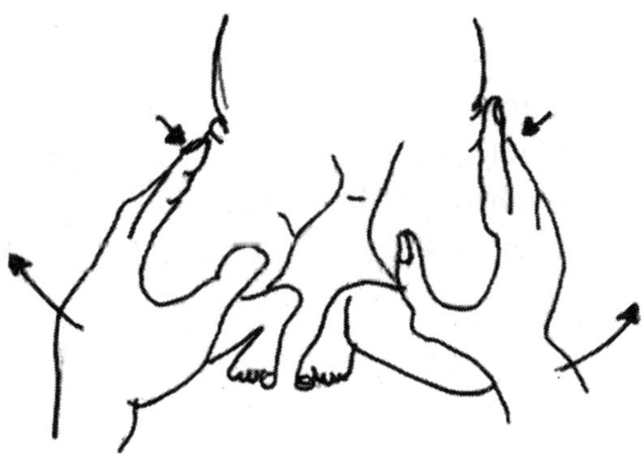

Fig. 41.9 Ortolani's test

Barlow test

In this test both hips are flexed at 90 degree while both knees are fully flexed. Now lower limbs are completely adducted and pressure is exerted downward along the axis of femur. Hand is kept in such a way that thumb remains at medial aspect of proximal thigh and fingers remain over greater trochanter. A sound of cluck can be heard in dislocatable femoral head while it rolls over posterior rim of acetabulum. Hip is dislocated. In second phase of this test hips are now gradually abducted from the position of full adduction. Greater trochanters are pushed inward by fingers over it. Femoral head can be felt to reduce with a sound of cluck into acetabulum.

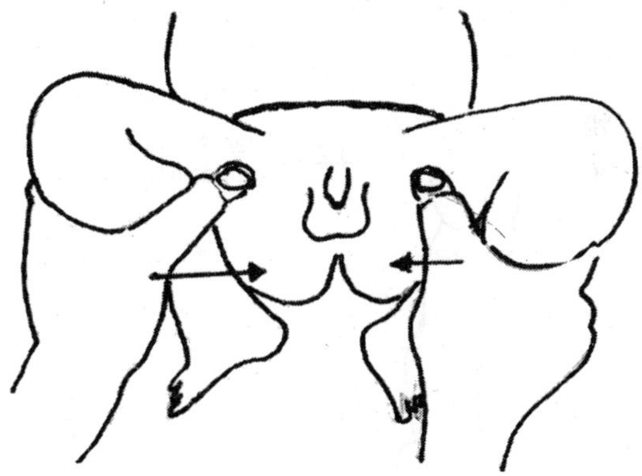

Fig. 41.10 Barlow test

Trendlenberg test

In standing position body weight is equally distributed on both legs. If one leg is lifted other leg will take entire weight of body and pelvis is raised on that side which is not taking weight. This happens due to pull of abductors of hip. This test becomes positive in failed abductor mechanism of hip. Patient is asked to stand on normal limb first. Buttocks on affected side will automatically rise. Now patient is asked to stand on affected limb. Now pelvis on opposite side which is normal sinks down. This test is positive in poliomyelitis, motor neurone disease, muscular dystrophies, congenital dislocation of hip, fracture neck femur, coxa vara, perthes disease etc.

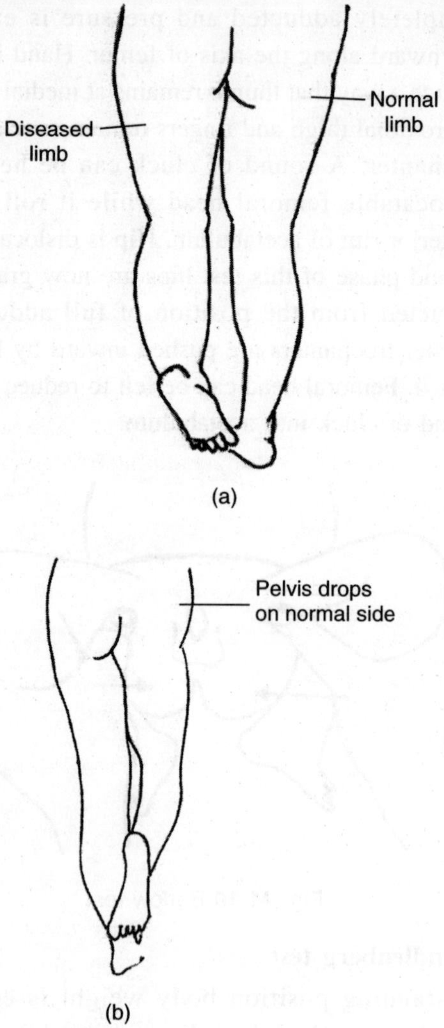

Fig. 41.11 Trendlenberg test

Galeazzi sign

This test is done to detect limb shortening in children. This can be done by flexing both hips and knees. Now levels of knees are compared.

Gauvain sign

This test was first performed by Sir Henry Gauvain. Early cases of tuberculous hip can be detected by this test. Patient is asked to lie supine. Now lower end of thigh is rotated inward and outward. Patient will complaint of pain at hip due to spasmodic contraction of muscle around hip.

EXAMINATION OF KNEE

Knee injuries are commonly seen among footballers and coal miners. A blow on lateral aspect of knee can result in injury to medial collateral ligament. A blow on medial side of knee which is very rare can stress lateral collateral ligament. Meniscus injuries are commonly seen in footballers. Internal rotation of femur on tibia can result in medial meniscus injury, while external rotation of femur on tibia causes lateral meniscus injury. Injured meniscus can lock the knee joint (bucket handle tear) i.e. knee cannot be extended beyond certain degree, but it can be flexed freely. Knee can also be locked due to presence of loose bodies. Bony injuries occur due to direct impact over knee.

Applied Anatomy

Knee joint is a compound synovial joint which is composed of 2 joints as follows:

1. Patellofemoral joint (saddle type)
2. Tibiofemoral joint (hinge type)

Common Clinical Conditions

1. Effusion (Haemarthrosis and traumatic synovitis are common causes).
2. Synovial thickening (inflammatory/infective pathology e.g. tuberculosis, rheumatoid arthritis etc.).
3. Bursitis (housemaid's knee, clergymen's knee.
4. Deformity (triple deformity is seen in tuberculosis of knee).
5. Bone tumors (GCT, Osteosarcoma).

Inspection

Patient should be examined in supine position with both limbs in identical position and completely exposed. Popliteal fossa can be exposed in standing position.

Attitude

Position of knees should be inspected whether it is adducted/abducted, hyperextended or posteriorly subluxated. Stiff knee will cause swinging of affected leg laterally during walking. In arthritis, joint is mildly flexed to accommodate maximum fluid within joint cavity (optimum position). Tripple deformity of knee (T.B. knee and rheumatoid knee) produces flexion, posterior subluxation and lateral rotation of tibia. It happens due to contraction of hamstring muscles. Other deformities e.g. genu valgum, genu varum and genu recurvatum should also be looked for. To find out the cause of genu valgum/varum, patient is asked to sit in squatting position. If deformity disappears, total fault lies in lower end of femur. If deformity does not disappear, fault lies in upper end of tibia.

Bow leg should be differentiated from genu varum. Anterior surface and position of patella tells about nature of existing deformity in lower limb.

Swelling

Bony injuries cause haemorrhagic effusion while ligamentous injuries cause serous or serosanguinous effusion in knee joint. Swelling becomes prominent at superior and lateral aspect of patella. Dislocated patella comes at lateral condyle of femur and it gives false impression of swelling. In cold cases bony swelling should always be looked for.

Wasting of muscle

Disuse of quadriceps muscle can cause muscle wasting in post-traumatic knee.

Palpation

Knee should be palpated for raised temperature and tenderness. Bony landmarks should be palpated (patella, lower end of femur, upper end of tibia and fibula).

Tenderness

Exact point of tenderness should be elicited as it can give indication of site of injury. Joint level tenderness over ligamentous area with no bony tenderness hints toward meniscus injury. If tenderness is present in between ligamentum patellae and tibial collateral ligament it will hint toward anterior horn of medial meniscus injury. If tenderness is posterior to tibial collateral ligament it will hint toward injury of posterior horn (medial meniscus). Gentle pressure should be applied from tip of thumb in between ligamentum patellae and tibial collateral ligament (in a 90 degree flexed knee) to detect injury of meniscus.

Patella

Patella should be palpated along its border to find out any gap. Bony irregularity and tenderness will confirm patellar fracture.

Supracondylar region of femur

In fracture of this region distal fragment is pulled by gastrocnemius muscle posteriory. Proximal fragment can be palpated easily because it projects anteriorly. Bony tenderness and irregularity at femoral condyle will confirm fracture. Dorsalis paedis artery should always be palpated in this fracture due to risk of injury to popliteal artery.

Upper End of Tibia and Fibula

Bony tenderness and irregularity at this area will confirm fracture. Springing test can be performed to detect fracture of upper end of fibula. Lower ends of tibia and fibula are squeezed. It will produce tenderness at fracture site.

Palpation of Swelling

Effusion of knee produces horse hoe shaped swelling. Bilateral effusion is seen in haemophillia, syphyllis (clutton's joint) and in bilateral knee injury. Extraarticular swelling is seen in bursitis. Prepatellar bursitis is seen in housemaid knee. Infrapatellar bursitis is seen in clergymen knee.

Morrant Baker's cyst can be palpated in popliteal fossa. This cyst is herniation of synovium posteriorly through fibres of oblique popliteal ligament. It becomes prominent on extension and disappears on flexion of knee.

Knee should also be palpated to look popliteal aneurysm and meniscus cyst.

Fluctuation test

Suprapatellar pouch is sqeezed with thumb and index finger of one hand and then impulse is felt with thumb and fingers of other hand placed on either side of patella or ligamentum patellae. This test is not helpful in small effusion.

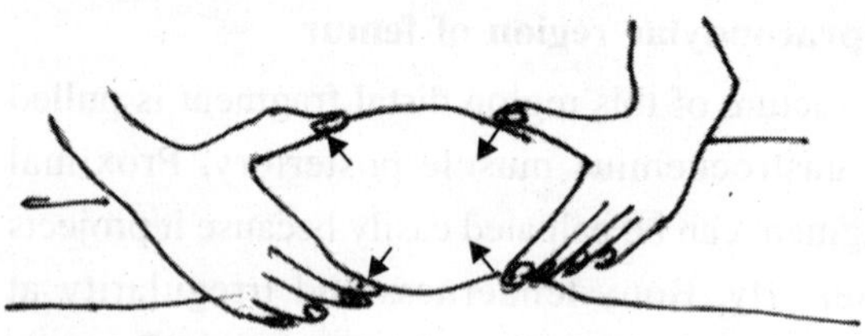

Fig. 41.12 Demonstration of fluctuation test

Patellar tap

Suprapatellar pouch is squeezed toward patella to bring whole of it's fluid into proper joint cavity. Now patella is pushed posteriorly toward femoral condyle with sharp and jerky movement. Patella is felt to strike on femur. This is known as patellar tap.

This test can also be done in standing position. Gentle pressure is applied over one of the obliterated hollows on both sides of ligamentous patellae. If pressure is released, hollow will refill slowly.

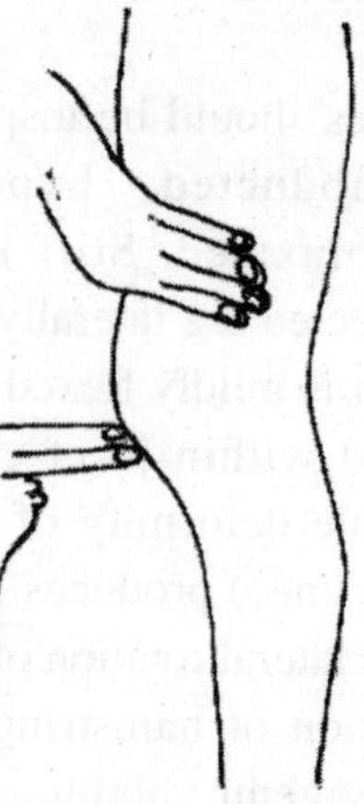

Fig. 41.13 Demonstration of patellar tap

Features of synovial swelling

Synovial thickening can be confirmed by a boggy feel sensation and absence of patellar tap. It also gives feel of earthworm-filled-in bag. This swelling is warm. Fluctuation occurs only in one axis. Edge of synovium can be rolled under finger. Transillumination test is negative. Synovial thickening can not be squeezed to another compartment of knee joint.

Movements

Knee can be flexed up to 135 degree while extension is possible from 135 to zero degree. In a semiflexed knee slight abduction and adduction movements are possible.

McMurray's test

In this test patient lies supine on a couch. Hip is flexed up to 90 degree. Now knee is flexed till heel touches thigh. Now limb is slowly extended by holding ankle in external rotation. Meanwhile valgus stress is given at knee during extension. Pain at medial aspect of knee during valgus stress indicates medial meniscus injury. This test can be repeated by holding ankle in internal rotation and giving varus stress at knee. If patient complaints of pain at lateral aspect of knee, it indicates lateral meniscus injury.

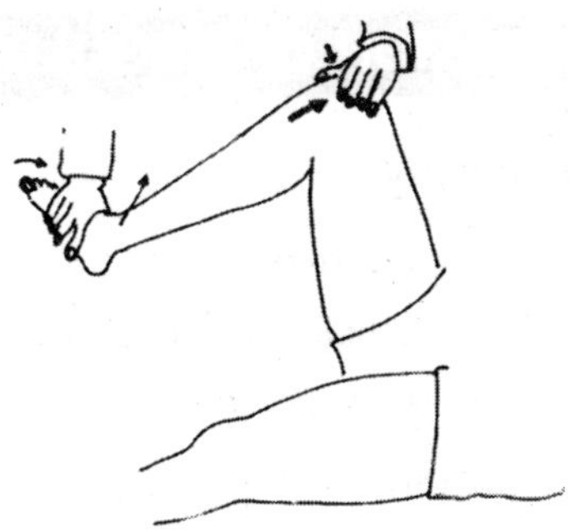

Fig. 41.14 McMurray's test

Apley's grinding test

This test is done in prone position. Examiner keeps his knee over patient's lower end of thigh. Knee is flexed up to 90 degree. Now distract leg upward and rotate it internally and externally. If patient has collateral ligamentous injury he will complaint of pain at corresponding site. Now leg is pushed downward and same rotatory movements are repeated. If meniscus is injured patient will complaint of pain at corresponding site.

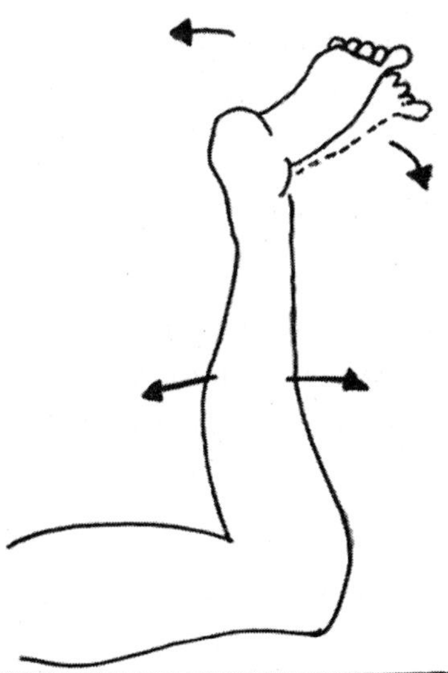

Fig. 41.15 (*a*) Apley's grinding test

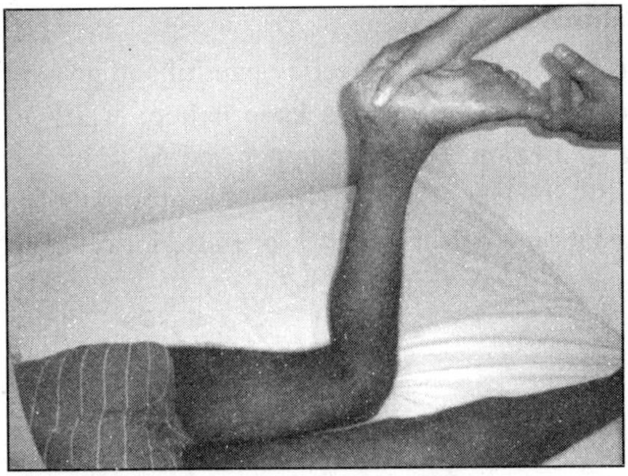

Fig. 41.15 (*b*) Apley's grinding test

Drawer's test

This test is done in supine position. Hip is flexed up to 45 degree and knee is flexed up to 90 degree. Examiner sits on patient's foot and holds his upper end of tibia and draws it antriorly and posteriorly. Anterior or posterior translation of tibia indicates anterior or posterior cruciate ligament injury respectively.

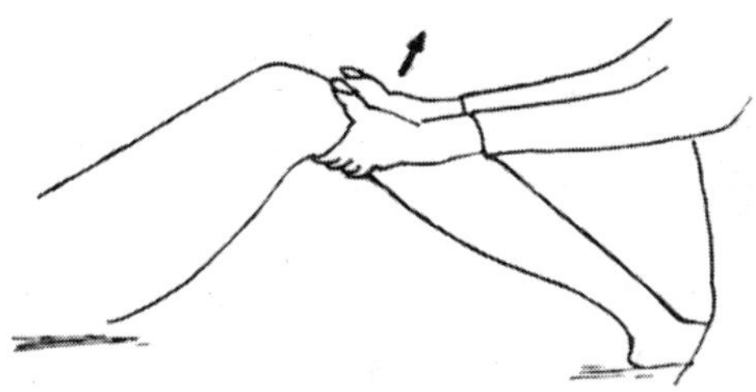

(*a*) Anterior Drawer test

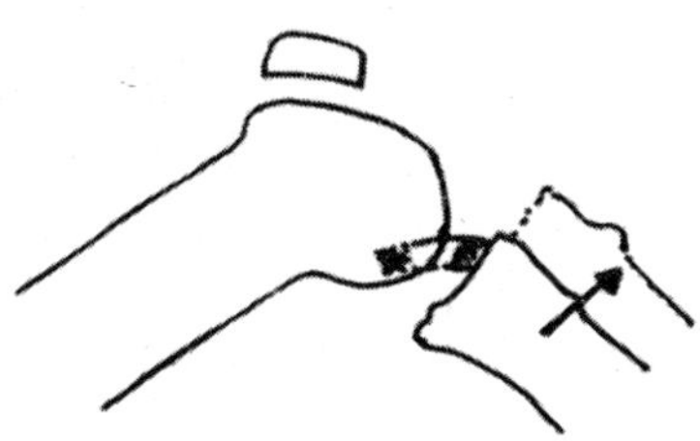

(*b*) Diagrammatic representation of anterior drawer test

Fig. 41.16

Lachman test

This test is done in a severley painful and grossly swollen knee. In this test knee is kept at 20–30 degree flexion. Hold the upper end of tibia and check its translation. Anterior or posterior translation confirms anterior or posterior cruciate ligament injury respectively.

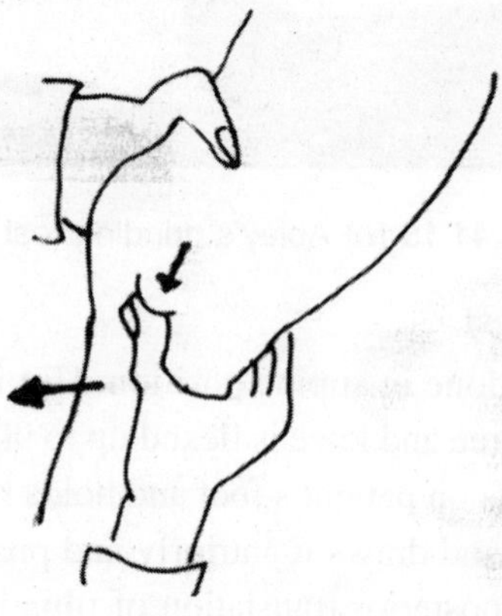

Fig. 41.17 Lachman test

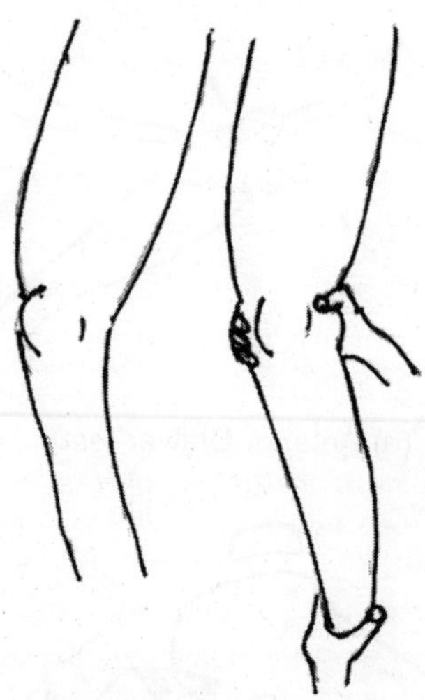

Fig. 41.18 Testing for collateral ligament

Measurements

Any muscle wasting around knee and thigh should be looked.

EXAMINATION OF SHOULDER

Applied Anatomy

Composition of Shoulder

Shoulder in itself is a ball and socket type of joint. It comprises of 4 joints as mentioned below:

1. Glenohumeral joint
2. Acromiaoclavicular joint
3. Sternoclavicular joint
4. Scapulothoracic joint

Rotator cuff and deltoid muscles have main role in glenohumeral function. Rotator cuff consists of four muscles, Subscapularis, Supraspinatus, Infraspinaus and teres minor. Teres minor and infraspinatus are external rotator while subscapularis depresses the head of humerus.

History

Patient may give history of pain, swelling and stiffness in shoulder joint. Pain may be localized in joint. It may radiate from acromian process down to lateral aspect of arm. It should be kept in mind that pain in shoulder may be reffered from other sites e.g. neck, chest and abdomen (due to irritation of diaphragm).

Inspection

Clothes of patient must be removed up to waist before starting examination for proper inspection and also to compare with opposite shoulder.

Attitude

Arm is held by the side of chest, internally rotated and slightly flexed. In traumatic cases arm is supported by other hand and kept slightly raised. Patient of anterior dislocation of shoulder and fracture clavicle supports the flexed elbow of injured side with the normal hand. Patient has the deformity of extension, abduction and external rotation at shoulder in anterior dislocation of shoulder.

Contour

Shoulder may be flattened or swollen. Flattening occurs due to wasting of deltoid muscle. Rheumatoid arthritis, tuberculous arthritis, osteoarthritis and rotator cuff lesion commonly cause wasting of deltoid. Swelling is seen in subacromial bursitis or effusion of joint. Subacromial bursitis shows swelling just beneath the deltoid muscle. In effusion of shoulder joint swelling may extend beyond anterior and posterior margin of deltoid and along the course of long head of biceps tendon. Swelling is always seen in fractures around shoulder joint.

Anterior dislocation of shoulder (subcoracoid type) will show abnormal swelling in deltopectoral groove. In this condition anterior axillary fold is lowered down, acromian process becomes unduly prominent and shoulder becomes flat. Anterior axillary fold is increased. Subcoracoid dislocation shows a bulge at deltopectoral groove.

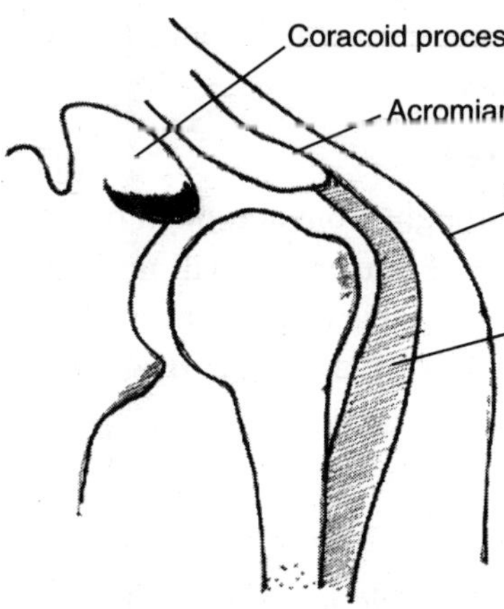

Fig. 41.19 Normal contour of shoulder

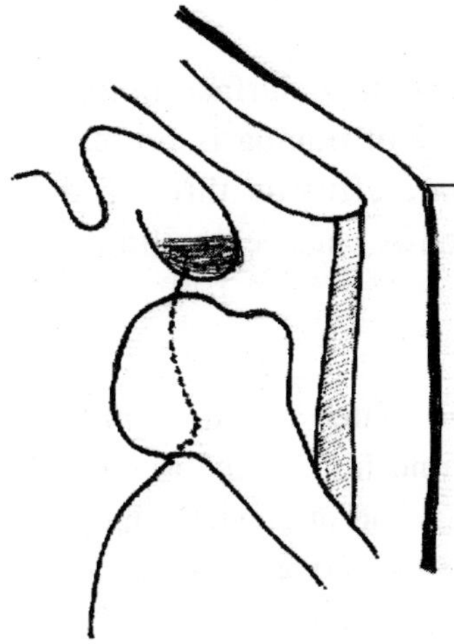

Fig. 41.20 Contour of shoulder after dislocation

In **fracture neck of humerus** roundness of shoulder is maintained but swelling appears below the acromian process. **Fracture of clavicle** will show abnormal prominence at fracture site. Any undue prominence at acromial or sternal end of clavicle hints toward dislocation of acromioclavicular and sternoccavicular joint respectively.

Fracture neck of scapula will show undue lengthening of arm and drooping of shoulder.

Bony arch of shoulder should be inspected to find out any irregularity or swelling.

Palpation

We should look for following points:

Tenderness

Arm should be kept by the chest wall with one hand and with the other hand shoulder should be palpated from all aspect to elicit tenderness.

Tenderness below the acromian process indicates supraspinatus tendinitis. Tenderness below acromian process with the arm in adducted position indicates painful arc syndrome. This tender spot disappears if arm is abducted. Crepitus can be felt in osteoarthritis.

Swelling

Swelling along the bony surface hints toward fracture (If history of trauma is present). It is difficult to palpate effusion through deltoid. Subacromial bursitis causes swelling beneath acromian process.

Clavicle

Patient should be seated on stool and Doctor should stand behind him. Palpation should be started from sternal end of clavicle and proceeds laterally on both sides along the entire length of clavicle. Anterior displacement of sternal end suggests sternoclavicular dislocation. Upward displacement of acromian end suggests acromioclavicular dislocation. A break in continuity of cortex of clavicle suggests fracture of clavicle.

Upper end of humerus

Palpation should be started from acromian process on both sides and fingers should be glided downward to palpate greater tuberosity. Absence of greater tuberosity from its place indicates dislocation of shoulder. Bony tenderness and irregularity at neck of humerus indicates fracture neck of humerus. Direction of head of humerus can be detected by direction of medial epicondyle. Direction of greater tuberosity can be detected by lateral epicondyle.

Loss of transmitted rotation of head of humerus, crepitus and pain at neck of humerus indicates fracture dislocation of shoulder.

Duga's Test

This test has significance in dislocation of shoulder. Ask the patient to touch his normal shoulder. If he is unable to do so it means shoulder is dislocated.

Scapula

Spine of scapula and acromian process should be palpated first. Medial and axillary border should also be palpated. Fracture neck of scapula is difficult to diagnose clinically due to resemblance with fracture upper end of humerus. If we apply axial pressure through a flexed elbow upward a crepitus will be felt which is suggestive of fracture neck of scapula. Along with this shoulder is drooped and tenderness is present medial to glenoid cavity.

3 Bony point's relationship

Shoulder has 3 bony points tip of coracoid process, greater tuberosity of humerus and acromial end of clavicle. If distance between tip of coracoid process and acromial end of clavicle is increased, clavicle comes closer to greater tuberosity and if clavicle becomes proment it means acromioclavicular joint is dislocated.

Measurements

Length of arm

It should be measured from angle of acromian to lateral epicondyle of humerus. Length of arm will be shortened in subcoracoid dislocationof shoulder and fracture neck of humerus. Length of arm will be increased in subglenoid dislocation of humerus (**Callaway's test**) and fracture neck of scapula.

Measurement of vertical circumference of axilla

Vertical circumference of axilla (anterior axillary fold) is increased in anterior dislocation of shoulder, fracture neck of scapula and fracture upper end of scapula.

Hamilton's ruler test

If we keep a ruler straight from acromian process to lateral epicondyle of humerus it will not touch both bony points at the same time. If it is possible it suggests dislocation of shoulder. It becomes possible due to medial displacement of greater tuberosity.

Arm Drop sign

In this test patient is unable to hold the abducted shoulder at 90 degree and shoulder drops by the side of trunk. This test indicates complete tear of rotator cuff.

Apprehension sign

This test is done to detect instability of shoulder. To check this sign passively abduct and externally rotate the shoulder. Patient becomes apprehensive and tries to resist further movement either by making his shoulder stiff or by using his hand.

Painful arc

This painful arc ranges between 60 to120 degree of abduction. Patient complaints of pain during abduction between range of 60 to120. This test is positive in painful arc syndrome. It happens due to impingement of rotator cuff under acromian.

Brayant's sign

Axillary fold is lowered down in dislocation of shoulder. This is known as Brayant's sign.

Movements

Shoulder

Flexion	0–90
Extension	0–45
Adduction	0–45
Abduction	0–180

External & internal rotation(arm in neutral position & held by the side of chest) 0–70

All the active and passive movements at shoulder should be checked.

In painful arc syndrome (supraspinatus tendinitis) initial abduction (0–60 degree) and terminal abduction (120–180 degree) is painless. Pain is felt during mid range of abduction (60–120 degree).

Shoulder joint moves 100–120 degree. Additional 60–80 degree of movement occurs by forward rotation of scapula and some movement of clavicle.

Glenohumeral joint contributes 15 degree and scapular movement contributes 5 degree of every 15 degree of elevation of arm.

EXAMINATION OF ELBOW

Applied Anatomy

Composition of Elbow Joint

Elbow is composed of following three joints as mentioned below in table:

Composition	Type	Function
Humeroulnar	Hinge	Flexion and extension at elbow
Humeroradial	Pivotal	Axial rotation of forearm
Superior radioulnar	Pivotal	Axial rotation of forearm

Examination of elbow should be done in following points:

Inspection

- Attitude
- Swelling
- Deformity
- Muscle wasting

Palpation

Local temperature and tenderness should be checked. Supratrochlear lymph nodes should also be palpated which indicates infective condition e.g., syphyllis.

Following bony landmarks should be palpated:

- Lower end of humerus
- Upper end of radius and ulna
- Olecranon process
- Relationship of 3 bony landmarks (2 epicondyles of humerus and tip of olecranon)

Fracture around elbow can be diagnosed by detecting following clinical signs:

- Local bony tenderness
- Local bony irregularity
- Abnormal bony mobility
- Bony crepitus

Measurements

Muscle wasting should be measured.

Movements

Flexion of elbow is checked from zero position or from the angle of deformity. Normal range of flexion at elbow is 145–0 degree. Elbow can be extended normally 0–145 degree.

Specific Test for Elbow

Cozen Test

This test is positive in tennis elbow. To perform this test, keep the elbow in full extension then extend the wrist against resistance. This will elicit pain at lateral condyle of humerus.

Test for Golfer's Elbow

Keep the elbow in extension and forearm in supination. Now ask the patient to make a fist and then to flex it against resistance. This will elicit pain at medial epicondyle. Pain aggravates by a valgus stress to elbow in extension.

EXAMINATION OF WRIST

Applied Anatomy

Composition of Wrist Joint

Wrist joint is composed of five joints which are mentioned below:

1. Inferior radioulnar joint
2. Radiocarpal joint
3. Ulnocarpal joint
4. Midcarpal joint
5. Intercarpal joint.

History

There are certain clinical entities which are commonly seen. So history should be taken from these points of views. Common clinical conditions around wrist joint are as follows:

1. Colles's fracture (in exam usually malunited case is given)
2. Giant cell tumor (This is common tumor around wrist joint which is kept in exam).
3. Carpal tunnel syndrome
4. Dequervain's disease
5. Madelung's disease
6. Radial club hand and rheumatoid arthritis are usually not kept in exam.

Patient usually presents with the following complaints:

1. Pain
2. Swelling
3. Deformity
4. Loss or restriction of movement at wrist joint.

Inspection

Wrist joint should be inspected on the basis of following points:

- Swelling
- Deformity
- Scar or sinus
- Wasting of muscle

Palpation

Findings which are seen on inspection are confirmed on palpation.

Palpation is done on the basis of following points:

- Local temperature
- Tenderness
- Swelling
- Bony deformity

Measurements

Length of arm and forearm should be measured. Muscle wasting should also be measured if present.

Movements

Wrist

Dorsiflexion	0–70
Palmarflexion	0–90
Radial deviation	0–20
Ulnar deviation	0–30

Specific Test of Wrist Joint

Phalen test

This test is also known as wrist flexion test. Patient is asked to flex the wrist. Patient will feel tingling numbness in distribution area of median nerve. These symptoms subside as soon as wrist is straightend.

Finkelstein test

This test is performed in Dequervain's disease. Patient is asked to pronate his forearm with flexed elbow. Now ask him to make a fist. After this, deviate his fist toward ulnar side. This will result in pain at the site of insertion of APL and EPB.

Finsterer's sign

This sign is positive in Keinbock's disease. Gentle percussion over 3rd metacarpal bone causes pain (provided arm is in pronation).

Maisonneuve sign

This sign is positive in malunited colles's fracture. Ask the patient to flex his elbow and pronate his forearm. If wrist joint shows marked hyperextension it means sign is positive.

EXAMINATION OF SPINE

Patient of spinal disorder may have following complaints:

1. Pain in spine (cervical, thoracic or lumbar).
2. Deformity in above mentioned area of spine.
3. Weakness or paralysis in upper or lower limbs.
4. Pain may be radiated to upper limb or lower limb according to site of lesion.

Inspection

Patient should be exposed up to iliac crest.

1. Check whether the patient can stand up?
2. Check posture of patient.
3. If patient can walk, examine his gait.
4. Whole of spine should be looked for swelling (cold abscess, lipoma etc.).
5. Deformity at spine should be examined from back and from lateral aspect.

Palpation

1. Local **temperature** should be checked.
2. Local **tenderness** can be checked by pressing the spinous process by thumb or by gentle hitting of spine by a fist.

Tenderness at spine can be performed by 3 following methods:

a. Direct pressure tenderness

b. Deep thurst tenderness

c. Twist tenderness.

Direct pressure tenderness

To elicit this tenderness you just directly apply firm pressure by thumb over spinous processes one by one from C-1 to L-5 vertebrae.

Deep thurst tenderness

To elicit this type of tenderness you just make a fist and apply a guarded thurst with proximal part of ulnar side of fist over the spinous process.

Twist tenderness

Apply a twisting pressure by thumb on the side of spinous process from C-1 to L-5 vertebrae.

Anvil test

In this test a sudden jerk is applied over the head of patient. Patient will feel pain at the site of lesion. This test can also be performed in another way. Ask the patient to jump down from a chair. Patient will feel pain at the site of lesion.

Movements

There are 3 movements to be checked at spine:

Flexion

Flexion at spine can be checked at spine by asking the patient to bend forward and touch his feet. Meanwhile examiner feels movement between two spinous processes.

Lateral flexion

This movement is tested by asking the patient to bend sideways. Any restricted movement should be examined.

Rotation of spine

This movement is tested in sitting position. Patient sits on a stool and asked to rotate his spine.

Specific Tests

Few specific tests associated with spinal disease are as follows:

1. SLR test
2. Lasegue test
3. Bragard test
4. Genslen test
5. Pump handle test

Above mentioned tests are discussed in the chapter of "Diseases of back".

Neurological Examination

Neurological examination should be done in following points:

1. Sensory examination
2. Motor examination
3. Reflex
4. Straight leg raising test
5. Lasegue test.

Limb length discrepancy

Both the lower limbs should be measured to check any discrepancy in limb length.

EXAMINATION OF BONY SWELLING

Most important aspect of bony swelling is its history. Most of the diagnosis of bony swelling are made, mainly by history and confirmed by X-ray and biopsy of local part.

Following points should be kept in mind while taking history:

1. Age of patient
2. Onset and course of symptoms
3. History of pain
4. Duration of bony swelling
5. Sinus or discharge from swelling
6. History of similar bony swelling elsewhere in body
7. History of constitutional symptoms
8. Past history
9. Family history.

Age of Patient

Certain bone tumors are seen during certain age: so age of patient is valuable.

Below mentioned table will be helpful in making diagnosis according to age group.

Age	Pathology
Since birth	Bony deformities of Osteogenesis imperfecta
Growing age	Osteoma, osteochondroma and acute osteomyelitis
5–15 years	Unicameral bone cyst
10–20 years	Osteosarcoma, ewingsarcoma, chondroblastoma (osteoblastoma)
10–25 years	Osteoid osteoma
10–30 years	Aneurysmal bone cyst and chondro-myxoid fibroma.
20–30 years	Synovial sarcoma
20–40 years	Giant cell tumor
20–60 years	Chondrosarcoma
30–50 years	Fibrosarcoma
After 40 years	Chordoma and paget's disease
40–60 years	Multiple myeloma
Young adults	Haemangioma

Onset of symptoms

Patient often gives history of trauma in case of osteosarcoma and acute osteomyelitis. But trauma only draws attention at patient toward swelling.

Histroy of high grade fever is found in acute osteomyelitis. Benign tumors grow slowly over a period of time; but malignant tumors grow very rapidly.

History of pain

As far as history of pain is concern, we should ask about site of pain, radiation to extremities, nature of pain, intensity of pain, its duration, its aggravating and relieving factors.

Bone tumors usually present with dull boring pain, whereas throbbing pain is characteristics of inflammation.

Duration of bony swelling

Benign bone tumors have history of long duration, while malignant tumors have very short duration. Acute osteomyelitis also presents within very short duration.

Sinus or discharge from swelling

We should also take history suggestive of sinuses. Discharge of pus or bony pieces suggest osteomyelitis.

Osteomyelitis

History of similar bony swelling

One should always take history of weight loss. We should always ask about similar bony swelling elsewhere in body. Diaphyseal aclasia presents with multiple bony swelling.

History of constitutional symptoms

We should always take history of weight loss fever, loss of appetite etc. There symptoms are suggestive of malignancy.

Past history

This is important in case of acute ostemoyelitis; as pneumonia, otitis media, typhoid fever and boils play a role in etiology of acute osteomyelitis.

Family History

This history must be taken in case of osteopetrosis, osteogenesis imperfecta, diaphyseal aclasia, achondroplasia etc.

First of all general examination should be done after that we should proceed for local examination.

LOCAL EXAMINATION OF SWELLING

Inspection

Following points should be kept in mind while describing a bony swelling:

1. Site

Certain bone tumors have their peculiar position as given in below mentioned table:

Bone tumors	Site of origin
Osteosarcoma	Lower end of femur, Upper end of tibia, Upper end of humerus
Osteoclastoma	Lower end of femur
	Upper end of tibia
Ewing Jarcoma	Diaphysis of Femur, tibia, fibula and humerus
Chondro sarcoma	Proximal end femur and humerus. Illium, ribs and scapula
Chondromyxoid fibroma	Femur and tibia
Multiple myeloma	Skull and trunk bones
Synovial sarcoma	Knee, ankle or wrist joint

2. Size

We should comment on vertical and horizontal dimension of swelling on inspection, as we can not see deeper dimension.

3. Shape

We should never say that swelling is circular, because we are unable to see its deeper dimension. Instead of this we can say that swelling is spherical. Otherwise this could be pearshaped or kidney shaped or avoid or irregular.

4. Surface

Benign tumors have smooth surface, while malignant tumors have irregular surface.

5. Edges of swelling

Edge of swelling can be sessile or pedunculated.

6. Pulsation

Bony tumors usually do not have pulsation. Telengiectatic osteosarcoma is exception. This is seen in aneurysm and vascular growth e.g. carotid body tumors.

7. Number of swelling

This is significant in case of diaphyseal aclasia, as this presents with more than one bony swelling.

8. Skin overlying swelling

Tense, glossy skin with venous prominence is a feature of sarcoma, we should also look for any healed scar mark, or sinus over swelling treated scar mark may hint toward previous operation, while sinus hints toward infection e.g. osteomyelitis.

9. Pressure effect

Oedema and wasting of muscle distal to tumor are pressure effects.

Palpation

1. Local temperature

This should be checked with dorsum of palm. This is raised in osteosarcoma and acute inflammatory condition.

2. Tenderness

Bone tumors are usually non tender. Tenderness is seen in inflammatory condition e.g. osteomyelitis

3. Site, size shape, surface and edge. These should be confirmed by palpation.

4. Consistency

Malignant tumors have bony hard consistency. Giant cell tumor has feel of egg sheel crackling. Diagnostic feature of osteosarcoma is its mixed consistency. Some where it is bony hard, somewhere it is soft and somewhere it is firm.

5. Pulsation

Pulsation can be felt in case of telangiectatic osteosarcoma.

6. Bony irregularity. Sinus/Ulcer

These are features of chronic osteomyelitis.

7. Pathological fracture

This can be present in metastatic carcinoma and bone cyst.

8. Pressure effect

Oedema and muscle wasting or sometimes features of nerve compression should be examined.

9. Fixity to deeper structure

Swelling can be fixed to skin, muscle, nerve, vessel or bone.

Early fixity to skin is a feature of malignant bone tumor.

It tumor is fixed to muscle, it will reduce its power as well as range of motion.

Features of neurovascular deficit may be seen if tumor is fixed to nerve and vessels.

10. Adjacent joints

Adjacent joint should be checked for range of motion.

11. Lymphnodes

Lymph nodes are enlarged in inflammatory condition as well as in late stage of malignancy.

Measurements

Measurement of length and circumference of limb should be done to rule out epiphyseal damage and muscle wasting respectively.

CHAPTER

42 Orthopaedic Viva

(Questions Commonly Asked in Orthopaedic Viva)

Q. 1. How will you define fracture?

Ans. Fracture is a breach in cortex of bone. OR Breach in continuity of lamellar pattern of bone is known as fracture.

Q. 2. What do you know about types of fracture?

Ans. Fractures have been classified into four types as follows:

1. **Aetiological**
   a. Traumatic
   b. Pathological
2. **Clinical**
   a. Simple
   b. Compound
3. **Displacement**
   a. Displaced
   b. Undisplaced
4. **Radiological**
   a. Transverse
   b. Oblique
   c. Spiral
   d. Segmental
   e. Comminuted
   f. Greenstick
   g. Butterfly

Transverse fracture

Fracture line is perpendicular to long axis of bone.

Oblique fracture

Fracture line runs obliquely.

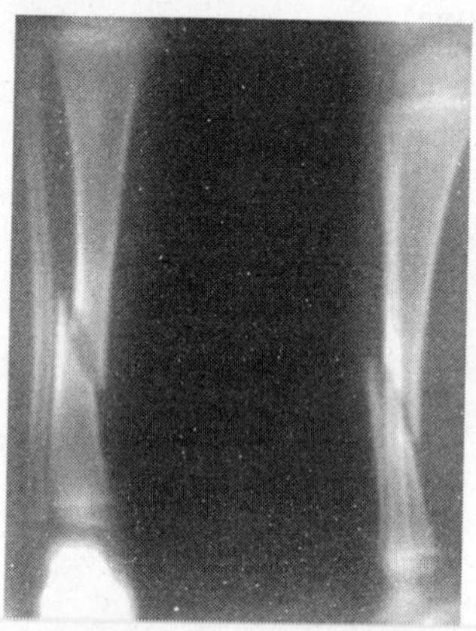

Fig. 42.1 Oblique fracture

Segmental fracture

Two or more fractures are present in a bone at different level.

Comminuted fracture

This type of fracture has more than two fragments in number.

Greenstick fracture

This fracture is commonly seen in children. Only one cortex is broken in this fracture.

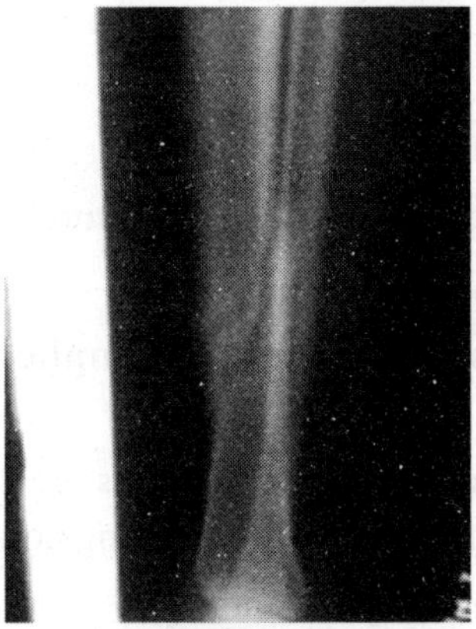

Fig. 42.2 Comminuted fracture

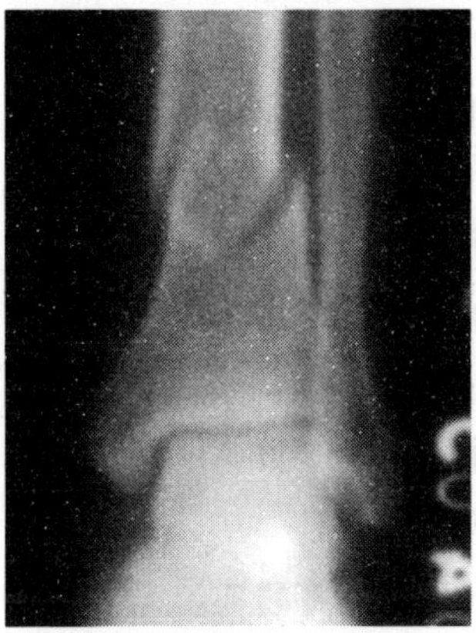

Fig. 42.3 Spiral fracture

Q. 3. What is compound fracture?

Ans. If fracture site or fracture haematoma communicates to external environment; it is known as compound fracture. Any associated abrasion or laceration away from fracture site will not be called compound fracture.

Q. 4. Do you know any compound fracture which does not have breach in skin?

Ans. There are such four fractures:

1. Fracture pelvis associated with injury to urethra or rectum.
2. Fracture ribs associated with rupture of pleural cavity.
3. Fracture mandible.
4. Fracture maxilla.

Q. 5. How will you classify the compound fractures?

Ans. Gustillo and Anderson have classified compound fractures into three types as follows:

Type 1 Wound is less than 1 cm size.

Type 2

- Wound ranges between 1–10 cm.
- Soft tissue is not devitalized
- Little contamination is present

Type 3

- Wound is more than 10 cm
- Soft tissue is devitalized and contaminated.

A. Extensive soft tissue injury but adequate soft tissue is available to cover the fracture site.

B. Extensive soft tissue loss. Bone is exposed and cannot be covered.

C. Compound fracture is associated with arterial injury.

Q. 6. Which injury is more dangerous inside out or outside in?

Ans. Inside out injury is more dangerous because fractured end takes contamination back inside the wound thus spreading infection deep inside the bone. These wound have small size which makes its drainage ineffective.

Q. 7. Why first 6 hours of a compound fracture is known as Golden period?

Ans. Compound fractures are usually contaminated by microorganism present in skin and environment. If such microorganism (bacteria) were allowed to grow, they will multiply their number. This multiplication needs at least 6 hours to reach a level which can establish infection in wound.

Q. 8. What do you understand by debridment?

Ans. Debridment is management of compound fracture in which whole wound is explored and all dead and devitalized tissue is excised. All foreign material is removed from wound. Wound margins are freshened till its edges start bleeding.

Q. 9. What are symptoms of fracture?

Ans. Patient usually presents with 4 symptoms

1. Pain
2. Swelling
3. Deformity
4. Loss of movement.

Q. 10. What are signs of a fracture?

Ans. Fracture has following signs:

1. Bony tenderness
2. Bony crepitus
3. Abnormal mobility
4. Loss of transmitted movement
5. Bony deformity

Q. 11. What are radiological features of good reduction?

Ans. A good reduction should have following features:

1. It should not have any angulation. (except shaft humerus in which 10–15 degree of angulation can be accepted as it is non weight bearing bone and deformity is not prominent).
2. There should not be any distraction or overriding.
3. Fracture should not be displaced.
4. Both the fractured ends should be in close contact to each other. (except in children where 50% contact is enough for fracture healing)

Q. 12. How do you manage fracture (principle of management)?

Ans. Fracture is managed on the following 3 principles:

1. Reduction of fracture
2. Retention of reduced fracture
3. Rehabilitation of limb.

Q. 13. What may be the complications of a fracture?

Ans. Apart from tetnus, gas gangrene and infection a fracture may following complications:

Immediate complications

1. Hypovolaemic shock
2. Neurovascular injury
3. Injury to soft tissue and joint

Early complications

4. Hypovolaemic shock
5. Crush syndrome
6. Fat embolism
7. Septicaemia
8. Compartment syndrome

Late complications

9. Delayed union
10. Nonunion
11. Malunion
12. Synostosis
13. Limb shortening
14. Joint stiffness
15. Avascular necrosis
16. Osteomyelitis
17. Traumatic myositis ossificans

Q. 14. Which are the common fractures to undergo malunion?

Ans. 1. Fracture lower end radius
2. Fracture supracondylar humerus
3. Fracture clavicle
4. Fracture intertrochanteric femur.

Q. 15. Which are the common fractures to undergo nonunion?

Ans. 1. Fracture scaphoid

2. Fracture lateral condyle humerus
3. Fracture lower end of tibia.

Q. 16. What do you understand by plaster of paris?

Ans. Plaster of paris is plaster power which is chemically known as calcium sulphate-hemihydrate. This converts to calcium sulphate dehydrate if water is added to it. This is an exothermic reaction.

$$2(CaSO_4\ ½\ H_2O) + 3H_2O = 2(CaSO_4.2H_2O) + Heat$$

Q. 17. How do you classify the joints?

Ans. Joints have been classified into 3 types as follows:

1. Fibrous Joint (Synorthosis)
2. Cartilaginous Joint (Amphorthosis)
3. Synovial Joint (Diarthrosis)

1. Fibrous Joint

Fibrous joints are immovable joints and further divided into three subtypes as follows:

a. Syndesmosis

b. Sutures

c. Gomphosis

a. Syndesmosis

This kind of joint has got dense fibrous membrane which holds the articular surface close and tight to each other. Distal tibiofibular joint is an example of such kind of joint.

b. Sutural joint

Sagital, coronal and lambdoid sutures of skull come under this type of joint. Bone margins are united by jagged interlocking process.

c. Gomphosis

This kind of joint has one socket into which conical part of bone fits itself e.g.,Teeth and socket of jaw bones.

2. Cartilaginous Joint

This kind of joint is made up of either hyaline cartilage (synchondrosis) or fibrous cartilage (symphysis). This joint provides slight movement. Symphysis pubis is an example of fibrocartilaginous joint whereas articulation between ribs and sternum is an example of synchondrosis.

3. Synovial Joint

Synovial joints are lined by synovial membrane which secretes synovial fluid that keeps joint lubricated and provides nourishment to articular cartilage. Synovial joints has fibrous capsule outside, holding the articulating bones together. These joints are most mobile joint in body. Synovial joints are divided into 3 types as follows:

a. Uniaxial

b. Biaxial

c. Multiaxial

a. Uniaxial joint

It provides movement in one axis; either in horizontal axis (elbow joint) or vertical axis (atlantoocipital joint) known as Hinge and Pivotal joints respectively.

b. Biaxial joint

It provides movements in two axis and two plain at 90 degree. These joints have two subtypes as follows:

(i) Saddle Joint

Articular surface of saddle joint are concave in one direction and convex in other direction whereas the articulating surface of opposite bone is exactly opposite. Carpophalangeal joint of thumb, joints between C1 and C2, the atlantoaxial joint are this kind of joint.

(ii) Condyloid Joint

It has one condyle that fits into a socket e.g., Radiocarpal joint.

c. Multiaxial joint

These joints provide movement in more than two axis. It is subdivided into two types as follows:

(i) Ball and Socket Joint

e.g., Hip, knee and shoulder joint.

(ii) Gliding Joint

This joint provides gliding movement in all planes. e.g., Joints between carpal bone and tarsal bone, joint between articular processess of vertebrae.

Q. 18. What are the different types of plasters and their extent?

Ans. Plaster and their extent have been discussed in Chapter 5 (Plaster, traction and splint)

Q. 19. What are the stages of fracture healing?

Ans. Fracture healing has been divided into five stages as follows:

1. Stage of haematoma
2. Stage of granulation tissue formation
3. Stage of callus formation
4. Stage of remodeling
5. Stage of modeling

Q. 20. What is fat embolism?

Ans. This is a clinical entity in which small vessels are occluded by fat globules. This is also known as post traumatic distress syndrome or acute respiratory distress syndrome. It occurs with in 72 hours of trauma and usually manifests within 24–48 hours.

Aetiology

1. Poly trauma
2. Fracture shaft femur
3. Fracture pelvis
4. Multisystem injuries.

Q. 21. What do you understand by deep vein thrombosis?

Ans. Virchov's triad is clinical presentation of deep vein thrombosis. It has following components.

1. Venous stasis
2. Vascular damage
3. Hypercoagulability.

Causes of DVT

1. Fracture pelvis
2. Fracture shaft femur
3. Fracture shaft tibia
4. Surgical procedure
5. Prolonged immobilization
6. Oestrogen intake
7. Pregnancy
8. Hypercoagulable conditions
9. Obesity
10. Behcet's disease
11. T.A.O.

Q. 22. What is crush syndrome?

Ans. Crushing of muscles due to prolonged compression leads to extensive muscle necrosis and release of large quantity of myoglobin and potassium into systemic circulation. This condition is known as Crush syndrome. This may become life threatening.

In this condition blood urea nitrogen is increased which leads to myoglobulin renal failure. (crush kidney)

Q. 23. What is compartment syndrome?

Ans. Raised pressure of more than 40 mm of water in osseofascial-compartment is known as compartment syndrome. This condition hampers the blood supply to muscles and nerves leading to ischaemia of muscle. Later muscles are grossly swollen.

Causes

1. Supracondylar fracture of humerus
2. Fracture both bones forearm
3. Crush injury of leg and forearm
4. Fracture of shaft tibia.

Q. 24. What is gas gangrene?

Ans. This is a fatal complication of road traffic accidents. This is mainly caused by Clostridium Welchii. Clostridium septicum and oedematiens are other organism which may cause gas gangrene. Clostridium is found in intestine and soil. Patient presents with pain in wound, grossly swollen muscle, toxaemia and vomiting. Crepitations can be felt over muscle. Exposed muscles become brick-red. Toxins released by clostridium act on adrenal glands leading to low blood pressure. X-ray is confirmatory which shows gas bubbles.

Q. 25. What do you understand by avascular necrosis of bone?

Ans. This is also known as aseptic necrosis of bone. Death of bone occurs due to lack of blood supply.

Aetiology

1. Fracture dislocation
2. Excessive stripping of periosteum from bone during surgery.
3. Caisson (Dysbaric) disease
4. Prolong intake of corticosteroid
5. Prolong intake of alcohol
6. Bone transplantation
7. Organ transplantation
8. Exposure to X-rays and radioactive substance
9. Metal erosion and ionization
10. Excessive reaming of intramedullary cavity, prior to insertion of nail.

Common Sites of AVN

1. Head of femur
2. Scaphoid
3. Talus

Other Sites of AVN

1. Capitellum
2. Segmental fractures

Q. 26. What is high radial nerve palsy?

Ans. Triceps and anconeus are spared in high radial nerve palsy. This is seen when radial nerve is injured in radial groove. Rests of the muscles (supplied by radial nerve) are paralysed. In very high radial nerve palsy all the muscles including triceps are paralysed.

Clinically patient presents with loss of wrist extension, digital extension, and loss of radial abduction of thumb, loss of accessory forearm flexion and loss of accessory supination. Sensation is lost at lateral 2/3rd of dorsal aspect of hand.

Q. 27. What is low radial nerve palsy?

Ans. All the muscles supplied by radial nerve in distal arm are paralysed except brachioradialis and extensor carpi radialis longus and brevis.

Q. 28. What is crutch palsy?

Ans. Radial nerve injury caused by improper use of crutch or due to fracture dislocation of upper end humerus is known as crutch palsy.

Q. 29. What is saturday night palsy?

Ans. This radial nerve palsy occurs when patient takes deep sleep on a chair under the influence of alcohol (with arm hanging at the edge of chair).

Q. 30. What is claw hand?

Ans. In this deformity hyperextension occurs at MP joint and flexion occurs at PIP and DIP joint. It occurs due to paralysis of interossei and lumbricals (which cause flexion at MP joint and extension at PIP and DIP joint). Claw hand is seen in ulnar nerve injury. If median nerve is also injured e.g., Klumpke's paralysis, it becomes more prominent.

Q. 31. What is Ulnar paradox?

Ans. High ulnar nerve palsy causes less deformity is known as Ulnar paradox. In high ulnar nerve palsy FDP (medial half) is paralyzed and does not work unopposed by interossei and lumbricals. This makes the deformity less obvious.

Q. 32. What is Volkman's ischaemia?

Ans. This is ischaemia of muscles and nerves of forearm (flexor compartment). Ischaemia occurs due to occlusion of brachial artery that causes reduced blood supply to flexor group of muscles of forearm. Flexor polices longus and Flexor digitorum profundus (medial half) are the commonly affected muscles in Volkman's ischaemia. It happens because these are supplied by an end artery; anterior interoseous artery. Ischaemia of these muscles causes **Compartment syndrome.**

Clinical Features of Volkman's Ischaemia

1. Pain in forearm.
2. Pallor (due to reduced capillary filling time).
3. Paresthesia.
4. Paralysis.
5. Pain on passive stretching of fingers.
6. Pulselessness
7. Swelling and tenderness over forearm.

Q. 33. What is Volkman's ischaemic contracture?

Ans. This is deformity of hand, wrist and forearm developing as a sequele to Volkman's ischaemia in which wrist and fingers go into flexion contracture.

Clinical features of VIC

1. Flexion contracture of forearm due to involvement of flexor digitorum profundus and flexor pollices longus.
2. Claw hand deformity may be present.
3. **Volkman's sign** is positive, i.e. extension of wrist exaggerate the deformity while flexion causes opposite to it. In other words fingers can be extended at interphalangeal joint only when wrist is flexed.
4. Contracture of joint and soft tissue with scarring of skin is also seen.
5. Bones are also deformed.
6. Sensory and motor loss may occur in forearm and hand due to peripheral nerve involvement.

Q. 34. What is pulled elbow?

Ans. If we lift a child by holding his wrist, head of radius may come out of annular ligament. This condition is known as pulled elbow.

Q. 35. What is Monteggia fracture?

Ans. Fracture of upper third of ulna with dislocation of head of radius is known as Monteggia fracture.

Q. 36. What is Galeazzi's fracture?

Ans. This is a fracture of shaft radius at the junction of middle and distal third, associated with subluxation or dislocation of distal radioulnar joint. This is also known as fracture of necessity i.e., open reduction and internal fixation is necessary if good result is to be achieved. This is also known as reverse of Monteggia fracture.

Q. 37. What is Colles's fracture?

Ans. This is a transverse fracture of lower end of radius within 3/4th of an inch from its distal articular margin at the corticocancellous junction occurring as a result of fall on outstretched hand leading to dinner fork deformity, commonly seen in post menopausal elderly females.

Q. 38. What is Jone's fracture?

Ans. This is fracture of base of 5th metatarsal. This is caused by pull of tendon of peroneus brevis muscle which is attached here.

Q. 39. What is Pott's fracture?

Ans. This was described by Sir Percivial Pott. This is bimalleolar fracture of ankle i.e. fracture of medial and lateral malleolus.

Q. 40. What is Cotton's fracture?

Ans. This was described by Cotton. This includes fracture of medial, lateral and posterior malleolus.

Q. 41. What is Aviator's fracture?

Ans. This is fracture of neck of talus caused by forced dorsiflexion of ankle, sustained in aircraft crash. It may be associated with posterior dislocation of body of talus.

Q. 42. What is rickets?

Ans. Rickets is a metabolic bone disease of children in which osteoid fails to mineralize due to faulty calcium metabolism. It is characterized clinically by softening of bone and development of bony deformity, radiologically by delayed appearance of epiphysis and widened epiphyseal plate, cupping and slipping of metaphysis (champagne glass appearance).

Q. 43. What is osteomalacia?

Ans. Osteomalacia is a clinical entitiy in which bones become soft due to excess of osteoid tissue and bone matrix fails to mineralize. It is adult counterpart of rickets.

Q. 44. What is osteoporosis?

Ans. When the rate of bone resorption (osteoclastic activity) exceeds the bone formation (osteoblastic activity) it results in deficiency of protein matrix in which calcium is laid down. This condition leads to diffuse reduction in bone density; known as osteoporosis. This is a metabolic bone disease commonly seen in old age people.

Q. 45. What is torticollis?

Ans. This is a rotational deformity of neck that produces turning and tilting deformity of head. This is also known as **wry neck**. Congenital torticollis is most common type of permanent torticollis.

Aetiology

1. Congenital
2. Traumatic
3. Infective (Tuberculosis of spine, Tonsillitis, labyrynthitis and infection of atlantoaxial joint)
4. Cervical disc prolapse
5. Spasmodic torticollis
6. Paralytic torticollis
7. Myositis
8. Neuritis of 11th nerve
9. Rheumatoid arthritis.

Q. 46. What is genu varum?

Ans. This is defined as lateral angulation of knee joint with medial deviation of longitudinal axis of femur and tibia.

Q. 47. What is genu valgum?

Ans. Medial angulation of knee with outward deviation of longitudinal axis of both femur and tibia is known as genu valgum deformity.

Q. 48. What is carpal tunnel syndrome?

Ans. This is compression neuropathy of median nerve while it passes beneath flexor retinaculum. This results due to narrowing of carpal tunnel. This is commonly seen in rheumatoid arthritis, pregnancy and as acomplication of Colle's fracture. Wowen of 40–60 years of age are commonly affected.

Aetiology

Idiopathic: This is most common cause.

Inflammatory

- Rheumatoid arthritis
- Osteoarthritis of wrist

Endocrinal

- Myxoedema
- Acromegaly

Post-traumatic

- Colles's fracture

Q. 49. What is ganglion?

Ans. This is pseudomucinous degeneration of tendon sheath or joint capsule. Patient presents with localized swelling which may or may not be painful. Common sites of ganglion are wrist, forearm and foot. This is multiloculated and can be relived by aspiration of cyst.

Q. 50. What is tennis elbow?

Ans. This is a clinical condition in which tendinous origin of common wrist extensor is affected that causes pain at the tip of lateral condyle of humerus. This is commonly seen in tennis players.

Q. 51. What is Golfer's elbow?

Ans. This is a clinical condition that affects tendinous insertion of common flexors of hand. This is also known as epitrochleitis.

Q. 52. What is Student's elbow?

Ans. This is a clinical condition in which olecranon bursa undergoes chronic inflammation. This is also known as olecranon bursitis.

Q. 53. What is trigger finger?

Ans. This is a clinical condition in which digital fibrous sheath is constricted in such a way that flexor tendon cannot glide freely. In this condition finger moves like trigger of a pistol. Finger is locked in flexed position and can only be extended by applying a force.

Q. 54. What is dequervain's disease?

Ans. This is tenovaginitis of common sheath of abductor pollices longus and extensor pollicis brevis tendons.

Clinical features

Patient presents with pain and swelling at radial styloid process. Tenderness is present at radial styloid.

Abduction of thumb across the palm and forced ulnar deviation causes pain at radial styloid process.

Q. 55. What is Dupuytren's contracture?

Ans. This is contracture of palmar aponeurosis which leads to flexion deformity of ring and little finger at MP and PIP joint. Palmaris aponeurosis is continuation of palmaris longus tendon.

Aetiology

Dupuytren's contracture can develop in following conditions:

1. Hereditary
2. Cirrhosis
3. Epilepsy
4. Drug induced: Phenylhydantoin
5. Chronic alcoholics
6. Trauma.

Q. 56. What is Tom-smith's arthritis?

Ans. Septic arthritis of infants is known as Tom-smith arthritis. It is clinically similar to congenital dislocation of hip.

Q. 57. What is Rolando's fracture?

Ans. Extraarticular fracture of base of first metacarpal is known as Rolando fracture. It can be managed by closed reduction followed by thumb spica for three weeks.

Q. 58. What is Bennett's fracture?

Ans. Edward Bennet was the first person to describe this fracture. This is an intraarticular fracture of base of first metacarpal of thumb. It may be associated with subluxation or dislocation of first metacarpophalangeal joint.

Q. 59. What is Barton's fracture?

Ans. This is fracture of distal articulating surface of radius. Barton fracture is treated by closed reduction followed by cast immobilization. If closed reduction fails, open reduction and internal fixation is done by buttress plate. Barton fracture is of **two subtypes** as follows:

Volar Barton Fracture

If fracture line passes through volar margin of distal articulating surface of radius, it is called as volar barton fracture.

Dorsal Barton Fracture

If fracture line passes through dorsal margin of distal articulating surface of radius, it is known as Dorsal Barton fracture.

Q. 60. What is Chauffer's fracture?

Ans. This is the fracture of radial styloid process and usually associated with scapholunate ligament tear, radial shortening and significant dorsal angulation. It is treated by closed reduction and percutaneous pin fixation.

[*Questions on other topics e.g. CTEV, chronic osteomyelitis, fracture neck femur/ intertrochanteric femur, radial nerve palsy, foot drop, non union, claw hand, bone tumors and cubitus varus (gunstock deformity) have been discussed under the chapter of clinical case presentation*]

CHAPTER

43 Clinical Case Presentation

- Congenital talipes equino varus
- Foot drop
- Radial nerve palsy
- Claw hand (Ulnar nerve injury)
- Chronic osteomyelitis
- Nonunion
- Fracture neck femur
- Cubitus varus
- Fracture intertrochanteric femur
- Giant cell tumor (Osteoclastoma)
- Osteosarcoma
- Ewing sarcoma

CONGENITAL TALIPES EQUINO VARUS

Q. 1. What are your findings on inspection?

Ans.

- Foot is small and bean shaped with a smaller heel.
- Tendoachillis is contracted.
- Splaying is seen in forefoot.
- Skin creases are present posteriorly above the heel and meadially at the forefoot and hindfoot junction.
- Callosities are present over dorsolateral aspect of foot.
- Bony prominence may also be seen at this place.
- Wasting of calf muscle is also seen.
- Following deformities are present at their corresponding joint:

Equinus (plantar flexion) at ankle joint

Inversion at Subtalar joint

Forefoot adduction at Midtarsal joint

Forefoot cavus at Midtarsal joint

(Talocalcaneal joint is called as subtalar joint. Talonavicular and calcaneocuboid joints are called as midtarsal joint.)

Q. 2. Apart from local examination did you examine spine, and why?

Ans.

- I examined spine to look any evidence of open neural tube defect, e.g., spina bifida, meningomyelocoele.
- I looked for tuft of hair or naevus or lipomatous mass at low back in case of spina bifida occulta.

- I looked for midline soft tissue mass which is suggestive of meningocoele or meningomyelocoele.
- I looked for other congenital anomalies e.g., cleft lip, supernumerary digits. I looked at limbs, face, chest and abdomen.
- I also looked for congenital dislocation of hip.

Q. 3. What did you find on palpation?

Ans. I confirmed my findings which I found on inspection.

Q. 4. Did you measure lateral and medial border of foot and what is its significance?

Ans. In this foot lateral to medial border ratio is reversed to 1.2. (normally medial to lateral border ratio is 1.2). This is known as B.N. Sinha index. This indicates severity of forefoot adduction.

Q. 5. How will you confirm that foot is normal?

Ans. If I dorsiflex the foot without any deviation, toes will touch the shin. It means foot is normal.

Q. 6. What is your diagnosis?

Ans. Congenital talipes equino varus (unilateral/ bilateral).

Q. 7. What is the meaning of talipes?

Ans. Talipes is a latin word which is also known as club foot. Talus means ankle bone while pes means foot.

Q. 8. What do you understand by varus?

Ans. Adduction and inversion deformity combinely is known as varus.

Q. 9. What is the cause of CTEV in your case?

Ans. Idiopathic (most common cause).

Q. 10. What are other causes of CTEV?

Ans. Aetiology of CTEV

1. Idiopathic is commonest cause.
2. Neurogenic
   a. Spina bifida occulta
   b. Meningocoele
   c. Meningomyelocoele
   d. Diastematomyelia
   e. Cerebral palsy
3. Myopathic
   Arthrogryposis multiplex congenita
4. Osteopathic
   Congenital absence of fibula is a common example.

Q. 11. What is acquired talipes equino varus?

Ans. This means that deformity develops later in life. It is not present since birth.

Q. 12. How will you differentiate between CTEV and acquired talipes equinovarus (ATEV)?

Ans.

	CTEV	ATEV
Duration	Since birth Most common cause is idiopathic.	Develops later in life. Polio is commonest cause. Other causes are LPN palsy, burn contracture, peroneal muscle dystrophy and Freidrich's ataxia.
History of polio	absent	present
Correction of deformities	Possible by manipulation before treatment	Possible if contracture has not established.
Medial skin crease	Peculiar feature	Absent
Muscle wasting	Absent	Present
Other features	of CTEV	of polio are seen

Q. 13. What do you understand by mobile and rigid CTEV?

Ans. Mobile CTEV

Deformities of foot can be partially corrected in mobile CTEV.

Rigid CTEV

Deformities can be hardly corrected or only one component of deformity can be corrected.

Q. 14. How to classify CTEV clinically?

Ans. Clinically it has been classified into following three types:

Resistant CTEV

If CTEV does not respond to treatment, it is known as resistant CTEV.

Relapse CTEV

If deformity reccurs inspite of getting adequate treatment it is called as relapse CTEV.

Neglected CTEV

If patient has not taken any treatment for a long time it is known as neglected CTEV.

Q. 15. What are indications of X-ray in CTEV?

Ans. Indications of X-ray

1. Neglected CTEV (To look for bony changes e.g., superior articulating surface of talus is partially out of ankle mortis that may change the preoperative planning of surgeon).
2. Tripple arthrodesis
3. To detect Kite angle (Angle between long axis of talus and calcaneum is called as Kite angle. Normally it is >35 degree. In CTEV this angle is reduced).

Q. 16. How will you manage this case?

Ans. One line answer for child of 1 month-3 years is repeated stretching and corrective manipulation followed by retention of correction in above knee POP cast till overcorrection is achieved.

Q. 17. Can you explain complete management of CTEV from day 1 to rehabilitation?

Ans.

1. Start the treatment as soon as possible or from the day one of seeing patient.
2. First 3 weeks since birth are called golden period for treatment because in this period relaxin hormone remains in circulation that keeps the ligaments relaxed. So ligaments are amenable to stretching.
3. In new born child skin is not mature enough for plaster so mother should be taught about repeated stretching and corrective manipulation of foot 5–6 times in a day or while at every time of feeding till 2–4 weeks.
4. Treatment for the age group of **1 month to 3 years is repeated stretching and corrective manipulation followed by retention of correction in AKPOP cast till over correction is achieved.** Knee is kept at 90 degree of flexion. To check over correction just tickle the sole. if dorsiflexion and adduction both are present it means over correction is achieved. BKPOP cast usually slips like a socks, so always apply AKPOP cast. It can also take care of internal tibial torsion deformity if present in child.
5. **Sequence of correction** starts from Adduction-Inversion-Equinus. If we do not follow this sequence, child will develop **Rocker bottom foot.** (convexity develops at sole of foot).
6. Aim of treatment is to provide painless, mobile and cosmetically normal appearing foot.
7. After achieving the correction Denis-Brown splint or Night shoes are prescribed to patient of less than walking age group. These shoes should be worn through day and night and can be removed 4-5 times in a day to clean and manipulate the foot. Both

the shoes are connected by a connecting bar which is connected in such a way that dynamic correction of deformity occurs while child kicks his leg.

8. Orthopaedic boot with straight and stiff border, with outside crooked and elongated heel are prescribed to child of more than walking age group. Forefoot adduction is corrected by straight and stiff medial border. Correction of varus is maintained by outside crooked and elongated heel. Denis Brown splint can be prescribed to these children during night time. These orthopaedic shoes should be used till bony maturity has achieved. (till 10–12 years of age)

Q. 18. What is extent of AKPOP cast in CTEV?

Ans. Proximally it is applied up to junction of upper and middle third of thigh. Distally on plantar aspect it is applied up to tips of toes to prevent curling of toes. Dorsally it is applied just proximal to MP joint. Medially it should extand till tip of great toe to maintain correction of adduction deformity.

Q. 19. How will you judge that deformity is over corrected?

Ans. If I tickle the sole of foot child will actively dorsiflex and evert his foot. It means overcorrection is achieved.

Q. 20. Are there any chances of complications of conservative treatment?

Ans. Conservative treatment can develop following complications:

1. Recurrence of CTEV
2. Plaster sore
3. Painful and stiff foot
4. Table top talus (Flat toped talus) can occur due to osteochondral compression fracture of talus.
5. Rocker bottom foot.
6. Neurovascular deficit of foot.

Q. 21. What are the surgical procedures if this conservative treatment fails?

Ans. There are several surgical methods, but following below mentioned methods are commonly performed, according to age group.

1. Posteromedial Soft Tissue Release (PMSTR)

This operation can be done up to 3 years of age.

Following **posterior structures** are released:

1. Lengthtening of tendoachilis by Z-plasty.
2. Posterior capsulotomy of ankle and subtalar joint.
3. Release of posterior talofibular and calcaneofibular ligament.

Following **medial structures** are released:

1. Lengthening of tendons of
   a. Tibialis posterior
   b. Flexor digitorum longus
   c. Flexor hallucis longus
2. Three ligaments are released:
   a. Talonavicular ligament
   b. Deltoid ligament (superficial ligament)
   c. Spring ligament
3. Capsule of naviculocuneiform and cuneiform-first metatarsal joint are released. Interosseous talocalcaneal ligament are also released.

2. Steindler's Release (Plantar release)

Extraperiosteal release of structure from medial calcaneal tuberosity is known as Steindler's release. Following structures are released:

1. Plantar apponeurosis
2. Flexor hallucis brevis
3. Abductor hallucis
4. Abductor digiti quinti minimi

3. Limited Soft Tissue Release

If only one component of deformity remains after conservative treatment, limited (selective) soft tissue release can be done e.g., posterior release for equinus, medial release for adduction and plantar release for cavus deformity.

4. Tendon Transfer

At the age of 5 years tendon transfer can be done. Tibialis anterior can be transferred to outer side of foot.

5. Dwyer's Osteotomy

This osteotomy is done **at the age of 3 years** to correct the varus at heel. Before the age of 3 years it is not recommended as the calcaneum is cartilaginous. This is an open wedge osteotomy of calcaneum by which varus of heel can be corrected.

6. Evan's Procedure

This surgery is performed **at the age of 4–8 years.** This procedure is indicated in neglected or recurrent CTEV. In this procedure calcaneocuboid fusion is done along with posteromedial soft tissue release. Calcaneocuboid fusion restricts the growth on lateral side of foot, leading to gradual correction of deformity.

7. Wedge Tarsectomy

This procedure is performed **at the age of 8–11 years**. Indication of this operation is neglected CTEV. In this operation triangular wedge of bone is removed from midtarsal area with it's base facing toward dorsolaeral side. After removing the wedge foot is brought in plantigrade position.

8. Triple Arthrodesis

This is indicated in patients of more than 12 years of age. In this procedure 3 joints are fused; subtalar, calcaneocuboid and talonavicular.

9. Joshi's External Stabilization System (JESS)

JESS frame is designed by Dr. B.B. Joshi (Bombay). The principle of controlled differential distraction is applied to correct all the aspect of deformities by gradual, sequential stretching of soft tissue by Kirschner wires anchored in bone. Jess is applied in children of more than 6 years age usually. But this frame is successfully used in all presentation of CTEV in children between the age of 3 months to their adulthood.

Advantages of JESS

1. It causes lengthening of all contracted tissue, preventing histogenesis without cutting and with minimal scaring of tissue.
2. No further shortening of foot in revision cases.
3. Magnitude of correction is controlled.
4. Results are much supplied as compared with surgical release.

Indications of JESS

1. All such cases of congenital and acquired talipes equino varus that cannot be corrected by conservative treatment.
2. Relapse cases of CTEV.
3. Arthrogryposis multiplex congenita.
4. Late presentation of cases.
5. Adjunct to surgical treatment for realignment of skeleton and to minimize bone resection and shortening of foot.

FOOT DROP

Q. 1. What are your findings on inspection?

Ans. My findings on inspection are as follows:

Patient walks with a high stepping gait.

1. **Deformity:** Foot drop is present in R/L foot.
2. **Muscle wasting:** Anterolateral aspect of leg shows wasting of muscle.
3. **Loss of motor power:** Certain groups of muscles are paralyzed.

A. Tibialis Anterior (main extensor of ankle)-active dorsiflexion at ankle is lost.

B. Extensor Hallucis Longus-active extension at great toe is lost.

C. Extensor Digitorum Longus-active extension at other toes is also lost.

D. Peroneus Longus and Brevis-active eversion is also lost.

Q. 2. What did you find on palpation?

Ans. I found anaesthesia over dorsum of foot (autonomous zone of nerve-central strip of skin at dorsum of foot). Skin at dorsum of foot is dry.

Q. 3. Which nerve is involved in this case?

Ans. Lateral popliteal nerve.

Q. 4. Why do you say so?

Ans. Because my findings are suggestive of lateral popliteal nerve palsy.

Q. 5. What is the other name of this nerve?

Ans. Common peroneal nerve.

Q. 6. Do you know the division of sciatic nerve?

Ans. Sciatic nerve divides into two division:

1. **Tibial division** (posterior tibial/medial popliteal nerve. This nerve divides further into 2 branches Lateral and medial plantar nerve.
2. **Peroneal division** (common peroneal/ lateral popliteal nerve). This nerve further divides into 2 branches:Superficial (musculocutaneous) and Deep peroneal (anterior tibial) nerve.

Q. 7. Can you tell me the area of distribution of lateral popliteal nerve?

Ans. Superficial nerve supplies:

1. Lateral aspect of leg.
2. Skin over lateral malleolus.
3. Skin over dorsum of foot.

Deep peroneal nerve supplies 1st web space over dorsum of foot.

Q. 8. What are other nerves which supply foot?

Ans. Medial border is supplied by saphenous nerve. Lateral border is supplied by sural nerve. Sole and tips of toes are supplied by posterior tibial nerve.

Q. 9. Can you enumerate the causes of lateral popliteal nerve palsy?

Ans.

1. Tight plaster application up to neck of fibula can cause LPN palsy.
2. Wrongy applied skin traction.
3. Thomas knee splint application without proper padding
4. Gross varus strain at knee due to fracture of medial condyle of tibia can also cause LPN palsy.
5. Dislocated knee is also a cause.
6. Leprosy.

Q. 10. What are the things that lead to foot drop?

Ans. Due to lateral popliteal nerve palsy extensors of ankle are lost. So combination of gravity and unopposed action of plantar flexors make dropping of foot.

Q. 11. Why is it not sciatic nerve palsy?

Ans. Because following additional features of medial popliteal (posterior tibial) nerve are absent:

1. Loss of plantar flexion at ankle and toes.
2. Paralysis of intrinsic muscles of foot
3. Anaesthesia over sole of foot.

Q. 12. How will you manage this case?

Ans. As nerve palsy has chances of recovery till 18 months. So I will wait for recovery but during this period I will give him toe raising appliance and below knee caliper with posterior check.

Q. 13. If recovery does not occur after 18 months?

Ans. Tendon transfer is the treatment of choice at this age.

Tibialis posterior can be transferred to substitute tibialis posterior muscle.

Incomplete foot drop can be managed by transfer of tibialis posterior to EHL along with peroneus brevis transfer that checks excessive valgus deformity due to excessive eversion.

RADIAL NERVE PALSY

Q. 1. What are your findings on inspection?

Ans. My findings on inspection are as follows:

1. **Deformity:** Patient has wrist drop and finger drop deformity.
2. **Muscle wasting** is present at extensor aspect of forearm.
3. **Loss of motor power**
   - Extensor muscles of wrist
   - Finger extensors
   - Thumb extensor
4. **Autonomic changes:** Hair loss is seen at hand and extensor aspect of forearm. Finger nails seems to be brittle.

Q. 2. What are your findings on palpation?

Ans. I found a zone of anaesthesia at first web space of hand. Skin of hand is dry. Nails are brittle.

Q. 3. What is your diagnosis?

Ans. –months/years old, post injection/post traumatic radial nerve palsy R/L with fracture shaft humerus (if present).

Q. 4. From where radial nerve takes its origin?

Ans. Radial nerve arises from posterior cord of brachial plexus.

Q. 5. What is the root value of radial nerve?

Ans. Its root value is C5,6,7.8 T1.

Q. 6. Can you explain its course?

Ans.

1. It descends behind the third part of axillary artery and infront of subscapularis, latisimus dorsi and teres major.
2. Before radial groove this nerve gives rise to branch to medial head of triceps and posterior cutaneous nerve of arm.
3. In radial groove it gives rise to branch to lateral head of triceps, anconeus, cutaneous branch to arm and forearm.
4. Radial nerve pierces the lateral intermuscular septum at the junction of middle and lower third of arm.
5. It reaches to anterior compartment between brachialis on medial side and extensor carpi radialis longus and brachioradialis on lateral side.

Q. 7. How does this nerve divide and supply to group of muscles?

Ans. Radial nerve divides into two branches before crossing elbow infront of lateral condyle.

Superficial sensory branches

This branch provides sensory supply to lateral part of dorsum of hand including lateral 3½ digits.

Deep branch (Posterior interosseous nerve)

This is primarily a motor nerve. Before piercing the supinator it gives rise branch to extensor carpi radialis brevis and supinator.

In posterior compartment of forearm it gives branches to following muscle:

1. Superficial muscles of back of forearm–ECRB, ED, EDM and ECU.
2. Deep muscles of back of forearm–supinator, APL, ERB, EPL and EI.

Q. 8. What do you understand by high radial nerve palsy?

Ans. High radial nerve palsy

Triceps and anconeus are spared in high radial nerve palsy (because branches to these muscles arise in axilla). This is seen when radial nerve is injured in radial groove. Rests of the muscles (supplied by radial nerve) are paralysed. In very high radial nerve palsy all the muscles including triceps are paralysed.

Q. 9. What is the clinical presentation of high radial nerve palsy?

Ans. Clinically patient presents with loss of wrist extension, digital extension, and loss of radial abduction of thumb, loss of accessory forearm flexion and loss of accessory supination. Sensation is lost at lateral part of dorsum of hand including lateral 3½ digits.

Q. 10. What is low radial nerve palsy?

Ans. Low radial nerve palsy

All the muscles (digital extensors and long abductors of thumb) supplied by radial nerve in distal arm are paralysed except brachioradialis and extensor carpi radialis longus and brevis.

Q. 11. What is crutch palsy?

Ans. Crutch palsy

Radial nerve injury caused by improper use of crutch or due to fracture dislocation of upper end humerus is known as crutch palsy.

Q. 12. What is night palsy?

Ans. Night palsy

This radial nerve palsy occurs when patient takes deep sleep on a chair under the influence of alcohol. (with arm hanging at the edge of chair)

Q. 13. Can you enumerate the causes of radial nerve palsy?

Ans. Causes of radial nerve palsy

1. Commonest cause of radial nerve injury is fracture shaft humerus.
2. Crutch palsy
3. Night palsy
4. Fracture dislocation of head radius (Posterior interoosseous nerve palsy)
5. Excision head radius (PIN palsy)
6. Monteggia fracture dislocation (PIN palsy)
7. During reduction of fracture shaft humerus
8. Post injection palsy.

Q. 14. How will you clinically examine the muscles supplied by radial nerve?

Ans. Clinical Examination of Muscles supplied by Radial Nerve.

Brachioradialis

Ask the patient to flex his elbow from 90 degree onward against resistance. Forearm should remain in mid prone position. During examination contracted brachioradialis becomes prominent which can be felt.

Triceps

Ask the patient to extend his elbow against resistance. Contracted triceps becomes prominent that can be felt by examiner.

Extensor digitorum

Ask the patient to extend his M.P. joint. In case of radial nerve palsy he will not be able to do so.

Extensor pollicis longus

Ask the patient to extend interphalangeal joint of thumb. In case of radial nerve palsy he will not be able to do so.

Wrist extensor

All the wrist extensors of wrist (except ECRL supplied by radial nerve itself) are supplied by posterior interosseous nerve branch of radial nerve. Patient will not be able to extend his wrist in this nerve injury.

Q. 15. How will you manage this case?

Ans. I would like to do following investigations prior to treatment:

1. Electromyography (EMG)
2. Nerve conduction velocity (NCV)
3. Strength duration curve.

Q. 16. What is electromyography?

Ans. In this procedure electrical activity of muscle is recorded on a graph during activity and rest.

Q. 17. What are the indications of EMG?

Ans. EMG is indicated in following condition:

1. To rule out nerve injury
2. To differentiate between complete and incomplete nerve injury
3. To find out regenerative changes in a nerve
4. To decide level of injury

Q. 18. What is nerve conduction velocity?

Ans. Measurement of conduction velocity of impulse generated between two points of nerve is known as nerve conduction velocity.

Q. 19. What is the normal conduction velocity?

Ans. Normal conduction velocity is approximate 70 meter/second.

Q. 20. What do you understand by strength duration curve?

Ans. In this investigation excitability of nerve and muscle is recorded on a graph.

Q. 21. What is Tinel sign?

Ans. This is a clinical sign of recovery of nerve function. If we gently percuss the skin by hammer along the course of nerve from distal to proximal, a tingling sensation will be felt by the patient in the area supplied by nerve (not at the percussion site). This tingling sensation usually persists for a few seconds and known as positive Tinel sign.

Q. 22. What kind of treatment you would like to start?

Ans. I would like to start following treatment:

1. Neurotropics should be started in the form of injection of methylcobalamine, Vitamin B1, B6, B12.
2. Gentle massage should be done at regular interval.
3. Dynamic cock up splint is most useful device. This splint prevents contractures by keeping wrist joint in functional position. (15–20 degree) While using dynamic cock up splint patient actively flexes wrist and fingers but extension is done passively by the springs attached to splint. It also maintains the tone and nutrition of paralyzed extensor muscle.

Q. 23. What are the indications of surgery?

Ans. Surgery is indicated in following conditions:

1. Perineural fibrosis
2. Sharp cutting injury of nerve
3. Nerve injury producing gap between 2 ends of nerve.

Q. 24. What kind of surgery can be done in fresh cases?

Ans. Following 3 types of surgeries can be done in fresh cases:

1. Neurolysis
2. Neurorrhaphy
3. Nerve grafting

Q. 25. What do you do in neurolysis?

Ans. Nerve is freed from adjacent fibrosis or callus.

Q. 26. What is neurorrhaphy?

Ans. In this surgical procedure both ends of nerve are sutured. Suturing can be done by three following methods:

a. Epineural suturing
b. Perineural suturing
c. Epiperineural suturing

Q. 27. What do you understand by nerve grafting?

Ans. Nerve graft can be taken from sural nerve to fill the gap between two ends of nerve.

Q. 28. What types of surgeries are required in old cases?

Ans. Old nerve injuries can be repaired by following tendon transfer:

Jones tendon transfer

Three types of tendon transfer have been described by Jones

1. Pronator teres (PT) can be transferred to extensor carpi radialis longus (ECRL) and brevis (ERCB).
2. Flexor carpi radialis (FCR) is transferred to extensor pollicis longus (EPL) and abductor pollicis longus (APL).
3. Flexor carpi ulnaris (FCU) can be transferred to extensor digitorum (ED) and extensor pollicis longus (EPL).

Modified Jones transfer (Zachary's method)

1. Pronator teres (PT) can be transferred to ECRL and ECRB.
2. Palmaris longus can be transferred to Abductor pollicis longus (APL).
3. FCU is transferred to extensor digitorum (ED) and extensor pollicis longus (EPL).

Other methods

1. Brand's transfer
2. Boye's transfer

CLAW HAND (ULNAR NERVE INJURY)

Q. 1. What are the points in favour of your diagnosis?

Ans. Sir, on examination I found following features suggestive of ulnar nerve injury:

1. Clawing Deformity

Patient has hyperextension at M.P. joint and flexion at interphalangeal joint of little and ring finger.

2. Muscle Wasting

Muscle wasting is seen at medial aspect of forearm, hypothenar eminence and at 1st dorsal interosseous muscle.

3. Sensory Deficit

Sensory deficit is present over autonomous zone of ulnar nerve i.e., tip of little finger.

4. Motor Deficit

- Card test is positive
- Froment test is positive
- Egawa test is positive
- Paralysis of FCU
- Weakness of abductor digiti minimi
- Paralysis of lumbricals and interosseosi. (Patient is unable to straighten his finger against resistance while holding his proximal phalanx)

Q. 2. How do you perform card test?

Ans. Card test

This test is done to check the function of palmar interossei. Insert a card in between 2 extended fingers and ask the patient to hold it tightly.

Meanwhile examiner tries to pull out the card. Card can be easily pulled out ia case of weakness of palmar interossei.

Q. 3. How do you detect froment sign?

Ans. Froment sign

This test is done to check the strength of adductor pollicis. Ask the patient to hold a book firmly with extended thumb and fingers. In case of weakness of adductor pollicis patient will hold the book with flexion of thumb at interphalangeal joint. This flexion is caused by flexor pollicis longus, supplied by median nerve.

Q. 4. How do you perform Egawa test?

Ans. Egawa test

This test is done to check the function of dorsal interossei. Dorsal interossei are abductors of middle finger. Ask the patient to keep his palm flat on table (palm facing downward). Now ask the patient to move his fingers sideways (abduction). In case of weakness of dorsal interossei he will not be able to do so.

Q. 5. How do you test for flexor carpi ulnaris?

Ans. Flexor carpi ulnaris

This muscle can be tested by asking the patient to palmar flex the wrist against gravity, Wrist will deviate toward radial side in case of weakness of FCU.

Q. 6. How do you test for abductor digiti minimi?

Ans. Abductor digiti minimi

To test this muscle, ask the patient to keep his hand flat on table, and then ask to abduct the little finger against resistance. In case of weakness of this muscle he will not be able to do so.

Q. 7. From where ulnar nerve takes its origin and what is its root value?

Ans. Ulnar nerve is a branch of medial cord of brachial plexus. It's root value is C_8 T_1.

Q. 8. What are the muscles supplied by ulnar nerve?

Ans. Muscular branches

1. Flexor carpi ulnaris and medial half of flexor digitorum profundus.
2. All interossei (Palmar and dorsal)
3. 3rd and 4th lumbricals
4. **Hypothenar muscles** (Palmaris brevis, Abductor digiti minimi, Flexor digiti minimi and Opponens digiti minimi.)
5. Adductor pollicis
6. Flexor pollicis brevis (Deep head)

Q. 9. What are the sensory areas in hand supplied by ulnar nerve?

Ans. Ulnar nerve gives sensory branches to following areas:

1. Medial side of hand
2. Whole of little finger
3. Medial side of ring finger.

Q. 10. What is high ulnar nerve palsy?

Ans. High ulnar nerve palsy

Following features are seen in high ulnar nerve palsy:

1. FCU and medial half of FDP are paralyzed.
2. Paralysis of muscles supplied by ulnar nerve in hand.
3. Clawing of little and ring finger is minimum or absent.
4. Sensory deficit is seen in skin of hand.

Q. 11. What is low ulnar nerve palsy?

Ans. Low ulnar nerve palsy

Following features are seen in low ulnar nerve palsy:

1. Only the muscles of hand supplied by ulnar nerve are paralyzed. Muscles of forearm are spared.
2. Clawing of little or ring finger is more prominent.
3. Sensory deficit occurs in skin of hand.

Q. 12. What is ulnar paradox?

Ans. Ulnar paradox

High ulnar nerve palsy causes less deformity this is known as Ulnar paradox. In high ulnar nerve palsy FDP (medial half) is paralyzed and does not work unopposed by interossei and lumbricals. This makes the deformity less obvious.

Q. 13. What actual difficulty patient is having in his day to day activities?

Ans. Patient has difficulty in grasping objects (due to paralysis of intrinsic muscles of hand). Along with this he has difficulty in pinching (due to paralysis of adductor pollicis and first dorsal interossei).

Q. 14. Can you enumerate the causes of ulnar nerve palsy?

Ans. Immediate palsy

1. Most common cause is fracture supracondylar humerus.
2. Fracture medial condyle of humerus.
3. Lacerated injuries at wrist can also cause ulnar nerve injury.

Late (Tardy) ulnar nerve palsy

1. Cubitus valgus deformity in fracture lateral condyle of humerus and fracture supracondylar humerus.
2. Entrapment of ulnar nerve by callus formation, commonly seen in fracture supracondylar humerus.

Other causes

Leprosy is commonest cause. Sometimes ulnar tunnel syndrome can also cause this nerve injury.

Q. 15. How will you manage this case?

Ans. Anterior transposition of nerve from behind medial epicondyle to the front. This will reduce tension and friction on nerve as well as it also reduces path of nerve.

Q. 16. How will you manage a case of entrapement of nerve?

Ans. For such case I will do neurolysis and free ulnar nerve from callus formation. After this procedure anterior transposition of nerve will be done.

Q. 17. Have you heard about tendon transfer for this nerve injury?

Ans. Two types of tendon transfer are commonly done:

1. Brand's transfer

This is also known as Zancolli's capsuldesis. In this procedure volar capsule of MP joint is shortened.

2. Bunnell's transfer

Flexor digitorum superficialis of ring finger is transferred to radial aspect of all 4 fingers by dividing FDS into 4 slips.

CHRONIC OSTEOMYELITIS

Q. 1. What are the points in favour of your diagnosis? (Chronic osteomyelitis of upper end of tibia)

Ans. I found classical features, which are suggestive of chronic osteomyelitis:

- History of chronic discharging sinus
- Mild to moderate pain
- History of bone pieces coming out of sinus tract.

Examination findings are as follows:

1. Upper end of tibia is thick, irregular and tender.
2. Discharging sinus is present which is fixed to bone. Its discharge is seropurulent (may be serous/yellowish/greenish)
3. Margins of sinus are inverted.
4. Sprouting granulation tissue is seen.
5. Skin surrounding the sinus is soft and pigmented.

6. Muscle atrophy is also seen at thigh and leg.
7. Stiffness is present at knee.

Q. 2. What is the significance of green colour pus?

Ans. Green colour pus is indicative of pseudomonas infection.

Q. 3. What is the significance of thick yellow pus?

Ans. Thick yellow pus is indicative of staph aureus infection.

Q. 4. What is osteomyelitis?

Ans. Osteomyelitis is an infection of bone and bone marrow. (Osteitis is infection of cortical bone.)

Q. 5. How do you classify osteomyelitis?

Ans. Classification

- Acute osteomyelitis
- Subacute osteomyelitis
- Chronic osteomyelitis
- Acute on chronic osteomyelitis

Q. 6. What are the criteria of calling it acute osteomyelitis?

Ans. When the duration of osteomyelitis is less than 2 weeks, it is called as acute osteomyelitis. Patient comes to hospital within 24–48 hours.

Q. 7. When do you call it chronic osteomyelitis?

Ans. If osteomyelitis persists for more than 3 weeks it is known as chronic osteomyelitis.

Q. 8. What is subacute osteomyelitis?

Ans. Subacute osteomyelitis is usually detected after 15 days of infection. Patient presents with pain with no other constitutional symptoms. It is caused by staphylococcus aureus. (ESR and leukocyte counts are raised. Blood culture is positive. It is treated by antibiotics)

Q. 9. What do you understand by primary and secondary acute osteomyelitis?

Ans. Acute osteomyelitis is subdivided into following two types:

Primary Acute Osteomyelitis

It is commonly seen in children. It spreads through haematogenous route.

Secondary Acute Osteomyelitis

When osteomyelitis develops following a compound fracture or operation it is known as secondary acute osteomyelitis. It is less severe than primary type.

Q. 10. Which is the commonest organism to cause osteomyelitis?

Ans. Haemolytic staphylococcus aureus is commonest organism to cause acute osteomyelitis. (Other organisms are streptococcus pneumococcus and *E.coli*.)

Q. 11. Which organism is responsible for osteomyelitis in patient of sickle cell anemia?

Ans. Salmonella causes osteomyelitis commonly in patients of sickle cell anemia and in diaphyseal osteomyelitis. It causes very severe osteomyelitis. Several bones including spine may be involved.

Q. 12. Which organism causes osteomyelitis in heroin addicts?

Ans. Pseudomonas causes osteomyelitis in heroin addicts. This is also seen commonly in puncture wounds.

Q. 13. Which organism is commonly seen during the ages of 6 months to 4 years?

Ans. Haemophillus influenza is commonly seen between the ages of 6 months to 4 years.

Q. 14. Which age is predominantly affected?

Ans. It is predominantly seen in infants and children.

Q. 15. Which part of bone is affected in osteomyelitis?

Ans. Metaphysis of long bones toward the growing ends is affected. Upper end of tibia and lower end of femur are common sites to be affected.

Q. 16. Where could be the foci of infection?

Ans. Foci of infections are usually seen in boils and tonsillitis.

Q. 17. Can you explain its pathogenesis in brief?

Ans. Acute osteomyelitis is most commonly spreads through haematogenous route from a pre existing foci of infection. (boils or tonsillitis) Infective embolus get lodged into small end arteries and capillaries situated in metaphysis. This metaphyseal area is highly vascularized part of bone. Here vessels are arranged in hair pin pattern which accounts for blood stasis. This blood stasis and hair pin arrangement of vessels allows bacteria to settle. This makes it potential area for getting infection.

Q. 18. Can you name a joint where metaphysis is intraarticular?

Ans. It is the hip joint where metaphysis is intraarticular and it leads to pyogenic arthritis.

Q. 19. Why do you say that knee is stiff in your patient?

Ans. On examination I found all the active and passive movements at knee are decreased. This is suggestive of stiffness.

Q. 20. What may be the causes of stiffness?

Ans. Stiffness can occur due to following reasons:

1. Prolonged immobilization of limb in a plaster.
2. Muscle is tethered around the joint leading to stiffness.

Q. 21. Can you enumerate the causes of chronic osteomyelitis?

Ans. Chronic osteomyelitis can be caused by following conditions:

1. Following an acute osteomyelitis
2. Postoperative
3. Garre's osteomyelitis
4. Brodies abscess
5. Tuberculosis, syphillis and fungal osteomyelitis.

Q. 22. Why this is not ankylosis? or what is the meaning of ankylosis?

Ans. This is not ankylosis because in ankylosis all the movements are lost at joint.

Q. 23. Do you know types of ankylosis?

Ans. Ankylosis is of 2 types, bony and fibrous.

Bony ankylosis	Fibrous ankylosis
This is painless	This is painful
No movement at the joint	Little movement is possible at the joint
Painful abductor spasm is absent	This is present in intra-articular (short fibrous) ankylosis. 0–10 degree of movement is possible in extraarticular (long fibrous) ankylosis
This is seen in arthrodesis of joint, ankylosing spondylitis (ankylosing spondylitis may have fibrous as well as bony ankylosis) and as a sequele of septic arthritis	This is commonly seen in tubercular arthritis

Q. 24. How acute osteomyelitis can convert into chronic osteomyelitis?

Ans. Acute osteomyelitis may convert into chronic osteomyelitis due to following reasons:

1. Inadequate and late treatment of acute osteomyelitis results into pus collection into medullary cavity and beneath the periosteum. Later sequestrum is formed that provides a seat for persistent infection.
2. High virulence of organism.
3. Poor immunity status of host.

Q. 25. What is sequestrum?

Ans. This is a dead separated piece of bone at the site of osteomyelitis which is surrounded by infected granulation tissue. Its inner surface is smooth, while outer surface is rough.

Q. 26. What are types of sequestrum?

A. Sequestrum is of following three types:

1. Ring Sequestrum

This is seen around pintrack and amputation stump.

2. Tubular Sequestrum

This is a tube like hollow, dead bone. It is seen in haematogenous osteomyelitis and segmental fractures.

3. Rice Grain Sequestrum

This is seen in tuberculosis.

Q. 27. What is involucrum?

Ans. Involucrum is a thick dense new bone formation overlying the sequestrum.

Q. 28. What are cloacae?

Ans. Cloacae are openings in involucrum through which pus; exudates, bone debris and sequestrum find their way out to surface.

Q. 29. How will you investigate this case?

Ans. I would like to do the following investigations:

- X-ray of local part.
- Pus culture and sensitivity.
- Sinogram is done to know the origin of sinus; from where it arises and also to localize the cavity that is not visible on X-ray.
- Hb, TLC, DLC, blood sugar and ESR.
- Bone scan can show the hot spot.

Q. 30. What is the method of sample collection for pus culture?

Ans. Local area should be cleaned first with normal saline. Now squeeze the local part to exclude few drops of pus. These initial drops of pus should not be taken for sample. Now press the local area again to collect the drops of pus. This should be sent for culture and sensitivity.

Q. 31. What do you know about sinogram?

Ans. This is radiological examination of sinus which is done after injecting a radio-opaque dye, commonly sodium iodide.

Q. 32. What are the indications of sonogram?

Ans. This is indicated in following conditions:

1. To detect origin of sinus. (from which part of bone it is arising.)
2. To see a cavity that is not visualized on X-ray.

Q. 33. O.K. what are the X-ray findings?

Ans. X-ray may show following findings:

- **Cortex of bone is thick and irregular.**
- Sclerosed cortex.
- Rarefaction of bone.
- **Sequestrum** is seen.
- **Involucrum** is a late finding.
- Cloacae are not easily seen in X-ray.
- Periosteal reaction.

Q. 34. What do you understand by periosteal reaction?

Ans. This is new bone formation which results due to stimulation of cambium layer of periosteum. (Pus comes out through Volkman's canal to subperiosteal area leading to stimulation of cambium layer.)

Q. 35. What radiological findings do you expect in case of acute osteomyelitis?

Ans. X-ray of acute osteomyelitis may show the following findings:

1. Periosteal reaction.
2. Patchy osteoporosis.

Q. 36. O.K. how will you manage this case?

Ans. I will manage this case by excision of sinus tract, sequestrectomy, curettage and saucerization. After this surgical procedure, limb will be kept on continous suction and irrigation system; in which an inlet tube goes into medullary cavity of bone carrying the irrigation fluid. This fluid comes out through an outlet tube.

Q. 37. When to perform sequestrectomy?

Ans. Followup X-rays are done to see the involucrum formation. If sufficient involucrum is formed sequestrectomy can be done.

Q. 38. Why to do sauccerization?

Ans. Bony cavity is converted into a saucer because pus collects inside the bony cavity and it does not come out of it. Pus is freely drained if sauccerization is done.

Q. 39. How long sauccerization should be done?

Ans. Curettage should be done until normal bone is seen and fresh bleeding starts from bone.

Q. 40. What do you do with this left cavity in bone?

Ans. Gentamicin impregnated beads can be used to fill the cavity.

Q. 41. What are the complications of osteomyelitis?

Ans. Osteomyelitis can have the following complications:

1. Damage to growth plate can lead to shortening.
2. If vascularity of growth plate is increased, it can cause lengthening of limb.
3. Deformity of limb can occur if growth plate is partially damaged.
4. Flare up of infection.
5. Pathological fracture.
6. Joint stiffness.
7. Squamus cell carcinoma at sinus tract.
8. Amyloidosis (can be diagnosed by rectal biopsy).

NONUNION

Q. 1. How to define non-union?

Ans. When the normal time of bone healing has passed still fracture dose not show any sign of clinical and radiological union, it is said to be non-union. In other words, biological process of bone healing has stopped in non-union.

Q. 2. What are the points in favour of your diagnosis?

Ans. I have following points in favour of my diagnosis:

1. Patient has history of trauma 2-3 months back.
2. Bony tenderness is not present at the fracture site.
3. Bony crepitus is absent.
4. I found frank painless abnormal mobility at fracture site.
5. Patient has loss of transmitted movements.

Following X-ray findings are also suggestive of non-union:

1. Sclerosis and smoothened fractured ends.
2. Breach in continuity of bone.
3. Bone marrow cavity is obliterated.
4. Area around the fracture site shows osteoporosis.

Q. 3. Could it be delayed union?

Ans. No, it could not be a case of delayed union because in delayed union bony tenderness will be present and frank abnormal mobility at fracture site will be absent. Bony crepitus will be absent.

Q. 4. Can you define delayed union?

Ans. When fracture has taken more than the expected time to unite, it is called as delayed union.

Q. 5. Can you enumerate the causes of non-union?

Ans. Common causes of non-union are as follows:

1. Inadequate immobilization
2. Inadequate blood supply
3. Infection
4. Poor internal fixation
5. Intact companion bone
6. Interposition of soft tissue.
7. Bone gap between fractured ends.

Q. 6. Do you know about Muller and Weber classification of non-union?

Ans. Muller and Weber classification of non-union

Muller has classified non-union into 2 types, which are further subdivided into subtypes.

1. Hypervascular Non-union
   a. Hypertrophic
   b. Horsehoof
   c. Oligotrophic
2. Avascular Non-union
   a. Torsion wedge non-union
   b. Atrophic non-union
   c. Defect (Gap) non-union
   d. Comminuted non-union

Hypervascular Non-union

This type of non-union has following characteristics:

1. In this type of non-union fractured ends are viable.
2. Biological reaction is seen at fracture site.
3. This type of non-union can be managed by stable internal fixation. Bone grafting is not required.

Hypertrophic non-union

This type of non-union occurs due to poor fixation of fracture and early weight bearing. Exuberant callus is formed in this type. This is also known as **elephant foot non-union.**

Horsehoof non-union

This is seen in inadequate fixation with plates and screws. Callus is formed in less quantity.

Oligotrophic non-union

Grossly displaced and distracted fractures are likely to undergo this type of non-union. Very poor callus is formed.

Avascular Non-union

This type may show following features:

1. Due to poor blood supply fracture ends undergo ischaemic necrosis.
2. This does not show any biological reaction.
3. This type of nonunion can be managed by rigid internal fixation with bone grafting.

Torsion wedge non-union

This is commonly seen in segmental fracture. Intermediate fragment has healed at one end and not at the other.

Atrophic non-union

Fracture ends become tapered, thin and sclerosed. A lot of scar tissue is formed in between the ends.

Defect (Gap) non-union

In this type bone fragment is lost. It is commonly seen in compound fracture and osteomyelitis.

Comminuted non-union

Proper callus is not formed in this non-union. It is commonly seen in comminuted fracture.

Q. 7. What is Paley's classification?

Ans. Paley's classification

Paley has classified non-union into two types, depending on amount of bone loss.

Type A

In this type bone loss is less than 1 cm.

Type B

In this type bone loss is more than 1 cm.

Q. 8. What is the significance of these classifications?

Ans. This has been classified for the management point of view. Because atrophic non-union requires bone grafting along with rigid internal fixation. Hypertrophic non-union can be managed by rigid internal fixation only.

Q. 9. What are the methods of rigid internal fixation?

Ans. Rigid internal fixation can be done by dynamic compression plate and screws in humerus, radius and ulna. Interlocking nail may be a better option for femur and tibia.

O.K. how will you manage this case if infection is persisting with it?

Ans. Definite surgery for non-union will be deferred till I see the signs of clearing up of infection.

O.K. what are the signs for that?

Ans. There should not be any discharge. Sinus should have healed. No tenderness should be present at local site.

Q. 10. How will you treat this infection?

Ans. I will excise the wound and sinus tract. I will do sequestrectomy and curettage of infected material.

Q. 11. Apart from rigid internal fixation with bone grafting, do you know any other method of treatment for non-union?

Ans. There are two other methods:

1. Electrical stimulation method. (not used now)
2. Illizarov method.

Q. 12. What is the principle of Illizarov method?

Ans. This acts on the basis on distraction histogenesis. This is a kind of ring fixator consisting of 1.5 mm diameter stainless steel wire. Corticotomy (cortex is cut in such a way that medullary cavity remains intact) is done followed by distraction of bone ends at the rate of 1 mm per day. Natural bone fills the gap (created by distraction of bone ends)

Q. 13. Which graft is most suitable?

Ans. Fresh autogenous, cancellous bone graft is most suitable for non-union.

Q. 14. What is the function of bone graft?

Ans. Graft induces osteogenesis. This is also useful in filling up bone gap and also provides stability.

Q. 15. What is autograft?

Ans. Autograft is taken from patient itself.

Q. 16. What is allograft?

Ans. Allograft is taken from genetically dissimilar person of same species. **(Homograft)**

Q. 17. What is xenograft?

Ans. Xenograft (Heterogeneous) is taken from other species.

Q. 18. What do you understand by cancellous bone graft?

Ans. Cancellous bone graft induces better osteogenesis. This graft can be taken from iliac crest and upper end of tibia (metaphyseal region).

Q. 19. What do you understand by cortical bone-graft?

Ans. This graft is used for the fracture of shaft of long bones. It can be used as single onlay graft (placed on one surface) or dual onlay graft (placed on both surface) or as a sliding graft. (bone graft is brought from above to fracture site in a sliding manner). Cortical bone graft is taken from middle third of medial surface of tibia and middle third of fibula.

Q. 20. What is corticocancellous graft?

Ans. This graft is taken from corticocancellous junction e.g., iliac crest, ribs and fibula.

Q. 21. How will you manage associated shortening of lower limb?

Ans. Less than 2 cm shortening can be compensated by body adjustment. This does not require surgery.

More than 2 cm shortening can be managed by epiphyseodesis and by Illizarov method.

Q. 22. What is epiphyseodesis?

Ans. In this method epiphyseal growth plate of opposite limb is closed by surgery.

CUBITUS VARUS

Q. 1. What are the points in favour of your diagnosis?

Ans. I have following points in favour of my diagnosis:

1. Cubitus varus deformity is present at elbow which is indicative of malunited fracture supracondylar humerus.
2. Relationship of 3 bony landmarks is not disturbed with respect to each other. This is disturbed in relation to long axis of humerus.
3. Supracondylar ridge is felt irregular on palpation.

Q. 2. What is gunstock deformity?

Ans. Gunstock deformity is cosmetic disability without functional impairment of elbow. In this condition carrying angle between extended long axis of arm and forearm is decreased in comparison to contralateral side. Normal carrying angle is 11 degree in male and 14 degree in female.

This is also known as cubitus varus deformity. This is most common complication of supracondylar humerus fracture. Distal fragment tilts medially during the union and goes into internal rotation either due to inadequate reduction or displacement of fracture.

Q. 3. When do you say that the fracture is malunited?

Ans. Fracture is said to be malunited if any of the below mentioned deformity is present:

1. Angulation.
2. Shortening (occurs due to overriding).
3. Rotation of fragments.
4. Side to side lateral displacement.

Q. 4. Apart from malunited supracondylar humerus is there any other cause of cubitus varus deformity?

Ans. Yes, it can occur due to disturbance in epiphyseal growth plate by trauma or any kind of infection.

Q. 5. What are other complications of this fracture?

Ans. Patient can have immediate, early and late complication as follows:

IMMEDIATE

- Vascular Injury
- Nerve injury

EARLY

Volkman's ischaemia

LATE

Cubitus varus deformity

Volkman's ischaemic contracture

Myositis ossificans

Q. 6. Which artery is most commonly injured in this fracture and why?

Ans. Brachial artery is most commonly injured in displaced fracture. Sharp edge of proximal fragment impinges the brachial artery, leading to vascular compromise of flexor group of muscle of forearm.

Q. 7. Which nerve is most commonly injured in this fracture?

Ans. Radial nerve is commonest nerve to be injured in this fracture. Other nerves to be injured are median and ulnar nerve in that order.

Q. 8. What is Volkman's ischaemia?

Ans. This is ischaemia of muscles and nerves of forearm (flexor compartment). Ischaemia occurs due to occlusion of brachial artery that causes reduced blood supply to flexor group of muscles of forearm. Flexor pollicis longus and Flexor digitorum profundus (medial half) are the commonly affected muscles in Volkman's ischaemia. It happens because these are supplied by an end artery; anterior interoseous artery. Ischaemia of these muscles causes compartment syndrome.

Q. 9. What are clinical features of Volkman's ischaemia?

Ans. Patient will present with the following clinical features:

1. Pain in forearm.
2. Pallor (due to reduced capillary filling time).
3. Paresthesia.
4. Paralysis.
5. Pain on passive stretching of fingers (earliest sign).
6. Pulselessness
7. Swelling and tenderness over forearm.

Q. 10. What is the treatment of Volkman's ischaemia?

Ans. Volkman's ischaemia can be treated on following measures:

1. Remove all the splint, bandage or slab/ plaster.
2. Elevate the forearm and advice to do active and passive movement of fingers.
3. Urgent fasciotomy should be done if no improvement occurs in response to above mentioned treatment. Fasciotomy is recommended when compartment pressure is more than 30 mmHg. In this method deep fascia is split longitudinally along it's entire length.

Q. 11. What is myositis ossificans and how does it develop?

Ans. Frequent and prolonged massage around a post traumatic elbow gives rise to ectopic new bone formation leading to stiff elbow.

Q. 12. How do you treat myositis ossificans?

Ans. This is treated by immobilization in above elbow POP slab for 3 weeks. Later gentle mobilization exercises can be started.

Q. 13. What is Volkman's ischaemic contracture?

Ans. This is deformity of hand, wrist and forearm developing as a sequele to Volkman's ischaemia in which wrist and fingers go into flexion contracture.

Q. 14. What are the clinical features of VIC?

Ans. Patient will present with the following clinical features:

1. Flexion contracture of forearm (due to involvement of flexor digitorum profundus and flexor pollicis longus).
2. Claw hand deformity may be present.
3. **Volkman's sign** is positive. i.e., extension of wrist exaggerate the deformity while flexion causes opposite to it. In other words fingers can be extended at interphalangeal joint only when wrist is flexed.
4. Contracture of joint and soft tissue with scarring of skin is also seen.
5. Bones are also deformed.

6. Sensory and motor loss may occur in forearm and hand due to peripheral nerve involvement.

Q. 15. What is the treatment of VIC?

Ans. VIC can be treated on following measures:

1. Volkman's splint is applied in mild case.
2. **Maxpage operation** is indicated in moderate cases. In this operation muscles of common flexor origin are released from medial epicondyle and ulna. This makes sliding of origin of muscles down thus releasing contracture.
3. Neurolysis, excision of scar and tendon transfer are other modes of treatment that can be applied for moderate cases.
4. **Seddon's carpectomy** is indicated in severe cases. In this operation proximal row of carpal bones is excised. This causes shortening of forearm thus masking the effect of contracture.
5. **Arthrodesis** of wrist joint in functional position can also be done in severe cases.
6. Amputation is done in very severe cases where wrist and hand show gangrenous changes.

Q. 16. Do you know about radiological signs of malunion?

Ans. There are 2 radiological signs:

1. **Fish tail sign.** Anterior border of proximal fragment is visible as a sharp spike due to rotation of distal fragment.
2. **Crescent sign.** It indicates varus or valgus tilt of distal fragment. Overlapping of capitulum over olecranon masks the normal radioluscent gap of elbow joint thus makes Crescent sign positive.

Q. 17. How will you manage cubitus deformity?

Ans. Corrective osteotomy (lateral close wedge osteotomy) is treatment of choice. This is also known as French osteotomy. (It should be done after the skeletal maturity, otherwise deformity can recur).

Q. 18. Can you explain French osteotomy in brief?

Ans. French Osteotomy

This is lateral closed wedge osteotomy of lower end of humerus. This procedure involves removal of lateral wedge of bone from supracondylar area and closing the osteotomy. In this osteotomy one screw is placed anteriorly in distal fragment and second screw is placed slightly posterior in proximal fragment. Now osteotomy is done in between these screws. Distal fragment is rotated in such a manner that both screws become parallel to each other. Both screws are tied by a stainless steel wire in figure of eight manner. This method fills the gap in between proximal and distal fragment. Drawbacks of this osteotomy are chances of non-union and lengthening of arm.

FRACTURE NECK FEMUR

Q. 1. What is your diagnosis?

Ans. My diagnosis is –days old fracture neck femur of R/L side.

Q. 2. What are the points in favour of your diagnosis?

Ans. I have following points in favour of my diagnosis:

1. Patient gives history of fall on ground due to trivial trauma.
2. R/L lower limb is externally rotated.
3. Pain and tenderness at the scarpa's triangle.
4. Axial tenderness of greater trochanter is present.
5. Movements at hip are restricted.
6. Minimal shortening of limb is present.

Q. 3. How will you confirm your diagnosis?

Ans. I would like to do X-ray of pelvis with both hip-A.P. view and affected hip-lateral view.

Q. 4. This is the X-ray. Can you tell me the findings in this X-ray?

Ans. Sir, this is the X-ray of pelvis with both hip-A.P. view showing both the hip joints. X-ray findings are as follows:

1. There is a breech in lamellar pattern of cortex of neck femur.
2. Shenton line is broken.
3. Greater trochanter is shifted upward.
4. Lesser trochanter becomes more prominent.
5. ASIS is shifted upward on same side.

Q. 5. What is shenton line?

Ans. If I draw a line from inferior border of superior pubic rami, continue this to inferior surface of head of femur, neck and medial border of shaft femur. It will make shenton line. A breach in this line indicates fracture neck femur.

Q. 6. How will you manage this case?

Ans. You should answer according to age of patient and duration of fracture.

Children (less than 16 years)

< 3 weeks old fracture

Undisplaced fracture can be treated by internal fixation by Austin Moore pins or POP hip spica.

Displaced fracture can be treated by closed reduction and internal fixation by Austin Moore pins.

> 3 weeks old fracture

This can be treated by **McMurray's osteotomy.** In this method osteotomy is done at the intertrochanteric region directed upward and medially, starting at the base of greater trochanter and finishing just above the lesser trochanter. This is a displacement abduction osteotomy. Advantage of this osteotomy is that it increases osteogenesis and blood supply at the local area. Most important advantage of this osteotomy is that it converts shearing forces into compressing forces.

Young Adults (16–60 years)

< 3 weeks old fracture

Undisplaced fracture can be fixed by **cancellous screws**, SP nail, Dynamic hip screws, Knowle's pins, Canulated bolt or Asnis screw.

Displaced fracture can be treated by closed/open reduction and internal fixation by above mentioned methods.

> 3 weeks old fracture

If neck is not absorbed it can be managed by internal fixation with bone graft like vascularised muscle pedicle graft. This graft is taken from quadratus femoris. This is known as **Meyer's procedure.**

If neck is absorbed, it can be managed by **McMurray's displacement osteotomy.**

Elder Patient (> 60 years)

< 3 weeks old Fracture

It can be treated by hemireplacement arthroplasty.

> 3 weeks old fracture

It can also be managed by hemireplacement arthroplasty. If osteoarthritic changes are seen in acetabulum, total hip replacement is the treatment of choice.

Q. 7. How will you manage a patient of 30–35 years of age?

Ans. I would like to closed reduction and internal fixation by cancellous screws.

Q. 8. Why not open reduction?

Ans. If we open the fracture site there is chances of damage to blood supply of femoral head. So we prefer closed reduction.

Q. 9. Which type of prosthesis is used in hemireplacement arthroplasty?

Ans. We commonly use following 3 types of prosthesis:

1. Austin Moore prosthesis

2. Thompson prosthesis
3. Bipolar prosthesis

Q. 10. Do you know basic principle of insertion of these prosthesis?

Ans. Prosthesis should be inserted in such a way that the distance between superior aspect of lesser trochanter and acetabulum is anatomically restored.

Q. 11. Can you explain in brief that which prosthesis is used where?

Ans. Austin Moore Prosthesis

This prosthesis is used when 1/2 to 1/4th of an inch of neck remains above lesser trochanter. It has got a small hole at the tip of stem which is used to extract the prosthesis. In its middle it has 2 holes through which bone grows thus helps in fixation of prosthesis in a better way. Bone cement is not used with this prosthesis.

Thompson Prosthesis

It is used in patients who have limited femoral neck. Before fixation of this prosthesis femoral neck is excised at the base. This prosthesis requires stabilization by bone cement. It is used in old fracture neck femur where neck is absorbed.

Bipolar Prosthesis

This is indicated when chances of acetabular erosion and protrusion are high (by a prosthesis). Advantage of bipolar prosthesis is that this can be easily converted into total hip arthroplasty.

Q. 12. What is Proxima hip?

Ans. This is a hip prosthesis which is used for primary hip arthroplasty. This is a latest prosthesis which is being used in India.

Q. 13. What are the indications of Proxima hip?

Ans. This is indicated when surgeon wants to conserve bone and soft tissue.This prosthesis provides physiological loading to proximal femur.

Do you have any idea about prerequisite for inserting proxima hip?

Ans. This prosthesis requires following prerequisite:

1. Metaphyseal area of femur should be of good quality.
2. Proximal femur should have supportive bone medially and laterally.
3. X-ray of hip A.P. view should be done in slight interal rotation.
4. True lateral view of hip should also be done to assess fitness of implant superiorly.

Q. 14. Can you name of surgical technique used in proxima hip?

Ans. Sir, this prosthesis is inserted through **"round the corner technique"**.

Q. 15. What are the complications of fracture neck femur?

Ans. Fracture neck femur can have following complications:

1. Most common complication is non-union.
2. Avascular necrosis of head femur
3. Limb shortening
4. Osteoarthritis

Q. 16. What is the cause of non-union?

Ans. Cause of non-union is inadequate immobilization and poor blood supply to head of femur. Absence of cambium layer in periosteum of femoral neck makes it prone to undergo non-union.

Q. 17. How will you treat a case of non-union? or what are the factors to be kept in mind while treating a case of ununited fracture neck femur?

Ans. Following three factors should be kept in mind while treating a case of non-union:

1. Viability of head
2. Degree of absorption of neck
3. Degree of osteoporosis

If patient has viable femoral head and adequate neck, it can be treated by McMurray's or

Dickson's geometric osteotomy in young adults. Elderly patients of more than 60 years of age can be treated by replacement arthroplasty.

Q. 18. What is the cause of avascular necrosis?

Ans. It is caused by disruption of retinacular vessels and vessels within the femoral neck in widely displaced fractures.

Q. 19. How will you treat avascular necrosis of femoral head?

Ans. Young patient can be treated by Meyer's procedure, bipolar arthroplasty or arthrodesis of hip. Replacement arthroplasty is reserved for older patients.

Q. 20. What is the cause of limb shortening in fracture neck femur?

Ans. Limb becomes short due to absrorption of neck and mismatch of size of prosthesis.

Q. 21. What is the cause of osteoarthritis in fracture neck femur?

Ans. Cause of arthritis is either faulty union or avascularity of femoral head.

FRACTURE INTERTROCHANTERIC FEMUR

Q. 1. Why this is not a case of fracture intertrochanteric femur?

Ans. This cannot be a case of intertrochanteric fracture due to following features:

1. Lower limb is not in complete external rotation.
2. Anteroposterior tenderness at greater trochanter is absent.
3. Greater trochanter is not broadened.

Q. 2. What are the complications of fracture intertrochanteric femur?

Ans. Most common complication is malunion (coxa vara) other complications are limb shortening and osteoarthritis.

Q. 3. What is the surgical treatment of intertrochanteric fracture?

Ans. Open reduction and internal fixation by dynamic hip screws is the treatment of choice.

GIANT CELL TUMOR (OSTEOCLASTOMA)

Q. 1. What is your diagnosis?

Ans. Sir, my diagnosis is osteoclastoma of lower end of femur (R/L).

Q. 2. Why do you say so? or what are the points in favour of your diagnosis?

Ans. Sir, I have following points in favour of my diagnosis.

1. Age 30 years. (normally 20–40 years age group patients are affected).
2. This swelling is present for last 6 months. (normally history is in months)
3. Lower end of femur is common site for this tumor.
4. Patient does not give history of significant pain.
5. I did not find any effusion in joint.
6. Skin overlying swelling is not shiny.
7. Skin overlying swelling does not show any dilated veins over it.
8. Swelling is smooth.
9. Mild tenderness is present over swelling.
10. Egg shell crackling is felt over swelling.
11. Joint movements are within normal limit.

Q. 3. What is osteoclastoma?

Ans. Osteoclastoma is a benign but locally malignant tumor. It is an osteolytic tumor which originates from epiphysis. This is also known as Giant cell tumor.

Q. 4. What is the site of origin of tumor?

Ans. GCT takes origin from epiphysis of long bones, e.g., lower end of femur, upper end of tibia/fibula, lower end of radius/ulna.

Q. 5. What is sex predilection in osteoclastoma?

Ans. This is commonly seen in males. Male to female ratio is 1.5:1.

Q. 6. What are other sites of origin of osteoclastoma?

Ans.

1. Upper end of tibia and fibula
2. lower end of radius
3. lower end of ulna

Q. 7. What is the pathological hallmark of this tumor?

Ans. Tumor gaint cells are seen under microscopy which is pathological hallmark of osteoclastoma.

Q. 8. How will you manage this case?

Ans. First of all I would like to confirm my diagnosis.

I would like to do X-ray of knee joint (A.P. and lateral), X-ray of chest P.A. view (to see secondaries).

After this I would like to do FNAC and biopsy to see the pathology of tumor.

I will do complete haemogram as a routine.

O.K. what are the findings you will get in above investigations?

Ans. X-ray of local part will show following findings:

- Eccentrically situated lytic lesion at upper end of tibia/lower end of femur/lower end of radius.
- Cortex is thin and expanded.
- Joint is not involved and joint lines are intact.
- No periosteal reaction is seen.
- Soap bubble appearance.
- Calcification is not seen within the tumor.

Pathology

Gross

Tumor is reddish brown, friable, ragged. Tissues are filled with blood clots.

Microscopy

Tumor giant cells are hallmark of GCT. Spindle cells are suggestive of malignant transformation.

Q. 9. What is the treatment for this tumor?

Ans. This tumor has a tendency of recurrence and along with that it is more invasive and aggrasive in nature. Surgery is the treatment of choice.

Q. 10. Which surgery you would like to perform in this case?

Ans. In this case I would like to excise the tumor and reconstruct the lower end of femur by turnoplasty.

O.K. what is turnoplasty?

Ans. This procedure is indicated in GCT of lower end of femur and upper end of tibia. In case of femur, after excision of GCT, required length of tibia is taken and split in two halves. One half is turned upside down and fixed with left stump of femur. Femur bone can be used for osteoclastoma of tibia.

Q. 11. Which bone is used for reconstruction of osteoclastoma of lower end radius?

Ans. Upper end of fibula is used because its shape resembles with lower end radius.

Q. 12. Is there any other option of surgery apart from turnoplasty?

Ans. Yes sir, there are two other options:

1. Arthrodesis
2. Reconstruction of joint after excision of tumor either by prosthesis or by filling auto/allograft.

Q. 13. What are other modalities of treatment?

Ans. Other modalities are as follows:

1. Curettage and cryosurgery with bone cementation
2. Curettage and bone cementation
3. Curettage and bone grafting
4. Enblock excision
5. Radiotherapy

Q. 14. What are the complications of cryosurgery?

Ans. Complications of this surgery are skin necrosis, neuropraxia, prolonged healing, infection and pathological fracture.

Q. 15. What are the indications of radiotherapy?

Ans. This is indicated when tumor is present in spine, vertebrae, sacrum or pelvis where excision of tumor is difficult. 1500–5000 rads can be given for 5-6 weeks.

Q. 16. What may be the harm of radiotherapy?

Ans. If radiotherapy is given to benign GCT it may produce malignant changes.

Q. 17. What is the nature of osteclastoma as far as malignancy is concern?

Ans. 1/3rd are benign, 1/3rd are locally malignant and 1/3rd are malignant.

Q. 18. What is your differential diagnosis?

Ans.

1. Chondroblastoma (benign)
2. Osteitis fibrosa
3. Aneurysmal bone cyst
4. Unicameral bone cyst
5. Non ossifying fibroma
6. Hyperparathyroidism
7. Chondromyxoid fibroma

OSTEOSARCOMA

Q. 1. What is your diagnosis?

Ans. My diagnosis is osteosarcoma of lower end of femur (R/L).

Q. 2. Why do you say so? or what are the points in favour of diagnosis?

Ans. Following points are in favour of my diagnosis:

1. Age of patient is 20 years. (normal age group for this tumor is 15–25 years).
2. Lower end of femur is involved. (common bone to be involved in this tumor).
3. Patient gives classical history of pain, followed by swelling. Pain is getting worse with the growth of tumor. This pain is more severe during night.
4. History of weight loss is present.
5. On examination this swelling is warm, tender and palpable. It's consistency varies firm to hard. Overlying skin is shiny and stretched. Premature veins are seen over skin.
6. Skin overlying swelling does not show any ulceration.
7. Movements at knee joint are restricted.
8. Patient seems to be anemic as his cunjuctiva shows pallor.

Q. 3. What is osteosarcoma?

Ans. Osteosarcoma is a highly malignant tumor of second decade, characterized by neoplastic osteoid formation and tumor tissue formation. This tumor arises from a common multipotential mesenchymal tissue and gives rise to fibroblastic, chondroblastic, osteolytic and osteoblastic type.

Q. 4. What is the site of origin of this tumor?

Ans. Osteosarcoma takes origin from metaphysis of long bones, e.g., lower end of femur, upper end of tibia and upper end of humerus.

Q. 5. What is the sex predilection in this tumor?

Ans. This tumor predominantly affects the male population.

Q. 6. What is secondary osteosarcoma?

Ans. Secondary osteosarcoma has following features:

- This osteosarcoma occurs when skeletal system is affected by benign tumors or if patient has generalized skeletal disorder.
- It is seen in Paget's disease, fibrous dysplasia, radiation exposure, multiple osteochondroma and multiple enchondromatosis.
- Secondary osteosarcoma is usually seen after 45 years of age.

Q. 7. How will you manage this case?

Ans. First of all I would like to confirm my diagnosis by doing following investigations:

1. X-ray of knee (A.P. and lateral)
2. X-ray of chest (P.A. view) to see secondaries.
3. Bone scan (to rule out skip lesion and intramedullary spread of tumor)
4. MRI (to detect spread of tumor in soft tissue)
5. FNAC (to see histopathological changes)
6. Biopsy (most confirmatory investigation)

Q. 8. What is the peculiar radiological feature of this tumor?

Ans. This tumor has following peculiar radiological features:

1. Codman's triangle
2. Sunburst appearance
3. Periosteal reaction

Q. 9. Can you explain that how these features develop?

Ans.

- Subperiosteal new bone formation occurs at the end of tumor in a triangular area which is known as **Codman's triangle.**
- New bone formation occurs along the Haversian canal which gives Sun-ray appearance.
- Periosteal reaction seen in osteosarcoma is different than seen in osteomyelitis because it is irregular in osteosarcoma and smooth in osteomyelitis.

Q. 10. What are other radiological features of this tumor?

Ans. Other radiological features of this tumor are as follows:

- Tumor arising from metaphysis shows irregular destruction of bone.
- Erosion of cortex is seen.
- Periosteal neoplastic new bone formation is seen.
- Pathological fractures may be seen in advanced cases.
- X-ray of chest shows pulmonary metastasis. CT-scan of chest is a better investigation to detect pulmonary metastasis.

Q. 11. What histopathological changes are seen in this tumor?

Ans. Area of destruction produces leg of mutton appearance. Tumor consistency varies from stony hard to soft gritty. Fibrous tumor is white, osseous tumor is yellowish white and tumor of cartilaginous origin is bluish white.

Malignant characteristics are seen in stromal cells e.g., anisocytosis, poikilocytosis, nuclear pyknosis, pleomorphism and polyhedral contour.

Q. 12. Is there any other investigation?

Ans. Few blood investigations are done:

1. Haemoglobin (low).
2. WBC, ESR (raised).
3. Serum alkaline phosphatase is markedely increased but it is not diagnostic. It's level falls after removal of tumor but it rises again if metastasis spreads in the body.

Q. 13. Do you know about any predisposing factors of osteosarcoma?

Ans. Osteosarcoma has following predisposing factors:

1. Oncogenic Virus

RNA virus which can produce bone tumor includes Harvey and Meloney mouse (murine) sarcoma virus. DNA viruses are polyoma virus and SV-40 virus.

2. Radiation

Radiation of more than 2000 rads may produce osteosarcoma. Tumor appears after 3-4 years of exposure.

3. Chemicals

Following chemicals may produce osteosarcoma:

- 20-methylcholanthrene
- Cupri chelated
  N-hydroxy2-acetylaminofluorene.
- Beryllium compound

Q. 14. How do you classify osteosarcoma?

Ans. Osteosarcoma has been classified in the following two types:

Clinical classification

1. Primary osteosarcoma
2. Secondary osteosarcoma

Pathological classification

1. Osteoblastic (sclerosing)
2. Osteolytic (telengiectatic or malignant bone aneurysm)
3. Chondroblastic
4. Fibroblastic

O.K. how will you treat this case?

Ans. Treatment Regimen

Following treatment regimen are applied for this tumor.

- Primary lesion is treated by amputation followed by high dose megavoltage therapy or vice versa.
- 1700 rads irradiation is given to lungs in 10 fractions in 15 days.
- Chemotherapy is started with Methotraxte, Adriamycin,Vincristine, Cyclophosphamide and Actinomycin-D.

Q. 15. How will you decide level of amputation?

Ans. First of all diagnosis should be confirmed by biopsy. Now level of amputation should be determined. Mid thigh thigh amputation is done if tumor involves lower end of femur (early case), and upper end tibia (early case). Disarticulation of hip or hind quarter amputation is done in tumor of upper end of femur. Fore quarter amputation is done in tumor of upper end of humerus. Time of surgery should be decided.

Q. 16. How will you treat pulmonary metastasis?

Ans. Pulmonary metastasis is treated on the following lines:

- Microemboli are treated by chemotherapy.
- Tumor mass of lung is treated either by lobectomy or wedge resection.
- After every 3 months CT-scan of lung is done.

Q. 17. What is Paget's sarcoma?

Ans. This is malignant transformation of Paget's disease. It is highly fatal and patient dies within 3 years.

Q. 18. What is parosteal sarcoma?

Ans. This is a low grade malignant tumor which takes origin within periosteum. It remains in intimate relationship to outer surface of periosteum. It is commonly seen between third and fourth decade.

Q. 19. What is the prognosis of osteosarcoma?

Ans. Prognosis

- This tumor is highly fatal. Patient dies within 2 years if he does not get any treatment.
- Pulmonary metastasis becomes evident usually 5-6 months after the onset of disease in 80% cases.
- Even after amputation 50% patients show pulmonary metastasis within 5 months.
- After detection of metastasis, death occurs within 6 months.
- 5–25% Patients show 5 years survival rate with or without metastasis.

EWING SARCOMA

Q. 1. What is your diagnosis?

Ans. My diagnosis is Ewing sarcoma of shaft of femur (R/L).

Q. 2. What are the points in favour of your diagnosis?

Ans. I have following points in favour of my diagnosis:

1. Patient age is 15 years. (normal range is 10–20 years)
2. This swelling is present in diaphyseal region of femur.
3. Patient gives history of painful localized swelling. Pain is intermittent and becomes worse at night.
4. Patient also gives history of intermittent fever.
5. This swelling is firm to hard.
6. Skin overlying swelling is red and oedematous and shows dilated veins.

Q. 3. What is ewing sarcoma?

Ans. Ewing sarcoma is a primary malignant bony tumor which arises from diaphysis of long bones.

Q. 4. Which are the common bones to be involved by this tumor?

Ans. This tumor commonly involve shaft of femur, tibia, fibula, and humerus in decreasing order of frequency.

Q. 5. What is peculiar feature of this tumor?

Ans. This tumor is extremely radiosensitive. During radiotherapy it melts like snow.

Q. 6. What is the radiological feature of this tumor?

Ans. Radiologically it is characterized by onion peel appearance.

Q. 7. Can you explain how does this feature develop?

Ans. New bone formation occurs around vessels that extend radially from periosteum to shaft.This subperiosteal new bone formation occurs in layers which produces onion peel appearance radiologically.

Q. 8. Are there any other conditions where you can get this onion peel appearance?

Ans. All of these 3 conditions may show onion peel appearance radiologically:

- Osteomyelitis
- Oseosarcoma
- Malignant lymphoma

Q. 9. How will you manage this case?

Ans. I would like to confirm my diagnosis first. I would like to do X-ray of local part (to see the type of tumor) as well as of chest (to see secondaries). Biopsy will confirm my diagnosis.

Q. 10. How does the metastasis spread in body?

Ans. Metastasis occurs through lymphatics and blood stream. Metastasis specially occurs in skull, vertebrae and ribs. **It metastasizes late to lungs.**

Q. 11. What do you expect from biopsy?

Ans. This tumor surrounds a central clear area with no central fibril thus creating **pseudorosette pattern.** Multiple layer of bones lie parallel to shaft.

Q. 12. Which is the stem cell for this tumor?

Ans. Stem cell for Ewing tumor is reticulum cell.

Q. 13. What are other investigations you would like to do for this tumor?

Ans. Hb (anemia), TLC (leukocytosis), urine examination (to see vanyllil mandelic acid VMA) and glycogen stain should be done.

O.K. how will you treat this case?

Ans. Treatment

Ewing sarcoma can be treated by following methods:

- This tumor is extremely radiosensitive. Tumor melts like snow. Radiation is treatment of choice. Recurrence is common.

Q. 14. What will you do for recurrence?

Ans. I will give combined local radiotherapy and systemic chemotherapy to decrease the chances of recurrence.

Q. 15. What is the dose of radiation?

Ans. 6000 rads exposure is given to local tumor and to control metastasis.

Q. 16. Can you tell me which chemotherapy is frequently given?

Ans.

1. Vincristine, cyclophosfamide or ifosfamide and adriamycin are given at every 3–4 weeks. Such 12–18 cycles are given.
2. New chemotherapy is used in the form of Ifosfamide, Cysplatinum and epipodophyllin toxin.

Q. 17. Do you have any idea of any surgical treatment for this tumor?

Ans. Yes, surgical treatment can be done in the form of debulking of tumor or limb preservation surgery.

Q. 18. What is the prognosis of this tumor?

Ans. Radiotherapy followed by amputation has 2 years survival rate.

Chemotherapy, radiotherapy and amputation combinedly increase survival rate upto 3–5 years in 50–75% cases.

Q. 19. What is your differential diagnosis?

Ans. I would like to keep following conditions in differential diagnosis:

- Osteomyelitis
- Oseosarcoma
- Malignant lymphoma.

CHAPTER

44 Orthopaedics Terminology

- Fractures with eponyms
- Important signs
- Dislocation with eponyms
- Clinical tests/signs
- Operations and their indications

FRACTURES WITH EPONYMS

Fracture of necessity

This is Galeazzi fracture i.e., fracture of lower end of radius with subluxation or dislocation of inferior radioulnar joint. Galeazzi fracture is also known as reverse monteggia fracture.

Chauffer's fracture

This is fracture of radial styloid process.

Bennet's fracture

This is an intraarticular fracture of base of first metacarpal bone.

Rolando fracture

This is an extra articular fracture of base of first metacarpal bone.

Essex-Lopresti fracture

This is fracture head of radius with dislocation of inferior radioulnar joint.

Night stick fracture

This is fracture of shaft of ulna.

Smith fracture

This is reverse of Colles's fracture. i.e., fracture of lower end of radius with palmar displacement.

Volar barton fracture

This is anterior marginal fracture of lower end radius.

Dorsal barton fracture

This is posterior marginal fracture of lower end of radius.

Base ball finger

This is also known as **Mallet finger.** This is an avulsion of extensor tendon of distal interphalangeal joint from it's insertion at the base of terminal phalanx.

Whiplash injury

This is a ligamentous injury of neck.

Malgaigne's fracture

This is disruption of pelvic ring associated with injury to pubic symphysis and sacroiliac joint on same side.

Holstein-Lewis fracture

This is an oblique fracture of distal third of humerus associated with radial nerve injury. Radial nerve is entrapped between fracture ends.

Mallet thumb

This is an avulsion of extensor pollicis longus insertion into base of disal phalanx, leading to flexion deformity of thumb.

Jersy finger

This fracture is seen in adolescent and young adults. Instead of more common avulsion of FDP from it's metaphyseal insertion on volar aspect of distal phalanx, a metaphyseal fragment with variable amount of physis may accompany the tendon.

Gamekeeper's thumb

This is also known as **Skier thumb.** This is partial or complete disruption of ulnar collateral ligament and volar plate, is caused by valgus stress applied to metacarpophalangeal joint of thumb.

Boxer's fracture

This is fracture neck of 5th metacarpal that is ventrally displaced. It is commonly seen in boxers.

Jefferson's fracture

This is fracture of first cervical vertebra.

Hangman fracture

This is fracture of second cervical vertebra that occurs through it's pedicle. This is not associated with any neurological deficit.

Chance fracture

This is a type of seat belt injury. This is a horizontal avulsion fracture of vertebral bodies.

Clay Shoveler's fracture

This is fracture of spinous process of first thoracic vertebra, caused by strong muscular action. It is commonly seen in shoveling by labourers.

Bumper's fracture

This is fracture of lateral condyle of tibia, occurs as a result of hit by bumper of a car of truck.

Dash board fracture

This is fracture of patella that occurs as a result of knee striking to dash board of a car due to sudden application of brake.

Pott's fracture

This is fracture of medial and lateral malleoli and also known as bimalleolar fracture.

Cotton's fracture

This is fracture of medial, lateral and posterior malleoli also known as trimalleolar fracture.

Aviator's fracture

This is fracture of neck of talus, caused by forced dorsiflexion of ankle and commonly seen in air craft crash.

Jone's fracture

This is fracture of base of 5th metatarsal.

March fracture

This is fatigue fracture of second metatarsal caused by repeated stress and commonly seen in soldiers.

Hoffa's fracture

This is fracture of femoral condyle in coronal plane.

Maisonneuve fracture

This is an ankle injury associated with fracture neck of fibula.

Jumper's knee

This is inflammation of patellar tendon which involves lower pole of patella. This is also known as Runner's knee (patellar tendinitis).

Dancer tendinitis

This is tendinitis of flexor hallucis longus. It is commonly seen among ballet dancers.

Facet syndrome

This is painful condition of spine. Patient has early morning stiffness in spine, chronic backache. Patient may have difficulty in sitting, standing and climbing upstairs and getting out of bed.

Pseudogout

This is arthropathy of larger joints (mainly knee joint) in which calcium pyrophosphate is deposited in joints. This condition is less severe than gout.

IMPORTANT SIGNS

Reisser's sign

This sign is seen in scoliosis.

Trethowan sign

This is seen in slipped capital femoral epiphysis.

Hawkin's sign

This sign is seen in avascular necrosis of talus.

Scottish terrier sign

This is seen in spondylolisthesis.

Aneurysmal sign

This is seen in anterior type of spinal tuberculosis.

DISLOCATION WITH EPONYMS

Otto pelvis

This is a pathological condition in which acetabulum gradually shifts into pelvis. It is commonly seen in osteomalacia.

Spondylolisthesis

(Spondylos=spine, olisthesis=to slip)

This is a slow anterior displacement of a vertebra at the lower lumbar spine. Interruption in continuity of pars interarticularis is essential lesion. It is commonly seen between L5-S1 and L4-5.

Perilunate dislocation

This is dislocation of carpal bones surrounding lunate bone. Lunate becomes stationary.

Lunate dislocation

This is dislocation of lunate which comes out, infront of carpal bones.

Divergent dislocation

This type of dislocation is seen in elbow where radius and ulna dislocates away from each other.

Luxatio erecta

This is subglenoid type of dislocation of shoulder. Patient comes with affected arm erected up in the air. This is uncommon type of dislocation.

Lisfranc's dislocation

This is dislocation through intertarsal joint.

Chopart's dislocation

This is dislocation through talonavicular joint.

CLINICAL TESTS/SIGNS

Apley's grinding test

This test is done to rule out injury to meniscus and collateral ligaments.

Apprehension sign

This test is done to detect instability of shoulder.

Anvil test

In this test a sudden jerk is applied over the head of patient. Patient will feel pain at the site of lesion. This test can also be performed in another way. Ask the patient to jump down from a chair. Patient will feel pain at the site of lesion

Allen's test

This is done to check the patency of radial and ulnar arteries. Ask the patient to clench his fist tightly. Now press his radial and ulnar arteries at wrist. Patient is asked to open his fist after one minute. Color of palm turns white. Now release pressure over radial artery. Normally color of palm will become normal. If it remains white that means radial artery is blocked. This test can be repeated and now pressure over ulnar artery is first released. If color of hand remains white that means ulnar artery is blocked.

Adson test

This test is positive in cervical rib and scalenius syndrome. In this test patient is asked to sit on a stool and to take a deep breath. Turn his face to affected side. Now feel pulsation of radial artery on wrist. Pulse will be obliterated.

Alli's test

This test is positive in congenital dislocation of hip.

Brayant's sign

Axillary fold is lowered down in dislocation of shoulder. This is known as Brayant's sign.

Barlow's test

This test is done in congenital dislocation of hip.

Cozen's test

This test is done in tennis elbow.

Callaway's test

This test is done in subglenoid dislocation of humerus (**Callaway's test**) and fracture neck of scapula.

Chovstek's sign

This is positive in tetany.

Coin test

This is positive in pott's spine.

Drawer test

Anterior or posterior translation of tibia indicates anterior or posterior cruciate ligament injury respectively.

Froment's sign

This test is done to check the strength of adductor pollicis. (median nerve)

Finkelstein test

This test is performed in Dequervain's disease.

Galleazzi's sign

This test is done to detect limb shortening in children.

Genslen's test

This test is done in ankylosing spodylitis.

Gower's sign

This sign is present in muscular dystrophy. Child stands up as if climbing upon his body by supporting it with his hand. Positive sign indicates weakness of pelvic girdle muscle.

Hamilton's ruler test

This test is done in dislocation of shoulder.

Kanavel's sign

This sign is positive in infection of ulnar bursa. Point of maximum tenderness is present in between transverse creases.

Ludloff's sign

This sign is positive in avulsion of lesser trochanter.

Lasegue test

This test is done in PIVD.

Lachman's test

This test is done in a severely painful and grossly swollen knee. Anterior or posterior translation confirms anterior or posterior cruciate ligament injury respectively.

McMurray's test

This is done to detect menisci injury.

Naffziger's sign

This sign is positive in prolapsed intervertebral disc. In this sign pressure on jugular vein is increased.

Ortolani's test

This test is done in congenital dislocation of hip.

Ober's test

This test is done in polio to see the tightness of ilio-tibial band.

O'Donoghue triad

This triad includes following three injuries:

1. Injury to medial structures
2. ACL injury
3. Medial meniscus injury

Policeman's tip hand

This is seen in Erb's palsy.

Sulcus sign

This sign is positive in inferior dislocation of shoulder.

Tinel's sign

This is sign of recovery of nerve injury.

Trendlenberg's test

This test is positive in poliomyelitis, motor neurone disease, muscular dystrophies, congenital dislocation of hip, fracture neck femur, coxa vara, perthes disease etc.

Volkman's sign

This sign is present in Volkman's ischaemic contracture.

OPERATIONS AND THEIR INDICATIONS

Operations	Indications
Bristow's procedure	Recurrent dislocation of shoulder
Bankart's procedure	Recurrent dislocation of shoulder
Dwyer's osteotomy	CTEV
Evan's procedure	CTEV
Girdlestone arthroplasty	Tuberculosis of hip
Grice-green procedure	Subtalar arthrodesis
Hauser's operation	Recurrent dislocation of patella
Jone's procedure	Correction of foot deformity in polio
Keller's procedure	Hallux valgus
Lambrinudi's procedure	Correction of equinus deformity
Meyer's procedure	Fracture neck femur
Putti-plat operation	Recurrent dislocation of shoulder
Steindler's release	CTEV
Soutter's release	Correction of flexion deformity of hip in polio
Turco's release	CTEV
Tension-band wiring	Fracture of patella, olecranon and medial malleolus
Yount's release	Flexion deformity of knee
Wilson's release	Flexion deformity of knee in polio

CHAPTER

45 Joint Replacement

- Hemireplacement arthroplasty of hip
- Total hip replacement
- Corail hip
- Total knee replacement
- Gender knee
- Shoulder arthroplasty
- Total elbow replacement
- Artificial disc replacement

Various implants are in use in different aetiology. Some of them are very common in use. A few implants are new in India e.g. proxima hip, artificial disc, telefix, ballon kyphoplasty and gender knee.

Here we will discuss different types of joint replacement.

HEMIREPLACEMENT ARTHROPLASTY OF HIP

Arthroplasty of hip can be performed by following prosthesis:

1. Austin-Moore prostheis
2. Thompson prosthesis
3. Bipolar hip prosthesis
4. Proxima hip.

Austin-Moore Prosthesis

This prosthesis is indicated for management of fracture neck femur in elderly patients. This prosthesis has 3 parts; head, neck and stem. Size of head varies from 35 mm to 59 mm. This prosthesis is used without cement because it has 2 holes in middle and use of bone cement will fix this prosthesis permanently in body. Through these 2 holes bone grows and helps in fixation of prosthesis. This prosthesis has a small hole at it's top through which a hook of extractor can be inserted to remove prosthesis.

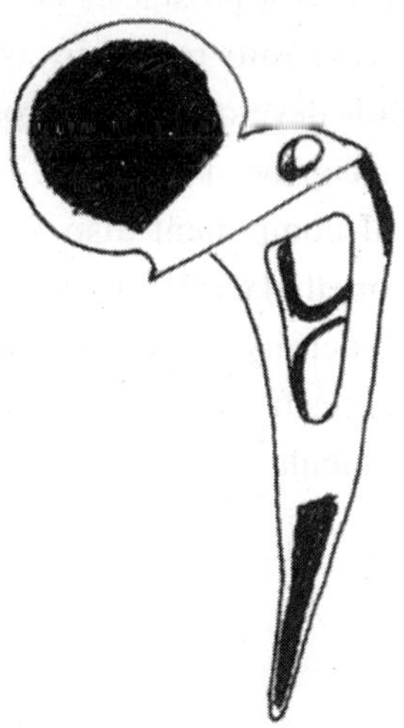

Fig. 45.1 Austin-Moore's prosthesis

Thompson Prosthesis

This prosthesis is used in old cases of fracture neck femur where neck is absorbed. This prosthesis can be used with or without bone cement. This prosthesis does not have fenestration holes in middle and hole at top for implant removal.

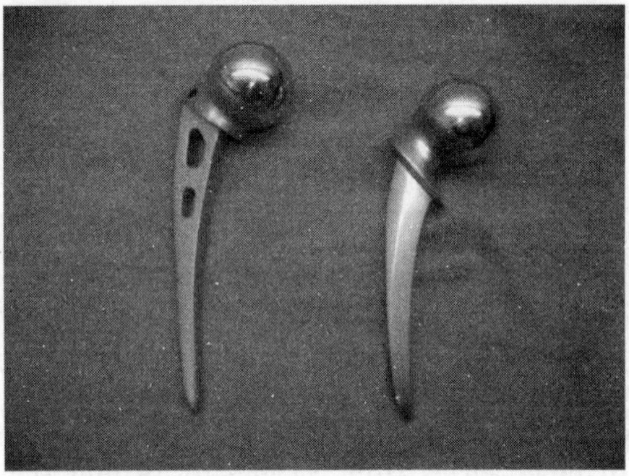

Fig. 45.2 Thompson's prosthesis (R) and Austin-Moore's prosthesis (L)

Bipolar Hip Prosthesis

This is indicated when chances of acetabular erosion and protrusion are high (by a prosthesis). This is usually done at or above 60 years of age. Advantage of bipolar prosthesis is that this can be easily converted into total hip arthroplasty if acetabular pain develops. This prosthesis had 3 parts: metallic cup, head and stem. This prosthesis has a femoral component also known as stem (made up of methylacrylate) and a metallic cup (lined by high density polyethylene). This bipolar prosthesis reduces friction and impaction forces at prosthesis-acetabular cartilage interface.

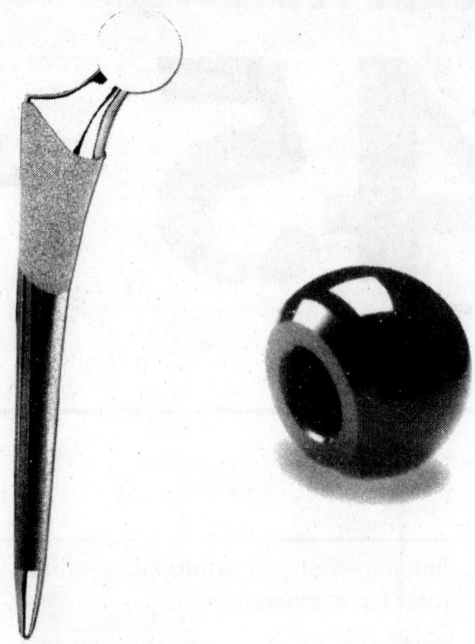

(*a*) Bipolar hip (*b*) Femoral head

Fig. 45.3

Proxima Hip

This is a hip prosthesis which is used for primary hip arthroplasty. This is latest prosthesis which is being used in India.

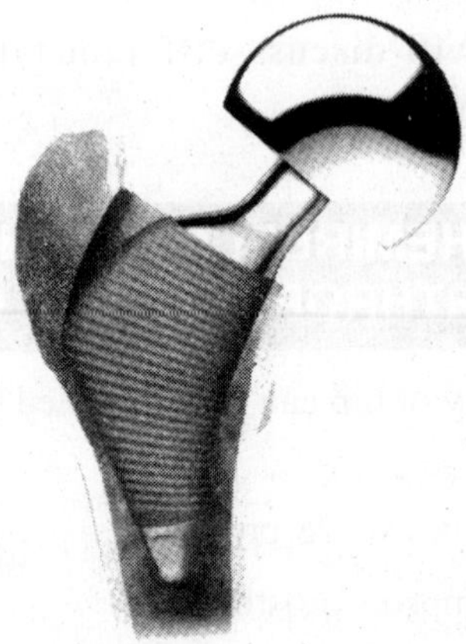

Fig. 45.4 Proxima hip

Indication

This is indicated when surgeon wants to conserve bone and soft tissue.This prosthesis provides physiological loading to proximal femur.

Pre-requisite

1. Metaphyseal area of femur should be of good quality.
2. Proximal femur should have supportive bone medially and laterally.
3. X-ray of hip A.P. view should be done in slight interal rotation.
4. True lateral view of hip should also be done to assess fitness of implant superiorly.

Technique

This prosthesis is implanted through **'round the corner technique'**. This is minimally invasive surgery. This can be done by anterior, anterolateral or posterolateral approach.

TOTAL HIP REPLACEMENT

Total hip replacement is done when patient presents with gross osteoarthritic changes in acetabulum and head of femur, severe pain in hip and difficulty in walking. Total hip replacement can be done by following prosthesis:

1. Charnley's total hip prosthesis
2. Muller's prosthesis
3. Corail hip prosthesis.

Charnley's Total Hip Prosthesis

This is a complete hip prosthesis by which damaged acetabulum and head of femur can be replaced. Acetabular component is made up of polyethylene while head is made up of steel. This prosthesis can be fixed with the help of bone cement. This is the total hip prosthesis which is most commonly used.

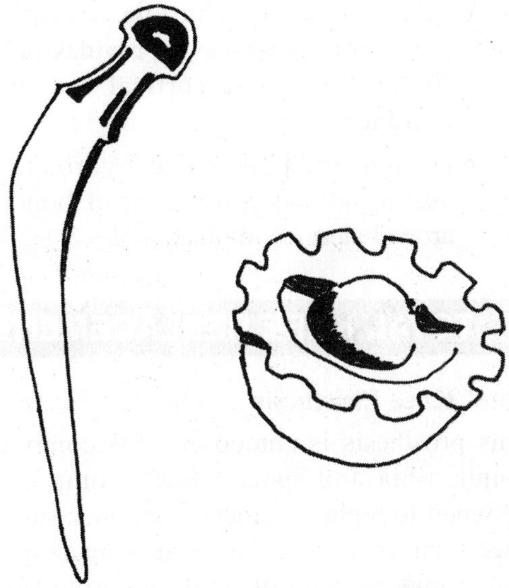

(*a*) Charnley's total hip prosthesis (*b*) Acetabular cup

Fig. 45.5

Muller Prosthesis

This prosthesis resembles with Charnley's prosthesis except it's head size is 32 mm size. Stem of this prosthesis is available in different sizes.

CORAIL HIP

This is a total hip prosthesis developed by international visitation centre Corail-France.

Indication

This is indicated in severe osteoarthritis of hip involving head of femur as well as acetabular cup.

Features

- It provides primary mechanical stability, secondary biological integration, bone preservation and harmonius stress transfer.
- This has hydroxyapatite coating which allows secondary biological integration.

- This surgical technique allows bone preservation because it provides optimum filling not a close cortical contact with implant.
- Design of implant and hydroxyapatite coating allows restoration of bone stock around stem of implant.

TOTAL KNEE REPLACEMENT

Total Knee Prosthesis

This prosthesis is composed of 3 components; femur, tibia and spacer. Each component is designed to replace damaged articular surface of knee joint. Femoral component is made of metal which may be with or without porous coating. Tibial component may be made of polyethylene or composed of metal tibial tray with or without porous coating and a polyethylene insert and locking component. Metal components may have modular stems or wedge. Patella component may be fully made of polyethylene or may be a metal backed polyethylene component. Patellar component is used only when, patella shows severe arthritic changes. Prosthesis is sterlised for 10 minutes at 270 degree F (132 degree C) by steam and prevaccum method.

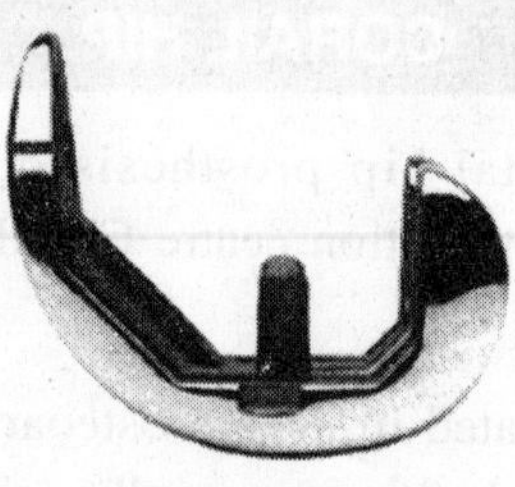

(*a*) Total knee prosthesis (Lateral view)

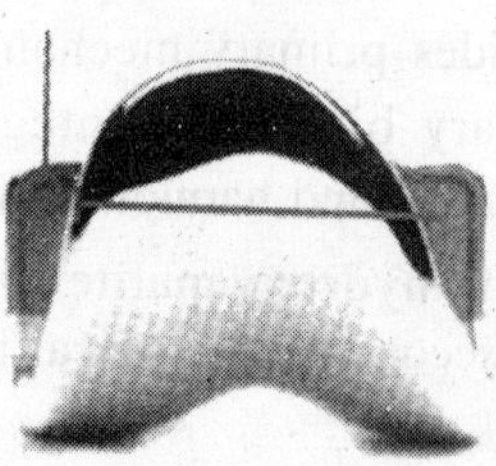

(*b*) Total knee prosthesis (A.P. view)

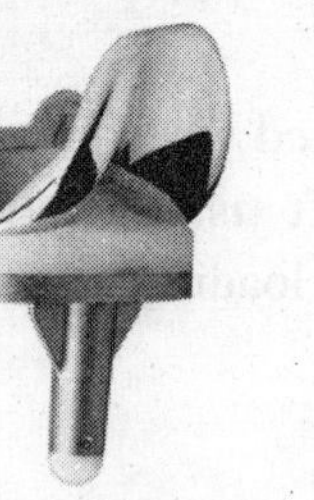

(*c*) Total knee prosthesis

Fig. 45.6

Titanium and polyethylene components are compatible with MRI.

Unicompartmental Knee Prosthesis

This is indicated when only one condyle of femur and tibia show gross arthritic changes. This is done when patient has more than 30 degree fixed valgus or varus deformity. Composition of prosthesis remains same.

Patellofemoral Prosthesis

This prosthesis is being used in U.K. This is a latest prosthesis which has also been started in India recently. This is indicated in isolated arthritis of patellofemoral area.

Indications

Primary goal of total/unicompartmental knee replacement is to provide pain free knee joint and to increase mobility by replacing damaged knee articulation. Knee replacement is indicated in following conditions:

1. Osteoarthritis
2. Post traumatic arthritis
3. Rheumatoid arthritis
4. Failed previous prosthesis.

Contraindications

Knee replacement should not be done in following conditions:

1. Active infection either local or systemic.
2. Osteoporosis
3. Loss of bone or musculature.
4. Neurovascular compromise.

5. Insufficiency of collateral ligaments.
6. Severely unstable knee due to loss of osteochondral structure.

Risk Factors

Following conditions can lead to failure of knee replacement:

1. Overweight patient
2. Excessive sport activity.
3. Alcohol or drug addiction.
4. Uncontrolled diabetes mellitus.
5. Intake of steroids and immunosuppressive drugs.
6. Active local or general infection.
7. Disability of other joint like hip and ankle.

Complications

Patient can have early and late post operative complications as follows:

Early Complications

1. Haematoma is a common complication.
2. Delayed wound healing.
3. Wound dehiscence.
4. Varus or valgus deformity.

Late Complications

1. Inadequate range of movements at knee joint.
2. Lossening of prosthesis.
3. Flexion contracture of knee.
4. Fracture of tibia or femur.
5. Myositis ossificans.
6. Allergic reaction to implant.

GENDER KNEE

This is a total knee replacement prosthesis which has been specially shaped for women's knee. This has been introduced recently in India. This has been shaped because of following reasons:

1. Anatomical differences in men's and women's knee.
2. Women's knee requires intraoperative adjustment.
3. Osteoarthritis is more commonly seen in women.

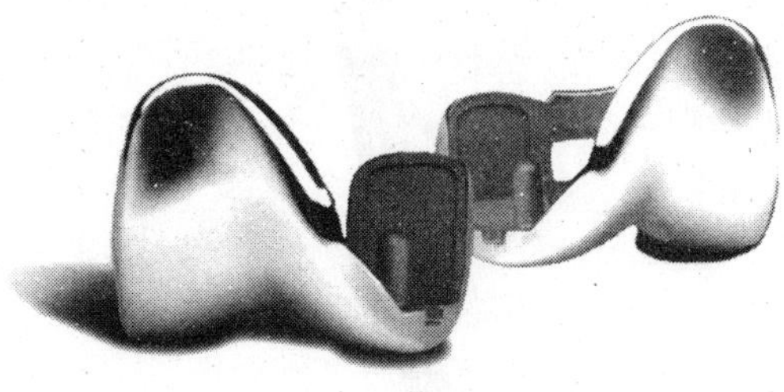

Fig. 45.7 Gender knee

Features

1. Modified anterior flange. Anterior flange thickness of implant has been reduced.
2. Patellar sulcus is recessed.
3. Anterior flange width is less in comparision to male.
4. Gender knee has increased trochlear groove.
5. This knee has modified mediolateral/ anteroposterior aspect ratio.

SHOULDER ARTHROPLASTY

Shoulder replacement is now becoming popular in our country. In hemireplacement of shoulder, we do not use glenoid prosthesis while in total shoulder replacement humeral head and glenoid cavity are replaced by prosthesis. Prosthesis is composed of humeral head, stem and glenoid components.

Indications

Total or hemireplacement of shoulder can be done in following conditions:

1. Severe osteoarthritis, traumatic arthritis or rheumatoid arthritis leading to severe painful and disabled shoulder joint.

CHAPTER 45

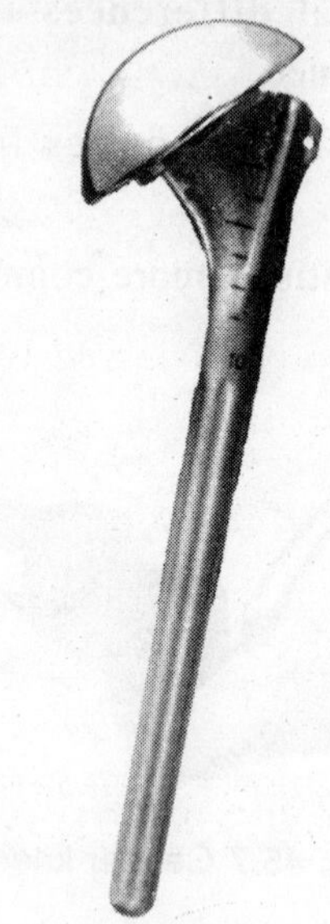

(*a*) Shoulder prosthesis

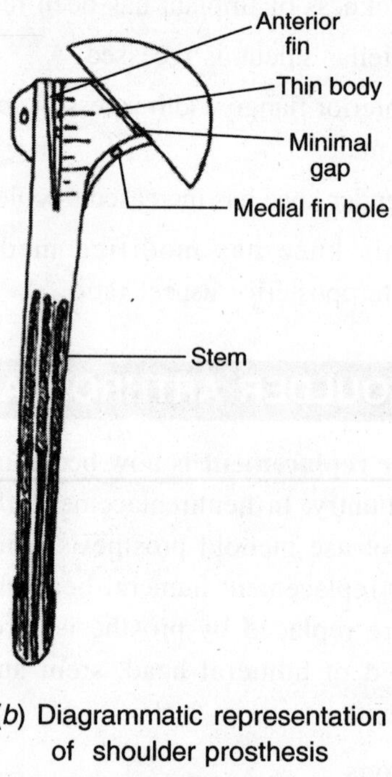

(*b*) Diagrammatic representation of shoulder prosthesis

Fig. 45.8

2. Fracture dislocation of proximal humerus with grossly comminuted articular surface, separated from it's blood supply.
3. Revision of failed primary prosthesis.

Hemi replacement of shoulder can also be done in following conditions:

1. Un united humeral head fracture.
1. Avascular necrosis of humeral head.
2. Rotator cuff tear arthropathy.

Contraindications

1. Active local or systemic infection.
2. Insufficient bone stock at proximal humerus or glenoid fossa to support the prosthesis.
3. Severe osteoporosis.
4. Total shoulder arthroplasty should not be done in absence of rotator cuff muscles or in case of nonfunctional/irreparable rotator cuff tear.

Complications

1. Postoperative haematoma
2. Infection
3. Lossening of prosthesis
4. Change in position of component.

TOTAL ELBOW REPLACEMENT

Elbow Prosthesis

Total elbow replacement is not such common as total knee replacement. However two types of prosthesis are being used for this purpose:

1. GSB III- Elbow prosthesis
2. Coonrad/Morrey elbow prosthesis.

GSB III-elbow prosthesis is much commoner than Coonrad/Morrey prosthesis.

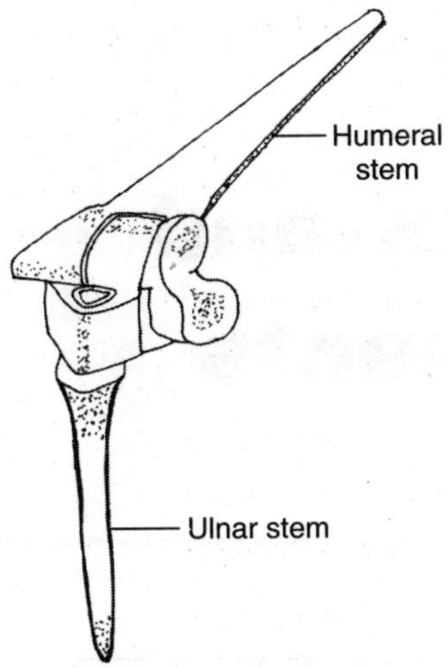

Fig. 45.9 (*a*) GSB III-elbow prosthesis

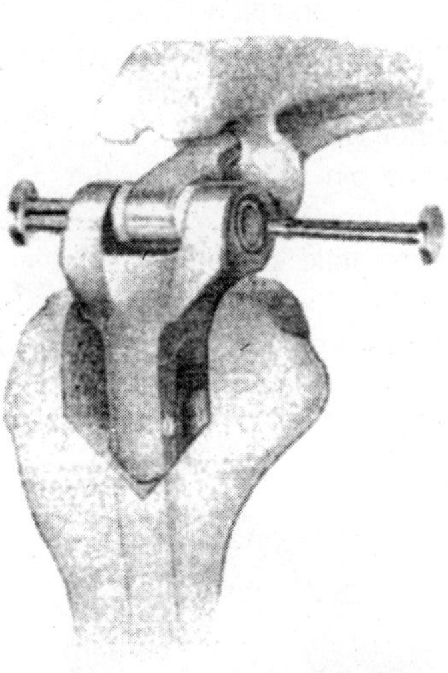

Fig. 45.9 (*b*) Coonrad/Morrey total elbow prosthesis

GSB III-Elbow Prosthesis

This is best prosthesis to replace elbow joint. This prosthesis is in use since 1971. This is indicated in grossly destroyed elbow joint where articular margins of humerus, radius and ulna are destroyed. This can also be performed in bony ankylosis of elbow.

Advantages

1. This prosthesis provides wide support plane on condyles.
2. Loose link connection between humerus and ulna allows an angle of 3-5 degree for axial deviation and rotation.
3. Anchoring of humerus and ulna is less strained.
4. Force is not transferred to the ends of anchoring shaft.

Other Elbow Prosthesis

1. Baksi's prosthesis
2. Soutter's prosthesis.

ARTIFICIAL DISC REPLACEMENT

Artificial disc replacement is indicated for spinal arthroplasty in skeletally mature patient who has discogenic pain with degenerative disc disease between L4 and S1. Disc replacement was **firstly** done by **Schellnack, Buttner and Janz** in Germany at charite hospital.

Indications

1. Mono or bisegmental degenerative disc disease with chronic backache.
2. Post discectomy syndrome.

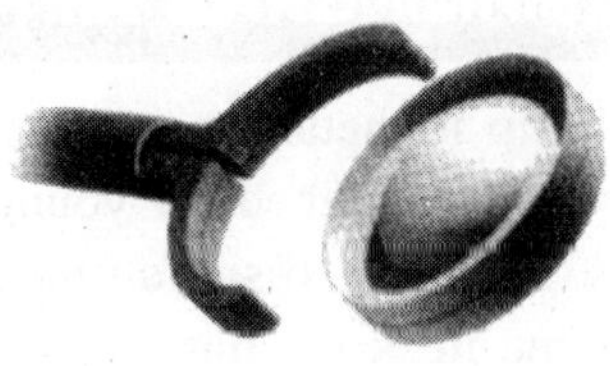

Fig. 45.10 Artificial disc

Contraindications

1. Lysis or lysthesis
2. Severe lumbar kyphosis
3. Lumbar canal stenosis
4. Multi level disc degeneration.

Implant position

It should be 2 mm posterior to midline.

CHAPTER

46 Implants and Instruments

- Hip resurfacing surgenry (Birmingham hip)
- Proximal femoral nail
- Distal femoral nail
- Management of fracture shaft femur
- Intramedullary 'V' nail
- Tibial interlocking nail
- Management of fracture shaft humerus
- Management of fracture both bones forearm
- Limited contact DCP
- Dynamic reconstruction plate
- Buttress plate
- Staples
- Semitubular plate
- Reconstruction plate
- Locking compression plate
- Versatile plate system
- Swanson hand prosthesis
- Kirschner wire
- Steinman pin
- Pedicle screw
- Vertebroplastic cement
- Telefix
- Balloon kyphoplasty

HIP RESURFACING SURGERY (BIRMINGHAM HIP)

Birmingham hip is metal on metal replacement which is specially designed for young patient of hip arthritis. This is a **resurfacing surgery** in which **head** and **neck** are **not removed.** Surface of femoral head is shaped to exactly fit the ball of femoral side of prosthesis.

Indication

This is indicated in young patient with arthritis of hip.

Advantages

Birmingham hip has following advantages over total hip replacement:

- This is long lasting.

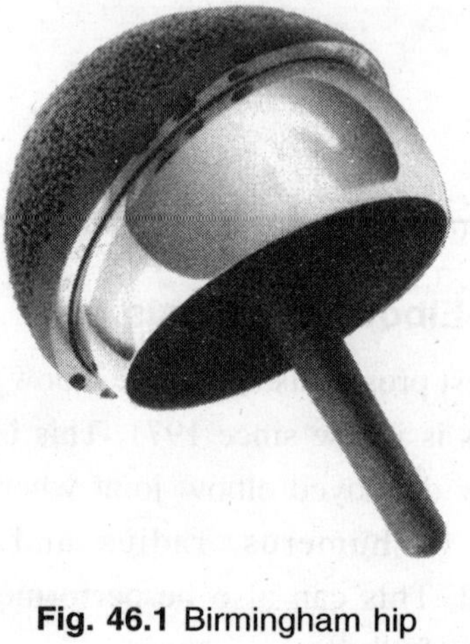

Fig. 46.1 Birmingham hip

- It resembles with normal anatomy of hip joint.
- This can restore same level of physical activity and quality of life in young patients.

- This prosthesis does not dislocate.
- Birmingham hip feels like normal hip.
- If revision surgery is required it can be performed with modular Birmingham hip replacement *(BHR)*.

Table 46.1: Differences between total and Birmingham hip replacement

THR	BHR
This is a metal on plastic prosthesis.	This is metal on metal prosthesis.
This requires excision of head and neck of femur.	This is conservative prosthesis and does not require same.
This is suitable for elderly patient with low activity.	This is suitable for young patient with hip arthritis.
This wears out rapidly and may require revision surgery.	This is usually long lasting and does not require revision surgery.
Activities are restricted due to fear of dislo-cation.	Patient can sit on floor, squat. He can use Indian toilet.
Patient is not advised sport activities.	Patient is encouraged for sport activities.
Polyethylene wears debries.	Osteolysis does not occur.

PROXIMAL FEMORAL NAIL (PFN)

This nail is indicated in fracture subtrochanteric femur and proximal fracture of shaft femur.

Features

PFN has 3 parts: nail, bolt and end cap. These parts have following features:

- This nail has various diameters: 9, 10, 11, 12, 13 mm.

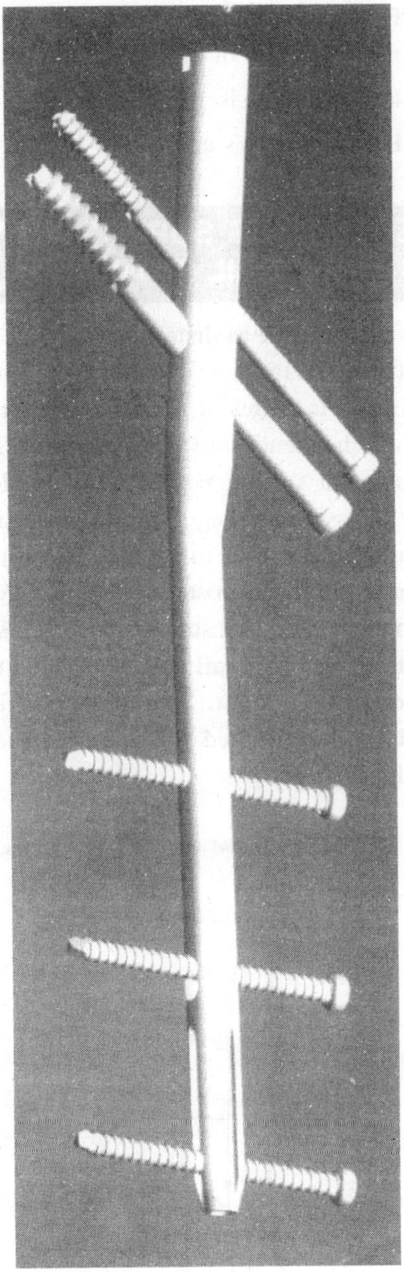

Fig. 46.2 Proximal femoral nail

- It's thread length are available in various sizes: 22, 24, 26 cm.
- It's bolt diameter is 7.5 mm and length is 50–120 mm.

- Bolts are cannulated with facility of guide wire insertion of 2.5 mm.
- It's nail angle is 135 degree
- Diameter of it's end cap is 14 mm.

INTERLOCKING SUPRACONDYLAR NAIL (DFN)

This is also known as distal femoral nail. This is an intramedullary nail which is used for comminuted fractures of supracondylar region of femur which extends into articular surface. Patient is positioned supine with knee flexed 30–40 degree across a sand bag support. Nail is inserted retrogradely through intercondylar notch just anterior to origin of posterior cruciate ligament. Placement of proximal screws should be superior to fracture line. This nail does not intend to carry full weight of patient. So full weight bearing should not be allowed till abundant callus is formed.

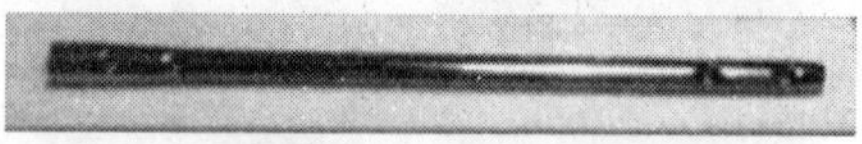

(*a*) Supracondylar nail

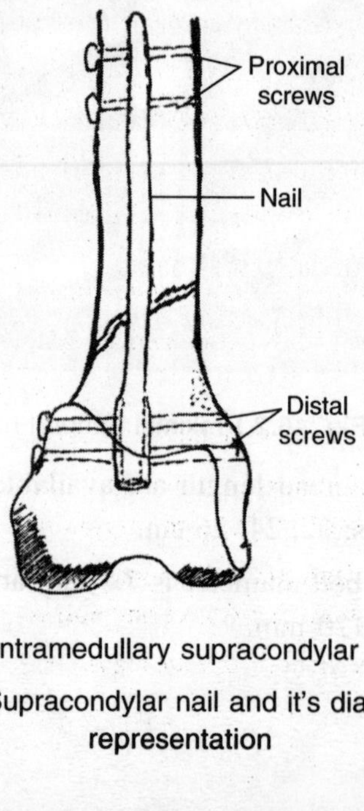

(*b*) Intramedullary supracondylar nail

Fig. 46.3 Supracondylar nail and it's diagrammatic representation

Indications

1. Fracture of distal third of femur (comminuted) which extends into articular area.
2. Pathological fracture at supracondylar region of femur.
3. Osteoporotic fracture of supracondylar region of femur.
4. Metaphyseal femoral fractures in obese and obstetric patients.
5. It can be used in patients with existing TKR but it depends on it's design.

Contraindications

1. Any acute infection.
2. In cases who has chance of crossing over epiphyseal plate.

Features

This nail has two types of locking system; spiral blade locking and standard locking.

Distal femoral nail has high purchase in osteoporotic metaphyseal fractures.

Advantages of Spiral blade locking

This provides angular stable locking of spiral blade.

It has got large bearing surface which provides optimized load distribution, high purchase in osteoporotic fractures.

This locking system has reduced risk of nail protrusion in knee joint.

It can be used for complex fractures and osteoporotic bone.

Advantages of standard locking

This has 2 locking screws of 6 mm size.

This system provides angular stable locking of distal locking screw.

It can be used for less complex fractures with high bone density.

TYPES OF DFN NAIL

This nail is of 2 types, short and long nail as follows:

Short nail

These nail have sizes of 160, 200, 240 mm. This can be used for distal femoral fractures with latero-medial locking.

Long nails

These nails have sizes of 300, 340, 380 and 420 mm. This nail can be used for metaphyseal or extensive femoral fractures with antero-posterior proximal locking. This nail has an option of immediate or secondary dynamisation.

MANAGEMENT OF FRACTURE SHAFT FEMUR

Fracture shaft femur can be managed by following implants:

1. Kuntscher intramedullary nail
2. Femur interlocking nail.
3. Expandable intramedullary nail (Isreal nail)
4. Proximal femoral nail **PFN** (for proximal fracture of shaft femur)

Kuntscher Intramedullary Nail

This nail has longitudinal gutter. This gutter makes the nail compressible. Along with this, endosteal callus can also grow inside it at the fracture site. Both the ends of nail have eye. This eye is used for extraction of nail. Distal eye can be used for

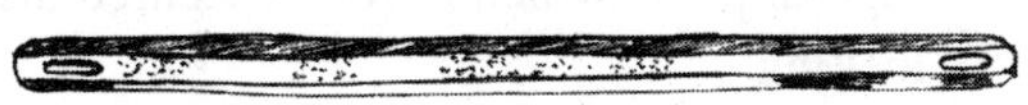

Kuntscher's cloverleaf intramedullary nail

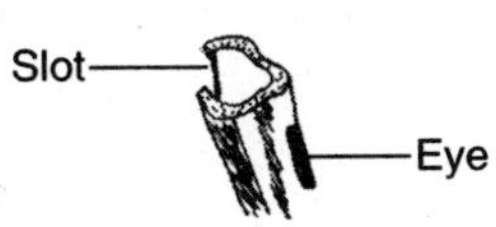

Fig. 46.4

extraction during retrograde nailing. This nail is trifoliate in cross-section. This trifoliate structure provides 3 point fixation in medullary cavity and nail does not rotate inside the marrow cavity.

Indications

Any fracture shaft femur traumatic/pathological/ segmental can be managed by KIM nail. Associated injuries (ipsilateral dislocation hip/ fracture both bones leg/case of polytrauma) also demand for KIM nail.

Absolute indication

Fracture shaft femur at the isthmus level is an absolute indication for KIM nail. Isthmus is part of femur where marrow is narrowest in diameter.

Femur Interlocking Nail

This nail is used for unstable fracture of shaft femur. This nail is available in various diameter (9, 10, 11, 12, 13 mm) and length (34, 36, 38, 40, 42, 44, 46, 48 cm).

Fig. 46.5 Femoral interlocking nail

MANAGEMENT OF FRACTURE SHAFT TIBIA

This fracture can be managed by following implants:

1. Intramedullary V nail.
2. Tibial interlocking nail
3. Broad DCP (*discussed later in this chapter*).

Intramedullary 'V' Nail

This nail is indicated for fracture shaft of tibia. Proximal end has an eye which is used for extraction of nail. Distal end is pointed while proximal end is normal. Proximal end has angulation for easy purchase of nail inside medullary cavity.

This nail is inserted from medial aspect of tibial tuberosity.

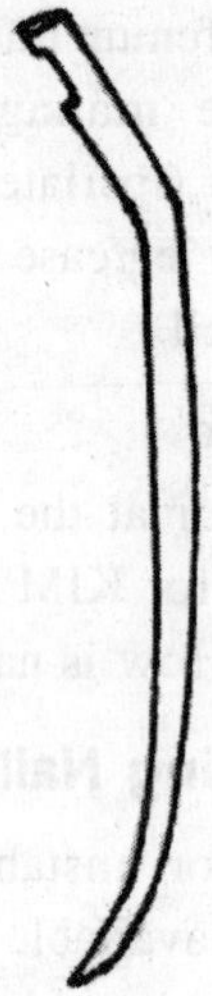

Fig. 46.6 'V' nail

TIBIAL INTERLOCKING NAIL

Tibial interlocking nails are of two types, solid tibial nail and cannulated tibial nail.

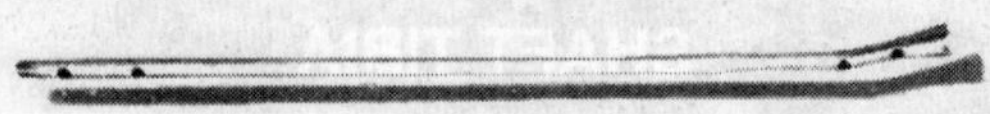

Fig. 46.7 Tibial interlocking nail

Indications (solid tibial nail)

1. It can be used in grade I and II compound fracture of shaft tibia.
2. It can also be used for unstable closed fractures of shaft tibia.
3. Narrow medullary canal.
4. Pre and postisthmic fractures of tibia.
5. It can also be used as a secondary procedure after removal of external fixator.

Indications (Cannulated Tibial Nail)

1. This nail can be used in simple and compound fractures of shaft of tibia.
2. Pre and postithmic fractures of tibia.
3. Malunited fractures of shaft tibia can be corrected.
4. Nonunion of shaft tibia.

Features (proximal end)

1. Proximal end of nail is flattened to prevent possible irritation of patellar tendon.
2. Proximal end has a curvature of 9 degree which fits the anatomy of tibia thus it provides a stabilizing effect.
3. Oblique locking hole provides stable interlocking of proximal third fracture.
4. Proximal end has a slot for dynamic or static locking depending on position of locking bolt.
5. Proximal end has a static transverse locking hole.

Features (distal end)

1. This end has 3 distal locking holes.
2. Two holes are in frontal plane and one in sagittal plane which provides secured distal locking.

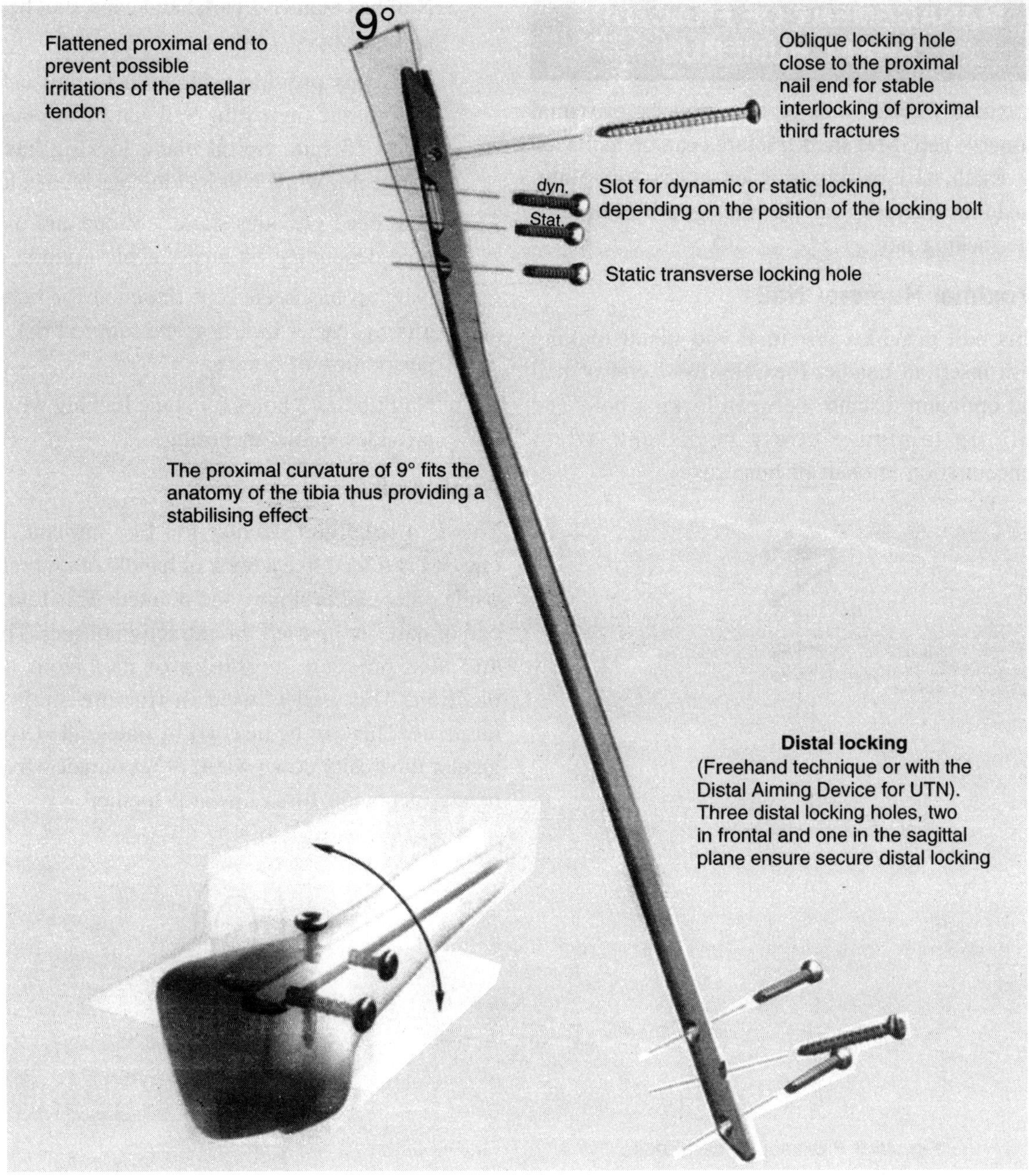

Fig. 46.8 Cannulated tibial nail

MANAGEMENT OF FRACTURE SHAFT HUMERUS

Proximal fracture can be managed by proximal humerus nail. Mid shaft fractures can be managed by Rush nail or dynamic compression plate. Unstable fractures can be managed by humerus interlocking nail.

Proximal Humeral Nail

This nail provides proximal and distal locking with insertion handle. Flexible distal end of nail and optimum distance between locking bolts and nail tip minimize stress peaks and stress concentration in shaft of humerus.

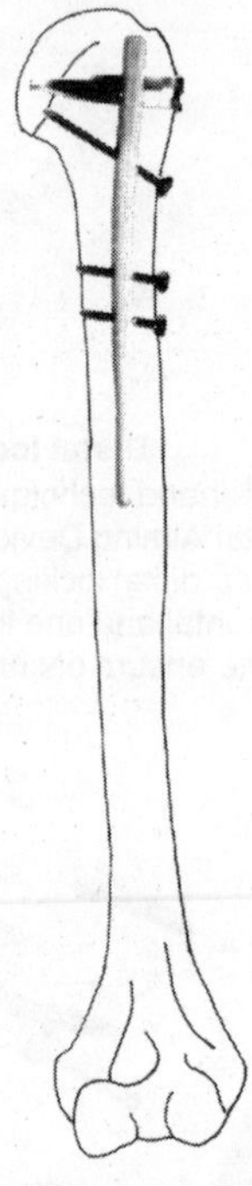

Fig. 46.9 Proximal humeral nail

Indications

1. Fractures at proximal end of humerus.
2. Subcapital humeral fractures in adults.

Features

1. This nail is made up of titanium alloy. TAN (Ti-6A-7Nb) provides high flexibility and excellent fatigue resistance.
2. Nail has mainly 3 parts; end caps, nail head and nail tip.
3. End caps provide protection to nail ends from tissue ingrowth. Nail can be extended up to 15 mm. Spiral blade locking has a gold color while bolt locking has blue color.
4. Nail head provides static, oblique and oval hole depending on anatomical variation.
5. Nail tip has been kept flattened for better gliding, easier insertion and reduced risk of perforation of cortex.
6. Nail tip has 3 holes for static locking which provides stable anchoring.

Rush Nail

This is a solid and circular rod like implant. Its one end is folded like a hook or handle of umbrella while other end is sloppy and pointed. This folded end of nail can be used for extraction of nail. This end also prevents migration of nail from it's position. This nail is used in fracture shaft of humerus. This can be inserted by antegrade (from greater tuberosity down ward) or retrograde (from below olecranon fossa upward) method.

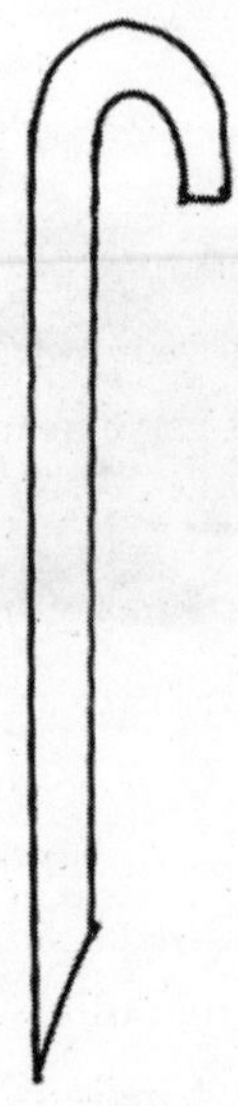

Fig. 46.10 Rush nail

EXPANDABLE INTRAMEDULLARY NAIL

This is called as expandable nail because it can be expanded by infusing saline into it's bars. This nail is not common in India. This is also known as **Isreal nail**. This nail has following features:

- This is made up of stainless steel.
- It has 4 longitudinal bars that combine a thin stainless steel wall of nail.
- It has got one way valve at proximal end of tube.
- Saline is used to expand diameter of nail. Saline in infused under controlled pressure with the help of pump through a one way valve.
- When pressurized saline is inserted into nail, membranes of bars become unfolded and nail expands. Nail can expand up to 160% of its initial reduced diameter. Nail does not collapse even if saline is removed from it because saline infusion causes plastic deformation of nail. There is no risk of nail explosion due to saline infusion.

Types

- Non interlocking nail
- Interlocking nail
- Proximal femoral nail (PFN).

Interlocking femoral nail can be inserted through knee prosthesis in a retrograde manner.

Indications

This nail can be used in following conditions:

1. Diaphyseal fractures of humerus, tibia and femur.
2. Acute fractures of humeri which are 5 cm below surgical neck and 5 cm proximal to distal end of medullary canal.
3. Non union and malunion.
4. Prophylactic nailing of impending pathological fracture.
5. Reconstruction of long bones following tumor resection.

MANAGEMENT OF FRACTURE BOTH BONES FOREARM

It can be managed by square nail as well as by dynamic compression plate.

Square Nail (Radial And Ulnar Nail)

Radial nail can be identified by its inverted spoon like structure at one end. This end looks like a "R". Ulnar nail is pointed. Other ends of these nails have thread which is used to hold the nail by an instrument.

These nails are square in their cross-section which prevents rotation of nail inside medullary cavity.

Indications

This can be used in fracture shaft of radius and ulna. This can also be used to fix the fracture of fibula and lateral malleolus.

Method of insertion

Radial nail is inserted through an entry point at lower end of radius (dorsal aspect) just lateral to lister tubercle.

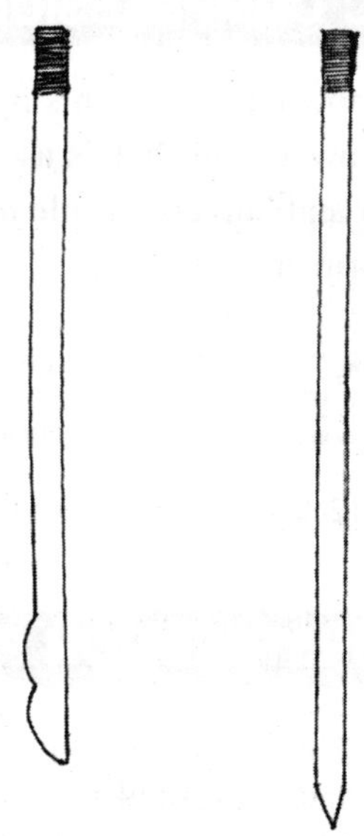

(*a*) Radial nail (*b*) Ulnar nail

Fig. 46.11 Square nail

Ulnar nail can be inserted through tip of olecranon.

LIMITED CONTACT DCP

This plate can be used in diaphyseal fractures of long bones. It has following peculiar features:

- This is also known as LC-DCP.
- This plate is made up of titanium.
- This is used to reduce dysvascularity and stress shielding under plate.
- This type of plate has only 50% contact with bone.

Advantages

- It allows vascularity under plate and synthesis of callus.
- It decreases cortical porosity of bone.
- It provides sequential compression between holes.
- Tissue compatibility is increased.
- LC-DCP has uniform material stiffness.

DYNAMIC COMPRESSION PLATE

This is also known as DCP. This is of two types, broad and narrow. Broad DCP is used for fractures of femur, tibia and humerus while narrow DCP is used for forearm fractures.

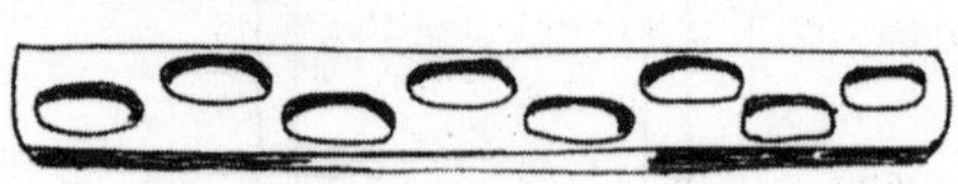

Fig. 46.12 Dynamic compression plate

RECONSTRUCTION PLATE

This type of plate has intermediate thickness between DCP and buttress plate. In between holes it has scallop like notches inside the plate. This plate is used in fractures of pelvis, humerus, calcaneum and ulna.

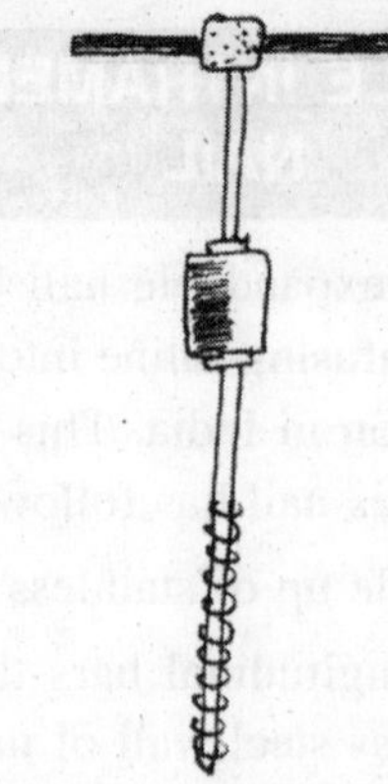

Fig. 46.13 Bone tap

STAPLES

Staples are thermally controlled compression device. These are used for physeal arrest, foot reconstruction, pott's fracture, arthrodesis of ankle/wrist joint, fracture of patella/trochanter, epiphyseodesis and valgus osteotomy of proximal tibia.

SEMITUBULAR PLATE

This is 1 mm thick selfcompressed plate. It has got oval holes and acts as buttress plate. This is of two types 1/3rd and 1/4th tubular plate. This is used in fibula, metatarsal, lower end of ulna and metacarpal.

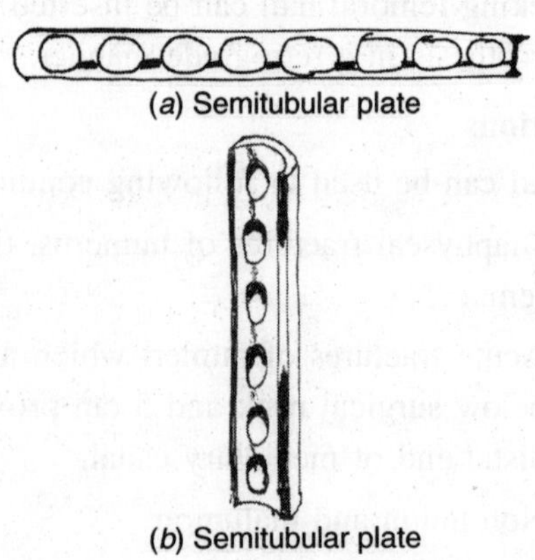

(*a*) Semitubular plate

(*b*) Semitubular plate

Fig. 46.14

BUTTRESS PLATE

This is a type of plate which provides support to fracture. It is used as rigid splint because it does not produce compression effect. Various types of buttress plates are in use e.g. C, H, L, T and S plate.

LOCKING COMPRESSION PLATES (LCP)

LCP provides angular stable fixation of fragments regardless of bone quality. This plate has minimum risk of primary and secondary loss of reduction, even under high dynamic loading. Limited plate contact causes reduced impairment of periosteal blood supply. This plate also has good purchase in osteoporotic bone and in multifragment fractures.

LCP have been classified into following types:

1. LCP metaphyseal plate
2. LCP 4.5/5.0 broad curved
3. LCP for proximal lateral tibia (PLT) and distal femur (DF)
4. LCP for distal radius
5. LCP compact hand.

1. LCP Metaphyseal Plate

This LCP is indicated for juxtaarticular fractures which extend into shaft area e.g. distal articular fractures of tibia and fibula, distal articular fracture of humerus.

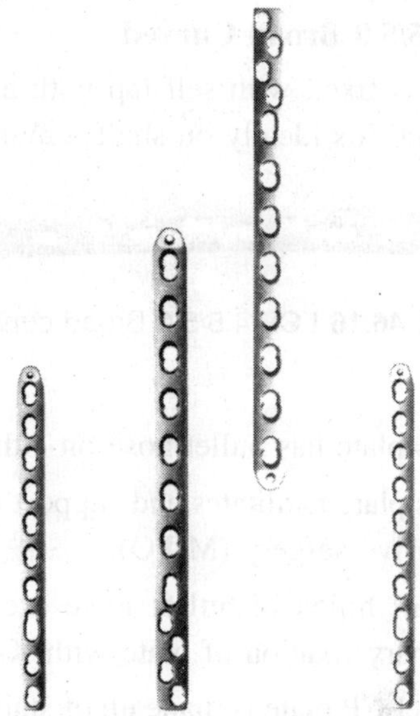

Fig. 46.15 LCP metaphyseal plate

Features

1. Distal part of this plate is flat which has got two holes for locking head screws in epiphyseal area. These holes are angled at 11 degree toward the centre of plate.
2. This plate has increased hole density which provides improved anchorage.
3. It has tapered round tip to be used for minimally invasive surgical technique. (**M**inimally **I**nvasive **P**ercutaneous **O**steogenesis)
4. Vascularity of periosteum is improved due to reduced plate to bone contact.
5. Elongated holes help in reduction of fracture in longitudinal axis.
6. Angle and axis stable locking head screws prevent loss of reduction under load.
7. This plate can be easily contoured due to its thinned plate profile.

2. LCP 4.5/5.0 Broad Curved

This plate is fixed with self tap with a radius of 1.5 m which fits ideally on shaft femur.

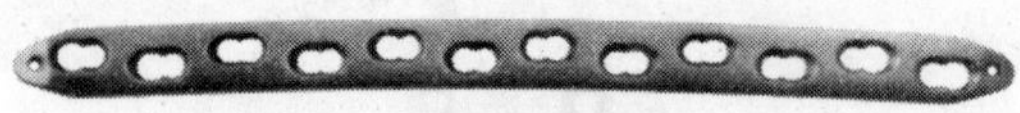

Fig. 46.16 LCP 4.5/5.0 Broad curved

Features

1. This plate has bullet nose on either side.
2. This plate facilitates and support minimally invasive surgery (MIPO).
3. Small holes in bullet nose are used for primary fixation of plate with K-wires.
4. This LCP plate is made up of stainless steel and titanium.
5. This plate may have 12–22 holes.
6. Small plates are straight.
7. This plate can be used with periprosthetic locking head screw or with circlage fix and circlage wiring altogether.

Indications

This plate is indicated for periprosthetic and shaft fracture of femur when nailing is contraindicated.

3. LCP, PLT and DF

These are LCP for **proximal lateral tibia** and **distal femur**. These are also anatomically precontoured plates which have combiholes and angular stability.

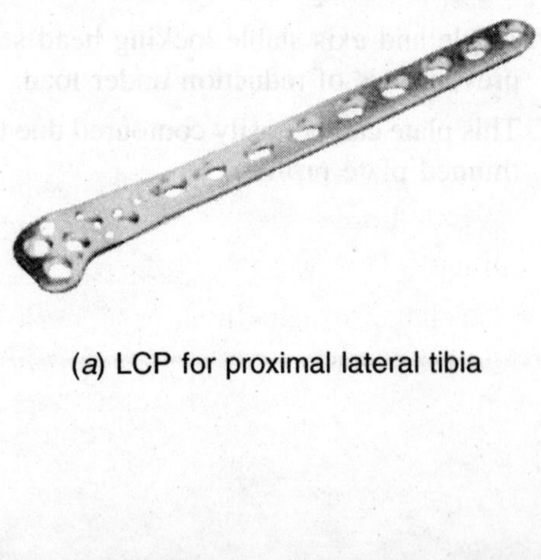

(*a*) LCP for proximal lateral tibia

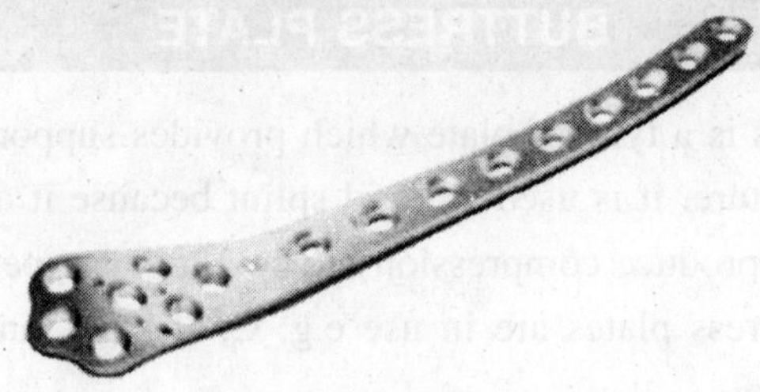

(*b*) LCP for distal femur

Fig. 46.17

Features

1. Angular stability prevents screw loosening and primary as well as secondary reduction.
2. Functional mobilization can be allowed early.
3. Purchase is improved in osteoporotic bones.
4. Bone vascularisation is preserved by this plate.
5. Spoon part of plate has guiding blocks which help in easy and correct mounting of threaded LCP drill guide.
6. This is a anatomically precontoured plate which has combi-holes.

Indications (PLT)

1. Proximal shaft fractures
2. Metaphyseal fractures
3. Intraarticular fractures
4. Periprosthetic fractures.

Indications (DF)

1. Distal shaft fractures of femur
2. Supracondylar fractures of femur.
3. Intraarticular fractures.
4. Periprosthetic fractures.

4. LCP for Distal Radius

These plates are used for fractures and osteotomies of distal radius.

Features

1. These plates are precontoured and do not require bending.
2. It causes minimum soft tissue injury.
3. This is a versatile plate system.
4. It has got combi-holes; angular stability and or compression.
5. Combi-holes allows internal fixation using standard screws, angle-stable locking head screws or combination of both.

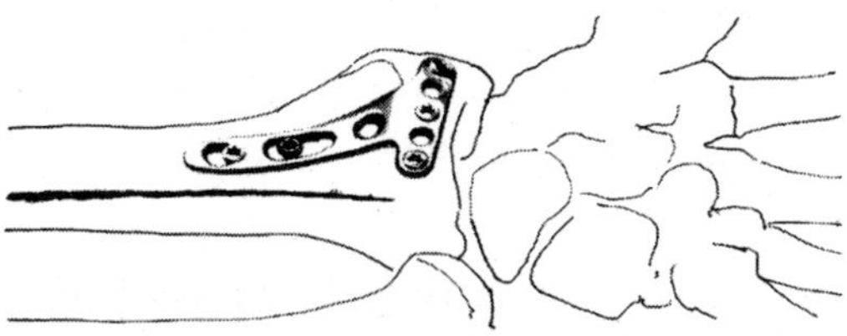

Fig. 46.18 LCP, distal radius

TYPES (LCD Distal radius)

This plate is of 2 types dorsal and volar plate as follows:

Dorsal plate

1. Locking and cortex screws can be inserted in the shaft.
2. Small plate and screw dimensions provide two plate technique.
3. This plate is applied on dorsal aspect of distal radius.

Volar plate

1. This plate is applied on volar aspect of distal radius.
2. Both locking and cortex screws can be inserted in shaft.
3. Plate is selected with juxtaarticular or extraarticular placement.

5. LCP Compact Hand

This system has wide range of anatomical and adaptable plates. These plates are available in titanium and stainless steel. Screw heads are completely buried in this plate.

Types of plate

1. LCP condylar plate
2. LCP straight plate
3. LCP-T plate
4. LCP-Y plate
5. Wrist fusion plate
6. Mini external fixator
7. Distal radius fixator.

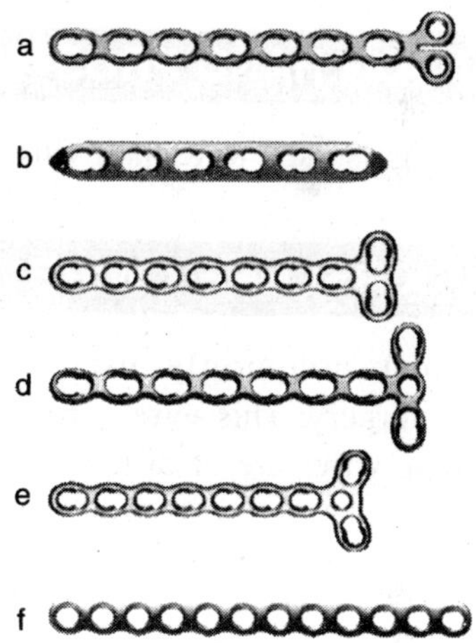

Fig. 46.19 LCP compact hand

Indications

1. Depressed fractures of DIP joint and refixation of bony extensor tendon tears of distal phalanges. (1 mm screw)
2. Fractures of distal and middle phalanges and refixation of bony ligament tears. (1.3 mm screw)
3. Fractures of phalanges, metacarpal and wrist bones and for arthrodesis of interphalangeal joint. (1.5-2 mm screw)
4. Fractures of metacarpals and wrist bones. (2.4 mm screw)

VERSATILE PLATE SYSTEM

This system has a wide range of dorsal and volar plates which can be used for individual fracture. These plates are in different sizes. It has different shapes e.g. T shape, L shape, extra long for treating distal radius fractures with extension into shaft.

Indications

This plate is indicated for dislocated extraarticular and intraarticular fractures and corrective osteotomies of distal radius.

SWANSON HAND PROSTHESIS

This prosthesis is used to replace finger joints.

KIRSCHNER WIRE

This is most commonly used implant in orthopaedic surgery. This wire is round in cross-section. These wires are of different size (1 mm-3 mm).

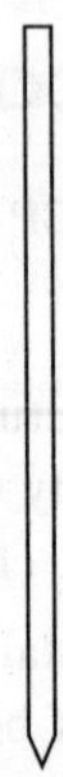

Fig. 46.20 K-wire

Indications

Most commonly it is used to fix the fracture supracondylar humerus in children, fracture lateral condyle of humerus and slipped capital femoral epiphysis.

This is also used to fix the fracture of metacarpals, metatarsals and phalanges.

STEINMAN PIN

This is a thicker implant in comparison to K wire (4 mm-6 mm). It's one end is sharply pointed. This is a circular rod like implant.

Indications

Steinman pin is most commonly used to apply tibial traction (upper/lower). This is used along with Bohler's stirrup.

Upper tibial traction is applied 2 cm below and behind the tibial tuberosity.

Stienman pin can also be used to apply skeletal traction through other bones as follows:

- Lower end of femur
- Calcaneum
- Olecranon

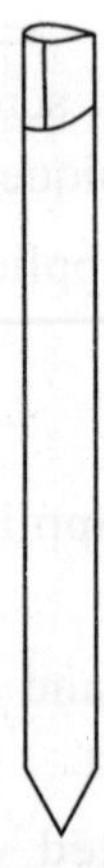

Fig. 46.21 Steinman pin

PEDICLE SCREW

This is designed to use for surgical stabilization of spine. This is either made of titanium or steel. Spine screws are available in monoaxial and polyaxial version. It can be used from anterior as well as from posterior aspect of spine.

Indications

Pedicle screws can be applied in following conditions:

1. Degenerative disc disease
2. Lumbar canal stenosis
3. Spondylolysthesis
4. Scoliosis
5. Kyphosis
6. Lordosis
7. Traumatic injuries of thoracolumar spine.

Contraindications

1. Infection or inflammation, fever leukocytosis.
2. Pregnancy.
3. Over weight patient.
4. Osteporosis is a relative contraindication.

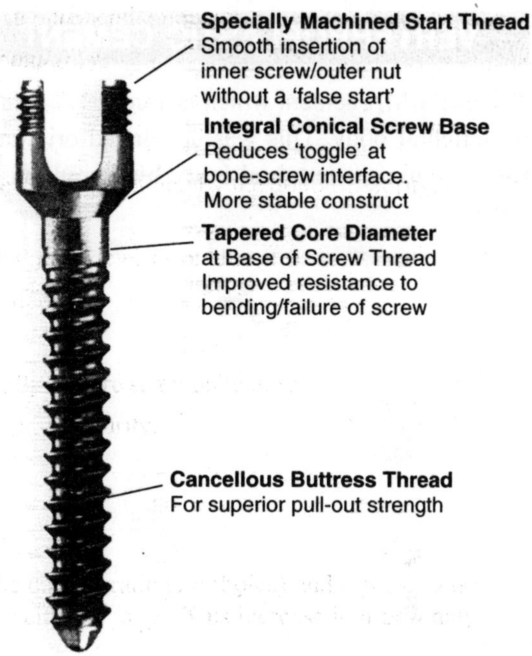

Fig. 46.22 (*a*) Pedicle screw

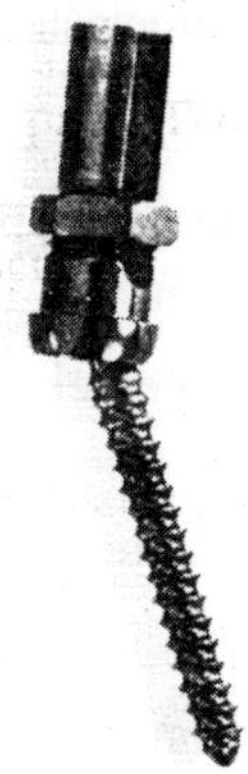

Fig. 46.22 (*b*) Spondylolisthesis reduction screw

VERTEBROPLASTIC CEMENT

This is PMMA cement which is used to fill defects of vertebral body. This was developed originally for angioma of vertebral body by Deramond in 1987.

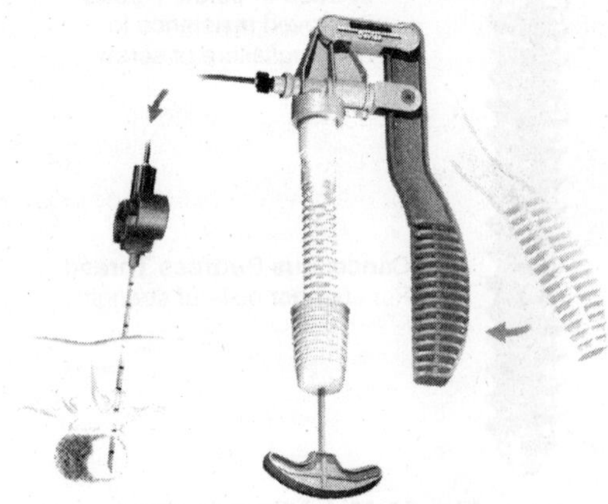

Fig. 46.23 Vertebroplastic cement insertion

Indications

1. Osteoporotic vertebral fracture with recalcitrant pain.
2. Angioma of vertebral body producing symptoms.
3. Symptomatic tumors of vertebral body.

Contraindications

1. Active infection.
2. Sensitivity to vertebroplastic cement.
3. Coagulation disorder.
4. Compromise of vertebral body and walls of pedicle.

MINIMALLY INVASIVE AND ENDOSCOPIC SPINAL SURGERY

Telefix

This is an implant system for anterior stabilization of thoracolumbar spine through **minimally invasive and endoscopic approach**. It has combined benefit of plates and rods in one implant. This is a pre assembled implant which works on telescopic mechanism for simple length adjustment and in situ compression or distraction. This has self locking screws for stable angular anchorage. Polyaxial bushings permit screw insertion tailored to individual anatomical situation. There is a ratchet mechanism which facilitates simple insertion of vertebral body replacement and subsequent in situ expansion.

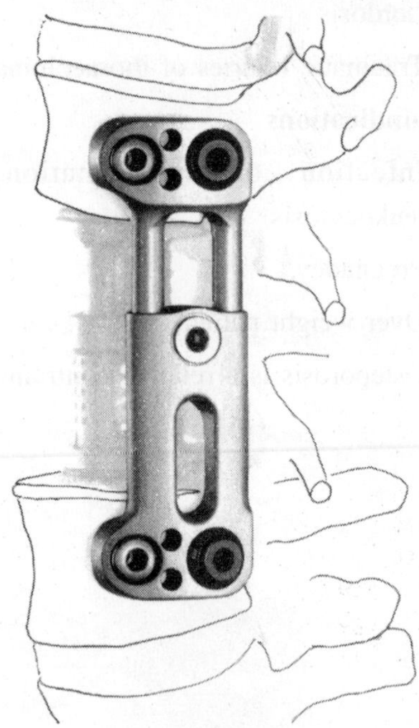

(*a*) Telefix

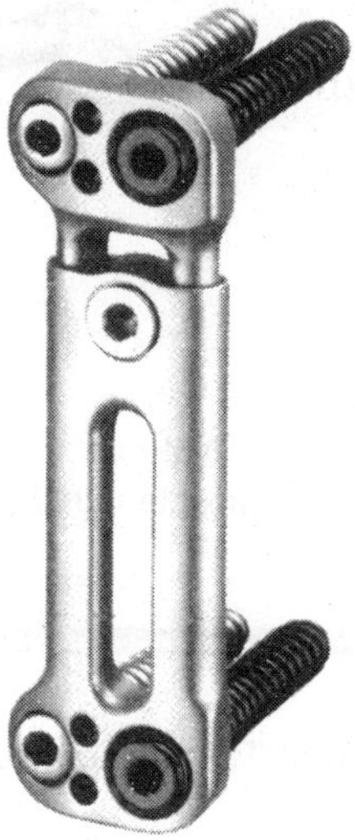

(*b*) Telefix

Fig. 46.24

Indications of Telefix

1. Fractures of thoracolumbar spine which can be adequately reduced and secured from an anterior approach.
2. Tumor and infection of spine.
3. Post traumatic kyphosis.
4. Posterior fixation of spine which equally requires additional anterior stabilization.

Contraindications of Telefix

1. Severe osteoporosis of spine
2. Scoliosis

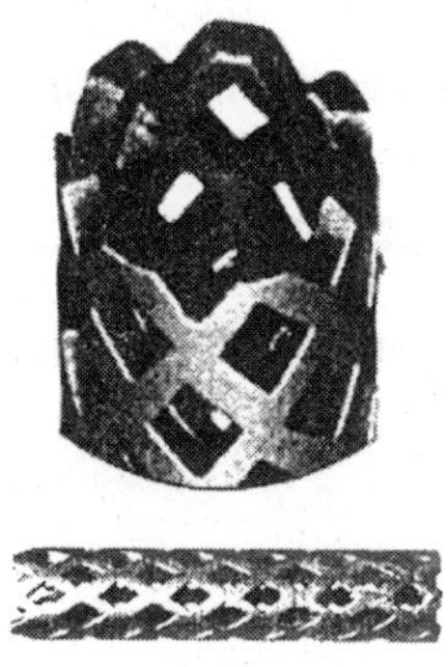

Fig. 46.25 Titanium mesh

BALLOON KYPHOPLASTY

This is an endoscopic spinal surgery which requires live fluoroscopy during surgery.

Indication

This is indicated in wedge compressed fracture of vertebrae which produce kyphosis.

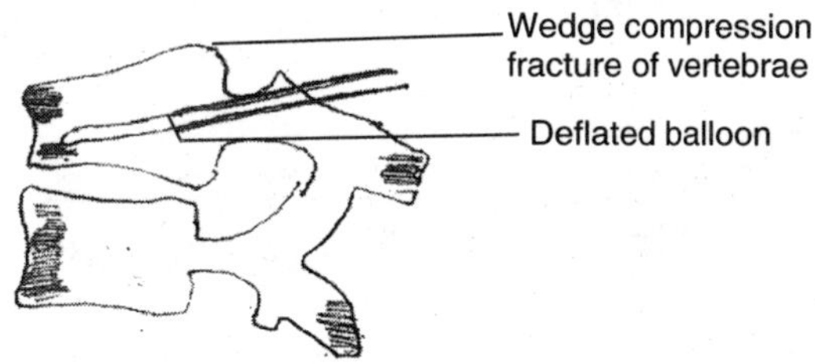

(*a*)

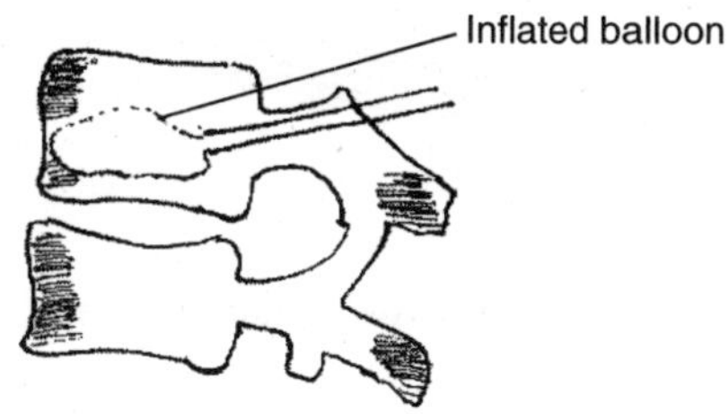

(*b*)

Fig. 46.26 Wedge compression fracture of vertebrae under balloon kyphoplasty

INSTRUMENTS

Fig. 46.27 Lag screw for barrel plates length 50 mm to 145 mm. Diameter 12.5 mm, Thread length 22 mm (Also available in short thread length 16 mm)

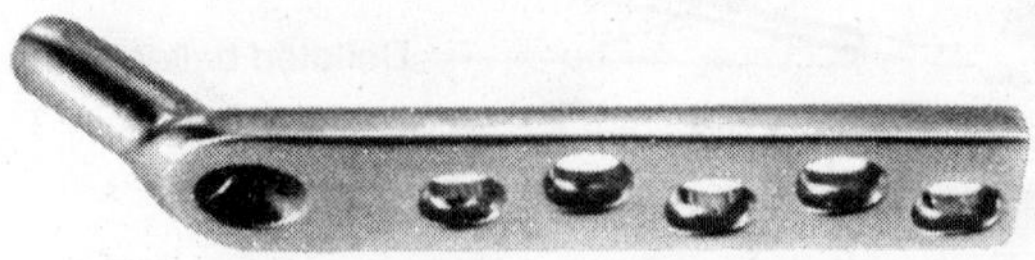

Fig. 46.28 Hip barrel plate 135° 2 holes to 18 holes, barrel length 38 mm (Also available in 130°, 140°, 145°, 150°)

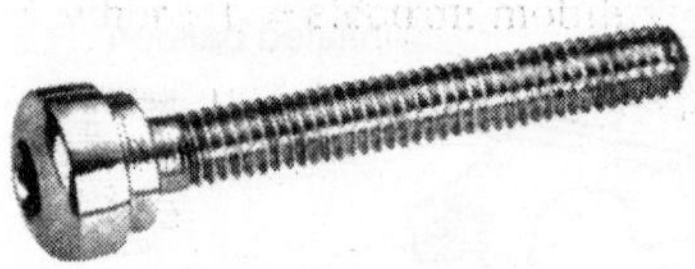

Fig. 46.29 Compression screw length 36 mm

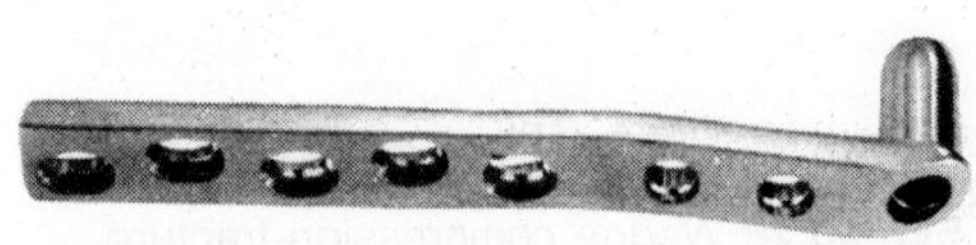

Fig. 46.30 Condylar barrel plate 95° 5 holes to 18 holes barrel length 25 mm

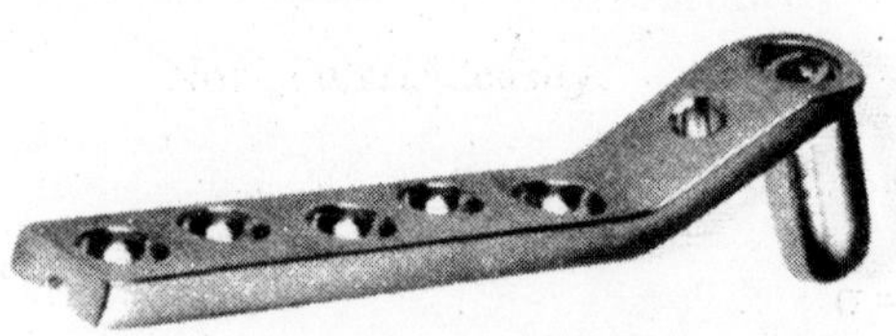

Fig. 46.31 Double angled barrel plate 120° 5 holes to 12 holes barrel length 25 mm

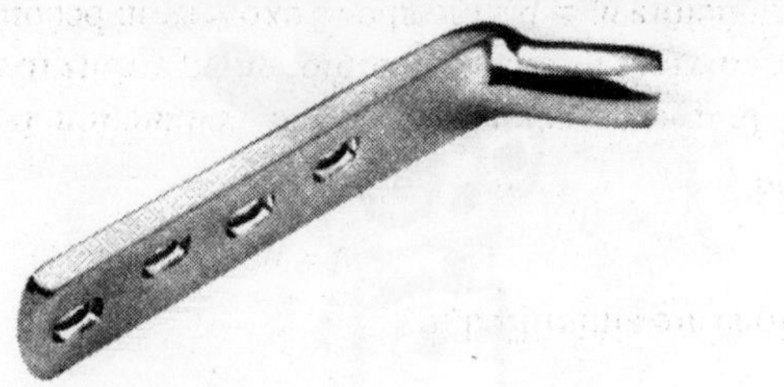

Fig. 46.32 Short barrel plate for hip 135° 4 holes to 10 holes barrel length 25 mm

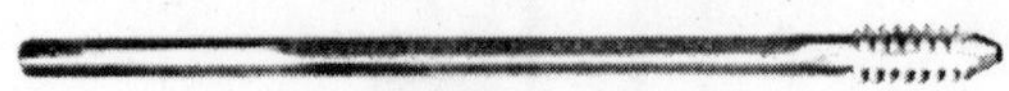

Fig. 46.33 Tap for lag screw

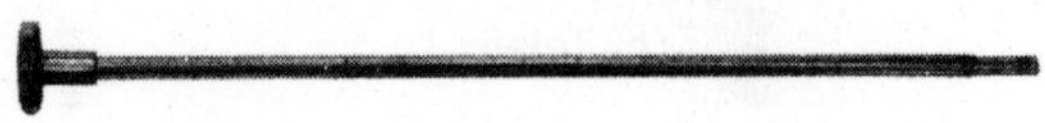

Fig. 46.34 Coupling screw for screw removal

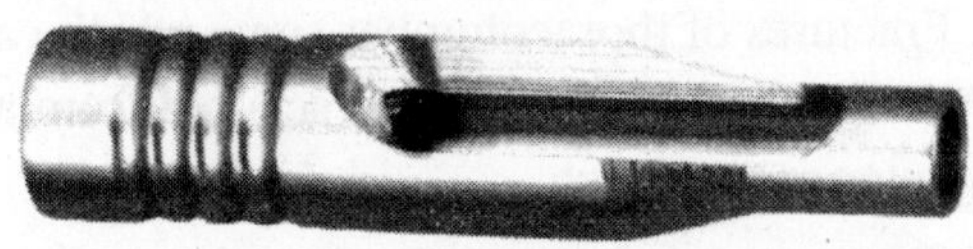

Fig. 46.35 Centering sleeve for tap

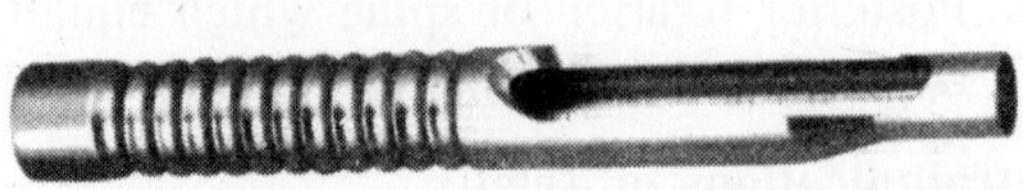

Fig. 46.36 Centering sleeve for wrench

Fig. 46.37 Guide shaft for coupling screw

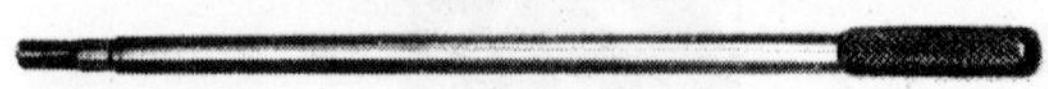

Fig. 46.38 Coupling screw for inserting screws

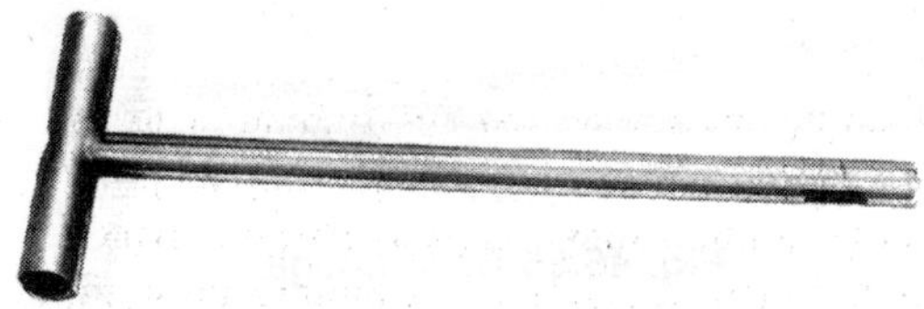

Fig. 46.39 Wrench for lag screw

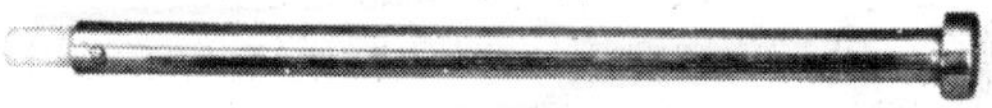

Fig. 46.40 Impactor

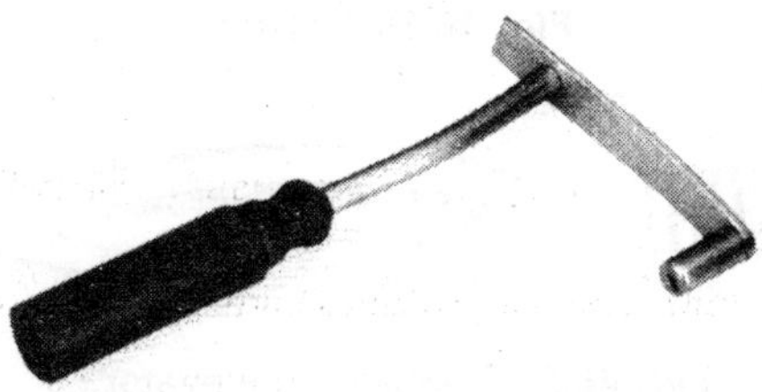

Fig. 46.41 Angle guide 95° for condylar barrel plate

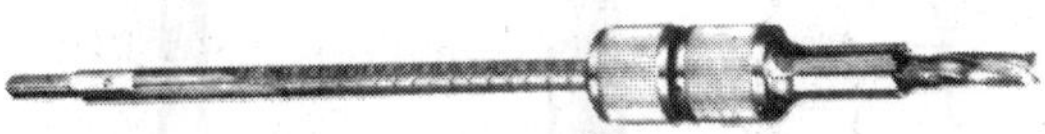

Fig. 46.42 Triple reamer for condylar screw plate complete

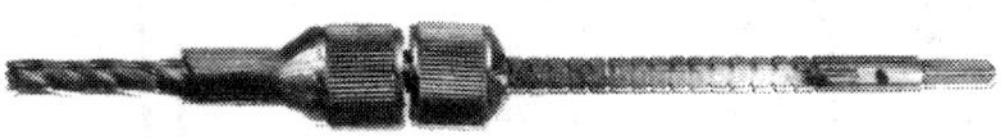

Fig. 46.43 Short barrel triple reamer

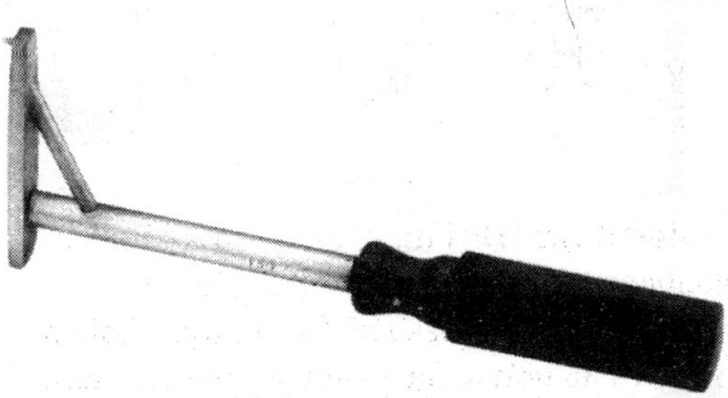

Fig. 46.44 Angle guide 150°

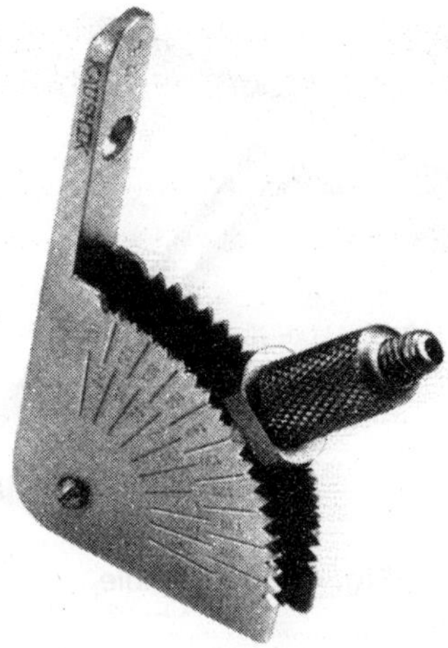

Fig. 46.45 Variable angle guide

Fig. 46.46 Threaded guide pin diameter 2.5 mm length 230 mm

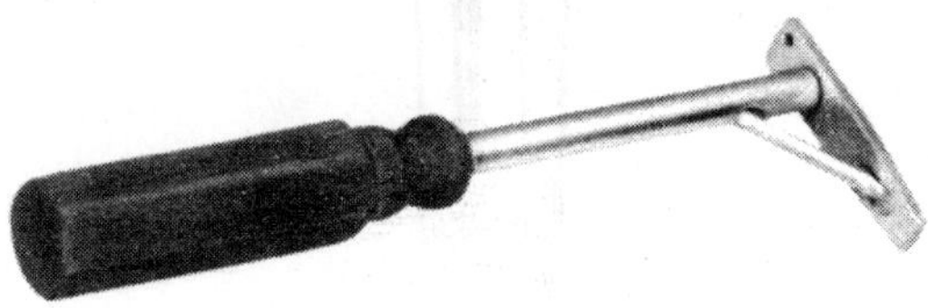

Fig. 46.47 Angle guide 135°

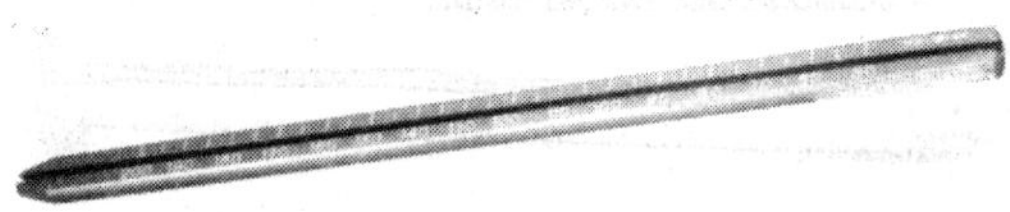

Fig. 46.48 Dirοct measuring device

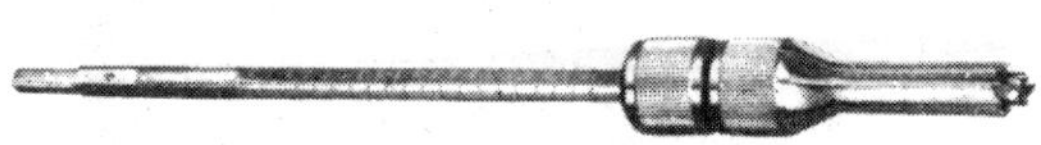

Fig. 46.49 Triple reamer for hip screw plate complete

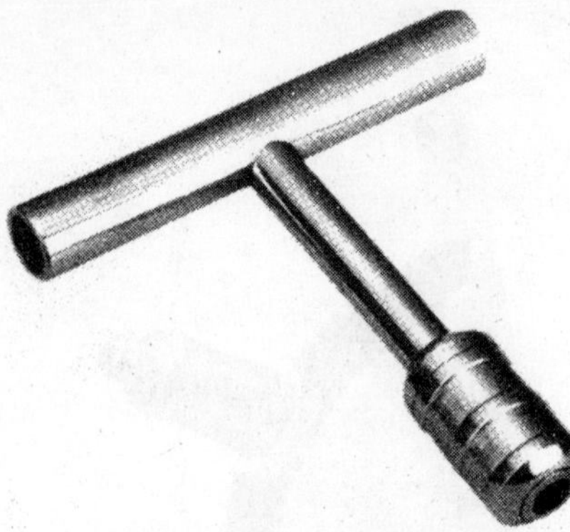

Fig. 46.50 T-handle

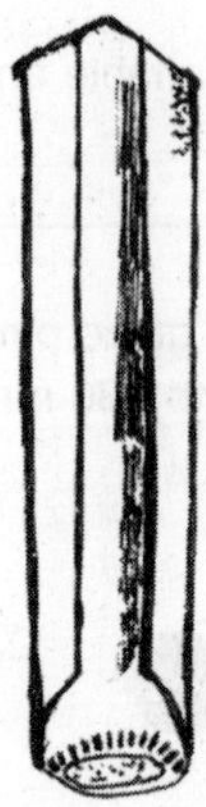

Fig. 46.51 Smith-Peterson nail (S.P. nail)

Cutting edge has an angle

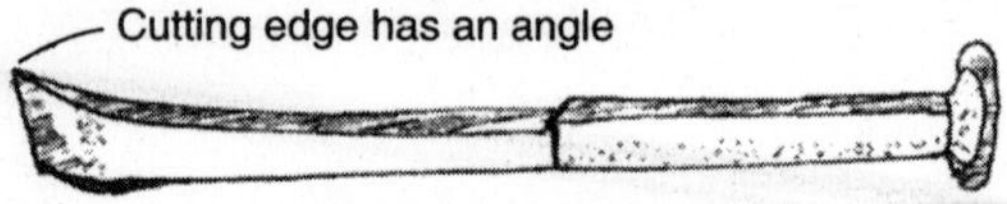

Fig. 46.52 Osteotome

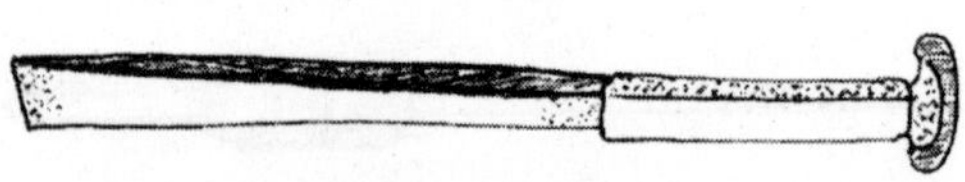

Fig. 46.53 Chisel

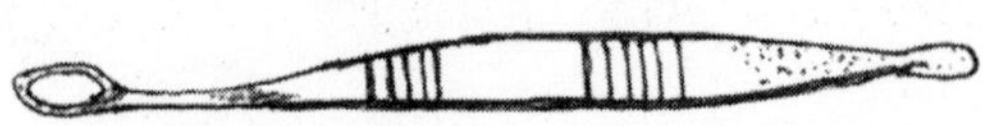

Fig. 46.54 Bone curette

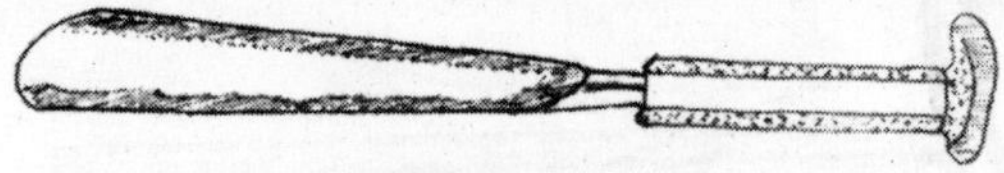

Fig. 46.55 Bone gouge

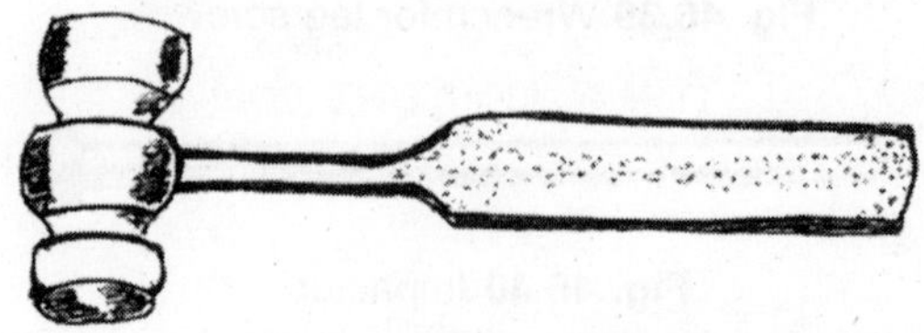

Fig. 46.56 Mallet

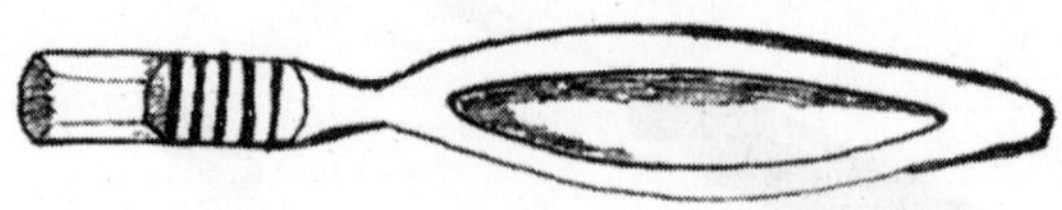

Fig. 46.57 Periosteum elevator

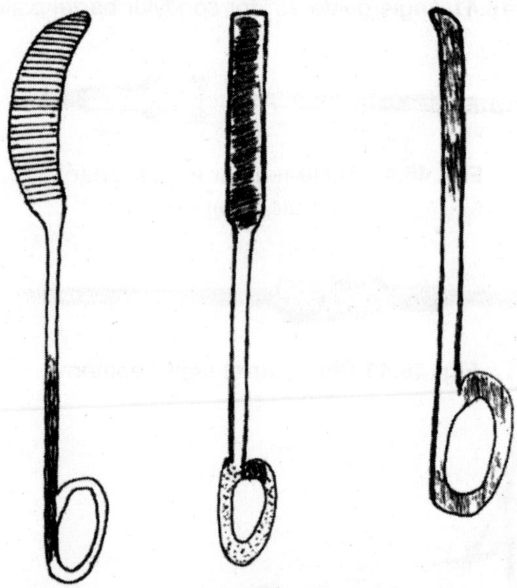

Fig. 46.58 Bone levers

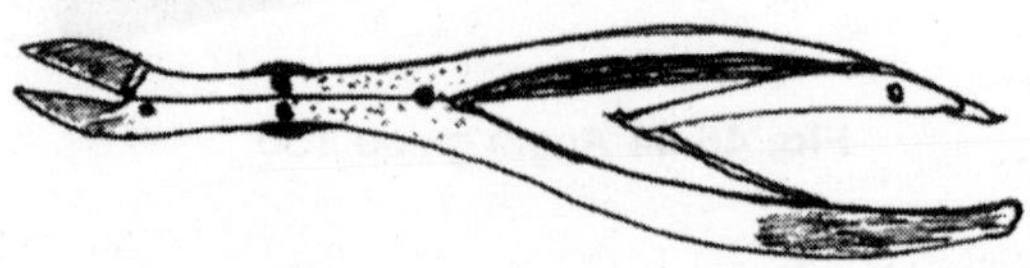

Fig. 46.59 Double action bone cutter

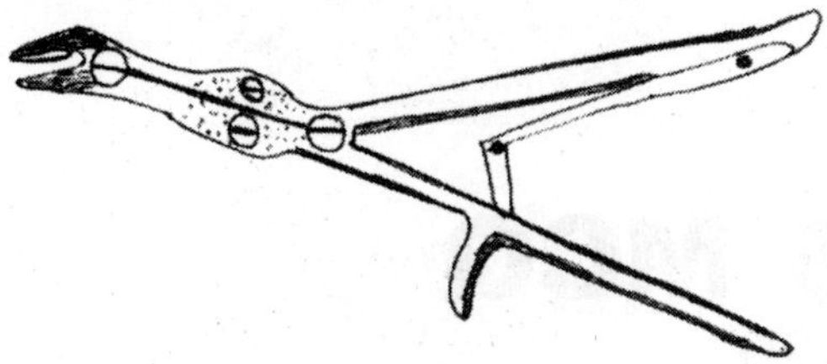

Fig. 46.60 Double action bone nibbler

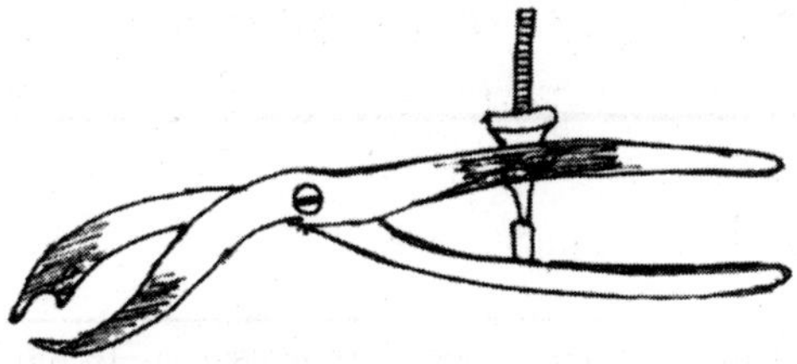

Fig. 46.61 A.O. forecep

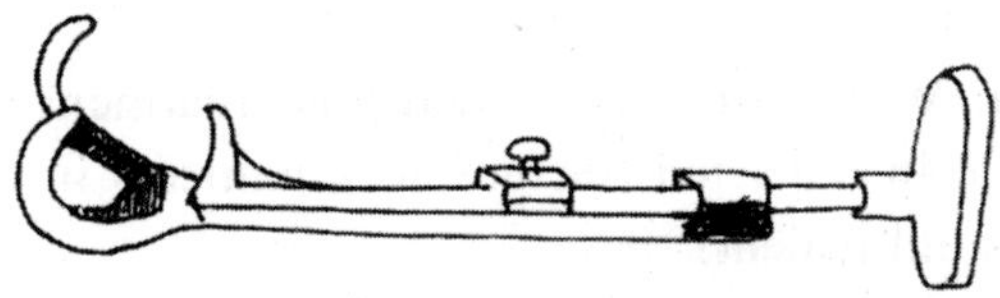

Fig. 46.62 Lowman's clamp

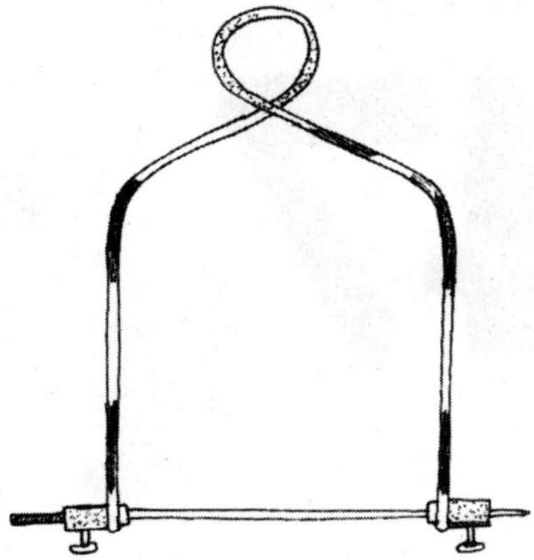

Fig. 46.63 Bohler's stirrup with steinman pin

CHAPTER

47 AIIMS MCQ

Following selected questions have been taken from AIIMS PG entrance examination. Students can assess themselves by doing these MCQ.

1999

Q. 1. A 65 year old female presented with fracture T12 vertebra with raised alkaline phosphatase and parathormone level along with low calcium and phosphate level. Most likely diagnosis is

a. vitamin D deficiency

b. osteoporosis

c. Paget's disease

d. primary hyperparathyroidism

Q. 2. A 40 years old patient presents with arthritis of PIP and DIP joint, along with carpometacarpophalangeal joint of thumb. Wrist and MP joints are spared. Most likely diagnosis is

a. osteoarthritis b. rheumatoid arthritis

c. psoriatic arthritis d. pseudogout

Q. 3. Traumatic anterior dislocation of shoulder with sensory loss in lateral side of forearm and weakness of elbow joint, most likely injured nerve is

a. radial b. ulnar

c. axillary d. musculocutaneous

Q. 4. Which of the following is treatment of choice in impacted fracture neck humerus in 65 years old patient?

a. Keep under observation

b. Arm to chest strapping

c. Arthroplasty

d. Triangular sling

Q. 5. Absolute indication of X-ray pelvis in case of CDH are all except

a. unstable hip

b. shortening of limb

c. breech presentation

d. positive family history

Q. 6. 6 years old child met an accident and had fracture elbow. After a gap of 4 years he presented with tingling and numbness at ulnar side of finger, fracture is

a. lateral condyle humerus

b. supracondylar humerus

c. dislocation of elbow

d. fracture olecranon

Q. 7. Fracture both bones forearm at same level, position of arm in plaster will be

a. mid-prone b. full supination

c. full pronation d. 10 degree supination

Q. 8. What will be the first line of action in case of cervical spine injury?

a. X-ray

b. Turn head to side

c. Stabilize cervical spine

d. Maintain airway

Q. 9. A 8 years old child presents with fracture humerus after a trivial trauma. X-ray shows lytic lesion. Most likely diagnosis is

a. aneurysmal Bone Cyst

b. unicameral Bone Cyst

c. osteoclastoma

d. osteomyelitis

Q. 10. A line joining ASIS to ischial tuberosity and passes to greater trochanter.

a. Perkin's line b. Chiene's line

c. Shoemakers line d. Nelaton's line

Q. 11. True about bone tumor is

a. osteoclastoma-5th decade

b. multiple myeloma->55 years age and above

c. chondrosarcoma-first decade

d. osteosarcoma 4th decade

Q. 12. Deformity in anterior dislocation of shoulder is

a. external rotation, abduction, flexion

b. external rotation, adduction, flexion

c. internal rotation, abduction, flexion

d. internal rotation, adduction, flexion

Q. 13. Stellate ganglion block is useful in

a. compound palmar ganglion

b. tenosynovitis

c. Sudeck's osteodystrohy

d. O.A. of I CMC joint

Q. 14. 10 year old boy presents with pain in left hip and limping. On examination abduction and internal rotation are restricted at hip. Most likely diagnosis is

a. perthes disease

b. CDH

c. tuberculous arthritis of hip

d. septic arthritis of hip

Q. 15. Most common cause of VIC in children

a. supracondylar humerus

b. lateral condylar humerus

c. medial condyle humerus

d. fracture both bones forearm

Q. 16. Commonest dangerous complication of posterior dislocation of knee is

a. femoral artery injury

b. popliteal artery injury

c. sciatic nerve injury

d. ischaemia of lower leg compartment

Q. 17. 3 year old child presents with progressive anemia, hepatospleenomegaly, osteomyelitis of jaw with pathological fracture. X-ray shows chalky white deposition on bone. Most likely diagnosis

a. osteopetrosis

b. osteopoikilocytosis

c. alkaptonuria

d. myositis ossificans progressiva

2000

Q. 18. Positive pivot shift test is done for injury of

a. ACL

b. PCL

c. MCL

d. lateral collateral ligament

Q. 19. A child falls on ground with fully outstretched hand. On examination pain and swelling is present at elbow. Most likely diagnosis is

a. posterior dislocation elbow

b. fracture supracondylar humerus

c. fracture both bones forearm

d. fracture olecranon

Q. 20. Which of the following deformity is seen in posterior dislocation of hip?

a. Flexion, adduction and internal rotation

b. Flexion, adduction and external rotation

c. Flexion, abduction and internal rotation

d. Flexion, abduction and internal rotation.

Q. 21. Which area is known as no man's land in hand surgery?

a. Between distal and proximal phalanx crease

b. Proximal phalanx

c. Distal phalanx

d. Wrist

Q. 22. True regarding mallet finger is

a. avulsion of tendon at the base of middle finger

b. avulsion of extensor tendon at the base of distal phalanx

c. fracture distal phalanx

d. fracture of proximal phalanx

Q. 23. Which of the following movements will be affected if greater tubercle of humerus is lost?

a. Abduction and lateral rotation

b. Abduction and flexion

c. Adduction and medial rotation

d. Flexion and medial rotation

Q. 24. A lady presents with swelling of hands with shiny skin. She had history of fracture radius and kept on POP cast for 4 weeks. Most likely diagnosis is

a. malunion

b. myositis ossificans

c. reflex sympathetic dystrophy

d. rupture of extendor pollicis longus tendon

Q. 25. A patient had history of fracture of tibia (left leg). Now he needs mobilization with a single crutch. He will use this crutch on

a. left side b. right side

c. any side d. both side

Q. 26. A 10 year old child with a mass on his left thigh. Mass seems to be arising from diaphysis of femur, and involving soft tissue of thigh. Child also has history of fever. Most likely diagnosis is

a. osteosarcoma

b. chondrosarcoma

c. Ewing sarcoma

d. malignant fibrous histiocytoma

Q. 27. Three point relationship is reserved in all, except

a. fracture medial epicondyle

b. fracture lateral epicondyle

c. fracture supracondylar humerus

d. posterior dislocation of elbow

Q. 28. Which is most common site of osteosarcoma?

a. Lower end of femur

b. Lower end of tibia

c. Upper end of humerus

d. Upper end of femur

Q. 29. Lytic bevelled lesions are seen in skull X-ray. Most likely cause of this is

a. metstasis

b. multiple myeloma

c. osteosarcoma

d. eosinophillic granuloma

Q. 30. A patient is unable to extend his MP joint. Most likely cause of this nerve injury is

a. radial nerve

b. ulnar nerve

c. median nerve

d. posterior interosseous nerve injury

Q. 31. A patient of leprosy presents with clumsiness of hand (ulnar nerve). Which of the following muscle is likely to be involved?

a. Extensor carpi ulnaris

b. Abductor pollicis brevis

c. Opponens pollicis

d. Interosseous muscle

Q. 32. Keinbock's disease is

a. osteochondritis of lunate

b. osteochondritis of neck femur

c. osteochondritis of navicular

d. osteochondritis of tibial condyle

Q. 33. A patient has osteoblastic lesion in spine and presents with paraplegia. Most likely diagnosis is

a. Ca thyroid b. Ca prostate

c. Ca breast d. Ca pancrease

Q. 34. A patient has backache. ESR is raised. X-ray shows multiple punched out lesions. Most important investigation to be done is

a. serum electrophoresis

b. whole body CT-scan

c. serum acid phosphatase

d. CT-scan head with contrast

Q. 35. Bankart lesion is seen at

a. anterior surface of glenoid labrum

b. posterior surface of glenoid labrum

c. anterior part of head of humerus

d. posterior part of head of humerus

Q. 36. A 20 year old boy presents with shortening of leg with adduction and internal rotation deformity following an accident. Most likely diagnosis is

a. posterior dislocation of hip

b. anterior dislocation of hip

c. fracture neck femur

d. trochanteric fracture

2001

Q. 37. 8 Year old child presents with gradually progressive swelling and pain for 6 months at upper end of tibia. X-ray show a lytic lesion with sclerotic margins at upper end of tibia. Most likely diagnosis is

a. Brodies abscess b. Ewing's sarcoma

c. osteoclastoma d. osteosarcoma

Q. 38. All are true regarding bone remodeling except

a. osteoclastic activity at compression site

b. osteoclastic activity at tension site

c. osteoclastic and osteoblastic activities are needed for bone remodeling in cortical and cancellous bone

d. osteoblasts transform into osteocytes

Q. 39. A child is spinned around by holding his hand. Suddenly child starts crying and does not allow to touch his elbow. Most likely diagnosis is

a. fracture olecranon

b. annular ligament tear

c. pulled elbow

d. radial head dislocation

Q. 40. A 18 year old suddenly twisted his knee on ankle while playing football and fell down. He got up after 10 minutes and started playing, but next day his knee was swollen and he could not move it. Most probable diagnosis is

a. medial meniscus tear
b. ACL tear
c. PCL tear
d. medial collateral ligament tear

Q. 41. Painful arc syndrome is seen in all except

a. supraspinatus tendonitis
b. subacromial bursitis
c. fracture greater tuberosity
d. fracture lesser tuberosity

Q. 42. Test for tight iliotibial band

a. Ober's test b. Osber's test
c. Simmond's test d. Charnley's test

Q. 43. A 19 year old boy presents with sclerotic lesion at diapysis. Diagnosis is

a. osteoid osteoma b. Ewing's sarcoma
c. osteoclastoma d. metastasis

2002

Q. 44. Most common site of adamantinoma of long bone is

a. femur b. tibia
c. ulna d. fibula

Q. 45. Chondroblastoma is commonly seen at

a. epiphysis b. metaphysis
c. diaphysis d. medullary cavity

Q. 46. 8 year old presents with pain in arm. X-ray shows expansile lesion in metaphseal area with breech of overlying cortex. Diagnosis is

a. ABC b. UBC
c. chondroblastoma d. osteoclastoma

Q. 47. A twisting injury of knee in flexed position would result in injury to all except

a. ACL tear
b. capsular tear
c. fibular collateral ligament tear
d. meniscus tear

Q. 48. Chondrocalcinosis is seen in

a. ochronosis
b. hypoparathyroidism
c. rickets
d. hypervitaminosis D

Q. 49. Most common injury due to torsion of knee

a. ACL
b. medial meniscus
c. tibial collateral ligament
d. fibular collateral ligament

Q. 50. Medial meniscus is more commonly injured than lateral meniscus because medial meniscus is

a. more mobile
b. less mobile
c. thinner
d. attached tightly to femur

Q. 51. Which activity will be difficult to perform for a patient with ACL injury?

a. Walk uphill
b. Walk down hill
c. Sit cross leg
d. Getting up from sitting

Q. 52. Which of the following is not a component of crush syndrome?

a. Bleeding diathesis
b. Acute tubular necrosis
c. Myohaemoglobinuria
d. Massive crushing of muscle

2003

Q. 53. Direct impact on bone will produce

a. transverse fracture b. spiral fracture

c. comminuted fracture d. oblique fracture

Q. 54. A 12 year old girl presents with persistent pain in leg for several weeks with low grade fever. X-ray shows a mass in diaphyseal region of femur with overlying cortical erosion and soft tissue extension. Biopsy shows numerous small round cells, rich in PAS positivediastase sensitive granules. Most likely diagnosis is

a. osteosarcoma b. osteoblastoma

c. Ewing sarcoma d. chondroblastoma

Q. 55. Whiplash injury is caused due to

a. a fall from height

b. acute hyperextension of spine

c. acute hyperflexion of spine

d. a blow on top of head

Q. 56. On 3 phase 99m Tc-MDP bone scan, which of the following bone lesions will show least osteoblastic activity?

a. Paget's disease b. Osteoid osteoma

c. Fibrous dysplasia d. Fibrous cortical defect

2004

Q. 57. A 44 year old man presented with acute onset of low backache radiating to right lower limb. Examination reveals SLRT<40 degree, weak EHL, sensory loss in first web space and brisk knee jerk on right side. Most likely diagnosis is

a. PIVD L4-5

b. spondylolysis L5-S1

c. lumbar canal stenosis

d. spondylolisthesis L4-5

Q. 58. A women of 45, known case of pemphigus vulgaris on a regular treatment with controlled primary disease presented with pain in right hip and knee. Examination reveals no limb length discrepancy but patient has tenderness at scarpa's triangle and limitation of abduction and internal rotation at right hip. Most likely diagnosis is

a. transient synovitis of hip

b. Perthe's disease

c. AVN head femur

d. stress fracture of neck femur

Q. 59. A 24 year old male, known epileptic, presented following a seizure with pain in right shoulder. Examination shows that right upper limb was adducted and internally rotated and movements could not be performed. Most likely diagnosis is

a. posterior dislocation of shoulder

b. luxatio erecta

c. intrathoracic dislocation of shoulder

d. subglenoid dislocation of shoulder

Q. 60. A 20 year old boy underwent excision of radial head. Later patient was unable to extend fingers and thumb. He does not have sensory deficit. Most likely cause is

a. injury to posterior interosseous nerve

b. iatrogenic injury to common extensor origin

c. injury to anterior interosseous nerve

d. high radial nerve palsy

Q. 61. A 10 year old boy presented with cubitus deformity and history of trauma 3 months back. Relationship of 3 bony landmarks is maintained. Most likely diagnosis is

a. old unreduced dislocation of elbow

b. nonunion lateral condyle humerus

c. malunited supracondylar humerus

d. malunited intercondylar humerus

Q. 62. Which of the following produces osteoblastic secondaries

a. Ca lung b. Ca prostate

c. Ca breast d. Ca urinary bladder

Q. 63. A 33 year old man presented with slowly progressive swelling in middle 1/3rd of right tibia. X-ray shows multiple sharply demarcated radiolucent lesion separated by areas of dense and sclerotic bone. Microscopic examination shows islands of epithelial cells in a fibrous stroma. Most likely diagnosis is

a. adamantinoma

b. osteosarcoma

c. osteofibrous dysplasia

d. fibrous cortical defect

2005

Q. 64. In a 1 year old child multiple fracture seen in various stage of healing. Most likely diagnosis is

a. survy

b. rickets

c. battered baby syndrome

d. fall from hight

Q. 65. Pathognomic features of Rheumatoid arthritis is

a. Rh factor b. Rheumatoid nodule

c. Morning stiffness d. Ulnar drift

2006

Q. 66. All of the following are cause of sudden increase in pain in osteochondroma except

a. sarcomatous changes b. fracture

c. bursitis d. degenerative changes

Q. 67. Rotator cuff interval is between

a. supraspinatus and teres minor

b. teres major and minor

c. supraspinatus and subscapularis

d. subscapularis and infraspinatus

Q. 68. Bankart's lesion involves .... of glenoid labrum

a. anterior lip b. superior lip

c. anterosuperior lip d. anteroinferior lip

Q. 69. Lesions associated with recurrent dislocation of shoulder includes all except

a. Hilsach's lesion b. Bankart's lesion

c. capsular laxity d. supraspinatus tear

Q. 70. Malunion of fracture supracondylar humerus leads to

a. flexion deformity b. cubitus varus

c. cubitus valgus d. extension deformity

Q. 71. All of the following are complications of fracture supracondylar humerus except

a. compartment syndrome

b. myositis ossificans

c. malunion

d. nonunion

Q. 72. True about posterior cruciate ligament is—attached to

a. lateral femoral condyle

b. intrasynovial

c. prevents posterior dislocation

d. relaxed in full flexion

Q. 73. All of the following are used for skeletal traction except

a. Steinman pin b. K-wire

c. Bohler stirrup d. Rush pin

2008

Q. 74. All of the following are markers of bone resorption except

a. hydroxyproline

b. deoxy pyridinoline

c. osteocalcin

d. Tartrate-resistant acid phosphatase

Q. 75. Which of the following nerve has best prognosis after repair?

a. Radial b. Ulnar

c. Medial d. Musculocutaneous

Q. 76. Most common cause of reactive arthritis.

a. Staph. aureus b. N. gonorrhea

c. S. flexneri d. *E. coli*

Q. 77. All of the following are features of osteopetrosis except

a. delayed fracture healing

b. pancytopenia

c. cranial nerve compression

d. osteomyelitis of jaw

2009

Q. 78. Tarsal tunnel syndrome is caused by

a. osteoarthritis

b. psoriatic arthritis

c. ankylosing arthritis

d. rheumatoid arthritis

Q. 79. Osteosclerotic bone lesion is found most commonly in which carcinoma

a. prostate b. kidney

c. thyroid d. lung

Q. 80. Kocher Langenback approach for emergency acetabular fixation is done in all except

a. recurrent dislocation inspite of closed reduction and traction

b. open fracture

c. progressive sciatic nerve compression

d. none of above

Q. 81. Earliest site of bone involvement in haematogenous osteomyelitis

a. diaphysis

b. metaphysis

c. at the point of entry of nutrient artery

d. epiphysis

Q. 82. 45 year old male, presents with abrupt onset of pain, weakness and muscle wasting of (L) shoulder on 5th day of immunization with tetanus toxoid is due to

a. thoracic outlet syndrome

b. radial nerve entrapement

c. hysterical

d. brachial neuritis

Q. 83. 3 months old child presents with fever and difficulty in abduction of hip for 2 days. His haemogram was normal, but ESR was raised. What is next line of management?

a. Admit and observe

b. Ambulatory observation

c. I/V antibiotics

d. USG guided aspiration of joint.

Q. 84. Cresentric fracture is

a. antero-posterior fracture pelvis

b. diastasis of pubis with pubic rami fracture

c. aritero-posterior instability with rotationally stability

d. fracture through S-1 8 rupture of iliac crest

Q. 85. Posterior glenohumeral instability can be tested by

a. Jene test b. Sulcus test

c. Fulcrum test d. Crank test

Following questions have been taken from various PG entrance examinations. Students can assess themselves by doing these MCQ.

INTRODUCTION

Q. 1. Pollicization is

a. reconstruction of thumb

b. reconstruction of index finger

c. reconstruction of middle finger

d. reconstruction of ring finger

Q. 2. Which of the following is not seen in tuberculous osteomyelitis?

a. Lymphadenopathy

b. X-ray shows honey-coomb appearance

c. Bone may show subperiosteal new bone formation

d. It is commonly seen in long bones

Q. 3. Myositis ossificans progressive can have the following except

a. congenital condition

b. normal living

c. only lab finding is raised eosinophil

d. ossification starts in trapezius and latissimus dorsi

Q. 4. Which of the following is most sensitive area of bone?

a. Cortex b. Epiphysis

c. Periosteum d. Epiphyseal cartilage

Q. 5. All of the following are true about traumatic myositis ossificans, except

a. injury to tendon over muscle

b. periosteal haematoma

c. elbow is commonest site

d. deposition of hydroxyappatite

Q. 6. All of the following are true about osteoclast except

a. resorption of bone

b. phagocytosis of foreign body

c. monocytes are precursor

d. stimulated by PTH

Q. 7. Ossification in foetus starts at

a. 3rd week b. 4th week

c. 5th week d. 3rd month

Q. 8. Normal angle of acetabulum is

a. 30–35 b. 30–32

c. 40–45 d. 45–50

Q. 9. Following movement takes place during extension of knee:

a. Lateral rotation of tibia

b. Medial rotation of tibia

c. Lateral rotation of femur on tibia

d. Medial rotation of femur on tibia

Q. 10. What is hydromyelia?

a. Fluid in subdural space

b. Fluid in subarachnoid space

c. Fluid in spinal canal

d. Fluid in extradural space

Q. 11. Following nerves supply to shoulder joint except?

a. Medial pectoral b. Lateral pectoral

c. Axillary nerve d. Suprascapsular nerve

Q. 12. Term orthopaedics was coined by

a. Nicholas andrey b. Hugh-Owen Thomas

c. Thomas brayant d. Sir Roberts jones

Q. 13. Which of the following is present in collagen?

a. Glycine b. Methionine

c. Hydroxyproline d. None of these

Q. 14. Which of the following is formed by osteoblast prior to osteoid formation?

a. Collagen

b. Mucopolysacchride

c. Mineral inducing enzymes

d. All of the above

Q. 15. Which of the following gives major blood supply to femoral head?

a. Foveolar vessels

b. Artery of ligamentum teres

c. Retinacular vessels.

d. Nutrient vessels.

Q. 16. Which of the following is first to ossify?

a. Mandible b. Lower end of femur

c. Upper end of tibia d. Os calcis

Q. 17. Which type of collagen is seen in tendon?

a. Type-I b. Type-II

c. Type-III d. Type-IV

Q. 18. Which is the earliest time for appearance of synovial tissue in a developing joint?

a. 6th week of IUL b. 12th week of IUL

c. 18th week of IUL d. 24th week of IUL

Q. 19. Which is the differentiating histological point of adult bone trabeculae to foetal bone trabeculae?

a. Different bone cells in both

b. Presence of certain staining pattern

c. Haversian system

d. Lamellar structure

Q. 20. Which of the following is produced by osteoblast?

a. Monosodium urate b. Pyrophosphate

c. Calcium d. Collagen

Q. 21. Knee is a

a. saddle joint

b. hinge joint

c. ball and socket joint

d. compound synovial joint (one joint between condyles of femur and tibia; another saddle joint between femur and patella)

Q. 22. Which of the following has maximum influence on bone growth?

a. Testosteron b. Thyroxine

c. Estrogen d. Growth hormone

Q. 23. Normal neck shaft angle in femur (adult male) is

a. 90 degree b. 100 degree

c. 120 degree d. 125 degree

Q. 24. Which angle is kept at M.P. joint in Jame's position?

a. 30 degree b. 60 degree

c. 90 degree d. 120 degree

Q. 25. At what age, calcification in costal cartilage takes place?

a. 20–25 years b. 25–30 years

c. 30–35 years d. 35–50 years

Q. 26. Distal femoral epiphysis becomes visible at the age of

a. Just after birth b. 14 weeks

c. 20 weeks d. 35 weeks (9 months)

Q. 27. Which of the following is known as best dressing?

a. Gauze piece b. Adhesive plaster

c. Skin d. Scab

Q. 28. Which of the following is responsible for longitudinal growth?

a. Epiphysis plate b. Metaphysis

c. Diaphysis d. None of these

Q. 29. Which of the following means arthroplasty?

a. Joint is excised and bones are kept as to avoid fusion

b. Plastic material is used in joint

c. Articular margins of bones are excised and made to fuse together

d. All of these

Q. 30. All of the following enzymes are present

in osteoblast except

a. alkaline phosphatase b. acid phosphatase

c. glycolate d. phosphorylase

Q. 31. Who is acclaimed globally for total joint replacement?

a. John charnley b. Paul brand

c. Paul Harington d. Huckstep

Q. 32. Which of the following stabilizes shoulder joint?

a. Capsule of joint b. Glenoid labrum

c. Rotator cuff tendon d. Rotator cuff muscles

Q. 33. Tensile strength of a tendon per square inch is

a. 1000 pounds b. 2000 pounds

c. 3000 pounds d. 5000 pounds

Q. 34. Where do you see a myofibroblast?

a. At wound margin

b. Normal connective tissue

c. Muscle septa

d. Bronchus

Q. 35. Which of the following is false about clavicle?

a. This is first bone to ossify

b. It has 2 primary ossification centre

c. It is commonly fractured at mid point

d. Fracture is commonly seen in children and young adults

Q. 36. True about shenton line

a. this is an arbitrary line from inferior border of superior pubic rami to inferior surface of femoral head and neck then medial border of shaft femur.

b. this is a line joining both ASIS

c. this is a line joining greater trochanter to ASIS.

d. none of the above

Q. 37. Which of the following is not a true flexor of elbow?

a. Biceps b. Brachialis

c. Brachioradialis d. Teres minor

Q. 38. Which of the following nerve is responsible for knee extension?

a. Femoral and obturator

b. Common peroneal and tibial nerve

c. Femoral nerve

d. Superficial and deep peroneal nerve

Q. 39. How many ossification centres are present at birth?

a. 2-3 b. 3-4

c. 4-5 d. 5-6

Q. 40. Which of the following is responsible for viscosity of synovial fluid?

a. Hyaluronic acid b. Heparin sulphate

c. Chondroitin sulphate d. All of these

Q. 41. Chondroblasts are

a. stable cells b. permanent cells

c. labile cells d. all of these

Q. 42. Which part of spine provides lateral flexion mostly?

a. Cervical b. Thoracic

c. Lumbar d. Sacral

Q. 43. Vascular cartilage is seen in

a. old age b. early childhood

c. early adulthood d. embryonic period

Q. 44. Normal atlantoaxial distance in an adult is

a. 2.5 mm b. 3.0 mm

c. 3.5 mm d. 4.5 mm

Q. 45. Which structure passes through spiral groove of humerus bone?

a. Radial artery

b. Radial nerve

c. Posterior interosseous nerve

d. Posterior circumflex humeral artery

Q. 46. Which part of cervical spine provides nodding movement?

a. Atlanto-axial joint b. Atlanto-occipital joint

c. C3-C4 d. C4-C5

Q. 47. Depth of ligamentum flavum from skin is

a. 1 cm b. 2 cm

c. 3 cm d. 4 cm

Q. 48. Distal extent of midpalmar space is

a. into the web space

b. into thenar space

c. along the digital sheath

d. into the flexor tendon sheath

Q. 49. Location of Babock's triangle is at

a. at lower part of thigh

b. at upper part of thigh

c. at inferior aspect of neck of femur

d. at lower part of back

Q. 50. Which of the following gives blood supply to femoral head at the age of 4–9 years?

a. Medial epiphyseal artery

b. Lateral epiphyseal artery

c. Lateral and medial epiphyseal and metaphyseal arteries

d. Lateral and medial epiphyseal arteries

Q. 51. Which artery is present in anatomical snuff box?

a. Radial artery b. Ulnar artery

c. Interosseous artery d. None of these

TRAUMA

Q. 52. AVN is commonly seen in all of the following except?

a. Tibia b. Talus

c. Scaphoid d. Neck of femur

Q. 53. Metaphyseal fracture is commonly seen in

a. rickets

b. scurvy

c. osteogenesis imperfecta

d. none of the above

Q. 54. Which movement should be avoided in anterior dislocation of shoulder?

a. Adduction and internal rotation

b. Abduction and external rotation

c. Extension

d. Flexion and internal rotation

Q. 55. Which is the last stage of fracture healing?

a. Callus formation b. Consolidation

c. Remodelling d. Haematoma formation

Q. 56. Collapse of L2-3 vertebrae with maintained disc space is indicative of

a. trauma b. tumor (malignancy)

c. tuberculosis d. congenital

Q. 57. Which of the following is best method of diagnosing fracture medial condyle in a child?

a. Arthroscopy

b. By taking history

c. By clinical examination

d. Comparing it with opposite side

Q. 58. Wringer injury is

a. side swipe injury

b. allergy to ringer lactate solution

c. road traffic accident

d. injury to upper extremity by its passage between 2 moving rollers (wringers of washing machine)

Q. 59. Which angulation is not accepted in fracture shaft tibia?

a. Anterior b. Posterior

c. Medial d. Lateral

Q. 60. Best management for fracture olecranon in an adult:

a. ORIF by TBW b. AEPOP cast

c. screw fixation d. excision of fragment

Q. 61. What is the cause of limb shortening in fracture neck femur?

a. Absorption of neck

b. Wrong size of prosthesis

c. Both of the above

d. None of the above

Q. 62. Which of the following is most serious complication of fracture pelvis?

a. Intra-pelvic haemorrhage

b. Urethral rupture

c. Bladder rupture

d. Rectum injury

Q. 63. Which technique is used to repair rupture of tendoachillis?

a. Bosworth technique

b. Mc Griffith technique

c. Both of above

d. None of these

Q. 64. Which of the following is true about neurological deficit in spinal injury?

a. More common in adult than children

b. More common in children than adult

c. Equally common in both

d. None of the above

Q. 65. Which is commonest injury around ankle?

a. Inversion injury

b. Eversion injury

c. External rotation injury

d. Internal rotation injury

Q. 66. Which joint is known for ligamentous injury?

a. Shoulder b. Elbow

c. Hip d. Ankle

Q. 67. Impacted fracture is usually not seen in

a. traction injury

b. simple fracture

c. compression fracture

d. fracture of vault of skull

Q. 68. What is normal period of healing in fracture shaft tibia in an adult?

a. 8 Weeks b. 12 Weeks

c. 16 Weeks d. 20 Weeks

Q. 69. Clay shoveller's fracture is

a. avulsion injury b. compound fracture

c. comminuted fracture d. green stick fracture

Q. 70. All of the following are complications of posterior dislocation of hip except

a. traumatic arthritis b. femoral nerve injury

c. myositis ossificans d. AVN of femoral head

Q. 71. Ideal time for reducing dislocation of ankle

a. immediately

b. after swelling subsides

c. after 2 days

d. after 1 week

Q. 72. A patient of fracture shaft radius with AEPOP cast presents after 4 weeks with swelling in hand and shiny skin. Most likely diagnosis is

a. malunion

b. myositis ossificans

c. reflex sympathetic osteodystrophy

d. rupture of extensor pollicis longus

Q. 73. A patient of anterior dislocation of shoulder presents with lack of sensation at lateral aspect of forearm and weakness of flexion at shoulder. Most likely diagnosis is

a. radial nerve

b. ulnar nevre

c. axillary nerve

d. musculocutaneous nerve

Q. 74. An old lady of 62 years falls on ground and presents with lower limb extended and externally rotated. She is unable to use lower limb. Most likely diagnosis is

a. anterior dislocation of hip

b. posterior dislocation of hip

c. trochanteric fracture

d. fracture neck femur

Q. 75. Pivotal test is done for

a. medial meniscus injury

b. lateral meniscus injury

c. ACL injury

d. PCL injury

Q. 76. Which of the following structure should be repaired first in hand injuries?

a. Nerve b. Tendon

c. Muscle d. Bone

Q. 77. During which movement of knee medial meniscus injury is least likely to develop?

a. Flexion b. Extension

c. Abduction d. Rotation

Q. 78. Gustillo-Anderson classification is known for

a. epiphyseal injuries

b. simple fracture

c. slipped capital femoral epiphysis

d. compound fracture

Q. 79. All of the following about Gustillo-Anderson classification (Type-3) are true except

a. wound is less than 10 cm

b. soft tissue is devitalized and contaminated

c. bone is exposed

d. it may be associated with an arterial injury

Q. 80. An adult patient of fracture shaft femur may lose

a. 500–600 ml of blood

b. 600–700 ml of blood

c. 800–1000 ml of blood

d. 1000–1500 ml of blood

Q. 81. An adult patient of fracture pelvis may lose

a. 1000–1200 ml of blood

b. 1200–1400 ml of blood

c. 1400–1600 ml of blood

d. 1500–2000 ml of blood

Q. 82. All of the following are subtypes of avascular nonunion except

a. oligotrophic nonunion

b. torsion wedge nonunion

c. atrophic nonuninon

d. gap nonunion

Q. 83. Allograft is taken from

a. other species

b. genetically dissimilar person of same species

c. from patient itself

d. none of the above

Q. 84. All of the following are features of cerebral type of fat embolism except

a. tachypnoea b. tachycardia

c. pyrexia d. bradycardia

Q. 85. All of the following are true about investigatory findings of fat embolism except

a. thrombocytopenia

b. ECG shows S wave

c. X-ray chest shows snow storm appearance

d. thrombocytosis

Q. 86. Virchov's triad includes all of the following except

a. venous stasis b. vascular damage

c. hypercoagulbility d. arterial stasis

Q. 87. Which of the following is drug of choice for DVT?

a. Low dose warferin

b. Low molecular weight dextran

c. Aspirin

d. Heparin

Q. 88. All of the following belongs to crush syndrome except

a. myglobin renal failure

b. highly acidic urine

c. hyperkalemic metabolic acidocis

d. hypokalemic metabolic acidocis

Q. 89. All of the following can be given in crush syndrome except

a. blood transfusion

b. manitol

c. injectable calcium gluconate

d. sodium lactate

Q. 90. Prussian disease is related to

a. myositis ossificans progressiva

b. pulmonary embolism

c. crush syndrome

d. traumatic myositis ossificans

Q. 91. All of the following are true about myositis ossificans progressive except

a. this is a congenital condition

b. death can occur due to intercurrent infection

c. blood chemistry is normal

d. significant thrombocytopenia

Q. 92. AVN may show the following radiological findings except

a. adjacent bone shows osteoporosis

b. zone of sclerois is seen at necrotic bone

c. bone is deformed

d. bone is not deformed

Q. 93. Whitman POP spica is applied in

a. post-operative phase of fracture neck femur where osteotomy has been done

b. fracture patella

c. fracture shaft femur

d. intertrochanteric fracture

Q. 94. Period of immobilization for Galeazzi fracture (in adult) is

a. 1 month b. 2 months

c. 3 months d. 4 months

Q. 95. Period of immobilization for surgical neck of humerus is

a. 1 week b. 2 weeks

c. 3 weeks d. 3-4 weeks

Q. 96. Period of immobilization for fracture head radius is

a. 1 week b. 2 weeks

c. 3 weeks d. 4 weeks

Q. 97. Period of immobilization for fracture shaft femur in new born is

a. 1 week b. 2 weeks

c. 2-3 weeks d. 4 weeks

Q. 98. Period of immobilization in greenstick fracture is

a. 45–60 days b. 60–75 days

c. 75–100 days d. 3 weeks

Q. 99. Nerve regeneration occurs at the rate of

a. 1 mm/day b. 1 inch/ month

c. both of the above d. none of these

Q. 100. All of the following are supplied by sciatic nerve except

a. lateral part of leg

b. skin over lateral malleolus

c. skin over dorsum of foot

d. first web space of foot

Q. 101. Seddon's classification is associated with

a. compound fracture

b. spinal injuries

c. epiphseal injuries

d. peripheral nerve injuries

Q. 102. All of the following are true about foot drop except

a. ankle plantarflexion is lost

b. active extension of great toe is lost

c. active extension of toes are lost

d. active eversion and inversion are lost

Q. 103. All of the following are supplied by radial nerve except

a. medial side of hand b. medial side of thumb

c. middle finger d. index finger

Q. 104. Which of the following is escaped in low radial nerve palsy?

a. Brachioradialis b. ECRL

c. ECRB d. All of these

Q. 105. All of the following are supplied by medial nerve except

a. abductor pollicis brevis

b. opponens pollicis

c. I and II lumbricals

d. III and IV lumbricals

Q. 106. Pen test is done for

a. opponens pollicis

b. flexor carpi radialis

c. flexor pollicis longus

d. abductor pollicis brevis

Q. 107. Which of the following anatomical relationship of ulnar nerve (in wrist) is correct?

a. It lies between pisiform bone on lateral side and ulnar artery on medial side

b. It lies between pisiform bone on medial side and ulnar artery on lateral side

c. Ulnar artery and pisiform bone lies medial to ulnar nerve

d. None of the above

Q. 108. All of the following are supplied by ulnar nerve except

a. abductor pollicis longus

b. adductor pollicis

c. all interossei

d. abductor digiti minimi

Q. 109. All of the following test are done for ulnar nerve except

a. Froment sign

b. Egawa test

c. Card test

d. Oschner's clasping hand

Q. 110. Allman classification stands for

a. fracture scapula

b. fracture of cervical spine

c. fracture clavicle

d. fracture shaft femur

Q. 111. Which of the following is not correct about panclavicular fracture?

a. This is also known as traumatic floating clavicle

b. There is no clavicle fracture

c. Two ligaments sternoclavicular & coraco-clavicular are disrupted

d. Clavicle is fractured

Q. 112. Billington-Yoke POP was used long ago for the fracture of

a. fracture humerus

b. fracture scapula

c. fracture clavicle

d. fracture lateral condyle humerus

Q. 113. Thompson classification is used for

a. fracture clavicle

b. fracture scapula

c. fracture medial condyle humerus

d. fracture intercondylar humerus

Q. 114. Holstein-Lewis fracture is

a. fracture mid shaft of humerus

b. fracture proximal humerus

c. fracture of distal third of humerus

d. fracture of distal third of humerus with radial nerve injury

Q. 115. Which of the following is seen in supracondylar fracture humerus?

a. Fish tail sign b. Fat pad sign

c. Crescent sign d. Tear drop sign

e. All of these

Q. 116. Smith traction is indicated in (fracture supracondylar humerus) following conditions except

a. threatened Volkman's ischaemia

b. failed closed reduction

c. grossly contaminated fracture

d. stable fracture

Q. 117. Miller's method of K-wire fixation is used for

a. fracture clavicle

b. fracture scapula

c. fracture supracondylar humerus

d. fracture proximal humerus

Q. 118. Which of the following is true about French osteotomy?

a. This is a medial closed wedge osteotomy

b. This is medial open wedge osteotomy

c. This is a lateral close wedge osteotomy

d. None of the above

Q. 119. All of the following are used for management of VIC except

a. Maxpage operation

b. arthrodesis

c. Seddon's carpectomy

d. none of these

e. all of the above

Q. 120. Tardy ulnar palsy is seen in

a. fracture supracondylar humerus

b. fracture intercondylar humerus

c. fracture lateral condyle humerus

d. fracture medial condyle humerus

Q. 121. Fracture lateral condyle humerus is known for following complications except

a. Cubitus varus

b. Nonunion

c. Cubitus valgus

d. Tardy ulnar nerve palsy

Q. 122. Riseborough and Radin classification is used for fracture of

a. medial condyle humerus

b. lateral condyle humerus

c. medial condyle femur

d. lateral condyle femur

Q. 123. All of the following are true about pulled elbow except

a. this is commonly seen between the age of 2–6 years.

b. head of radius comes out of annular ligament

c. child presents with forearm in pronation

d. head of radius is fractured

Q. 124. All of the following are true about dislocation of elbow except

a. this is caused by fall on outstretched hand

b. Stimson's classification is used

c. it can be reduced by Puller's technique

d. tear drop sign is seen on X-ray

Q. 125. All of the following are true about fracture olecranon except

a. this is uncommon in children

b. this is classified by Colton

c. this can be managed by Leinbach screw

d. AEPOP cast is applied in full extension

Q. 126. Laugier fracture is fracture of

a. trochlea b. capitullum

c. medial epicondyle d. head radius

Q. 127. Which of the following is true about Kocher fracture?

a. This is fracture of capitullum

b. This is also known as uncapping of condyle

c. ORIF is very difficult

d. This is of 2 types

e. All of the above

Q. 128. Maclaughlin's criteria has all of the following except

a. angulation >30 degree

b. displacement >3 mm

c. >1/3rd head is involved

d. none of the above

e. all of the above

Q. 129. Which of the following is true about fracture head radius?

a. Mason has classified this fracture into 3 types

b. This is an intra-articular fracture

c. Type-3 fracture can be managed by excision of head radius and replaced by silicon prosthesis

d. All of the above

Q. 130. Terible triad stands for

a. fracture coronoid

b. fracture head radius

c. gross instability of elbow

d. all of the above

Q. 131. Which of the following statements are true?

a. Monteggia fracture is fracture of upper third of ulna with dislocated head radius

b. Galeazzi fracture is fracture of shaft of radius at the junction of middle and distal third; associated with subluxation/dislocation of inferior radioulnar joint

c. Frykman's classification is used for colles's fracture

d. None of the above

e. All of the above

Q. 132. Which of the following deformity is not seen in colles's fracture?

a. Impaction b. Pronation

c. Doral displacement d. Dorsal tilt

Q. 133. Darrach's procedure is

a. excision of head radius

b. excision of lower end of ulna 2.5 cm including head and periosteum is left behind

c. excision of styloid process of ulna

d. none of the above

Q. 134. Which of the following statement is true?

a. Fernandes osteotomy is dorsal wedge osteotomy

b. Campbell osteotomy is lateral wedge osteotomy

c. Above mentioned procedures are cosmetic surgeries

d. All of the above

e. None of the above

Q. 135. Which of the following is true about scaphoid fracture?

a. 65% fractures occur through its waist

b. 15% occur through proximal pole

c. AVN of entire scaphoid is known as Preiser disease

d. Vascular bone graft is used for nonunion

e. All of the above

f. None of the above

Q. 136. Which of the following is true about Bennet's fracture?

a. This is an intra-articular fracture of base of first metacarpal

b. Failed closed reduction should be managed by percutaneous K-wire fixation

c. Excess hyperextension should be avoided at MP joint while applying cast

d. All of the above

Q. 137. Which of the following statement is true?

a. Chauffer's fracture is fracture of radial styloid process

b. Essex-Lopresti fracture is fracture head radius plus subluxation of ine inferior radioulnar joint

c. Keinbock disease is fracture of lunate bone

d. All of the above

e. None of the above

Q. 138. Which of the following is true about Kaplan's lesion?

a. Complex dislocation of MP joint is known as Kaplan's lesion

b. This is also known as button-holing of metacarpal head into palm

c. Patient presents with flexed IP joint and mildly hyperextended MP joint

d. All of the above

e. None of the above

Q. 139. Which of the following is true about fracture pelvis?

a. Straddle fracture is double vertical fracture of pubis

b. Malgaigne's fracture is ipsilateral pubic rami fracture plus ipsilateral sacroiliac joint dislocation

c. Undisplaced fracture can be treated by absolute bed rest for 3-4 weeks

d. All of the above

Q. 140. Which of the following about dislocation of hip is true?

a. Thompson-Epstein has classified this dislocation

b. Pipkin has classified this dislocation

c. Biglow's 90-90 method is most commonly used method for reduction

d. All of the above

Q. 141. True about subcapital fracture neck femur is

a. fracture line passes through femoral neck

b. fracture line is present at the base of neck

c. fracture line occurs just beneath the articular surface of femoral head

d. none of the above

Q. 142. True about cervicotrochanteric fracture

a. fracture line is seen between neck and shaft

b. fracture line is between neck and head

c. fracture line is between greater and lesser trochanter

d. fracture line is present at trochanteric area

Q. 143. True about intertrochanteric fracture

a. it can be managed by closed reduction and AK skin traction on TK splint

b. it can be managed by ORIF by DHS

c. it can be managed by Sarmeinto osteotomy

d. it can be managed by Dimon-Hughston osteotomy

e. none of the above

f. all of the above

Q. 144. Which of the following is most accurate about Bumper's fracture?

a. Fracture of lateral condyle tibia

b. Fracture of proximal tibia

c. Fracture of medial condyle of tibia

d. None of the above

Q. 145. Fracture patella can be managed by

a. TBW

b. Martin's wiring

c. Manuson's method

d. Shaeuwacker's method

e. all of the above

f. none of the above

Q. 146. Triad of Donoghue includes except

a. medial meniscus injury

b. ACL injury

c. injury to medial structure

d. PCL injury

Q. 147. Superficial part of deltoid ligament includes all of the following except

a. anterior tibiotalar ligament

b. tibionavicular ligament

c. tibiocalcaneal ligament

d. posterior tibiotalar ligament

Q. 148. All of the following constitute syndesmotic ligament except

a. anterior and posterior interosseous ligament

b. interosseous ligament

c. inferior transverse ligament

d. superior transverse ligament

Q. 149. Leforte-Wagstaffe fracture is

a. avulsion fracture of anterior margin of fibula at the insertion site of anterior tibiofibular ligament

b. fracture of lower end of fibula

c. fracture of lower end of tibia

d. none of the above.

Q. 150. Bosworth fracture is

a. fracture of lower end of tibia

b. fracture of lower end of fibula which is displaced behind tibia

c. this is burst fracture of talus

d. fracture of upper end of fibula

Q. 151. All of the following are true about talus except

a. fracture of lateral tubercle of posterior process of talus is known as Shephard fracture

b. Hawkin's sign is positive in X-ray

c. AVN of talus can be managed by Blair's fusion

d. undisplaced fractures can be managed by BKPOP cast for 1 month

PATHOLOGICAL

Q. 152. Persistant transverse looser's zone and demineralization are radiological findings of

a. osteoporosis b. osteopetrosis

c. osteomalacia d. scurvy

Q. 153. Codfish spine is a radiological findings of

a. osteomlacia b. osteoporosis

c. both of them d. none of these

Q. 154. Singh index is used in

a. osteoporosis b. osteomalacia

c. osteopetrosis d. scurvy

Q. 155. All of the following are radiological features of osteoporosis except

a. lumbar vertebrae are biconcave and lumbar discs are ballooned out

b. compression fracture of vertebrae

c. anterior wedge compression of thoracic vertebrae

d. triradiate pelvis

Q. 156. All of the following are radiological features of osteomalacia except

a. protrusio acetabuli

b. triradiate pelvis

c. Milkman pseudofracture

d. Pelcun spur

Q. 157. Which of the following is not a feature of scurvy?

a. Wimberger line

b. Scurvy line

c. White line of frankel

d. Subperiosteal haemorrhage

e. Blood level of vitamin C is >1 mg/dl

Q. 158. Which of the following is correct statement?

a. Serum alkaline phosphatase is low in osteomalacia

b. Serum alkaline phosphatase is high in osteoporosis

c. Sreum alkaline phosphatase is high in osteomalacia

d. Serum alkaline phosphatase is normal in osteomalacia

Q. 159. Which of the following statement is true?

a. Urine phosphorus level is decreased in osteomalacia

b. Urine phosphorus level is increased in osteomalacia

c. Urine phosphorus level is normal in osteoporosis

d. Urine phosphorus level is low in osteoporosis

Q. 160. Which of the following statement is true?

a. 24 hours urine calcium level is increased in osteomalacia

b. 24 hours urine calcium level is normal in osteomalacia

c. 24 hours urine calcium level is decreased in osteomalacia

d. Urinary excretion of calcium is slightly lower than uptake

Q. 161. Which of the following is confirmatory diagnostic tool for osteomalacia?

a. Clinical features

b. X-ray findings

c. Serum alkaline phosphatase level

d. Bone biopsy taken from iliac crest

Q. 162. All of the following are given in the treatment of osteomalacia except?

a. Vitamin D

b. Calcium

c. High protein diet

d. Estrogen and androgens

Q. 163. Champagne glass appearance of lower ends of bone is a feature of

a. scurvy b. rickets

c. osteoporosis d. osteomalacia

Q. 164. Alendronate is used for the treatment of

a. osteomalacia b. osteoporosis

c. rickets d. scurvy

Q. 165. Barton's disease is

a. scurvy b. rickets

c. combination of both d. none of these

Q. 166. Subperiosteal resorption of phalanx is a feature of

a. primary hyperparathyroidism

b. hypoparathyroidism

c. hypophosphatasia

d. osteoporosis

Q. 167. Which of the following drug can be used as a diagnostic test for gout?

a. Colchicine b. Allopurinol

c. Suphinpyrazone d. Probenecid

Q. 168. Which of the following is not a feature of fluorosis?

a. Raised serum fluoride level

b. Raised level of fluoride in bone biopsy

c. Raised urine and drinking level of fluoride

d. Raised uric acid level

CONGENITAL, DEVELOPMENTAL AND REGIONAL DISEASES

Q. 169. All of the following structures are released in Steindler's release except

a. plantar apponeurosis

b. abductor hallucis

c. flexor halluc7is longus

d. abductor digiti minimi

Q. 170. Dwyer's osteotomy is done at the age of

a. 1 year b. 2 years

c. 3 years d. 4 years

Q. 171. Evan's procedure is done at the age of

a. 2–4 years b. 4–6 years

c. 6–8 years d. 4–8 years

Q. 172. Wedge tarsectomy is done at the age of

a. 2–5 years b. 5–8 years

c. 8–11 years d. 11–14 years

Q. 173. Tripple arthrodesis for CTEV is done at the age of

a. 4 years b. 8 years

c. 12 years d. 1 year

Q. 174. Which of the following is not a feature of CDH?

a. Perkin's line

b. Von-rosen line

c. Distorted shenton line

d. Wimberger line

Q. 175. Undescended scapula is known as

a. cleidocranial dysostosis

b. congenital torticollis

c. sprengel deformity

d. congenital coxa vara

Q. 176. Which of the following is not a feature of Madelung deformity?

a. Common at the age of 10–15 years

b. Male to female ratio is 1 : 4

c. Majority of cases have bilateral deformity

d. Common at the age of 30–45 years

Q. 177. All of the following are related with Kleippel-feil syndrome except

a. brevicollis b. pterigeum colli

c. it is treated by traction and immobilization by cervical collar or cast

d. this is a developmental condition

Q. 178. Which of the following is true about marble bone disease?

a. Medullary canal is not obliterated

b. Haversian canals are abundant

c. Mandible is involved

d. Shallow pituitary fossa

Q. 179. Which of the following is congenital disease?

a. Mafucci disease

b. Olier disease

c. Osteopoikilosis

d. Proximal femoral focal deficiency

Q. 180. Osteopathia condensans disseminate is also known as

a. pyknodysostosis b. Engelmann's diseae

c. osteopikilosis d. melorheostosis

Q. 181. Mandible is affected in

a. Engelmann's disease b. pynodysostosis

c. both of them d. none of these

Q. 182. Epiphyseal stapling is recommended in genu varum at the age of

a. 4 years b. 4–10 years

c. 10–14 years d. >16 years

Q. 183. 15 years old child presents in OPD with genu varum. Which of the following treatment you would like to recommend?

a. Epiphyseal stapling b. Medial heel raise

c. Wait and watch d. Osteotomy

Q. 184. Which of the following is commonest cause of genu recurvatum?

a. Quadriceps contracture

b. Polio

c. Congenital disorder

d. Malunited fracture of knee

Q. 185. Which of the following is not related with tibia vara?

a. Blount's disease

b. Erlacher's disease

c. Osteochondrosis deformans tibia

d. 50% infantile type cases are unilateral

Q. 186. Which of the following is most effective surgical method for recurrent dislocation of patella?

a. Galeazzi procedure

b. Hauser method

c. Elmslie-Trillat method

d. Campbell operation

Q. 187. Larson-Johanson disease is

a. osteochondritis of tibial tubercle

b. osteoarthritis of lower pole of patella

c. softening of articular cartilage of patella

d. none of the above

Q. 188. Chondromalacia patellae is

a. osteochondritis of tibial tubercle

b. osteoarthritis of lower pole of patella

c. softening of articular cartilage of patella

d. none of the above

Q. 189. Osgood schlatter disease is

a. osteochondritis of tibial tubercle

b. osteoarthritis of lower pole of patella

c. softening of articular cartilage of patella

d. none of the above

Q. 190. Which of the following is related with chondromalacia patellae?

a. Cinema sign

b. Outerbridge's grading

c. Blistering of cartilage

d. All of the above

e. None of the above

Q. 191. Slipped capital epiphysis means

a. AVN of ossification centre of capital femoral epiphysis

b. AVN of femoral head and chondrolysis

c. this is also known as coxa plana

d. none of the above

Q. 192. Gage sign is seen in

a. Perthes disease

b. slipped capital femoral epiphysis

c. Osgod schlatter disease

d. none of the above

Q. 193. Restricted abduction and internal rotation at hip, antalgic gait and limp are features of

a. slipped capital femoral epiphysis

b. leg-calve-perthes disease

c. both of above

d. none of the above

Q. 194. Perthes disease is seen at the age of

a. 3–12 years b. 10–17 years

c. 15–20 years d. 20–25 years

Q. 195. Slipped capital femoral epiphysis is seen at the age of

a. 3–12 years b. 10–17 years

c. 15–20 years d. 20–25 years

Q. 196. Which of the following is a feature of perthes disease?

a. Waldenstorm sign

b. Gage sign

c. Teardrop phenomenon

d. Thickened epiphyseal plate

e. All of the above

f. None of the above

Q. 197. Which of the following statement is correct?

a. Dorsiflexion of I metatarsal and plantarflexion of great toe is seen in Dorsal bunion

b. Great toe is deflected laterally with prominence of metatarsal head and neck medially (Bunion)

c. Both of above

d. None of the above

Q. 198. Which of the following nerve is involved in elbow tunnel syndrome?

a. Radial nerve

b. Ulnar nerve

c. Medial nerve

d. Musculocutaneous nerve

Q. 199. Dequervain's disease is tenovaginitis of

a. abductor pollicis longus

b. extensor pollicis brevis

c. both of above

d. none of the above

Q. 200. Which of the following is most commonly affected by tuberculosis?

a. Spine b. Hip

c. Knee d. Elbow

Q. 201. Which of the following is earliest sign of pott's spine?

a. Paravertebral shadow

b. Collapse of vertebra

c. Paresis

d. Reduced disc space

Q. 202. Tuberculosis hip constitutes

a. 5% of cases of skeletal tuberculosis

b. 10% of cases of skeletal tuberculosis

c. 15% of all cases of skeletal tuberculosis

d. 20% of cases of skeletal tuberculosis

Q. 203. Stage of apparent lengthening (T.B. hip) is known as

a. stage of synovitis b. stage of arthritis

c. stage of erosion d. stage of subluxation

Q. 204. Spina ventosa is

a. tuberculosis of phalanx

b. tuberculosis of metacarpal

c. tuberculosis of carpal bone

d. none of the above

Q. 205. All of the following are true about cerebral palsy except

a. mask facies

b. thumb in palm deformity

c. clonus is present

d. elbow is extended and forearm is supinated

Q. 206. Which is the commonest organism responsible for acute osteomyelitis?

a. Streptococcus b. *E. coli*

c. Salmonella

d. Staphylococcus aureus

Q. 207. Diaphyseal osteomyelitis is caused by

a. streptococcus b. *E. coli*

c. salmonella

d. staphylococcus aureus

Q. 208. Which of the following is complication of chronic osteomyelitis?

a. Amyloidosis

b. Squamus cell carcinoma at sinus tract

c. Damage to growth plate

d. All of the above

Q. 209. Which of the following is true about Salmonella osteomyelitis?

a. Ulna, tibia and vertebrae are commonly affected.

b. Agglutination test is diagnostic

c. Chloremphenicol is drug of choice

d. Children of sickle cell anemia are commonly affected.

e. All of the above

Q. 210 Which of the following is not true about Garre's osteomyelitis

a. Non suppurative sclerosing osteomyeltis

b. Subperiosteal area is commonly affected

c. Blood culture is normal

d. It does not responds to antibiotics

Q. 211. Which of the following is true about Tomsmith arthritis?

a. This is septic arthritis of infants

b. X-ray shows complete absence of head and neck of femur

c. Telescopy test is positive

d. All of the above

Q. 212. All of the following is true about septic arthritis except

a. polymorphonuclear leukocytosis (10000-20000)

b. raised ESR >20 mm/hr

c. clinical methods-reactive protein is positive.

d. gram stain is positive

Q. 213. Which of the following is true about gonococcal arthritis?

a. Fibrous ankylosis is common

b. Bony ankylosis is common

c. Both are common

d. None of the above

Q. 214. Parrot's pseudoparalysis is also known as

a. late congenital syphyllis

b. adult syphillis

c. early congenital syphilis

d. gonococcal arthritis

Q. 215. All of the following are true about deep palmar abscess except

a. it looks like frog hand

b. extension at IP joint is painless

c. extension at MP joint is painful

d. it constitutes >5% of all infection of hand

Q. 216. Diagnostic features of rheumatoid arthritis includes

a. swelling in atleast one joint continuosly for not less than 6 weeks

b. subcutaneous nodule

c. symmetrical joint swelling

d. finger shows ulnar drift

e. all of the above

Q. 217. Which of the following is drug of choice among all DMARD?

a. Gold　　b. d-pencilamine

c. Chloroquine　　d. Leflunomide

BONE TUMOR

Q. 218. Which is commonest benign bone tumor?

a. Chondroma　　b. Osteochondroma

c. Osteoma　　d. Osteoid osteoma

Q. 219. Soap bubble appearance is seen in

a. GCT　　b. osteosarcoma

c. Ewing tumor　　d. chondrosarcoma

Q. 220. GCT is commonly seen at the age of

a. 10–20 years　　b. 5–10 years

c. 20–40 years　　d. 20–30 years

Q. 221. Osteosarcoma is seen at the age of

a. 5–10 years　　b. 10–15 years

c. 15–25 years　　d. 20–40 years

Q. 222. All of the following are features of GCT except

a. severe painful swelling

b. effusion is not seen in joint

c. egg shell crackling

d. joint movements are normal

Q. 223. Which of the following is hallmark of GCT?

a. Tumor giant cell　　b. Spindle cell

c. Periosteal reaction　　d. Effusion

Q. 224. All of the following are features of osteosarcoma except

a. Codman's triangle

b. Sun-ray appearance

c. Periosteal reaction

d. Soap bubble appearance

Q. 225. Which of the following is not true about parosteal osteosarcoma?

a. Radiotherapy is treatment of choice

b. This is a low grade malignant tumor

c. Commonly seen between 30–40 years of age

d. Painless localized bony hard swelling

Q. 226. All of the following are true about Ewing sarcoma except

a. metastasizes early to lung

b. pseudorosette pattern

c. affects diaphysis of bone

d. it is commonly seen between 10–20 years of age

Q. 227. Chondrosarcoma is seen at the age of

a. 5–10 years b. 10–20 years

c. 20–30 years d. 20–60 years

Q. 228. All of the following are true about chondrosarcoma except

a. metstasis occurs through lymphatics to prostate

b. diagnosis is confirmed by biopsy

c. pain is not prominent feature

d. it is a palpable mass which is fixed to bone

Q. 229. Popcorn or breadcrumb appearance is seen in

a. osteosarcoma b. Ewing sarcoma

c. chondrosarcoma d. osteoma

Q. 230. Aneurysmal bone cyst is seen at the age of

a. 20–30 years b. 30–40 years

c. 5–10 years d. 10–30 years

Q. 231. Unicameral bone cyst is seen at the age of

a. 5–15 years b. 10–20 years

c. 20–30 years d. 30–40 years

Q. 232. All of the following are true about unicameral bone cyst

a. calcar is not involved

b. pathological fractures are seen

c. fracture heals rapidly within a few week

d. it originates from diaphysis of long bone

Q. 233. Osteoid osteoma is seen at the age of

a. 5–10 years b. 10–25 years

c. 20–40 years d. 30–40 years

Q. 234. Which of the following is classical feature of osteoid osteoma?

a. Tibia and femur are commonly involved

b. Overlying skin is not stretched

c. Predominantly seen in male

d. It quickly responds to Aspirin

Q. 235. All of the following are true about chondroblastoma except

a. commonly seen at the age of 10–20 years

b. this is a malignant cartilaginous tumor

c. males are predominantly affected

d. multiple calcium deposits are seen within the tumor

Q. 236. Chondromyxoid fibroma is seen at the age of

a. 10–20 years b. 20–30 years

c. 30–40 years d. 40–50 years

Q. 237. Which of the following is least common benign cartilaginous tumor?

a. Chondroma

b. Chondroblastoma

c. Osteochondroma

d. Chondromyxoid fibroma

Q. 238. Which of the following is commonly seen in spine and jaw?

a. Osteoblastoma b. Chondroma
c. Osteochondroma d. Chondroblastoma

Q. 239. Which of the following is not true about reticulum cell sarcoma?

a. This is highly radiosensitive tumor
b. Commonly seen in long bones
c. X-ray shows moth eaten appearance
d. Commonly seen at the age of 10–20 years

Q. 240. All of the following are related to Mafduci syndrome except

a. dyschondroplasia
b. cavernous haemangioma
c. hereditary condition
d. commonly seen in India

Q. 241. Synovial sarcoma commonly metastasizes to

a. brain b. prostate
c. bladder d. lung

Q. 242. All of the following are related to synovial sarcoma except

a. sarcomesothelioma
b. cancerous synovial tumor
c. commonly seen around knee joint in the soft tissue
d. commonly seen at the age of 40–60 years

Q. 243. All of the following are synonyms of multiple myeloma except

a. monoclonal gammopathy
b. solitary myeloma
c. myelomatosis
d. hamartoma

Q. 244. All of the following are true about multiple myeloma except?

a. Serum globulin is raised
b. Serum calcium is raised
c. ESR is raised
d. Serum alkaline phosphatase is raised

Q. 245. Biconcave vertebrae can be found in all of the following except

a. multiple myeloma b. osteomalacia
c. osteoporosis d. synovial sarcoma

Q. 246. Shepherd crook deformity is seen in

a. osteochondroma b. multiple myeloma
c. fibrous dysplasia d. synovial sarcoma

Q. 247. All of the following are true about fibrous dysplasia except

a. serum alkaline phosphatase is raised
b. serum calcium is normal
c. serum phosphorus is normal
d. pituitary fossa is normal

Q. 248. Most common site for origin of chordoma is

a. cervical spine b. thoracic spine
c. lumbar spine d. sacrococcygeal region

Q. 249. All of the following are related with PIVD except

a. Schmorl node
b. Brown degeneration
c. commonest level is L4-5
d. commonly seen at the age of 40–50 years

Q. 250. All of the following statements are true about cauda equina syndrome except

a. bilateral ankle jerks are absent
b. bowel and urinary incontinence is present
c. sensation are reduced along the course of L4-5 dermatome
d. this is upper motor neurone type paralysis

Q. 251. Bragard test is related to

a. ankylosing spondylitis
b. PIVD

c. Scheurmann's disease

d. none of the above

Q. 252. Which of the following is used in chemonucleosis?

a. Chymotrypsin b. Chymopapin

c. Trypsinogen d. None of these

Q. 253. All of the following are true about Scheurmann's disease except

a. this is osteochondritis of lower thoracic spine

b. kyphosis is present

c. this is seen in adolescent period

d. patient should lie in bed with flexed spine

Q. 254. Calves disease of spine is also known as

a. Scheurmann's disease

b. PIVD

c. spondylolisthesis

d. vertebra plana

Q. 255. All of the following are true about Scottish dog sign except

a. seen in spondylolisthesis

b. visible in oblique view of spine

c. neck of dog represents defect in isthmus

d. head of dog represents defect in isthmus

Q. 256. Ullaman sign is positive in

a. ankylosing spondylitis

b. Scheurmann's disease

c. spondylolisthesis

d. PIVD

Q. 257. Most common cause of scoliosis

a. congenital b. neuromuscular

c. idiopathic d. trauma

Q. 258. Risser's sign indicates

a. fusion of iliac apophysis with iliac bone

b. sepration of iliac apophysis from iliac bone

c. indicates growth is incomplete

d. indicates more chances of curve worsening

Q. 259. All of the following are true about diastematomyelia except

a. this is longitudinal division of spinal cord

b. this is congenital malformation

c. commonly seen in lower thoracic and upper lumbar vertebra

d. laminectomy is not effective

Q. 260. Which of the following is true about Duchenne's muscular dystrophy?

a. Autosomal dominant

b. Autosomal ressesive

c. Abnormal deletion gene is present at x-chromosome in cytogenetic band xp-21

d. Gower sign is negative

Q. 261. All of the following about Werdnig Hoffman disease are true except

a. deep tendon reflexes are absent

b. tone is increased

c. muscle biopsy is diagnostic

d. autosomal recessive

Q. 262. Landouzy-Dejerine dystrophy is

a. x-linked recessive b. autosomal dominant

c. autosomal recessive d. none of these

MISCELLANEOUS

Q. 263. Excision of head radius in children may lead to

a. valgus deformity b. varus deformity

c. restricted supination d. lengthening of limb

Q. 264. Below elbow amputation is done

a. 5 inches from olecranon

b. 6 inches from olecranon

c. 7 inches from olecranon

d. 8 inches from olecranon

Q. 265. Above elbow amputation is done:

a. 5 inches from acromian

b. 6 inches from acromian

c. 7 inches from acromian

d. 8 inches from acromian

Q. 266. Above knee amputation is done

a. 6 inches from greater trochanter

b. 7 inches from greater trochanter

c. 8 inches from greater trochanter

d. 9 inches from greater trochanter

Q. 267. Below knee amputation is done

a. 4.5 inches from knee joint

b. 5.5 inches from knee joint

c. 6.5 inches from knee joint

d. 7.5 inches from knee joint

Q. 268. Which of the following requires lumbar spine posteotomy?

a. Pott's spine

b. Lumbar canal stenosis

c. Ankylosing spondylitis

d. Spondylolisthesis

Q. 269. Which of the following is surgery of choice in Pott's spine?

a. Anterolateral decompression

b. Costotransversectomy

c. Laminectomy

d. Spinal fusion

Q. 270. Which of the following require Meyer's procedure?

a. Fracture neck femur

b. Fracture patella

c. Fracture shaft femur

d. Fracture shaft humerus

Q. 271. Which of the following radioactive dye is used in bone scan?

a. Gallium b. 99m Tc

c. Strontium 99 d. I 131

Q. 272. Which of the following statement is correct?

a. Nerve should be repaired before tendon

b. Tendon should not be repaired

c. Tendon should be repaired before nerve

d. None of the above

Q. 273. The maximum weight that can be applied through skin traction is

a. 4 kg b. 5 kg

c. 6 kg d. 7 kg

Q. 274. Which of the following is not a radiological sign of perthes disease?

a. Reduced joint space

b. Coxa magna

c. Irregular epiphyseal line

d. Flattening of capital femoral epiphysis

Q. 275. Charcot-Marie-tooth disease is also known as

a. peroneal muscular atrophy

b. carries tooth

c. syphyllis

d. dental carries

Q. 276. Which of the following is known as mirror hand?

a. Congenital absence of radius

b. Reduplication of ulna

c. Injury with a piece of glass

d. None of the above

Q. 277. Still's disease is also known as

a. rheumatic fever

b. viral fever

c. rheumatoid arthritis in children

d. rheumatoid arthritis in adults

Q. 278. Which of the following is commonest cause of low backache in old age?

a. Spondylosis

b. Spondylolisthesis

c. PIVD

d. Ankylosing spondylitis

Q. 279. Most important step in management of gas gangrene

a. Blood transfusion

b. Pencillin injection

c. A.G.G.S.

d. Surgical debridement of wound

Q. 280. Most likely cause of intermittent claudication in lower limb is

a. arterial insufficiency

b. venous occlusion

c. peripheral neuropathy

d. toxaemia

Q. 281. Calcification of menisci is seen in

a. tuberculosis b. pseudogout

c. hyperparathyroidism d. renal osteodystrophy

Q. 282. Which of the following drug can cause osteomalacia?

a. Steroid b. Phenytoin

c. Procainamide d. Hydralazine

Q. 283. Alli's sign is seen in

a. Osteoarthritis b. Osteomalacia

c. CDH d. Marfan's syndrome

Q. 284. Which of the following is commonest cause of paraplegia?

a. Trauma b. Tumor

c. Tuberculosis d. Transverse myelitis

Q. 285. Which of the following can cause osteitis?

a. Syphillis b. Toxoplasma

c. Rubella d. CMV

Q. 286. Which of the following is involved in Kashin-Beck disease?

a. Ankle b. Knee

c. Phalanges d. Wrist

Q. 287. Which of the following test can assess integrity of palmar arch?

a. Schwartz test b. Paget's test

c. Allen's test d. Homan's test

Q. 288. Most common deformity in rickets is

a. genu varum b. genu valgum

c. genu recurvatum d. bow legs

Q. 289. Which of the following can increase bone density?

a. Estrogen in postmenopausal women

b. Parathyroid hormone

c. Immobilization

d. Postmenopausal

Q. 290. Which of the following posture provides least intradiscal pressure?

a. Lying supine b. Standing

c. Sitting d. Lying by side

Q. 291. Commonest joint to be involved in Behcet's syndrome

a. Ankle b. Knee

c. Wrist d. Hip

Q. 292. Heberden nodes are seen in

a. Osteoarthritis b. Rheumatoid arthritis

c. Rheumatic arthritis d. Psoriatic arthritis

Q. 293. Patchy calcification is seen in

a. GCT b. Osteosarcoma

c. Chondrosarcoma d. Ewing's tumor

Q. 294. All of the following can cause painful limp except

a. T.B. hip

b. perthes disease

c. congenital coxa vara

d. slipped capital femoral epiphysis

Q. 295. Which of the following is true about synovial membrane of knee joint?

a. Pierced by cruciate ligament posteriorly

b. Continuous with prepatellar bursa

c. Continuous with intrapatellar bursa

d. Covers under surface of menisci

Q. 296 Which of the following is involved in SLE?

a. Cervical spine b. Thoracic spine
c. Lumbar spine d. Sacrum

Q. 297. Which age group (years) is affected in Osggod-schlatter's disease?

a. 4–8 b. 8–12
c. 12–16 d. 10–14

Q. 298 Which of the following shows Sausage toe?

a. Gout b. Pseudo gout
c. Psoriatic arthritis d. Reactive arthritis

Q. 299. Which type of osteogenesis imperfecta commonly show blue sclera?

a. 1 b. 2
c. 3 d. 4

Q. 300. Which of the following subtype of osteogenesis imperfecta is autosomal dominant?

a. 1 b. 2
c. 3 d. 4

Q. 301. Smith fracture unites in

a. 6 weeks b. 12 weeks
c. 4 weeks d. 3 weeks

ANSWERS (AIIMS MCQ)

1. (*a*)	**2.** (*a*)	**3.** (*d*)	**4.** (*d*)	**5.** (*c*)	**6.** (*a*)
7. (*a*)	**8.** (*c*)	**9.** (*b*)	**10.** (*d*)	**11.** (*b*)	**12.** (*a*)
13. (*c*)	**14.** (*a*)	**15.** (*a*)	**16.** (*b*)	**17.** (*a*)	**18.** (*a*)
19. (*b*)	**20.** (*a*)	**21.** (*a*)	**22.** (*b*)	**23.** (*a*)	**24.** (*c*)
25. (*b*)	**26.** (*c*)	**27.** (*c*)	**28.** (*a*)	**29.** (*b*)	**30.** (*d*)
31. (*d*)	**32.** (*a*)	**33.** (*b*)	**34.** (*a*)	**35.** (*a*)	**36.** (*a*)
37. (*a*)	**38.** (*a*)	**39.** (*c*)	**40.** (*a*)	**41.** (*a*)	**42.** (*a*)
43. (*a*)	**44.** (*b*)	**45.** (*a*)	**46.** (*a*)	**47.** (*c*)	**48.** (*a*)
49. (*b*)	**50.** (*b*)	**51.** (*a*)	**52.** (*a*)	**53.** (*a*)	**54.** (*c*)
55. (*b*)	**56.** (*d*)	**57.** (*a*)	**58.** (*c*)	**59.** (*a*)	**60.** (*a*)
61. (*c*)	**62.** (*b*)	**63.** (*a*)	**64.** (*c*)	**65.** (*b*)	**66.** (*d*)
67. (*c*)	**68.** (*d*)	**69.** (*d*)	**70.** (*b*)	**71.** (*d*)	**72.** (*c*)
73. (*d*)	**74.** (*c*)	**75.** (*a*)	**76.** (*c*)	**77.** (*a*)	**78.** (*a*)
79. (*a*)	**80.** (*d*)	**81.** (*b*)	**82.** (*d*)	**83.** (*c*)	**84.** (*d*)
85. (*a*)					

ANSWERS (PG ENTRANCE)

1. (*a*)	**2.** (*d*)	**3.** (*b*)	**4.** (*c*)	**5.** (*a*)	**6.** (*b*)
7. (*a*)	**8.** (*b*)	**9.** (*d*)	**10.** (*c*)	**11.** (*d*)	**12.** (*a*)
13. (*c*)	**14.** (*a*)	**15.** (*c*)	**16.** (*a*)	**17.** (*a*)	**18.** (*b*)
19. (*d*)	**20.** (*d*)	**21.** (*d*)	**22.** (*a*)	**23.** (*d*)	**24.** (*c*)
25. (*d*)	**26.** (*d*)	**27.** (*c*)	**28.** (*a*)	**29.** (*a*)	**30.** (*b*)
31. (*a*)	**32.** (*d*)	**33.** (*d*)	**34.** (*a*)	**35.** (*c*)	**36.** (*a*)
37. (*d*)	**38.** (*c*)	**39.** (*d*)	**40.** (*d*)	**41.** (*a*)	**42.** (*b*)
43. (*d*)	**44.** (*b*)	**45.** (*b*)	**46.** (*b*)	**47.** (*c*)	**48.** (*a*)
49. (*c*)	**50.** (*d*)	**51.** (*a*)	**52.** (*a*)	**53.** (*c*)	**54.** (*b*)
55. (*c*)	**56.** (*b*)	**57.** (*d*)	**58.** (*d*)	**59.** (*c*)	**60.** (*a*)

61. (*c*) 62. (*a*) 63. (*c*) 64. (*a*) 65. (*a*) 66. (*d*)
67. (*a*) 68. (*c*) 69. (*a*) 70. (*b*) 71. (*a*) 72. (*c*)
73. (*d*) 74. (*c*) 75. (*c*) 76. (*d*) 77. (*d*) 78. (*d*)
79. (*a*) 80. (*a*) 81. (*d*) 82. (*a*) 83. (*b*) 84. (*d*)
85. (*d*) 86. (*d*) 87. (*d*) 88. (*d*) 89. (*a*) 90. (*d*)
91. (*d*) 92. (*d*) 93. (*a*) 94. (*c*) 95. (*d*) 96. (*c*)
97. (*c*) 98. (*a*) 99. (*c*) 100. (*d*) 101. (*d*) 102. (*a*)
103. (*a*) 104. (*d*) 105. (*d*) 106. (*d*) 107. (*a*) 108. (*a*)
109. (*d*) 110. (*c*) 111. (*d*) 112. (*c*) 113. (*b*) 114. (*d*)
115. (*e*) 116. (*d*) 117. (*c*) 118. (*c*) 119. (*d*) 120. (*c*)
121. (*a*) 122. (*b*) 123. (*d*) 124. (*d*) 125. (*d*) 126. (*a*)
127. (*e*) 128. (*e*) 129. (*d*) 130. (*d*) 131. (*e*) 132. (*b*)
133. (*b*) 134. (*d*) 135. (*e*) 136. (*d*) 137. (*d*) 138. (*d*)
139. (*d*) 140. (*d*) 141. (*c*) 142. (*a*) 143. (*f*) 144. (*a*)
145. (*e*) 146. (*d*) 147. (*a*) 148. (*d*) 149. (*a*) 150. (*b*)
151. (*d*) 152. (*c*) 153. (*c*) 154. (*a*) 155. (*d*) 156. (*d*)
157. (*e*) 158. (*c*) 159. (*a*) 160. (*c*) 161. (*d*) 162. (*d*)
163. (*b*) 164. (*b*) 165. (*c*) 166. (*a*) 167. (*a*) 168. (*d*)
169. (*c*) 170. (*c*) 171. (*d*) 172. (*c*) 173. (*c*) 174. (*d*)
175. (*c*) 176. (*d*) 177. (*d*) 178. (*d*) 179. (*d*) 180. (*c*)
181. (*c*) 182. (*c*) 183. (*c*) 184. (*a*) 185. (*d*) 186. (*b*)
187. (*b*) 188. (*c*) 189. (*a*) 190. (*d*) 191. (*b*) 192. (*a*)
193. (*c*) 194. (*a*) 195. (*b*) 196. (*e*) 197. (*c*) 198. (*b*)
199. (*c*) 200. (*a*) 201. (*d*) 202. (*c*) 203. (*a*) 204. (*a*)
205. (*d*) 206. (*d*) 207. (*c*) 208. (*d*) 209. (*e*) 210. (*d*)
211. (*d*) 212. (*a*) 213. (*a*) 214. (*c*) 215. (*d*) 216. (*e*)
217. (*d*) 218. (*b*) 219. (*a*) 220. (*c*) 221. (*c*) 222. (*a*)
223. (*a*) 224. (*d*) 225. (*a*) 226. (*a*) 227. (*d*) 228. (*a*)
229. (*c*) 230. (*d*) 231. (*a*) 232. (*d*) 233. (*b*) 234. (*d*)
235. (*b*) 236. (*b*) 237. (*d*) 238. (*a*) 239. (*d*) 240. (*d*)
241. (*d*) 242. (*d*) 243. (*d*) 244. (*d*) 245. (*d*) 246. (*c*)
247. (*a*) 248. (*d*) 249. (*d*) 250. (*d*) 251. (*b*) 252. (*b*)
253. (*d*) 254. (*d*) 255. (*d*) 256. (*c*) 257. (*c*) 258. (*a*)
259. (*d*) 260. (*c*) 261. (*b*) 262. (*b*) 263. (*a*) 264. (*c*)
265. (*d*) 266. (*d*) 267. (*b*) 268. (*c*) 269. (*a*) 270. (*a*)
271. (*b*) 272. (*c*) 273. (*a*) 274. (*a*) 275. (*a*) 276. (*b*)
277. (*c*) 278. (*a*) 279. (*d*) 280. (*a*) 281. (*b*) 282. (*b*)
283. (*c*) 284. (*a*) 285. (*a*) 286. (*c*) 287. (*c*) 288. (*b*)
289. (*a*) 290. (*a*) 291. (*b*) 292. (*a*) 293. (*c*) 294. (*c*)
295. (*a*) 296. (*a*) 297. (*d*) 298. (*d*) 299. (*a*) 300. (*a*)
301. (*a*)

Index

A

B

R

S